T0293382

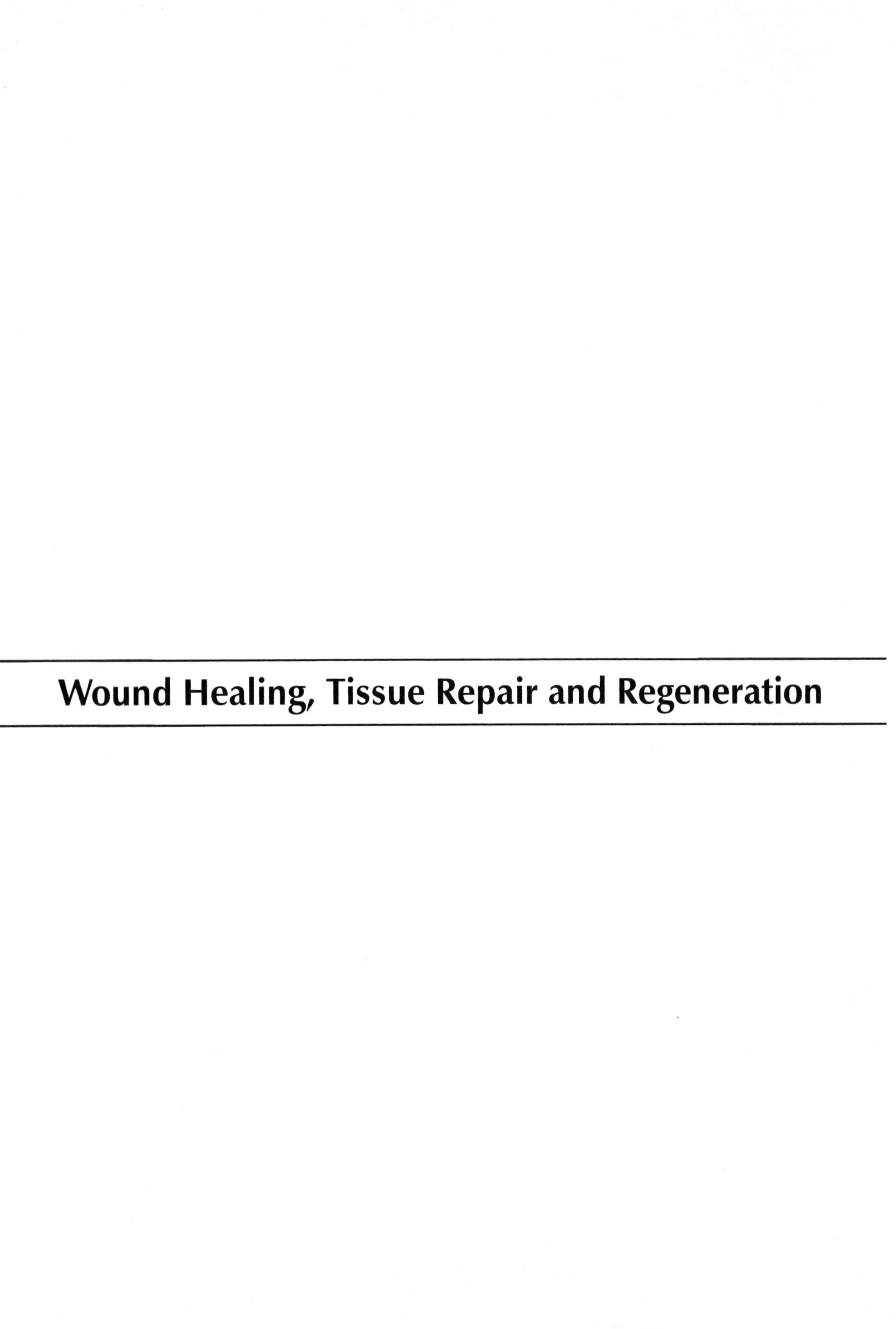

Wound Healing, Tissue Repair and Regeneration

Wound Healing, Tissue Repair and Regeneration

Editor: Adelina Cooper

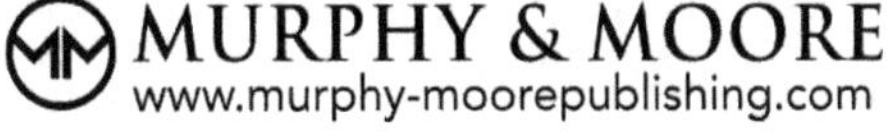

www.murphy-moorepublishing.com

MURPHY & MOORE

Cataloging-in-Publication Data

Wound healing, tissue repair and regeneration / edited by Adelina Cooper.
p. cm.
Includes bibliographical references and index.
ISBN 978-1-63987-765-2
1. Wound healing. 2. Wounds and injuries. 3. Wounds and injuries--Treatment. I. Cooper, Adelina.
RD94 .W68 2023
617.1--dc23

Murphy & Moore Publishing
1 Rockefeller Plaza,
New York City,
NY 10020, USA

ISBN 978-1-63987-765-2

Contents

Preface

A wound is an injury that damages the outermost layer of the skin, also known as the epidermis. It involves punctured and lacerated skin, or a contusion caused by a blunt force compression or trauma. Wounds are classified into two major categories, namely, open wounds and closed wounds. Open wounds include incisions, lacerations, abrasions, puncture and avulsions, while closed wounds encompass contusions, hematomas and crush injury. The healing of a wound involves replacement of the damaged or destroyed tissue by a new tissue. Wound healing involves a controlled sequence of biochemical events, which are set into action for repairing the damage. The process of healing takes place in phases, which include blood clotting, inflammation, tissue growth and tissue remodeling. This book contains some path-breaking studies on wound healing as well as tissue repair and regeneration. It consists of contributions made by international experts. The book will provide comprehensive knowledge to the readers.

This book is a result of research of several months to collate the most relevant data in the field.

When I was approached with the idea of this book and the proposal to edit it, I was overwhelmed. It gave me an opportunity to reach out to all those who share a common interest with me in this field. I had 3 main parameters for editing this text:

1. Accuracy - The data and information provided in this book should be up-to-date and valuable to the readers.

2. Structure - The data must be presented in a structured format for easy understanding and better grasping of the readers.

3. Universal Approach - This book not only targets students but also experts and innovators in the field, thus my aim was to present topics which are of use to all.

Thus, it took me a couple of months to finish the editing of this book.

I would like to make a special mention of my publisher who considered me worthy of this opportunity and also supported me throughout the editing process. I would also like to thank the editing team at the back-end who extended their help whenever required.

Editor

1

Selection of Appropriate Wound Dressing for Various Wounds

Chenyu Shi[1,2], Chenyu Wang[3], He Liu[2], Qiuju Li[2], Ronghang Li[2], Yan Zhang[2], Yuzhe Liu[2], Ying Shao[2,3] and Jincheng Wang[1,2]**

[1] School of Nursing, Jilin University, Changchun, China, [2] Orthopaedic Medical Center, The Second Hospital of Jilin University, Changchun, China, [3] Department of Plastic and Reconstructive Surgery, The First Hospital of Jilin University, Changchun, China

There are many factors involved in wound healing, and the healing process is not static. The therapeutic effect of modern wound dressings in the clinical management of wounds is documented. However, there are few reports regarding the reasonable selection of dressings for certain types of wounds in the clinic. In this article, we retrospect the history of wound dressing development and the classification of modern wound dressings. In addition, the pros and cons of mainstream modern wound dressings for the healing of different wounds, such as diabetic foot ulcers, pressure ulcers, burns and scalds, and chronic leg ulcers, as well as the physiological mechanisms involved in wound healing are summarized. This article provides a clinical guideline for selecting suitable wound dressings according to the types of wounds.

Keywords: wound, wound healing, wound dressing, clinical application, physiological mechanism

***Correspondence:**
Ying Shao
13844880131@163.com
Jincheng Wang
jinchengwang@hotmail.com

INTRODUCTION

Physical or thermal damage can cause defects or interruptions in the epidermis of the skin or mucous membranes, forming a wound (Singh et al., 2013). Wounds are classified as acute or chronic wounds. Acute wounds can recover in a short period of time. The size, depth, and degree of injury of the wound are factors that influence the healing process. However, the healing process of chronic wounds is longer and different from that of acute wounds (Schreml et al., 2010). The healing of acute wounds occurs in a normal, orderly and timely manner throughout the entire process. However, the repair of chronic trauma in this fashion is challenging, and it is difficult to restore normal anatomical structure and function (Tarnuzzer and Schultz, 1996; Borda et al., 2016).

There are many factors involved in wound healing (Guo and Dipietro, 2010). The healing process is not static and growth involves four different phases, namely coagulation and hemostasis, inflammatory, proliferation, and remodeling. These phases are not independent but partially overlap on the basis of a sequence by hemostasis, inflammatory, proliferation, and remodeling (Kasuya and Tokura, 2014; Wilhelm et al., 2017). After skin injury, the wound or tissue fracture is filled with blood clots, followed by acute inflammation of the surrounding tissue. The release of inflammatory mediators and infiltration of inflammatory cells cause tissue swelling and pain. Proliferative fibroblasts, endothelial cells, and newly formed capillaries interact to form granulation tissue filling the crevices. During the shaping period, the scars are softened without affecting the tensile strength through the action of various enzymes and stress, thereby adapting to physiological functions (Jeffcoate, 2012; Harper et al., 2014; Nuutila et al., 2016; Ascione et al., 2017a,b).

Medical dressings are essential devices in healthcare. According to the types and stages of wounds, dressings can be applied to their surface and promote healing. The therapeutic effects

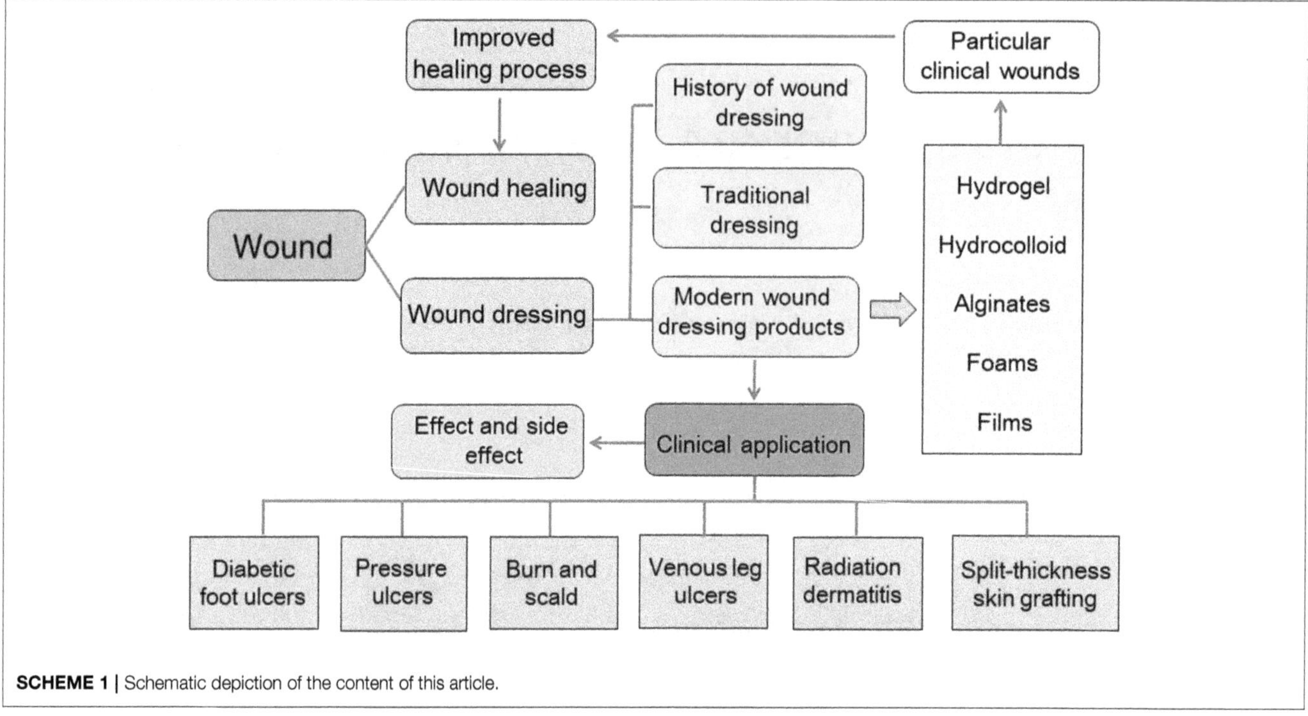

SCHEME 1 | Schematic depiction of the content of this article.

of traditional dry dressings and modern wet dressings in the clinical management of wounds are documented. Although dressings commonly used in clinical practice (gauze, sterilized absorbent cotton, and bandages) are economical, they can only offer physical protection and have limited benefit on wound healing and prevention of infection. Adherence of the dressing to the wound will cause secondary damage when the two are eventually separated. The generation and development of modern dressings are based on the healing theory of the moist environment and have numerous advantages compared with traditional dressings (Skorkowska-Telichowska et al., 2013; Vowden and Vowden, 2014). For example, modern dressings are conducive to the dissolute and abort necrotic tissue and fibrin, as well as play a role in autolysis and debridement. Moreover, they are beneficial in maintaining a relatively constant local temperature and humidity of the wound, providing the wound with conditions similar to those of the body's internal environment (Richetta et al., 2011; Heyer et al., 2013). Furthermore, modern dressings avoid re-injury of new granulation tissue due to scarring and promote cell proliferation, differentiation, and epithelial cell migration. Particularly, they may play a role in avoiding wound contact with external bacteria and effectively prevent cross-infection (Murakami et al., 2010; Horn, 2012). Although various advanced wound dressings have been developed and applied in the clinical setting, there is no relevant study investigating the reasonable selection of dressing for a certain type of wound (Powers et al., 2016).

In this review, we summarized the mechanisms of wound healing, traditional and modern wound dressings, and the advantages and disadvantages of both types of dressings. In particular, the clinical application of commercialized modern dressing products in various pathological wounds (diabetic foot ulcers [DFUs], pressure ulcers, burns and scalds, chronic leg ulcers, radiation dermatitis, and skin grafts) is described in detail to provide insight into the care of wounds. The content of this article is shown in **Scheme 1**.

WOUND DRESSINGS

With the gradual acknowledgment of wound healing theories, the development of wound dressings also evolved considerably. At present, wound dressings are expected to cover the wound and accelerate the healing process (Vowden and Vowden, 2014). Traditional dressings, also termed inert dressings (gauze, cotton pads, and bandages), are the most widely used clinical dressings owing to their low cost and simple manufacturing process (Broughton et al., 2006). However, several shortcomings limit their application, such as difficulty to maintain the wound bed moist and proneness to adhesion to granulation tissue (Moore and Webster, 2013). Modern dressings may be more suitable candidates owing to their properties providing a moist environment for wound healing (Heyer et al., 2013; Moura et al., 2013). Compared with traditional dressings, modern dressings are characterized by better biocompatibility, degradability, and moisture retention. These advantages of modern dressings relieve pain and improve the hypoxic or anaerobic environment (Hopper et al., 2012; Thu et al., 2012; Okuma et al., 2015). The most commonly used modern dressings in clinical practice are hydrogels, hydrocolloid, alginates, foams, and films (**Table 1**).

Hydrogels have a three-dimensional structure composed of hydrophilic substances (Tsang and Bhatia, 2004). They are insoluble in water and subsequently absorb water from 10%

TABLE 1 | Modern dressings used in clinical practice.

Variety	Description	Characteristics	Suitable conditions
Hydrogel	Three-dimensional network of hydrophilic polymers	Moisturizing, removal of necrotic tissue, and monitoring of the wound without removing the dressing	Pressure ulcers, surgical wounds, burns, radiation dermatitis
Hydrocolloid	Hydrogel mixed with synthetic rubber and sticky materials	Excellent exudate absorption properties	Severe exudative wound
Alginate	Consists of polysaccharides derived from brown seaweed	Excellent exudate absorption properties, hemostasis	Infected and non-infected wounds with a large amount of exudate
Foam	Consists of polyurethane or is silicone-based	Semipermeability, thermal insulation, antimicrobial activity	Infected wounds
Film	Consists of adhesive, porous, and thin transparent polyurethane	Autolytic debridement properties, impermeable to liquids and bacteria	Epithelializing wounds and superficial wounds with limited exudate

to thousands fold their equivalent weight (Goodwin et al., 2016). Owing to their excellent moisturizing ability, hydrogels maintain the wound moist and play a positive role in the cleansing of necrotic tissue. In addition, a wound covered with a dressing can be monitored, as the hydrogels are typically transparent (Hunt, 2003; Scanlon, 2003; Kamoun et al., 2017). Based on these characteristics, hydrogels are primarily used on pressure ulcers, surgical wounds, burns, radiation dermatitis, etc. (Francesko et al., 2017; Shamloo et al., 2018). They are suitable for wounds with minimal-to-moderate exudate. The degradation rate of the hydrogel can also be adjusted, which renders this material appropriate for use as a drug carrier and biologically active substance (Gil et al., 2017). For example, silver nanoparticles (Ag NPs) and ZnO NPs loaded hydrogels can maintain antibacterial activity for a long period of time (Li S. et al., 2018). Recently, a study prepared a multifunctional hydrogel for diabetic wounds. This hydrogel can be used on wounds to collect wound photos via mobile phone and transformed into RGB signals to monitor the pH and glucose levels of diabetic wounds in real time (Zhu et al., 2019). Hydrocolloid and hydrofiber dressings are composed of the same materials in nature. Notably, the latter type is a variant of hydrocolloid dressing appropriate for use as a secondary dressing, which can absorb >25-fold its own weight in fluid while maintaining its integrity (Hobot et al., 2008; Richetta et al., 2011).

Sodium alginate (SA) dressings are fibrous products derived from brown seaweed, which can form a gel after binding to wound exudate (Dumville et al., 2013c; O'Meara and Martyn-St James, 2013). The SA dressings used in the clinic are generally made into sheet fibers, which can be freely cut according to the shape of the wound. SA is also often used to synthesize hydrogels. The SA dressings also possess excellent exudate absorption properties; hence, they can be used in infected and non-infected wounds with a large amount of exudate (Hess, 2000). Owing to the strong absorption property of alginates, their use in the treatment of dry wounds or wounds with minimal exudate should be avoided. Meanwhile, A study developed an alginate hydrogel contained both bioglass and desferrioxamine, which better facilitated diabetic skin wound healing. The results demonstrated that combination use of BG and DFO improved the migration and tube formation of HUVECs as compared with the use of either BG or DFO alone as BG and DFO could synergistically upregulate VEGF expression (Kong et al., 2018).

Foam dressings are semipermeable and either hydrophilic or hydrophobic with a bacterial barrier (Sedlarik, 1994). They are composed of polyurethane or silicone-based, rendering them suitable for handling moderate-to-high volumes of wound exudate (Marks and Ribeiro, 1983). Foam dressings provide thermal insulation and maintain moisture to the wound, and prevent damage to the wound at the time of removal. These dressings may also be used as secondary dressings with hydrogel or alginate dressings, in conjunction with a topical antimicrobial agent for infected wounds (Davies et al., 2017)Moreover, polyaniline/polyurethane foam dressing carried an anti-biofilm lichen metabolite usnic acid indicated an improved antibiofilm activity of conducting polymer (dos Santos et al., 2018).

Film dressings are composed of adhesive, porous, and thin transparent polyurethane. Oxygen, carbon dioxide, and water vapor from the wound pass through the dressing, whereas liquids and bacteria are well-isolated. Furthermore, film dressings possess autolytic debridement properties (Thomas, 1990; Fletcher, 2003), and are suitable for use on epithelializing wounds and superficial wounds with few exudates (Imran et al., 2004). The various types of dressings described above have their own characteristics; thus, the selection of the dressing should be based on the specific conditions of the wound.

CLINICAL APPLICATIONS OF MODERN WOUND DRESSING PRODUCTS

Wound healing involves four different phases, namely coagulation and hemostasis, inflammatory, proliferation, and remodeling (Amini-Nik et al., 2018). Different types of dressings have different characteristics; different pathological types of wounds also have their own characteristics (**Table 2**). For example, DFUs are prone to infection and cause unsatisfactory wound healing. The prevention of pressure ulcers is focused on the reduction of the shear force and pressure in the hazardous area. Following the formation of the ulcer, it is equally important to prevent further pressure on the ulcer and apply the dressing.

TABLE 2 | Overview of various wounds and appropriate clinical dressings.

Variety	Description	Characteristics	Appropriate dressing
Diabetic foot ulcer	Caused by neuropathy and lower extremity vascular disease	Lack of supply of oxygen and blood in the wound bed; long-term stagnation in the inflammatory phase	Silver ion foam dressing, hydrofiber dressing, UrgoStart Contact dressing, Mepilex® Lite Dressing, hyaluronic acid, Biatain® Non-adhesive Dressing
Pressure injury	Caused by stress and tissue tolerance	A local injury to the skin or subcutaneous soft tissue occurring at the site of the bone prominence or the compression of the medical device	Foam dressing, hydrocolloids dressing, multi-layered soft silicone foam dressings, polyurethane film, Mepilex® Ag dressing, polyurethane foam dressing
Burn and scald	Tissue damage caused by heat	A large amount of exudate; prone to infection; severe cases can injure subcutaneous and submucosal tissues	Moist occlusive dressing (AQUACEL® Ag), ACTICOAT™ with nano silver
Chronic venous leg ulcer	Caused by high pressure of the blood in the leg veins	Lack of blood supply to the wound; a large amount of necrotic tissue and abnormal exudate on the surface of the ulcer, accompanied by multiple bacterial infections	Alginate dressing, AQUACEL® Ag dressing, Urgotul® Silver dressing, ALLEVYN® Hydrocellular foam dressings, Mepilex® foam dressing
Radiation dermatitis	Local skin lesions caused by radiation	Slow cell proliferation; decreased cytokine activity; decreased collagen content	Film dressing (Airwall), silver-containing hydrofiber, film dressing (3M™ Cavilon® No Sting Barrier Film), Mepilex® Lite dressing
Split-thickness skin grafting	None	Hypertrophic scars; hypopigmentation; hyperpigmentation	Polyurethane foam (ALLEVYN™), calcium alginate (Kaltostat®), AQUACEL® Ag (Convatec), Alginate Silver (Coloplast)

Lower extremity chronic ulcers are associated with exudation from wounds due to lower limb edema. Acute wounds, such as burns and scalds, also have their own characteristics. The application of different dressings to different pathological types of wounds in the clinical setting is illustrated in **Table 2**.

DFUs

In diabetics, the incidence of DFUs is approximately 5–10%. It is one of the most common chronic complications and the cause of lower extremity amputation in patients with diabetes mellitus (Brennan et al., 2017). DFUs as a common type of non-healing or chronic wounds are attracting considerable attention in the medical field (Khanolkar et al., 2008). Currently, the selection of the most appropriate treatment is challenging. During this process, multiple types of dressings are applied to the treatment of DFUs (Saco et al., 2016). One such method is the application of various kinds of modern dressings. Treatment with suitable dressings is an important part of the management of DFUs.

DFU is defined as foot pain, foot ulcer, and foot gangrene caused by neuropathy and lower extremity vascular disease. The pathogenesis of DFU is very complicated, and its clinical manifestations are heterogeneous (Acosta et al., 2008; Blakytny and Jude, 2009). Therefore, the treatment strategy for DFU is a multi-disciplinary, long-term combination therapy process. Application of dressings is an integral part of long-term treatment options. In the diabetic state, multiple factors cause stagnation in one or more stages of the normal healing process. Microvascular disease results in a reduced supply of oxygen and blood in the wound bed, which delays healing and increases the risk of infection (Rathur and Boulton, 2005; Snyder and Waldman, 2009). Bioactive dressings are a good choice for the repair of diabetic wounds. As shown in **Figure 1**, researchers have prepared an injectable adhesive thermosensitive multifunctional polysaccharide-based dressing (fluorinated ethylenepropylene) that can continuously release exosomes to promote angiogenesis at the wound site and accelerate the healing process (Khanolkar et al., 2008; Wang et al., 2019). The silver ion foam dressing used in patients with diabetic foot maintains the wound moist. Studies have shown that a better extracellular matrix environment is a vital factor in promoting the migration of keratinocytes and fibroblasts, and synthesis of collagen (Alvarez, 1988; Morton and Phillips, 2012). In addition, silver ions prevent wound infection, thereby avoiding long-term stagnation in the inflammatory phase due to recurrent infections (Barnea et al., 2010).

Several studies have applied modern dressings containing silver ions to the treatment of DFUs. Jude et al. reported the effect of AQUACEL® Hydrofiber® (E. R. Squibb & Sons, L.L.C., Princeton, NJ, USA) dressings containing ionic silver and Algosteril® (Les Laboratoires Brothier, S.A., Nanterre, France) calcium alginate (CA) dressings in patients with diabetes mellitus and non-ischemic Wagner Grade 1 or 2 DFUs. The study found that the clinical effect of ionic silver dressings was better compared with that of CA dressings, especially for the reduction of ulcer depth and healing of infected ulcers. Ionic silver-treated ulcers reduced in depth nearly twice as much as CA-treated ulcers (Jude et al., 2007). Another study used Contreet Foam (Coloplast A/S, Humlebaek, Denmark), a foam dressing containing silver ions to manage patients with diabetic foot. The study showed that Contreet Foam is safe and easy to use, and effectively accelerates the wound healing process (Rayman et al., 2005). A study evaluated the efficacy of hydrofiber dressings and wound healing in DFUs, comparing the safety, final outcome, and patient

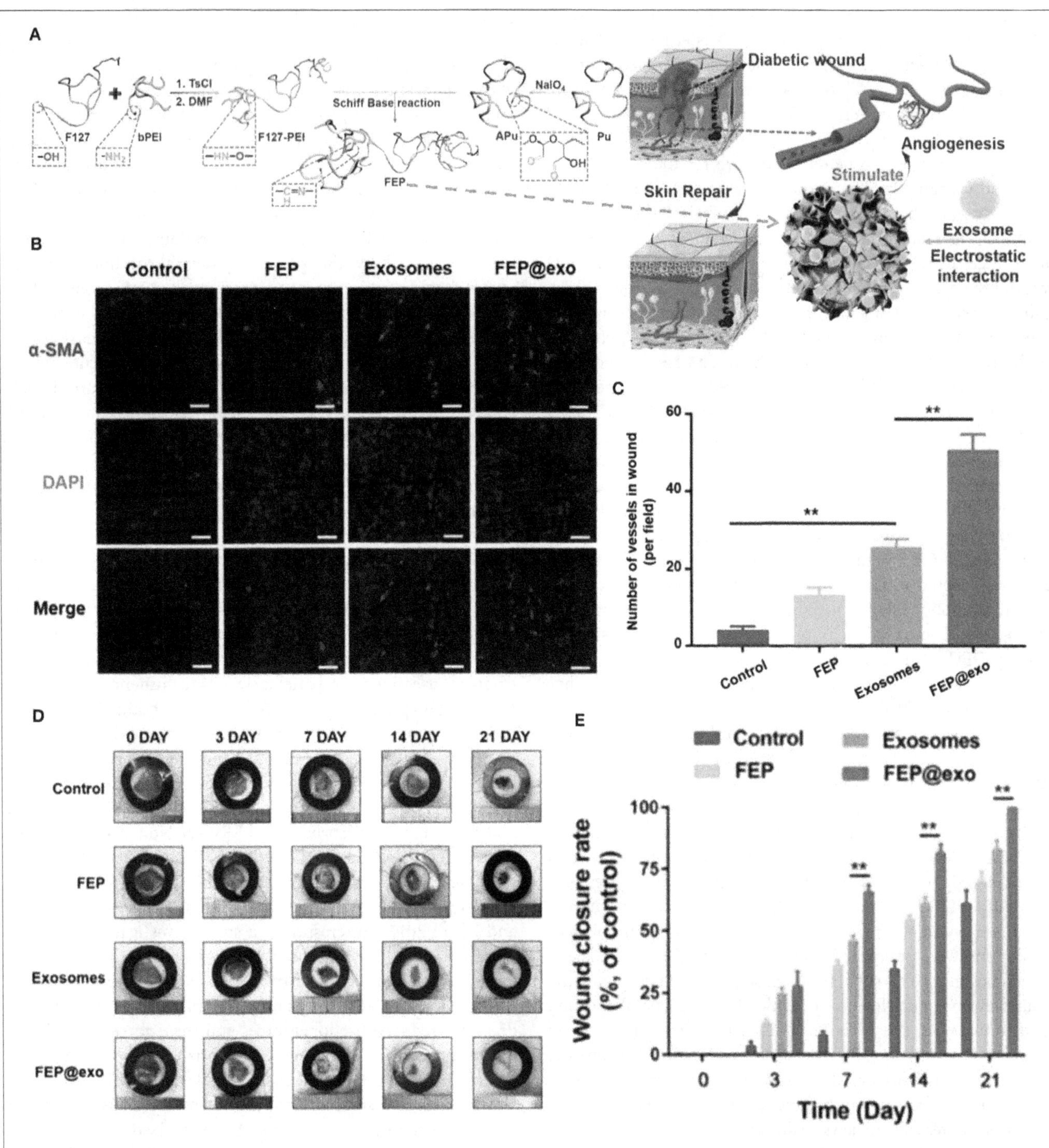

FIGURE 1 | Bioactive dressing promoted angiogenesis in DFU. **(A)** Synthesis and biological function of the fluorinated ethylenepropylene (FEP) hydrogel scaffold containing exosomes. **(B)** Immunofluorescence images of the wound bed stained withα-smooth muscle actin(α-SMA) at day 7. **(C)** The number of new blood vessels at day 7. **(D)** Images of wound healing in mice in different groups. **(E)** Wound closure rate in different groups during wound healing (**$P < 0.01$). Reproduced with permission from Wang et al. (2019).

compliance. Following treatment, hydrofiber dressing showed better healing of the foot ulcer vs. the povidone dressing (Suvarna et al., 2016). Richard et al. studied the effect, tolerance, and acceptability of UrgoStart Contact dressing (Laboratoires Urgo, Chenove, France) in diabetic patients with a neuropathic foot ulcer. The results indicated that the UrgoStart Contact dressing is linked to good tolerance and acceptability, which can effectively promote the healing of neuropathic DFU (Richard et al., 2012).

Zhang et al. compared the efficacy of Mepilex® Lite Dressings (Mölnlycke Health Care, Gothenburg, Sweden) with Vaseline Gauze in the treatment of DFU. The results showed that the study group (Mepilex® Lite) was significantly different from the control group in terms of the mean healing time and wound area. The investigators concluded that the Mepilex® Lite dressing provides a better alternative for the treatment of DFU and warrants further research (Zhang and Xing, 2014). In one study, pure hyaluronic acid was applied to the treatment of DFUs. The results showed that pure hyaluronic acid without other ingredients significantly promotes the healing of DFU without the occurrence of adverse reactions (Lee M. et al., 2016). Lohmann et al. investigated the effect and safety of Biatain® Non-adhesive Dressing (Coloplast A/S, Humlebaek, Denmark) in the treatment of patients with DFU. The results indicated that the average wound area was reduced by more than half in patients treated with the Biatain® dressing (Lohmann et al., 2004). In addition to the common dressings mentioned above, there are other dressings that promote the healing of DFU. A study used sucrose octasulfate dressing treating neuroischemic DFU for 20 weeks, result indicated this dressing significantly improved wound closure without affecting safety (Edmonds et al., 2018). Other study compared bioimplant dressing, a tissue-engineered form of wound dressing containing acellular human amniotic collagen membrane (Life Patch, International Bioimplant Company, Tehran, Iran) with wet dressing in treating DFU. The results show that bio-implantable dressings promote wound healing in DFU better than wet dressings (Edmonds et al., 2018).

DFU is a prevalent and serious global health issue. Wound dressings are regarded as important components of treatment system, with clinicians and patients having many different dressing types to choose from, including hydrogel, foam, hydrocolloid, alginate. The effectiveness of these dressings in DFU has been systematically evaluated, but the conclusions indicated only hydrogels are superior to other types of dressings in healing of DFU (Dumville et al., 2013a,b,c,d). It is worth noting that these systematic reviews included a very small number of studies and were performed several years ago. Decision makers can consider aspects such as the cost of the dressing and the wound management features provided by each type of dressing to determine its use (Wu L. et al., 2015). The effectiveness of these dressings in DFU has been systematically evaluated, but only conclusions are that only hydrogels are superior to other types of dressings in healing of DFU. It is worth noting that these systematic reviews included a very small number of studies and were performed several years ago. Decision makers can consider aspects such as the cost of the dressing and the wound management features provided by each type of dressing to determine its use. It is suggested that more higher quality clinical dressing studies and more comprehensive systematic reviews of the effects of dressings will be conducted in the future.

Pressure Injury

Pressure injury is local injury to the skin or subcutaneous soft tissue, manifested as intact skin or an open ulcer, possibly accompanied by pain. It usually occurs at the site of bone prominence or compression of the medical device (Webb, 2017). Stress injuries often occur in patients who are unable to change their position (Pancorbo-Hidalgo et al., 2006; Pieper et al., 2009). The application of dressings is one of the preventive strategies employed in such cases; however, this approach also increases the total cost of treatment. Therefore, it is necessary to determine whether the use of these dressings provides potential benefit to patients (Sebern, 1986). The main factors in the occurrence of injury are stress and tissue tolerance. Stress factors include compressive strength and duration; tissue tolerance is usually affected by the patient's patient's condition and the external microenvironment (Tirgari et al., 2018; Weller et al., 2018). Since the formation of stress injuries can be avoided, prevention is the main task in the clinic. Foam dressings help to reduce the vertical pressure, shear, and friction of the skin, effectively preventing the occurrence of pressure damage (Bolton, 2016; Truong et al., 2016). As shown in **Figure 2**, researchers have evaluated the effects of the structural and mechanical properties of different dressings to the soft tissue around the wound. These three dressings were Mepilex® Border Sacrum, hypothetical isotropic stiff dressing, and hypothetical isotropic flexible dressing. The anisotropic stiffness feature of the Mepilex® Border Sacrum dressing is essential in wound healing (Schwartz and Gefen, 2019). Studies have shown that excessive skin moisture leads to excessive hydration and damage to the normal barrier function of the skin, hence increasing the risk of ulceration (Demarre et al., 2015). Hydrocolloids or foam dressings for patients with incontinence protect the skin of the appendix from infestation, maintain the skin dry, provide a good microenvironment, and improve tissue tolerance (Williams, 2000). A study assessed the pressure-reducing effect of 10 dressing products, consisting of five types of material (polyurethane foam, hydropolymeric, hydrofiber, hydrocolloid, and low-adherent absorbent). ALLEVYN Non-Adhesive(Smith & Nephew Healthcare, London, UK) exhibited the lowest pressure, while DuoDERM® Extra Thin CGF (ConvaTec Inc., Princeton, NJ, USA)showed the highest pressure (Matsuzaki and Kishi, 2015). Interestingly, a study investigated the modes of action preventing the occurrence of pressure ulcer, such as shear and friction force redistribution, and pressure distribution. The results revealed that the use of Mepilex® and ALLEVYN® dressings reduced frictional forces and shear forces at high-risk areas. In addition, dressings with horizontal fabric structures transferred load over a greater area (Call et al., 2015).

Many clinical studies show that foam dressings can reduce the incidence of pressure ulcers. A randomized controlled trial investigated the role of Mepilex® Border Sacrum and Mepilex® Heel dressings in preventing stress injuries in critically ill patients prior to transfer to the intensive care unit (ICU). The results showed significant differences in the incidence of pressure injuries between the two groups ($\leq$10%). Thus, the study concluded that the application of multi-layered soft silicone foam dressings reduces the incidence in patients prior to transfer to the ICU (Santamaria et al., 2015). A study reported the preventive effect of a five-layer soft silicone border dressing in patients undergoing cardiac surgery in the ICU. The results indicated that there are differences in the occurrence of pressure

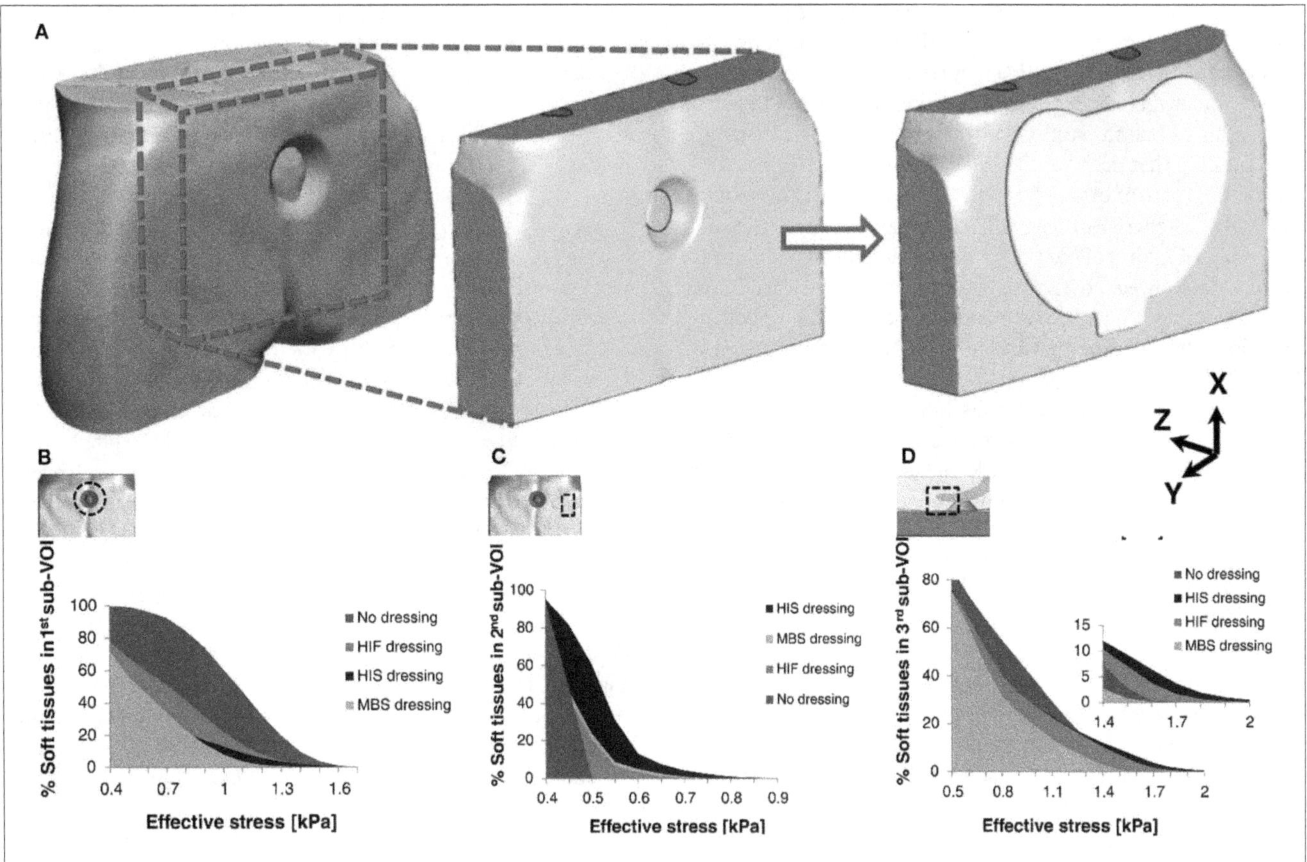

FIGURE 2 | Cumulative volumetric exposures to effective stresses in different parts of the buttocks under combined compression and shear loading. **(A)** Models of the buttock under pressure and coated dressing. **(B)** On the skin surface near the perimeter of the pressure ulcer. **(C)** On the skin surface near the border of the dressing. **(D)** On the skin surface near the tip of the coccyx. Reproduced with permission from Schwartz and Gefen (2019).

injury; however, the difference was not significant (Brindle and Wegelin, 2012). Chaiken et al. applied a silicone border foam dressing to the appendix of patients in the ICU to examine whether the dressing reduces sacral pressure injury. The results showed that the incidence of pressure ulcers decreased from 13.6 to 1.8% after application of the dressing, indicating that this type of dressing effectively reduces the incidence of sacral pressure injury in the ICU (Chaiken, 2012). Furthermore, Walsh et al. applied a silicone border foam dressing to the tibia region of patients in the ICU. The results showed that the incidence of hospital-acquired pressure injury in the ICU decreased from 12.5% in 2009 to 7% in 2010, and the number of sacral pressure injury cases decreased from 50 to 13, respectively (Walsh et al., 2012). Nakagami et al. reported a new dressing containing ceramide 2, which can improve the water-holding capacity. The results indicated that the incidence of persistent erythema was significantly lower in the intervention area compared with the control area. The study concluded that the dressing may be applied to patients with thin and dry skin for the prevention of pressure injury (Nakagami et al., 2007). Another study reported the effect of a polyurethane film in preventing postoperative pressure ulcers. The study found that the polyurethane film patch effectively prevented the occurrence of erythema in the sacral area immediately after surgery (Imanishi et al., 2006). A retrospective study investigated the effectiveness of Mepilex® Ag dressings in decreasing post tracheotomy pressure injury. Another retrospective study reported the effectiveness of Mepilex® Ag dressings in preventing stress injuries in children after thoracotomy. Prior to the application of Mepilex® Ag, the incidence of skin rupture during replacement of the first tracheostomy tube was 11.8%. When Mepilex® Ag was applied, there was no occurrence of skin rupture around the stoma. The study concluded that use of Mepilex® Ag reduces the occurrence of postoperative peristomal pressure injury (Kuo et al., 2013). A systematic review evaluated the effectiveness of dressings and topical preparations in preventing pressure ulcers. Nine dressing studies were included in the 18 included studies. It is concluded that silicone dressings can reduce the incidence of pressure ulcers, but the certainty of the evidence is still low and further research is needed to confirm it. At the same time, the role of polyurethane foam dressings and conventional treatments or hydrocolloids in the prevention of pressure ulcers was also compared. Although the results showed no significant difference, the level of evidence in these studies was very low, and more high-quality studies are needed in the future (Moore and Webster, 2018).

Dressings are widely used to treat pressure ulcers and promote healing, and there are many options, including alginates, hydrocolloids, etc. In 2017, a network meta-analysis of dressings and topical medications for pressure ulcers has been performed. This work concluded that there is currently insufficient evidence to determine whether any dressing or topical treatment promotes the healing of pressure ulcers over other methods. However, it is worth noting that many of the trials in this review are small and carry a high risk of bias (Westby et al., 2017). Only one of these studies had a low risk of bias, which compared the effects of local collagen and hydrocolloids on pressure ulcer healing. Although the results showed no significant difference in healing results between collagen and hydrocolloids, the cost of using collagen was more than double that of hydrocolloids (Graumlich et al., 2003).

Although some research results have demonstrated the role of dressings in the prevention and treatment of pressure ulcers. At the same time, the network meta-analysis also revealed generally poor quality of randomized controlled trials of pressure ulcer dressings, which indicates that the trial plan in this field needs to be improved and perfected. Given the uncertainty of the effectiveness of dressing interventions, any investment in future research must maximize its value to decision makers. Any evaluation of future interventions for the healing of compression ulcers should focus on the dressings most widely used by health professionals. In addition, for people with pressure ulcers, faster recovery is as important as whether recovery occurs, so future research should consider the time to recover from pressure ulcers.

Burns

Burns, generally caused by heat (i.e., hydrothermal fluids, vapors, hot gases, flames, hot metal liquids or solids) cause tissue damage, mainly on the skin and mucous membranes. Severe cases may also injure subcutaneous and submucosal tissues, such as muscles, bones, joints, and even internal organs (Park, 1978). Acute burns are divided into surface, partial, and full thickness burns (Stavrou et al., 2014). Full-thickness burns involve the entire structure of the skin, and even affect the muscles and bones in severe cases. Despite causing considerable pain and suffering, these types of burns heal easily without surgical intervention. Accurate assessment of the depth of burns is crucial for treatment decision-making. In the presence of infection, superficial and partial thickness wounds can deteriorate into deeper burns. A large amount of exudate causes the patient to lose water and nutrients, and provides the appropriate conditions for bacterial growth. Exudation continues to increase in the inflammatory phase, eventually leading to delayed wound healing. Therefore, most of the dressings (e.g., Ag foam dressings) have the ability of osmotic absorption and prevention of infection. Modern dressings used in the remodeling stage reduce the formation of scars and maximize functional recovery at the wound area. Researchers have prepared a new type of hydrogel, termed HA-az-F127 hydrogel. It is formed by the reaction of a hydrazide-modified hyaluronic acid with a F127 triblock copolymer terminated with a benzaldehyde, as shown in **Figure 3**. The excellent physical properties of this hydrogel and the action of aspiration drainage promote healing of burn wounds (Li Z. et al., 2018).

Mabrouk et al. compared the effects of two moist wound management methods, AQUACEL® Ag (ConvaTec Inc., Princeton, NJ, USA), a moist occlusive dressing, and MEBO® (Beijing, China), a moist open dressing, in children with facial partial thickness burns. The results showed that the AQUACEL® Ag group had a faster re-epithelialization rate, a lower frequency of dressing change, and less pain, compared with the MEBO® group. The study concluded that the healing rate and long-term outcomes of the moist occlusive wound dressing was better than those of the moist open dressing for the repair of facial partial thickness burns (Mabrouk et al., 2012). A study reported the effectiveness of two commonly used silver dressings, ACTICOAT™ (Smith & Nephew, Hull, UK) and AQUACEL® Ag, in the treatment of partial burns. The results showed that the healing time and bacterial control of the two silver dressings was similar. However, AQUACEL® Ag dressings have advantages over ACTICOAT™ dressings in terms of patient comfort and cost-effectiveness (Verbelen et al., 2014). Bugmann conducted a study to compare the effects of Mepitel® (Mölnlycke Health Care, Gothenburg, Sweden) and silver sulfadiazine for the treatment of pediatric burns. The results indicated that the Mepitel® group achieved a faster healing process (Bugmann et al., 1998). Huang et al. reported the efficacy and safety of the ACTICOAT™ Ag dressing and silver sulfadiazine for the treatment of burn wounds. The study concluded that ACTICOAT™ with nano silver effectively promoted the healing process of residual wounds after burns without the occurrence of adverse effects (Huang et al., 2007).

A study investigated the degree of pain experienced by the patient when using two different dressings: ACTICOAT™ dressing and silver sulfadiazine. The results demonstrated that the use of the ACTICOAT™ dressing for burn wound care is less painful than the use of silver sulfadiazine in patients with partial thickness burns (Varas et al., 2005). A study reported the pain-reducing function of a silver dressing (AQUACEL® Ag) in patients with partial thickness burns. The results indicated that the wound healing time in the AQUACEL® Ag group was significantly shorter compared with that observed in the silver sulfadiazine group. In addition, the patient's pain was also significantly reduced (Muangman et al., 2010). Another study reported the efficacy of an alginate silver dressing, Askina Calgitrol Ag® (B. Braun Hospicare Ltd, Collooney Co. Sligo, Ireland), and 1% silver sulfadiazine in the management of partial-thickness burn wounds. The results indicated that the average pain score and wound healing time in the Askina Calgitrol Ag® group was significantly lower/shorter than those reported in the silver sulfadiazine group (Opasanon et al., 2010).

Similar to DFUs, burns and scalds are generally larger and prone to infection. Therefore, some antibacterial dressings are often used. Silver sulfadiazine is a commonly used wound management method for burns; however, it can easily cause pain in patients. A recent systematic review evaluated the effectiveness of silver-containing foam dressings and traditional SDD dressings in treating partial thickness burns. This work concluded that there is no significant difference in wound healing

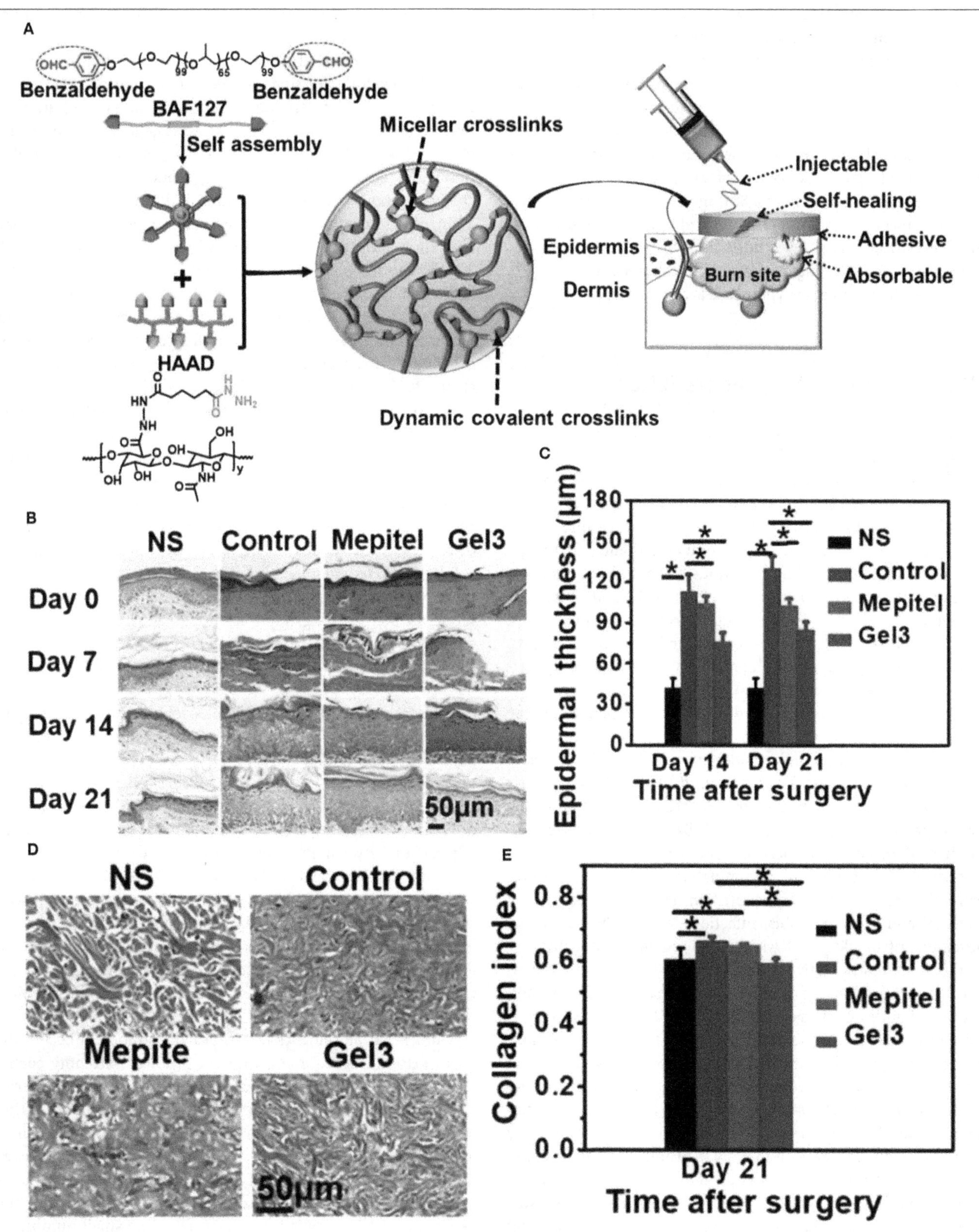

FIGURE 3 | HA-az-F127 hydrogel promotes healing of burn wounds. **(A)** Synthesis and physical characteristics of the HA-az-F127 hydrogel. **(B)** H&E staining at different days after treatment. **(C)** Epidermal thickness in different treatment groups at days 14 and 21. **(D)** Masson's trichrome staining of wounds at day 21. **(E)** Quantification of collagen content in different treatment groups at day 21 (*$P < 0.05$). Reproduced with permission from Li Z. et al. (2018).

between silver-containing foam dressing and SSD dressing, but silver-containing foam dressing reduced pain during the early treatment phase and potentially decreased infection rates. Excessive pain may severely affect the patient's mental and physiological state. Therefore, most studies select the severity of pain as one of the outcome variables to compare these two dressings. Rapid healing of wounds and the prevention of hyperplasia of scars in advanced stages of healing are important aspects for patients with burns. Scar hyperplasia in key areas will seriously affect the patient's physiological function and quality of life. Nevertheless, very few studies have focused on this aspect. Future studies including larger sample sizes and follow-up of patients with wound scar hyperplasia are warranted.

Chronic Venous Leg Ulcers (VLU)

Venous leg ulcers (VLU) are chronic ulcers caused by excessive venous pressure in the lower extremities and abnormal venous blood flow, eventually leading to the formation of an ulcer on the skin of the lower leg (Palfreyman et al., 2007; Chapman, 2017). It is one of the clinical manifestations of chronic venous insufficiency at the most severe stage. The underlying causes of the disease are venous valve incompetence and calf muscle pump insufficiency, leading to venous stasis and hypertension (Gianfaldoni et al., 2017). In this case, the local blood circulation is altered, and the blood supply to the local tissue is insufficient (Serra et al., 2016). Prolonged care leads to high treatment costs. Moreover, the quality of life of patients with chronic VLU is severely affected (Salome et al., 2016).

The venous regurgitation disorder, insufficiency of the vascular function, weak venous wall, and incomplete systolic muscle pump function are considered to be the main causes of VLU formation (Lozano Sanchez et al., 2014). The inflammatory response of leukocytes and endothelial cells is important in the development of VLU (Raffetto, 2009). Based on the above, skin capillary damage, local microcirculation and tissue absorption disorders, fibrin exudation, accumulation of metabolites, lower extremity edema, and skin nutrition changes, followed by bacterial and other microbial infections, eventually lead to the development of ulcers (Dawkins, 2017). Compression therapy is the main conservative treatment of VLU. The treatment mainly includes bandages, elastic stockings, and inflation and compression devices (Rajendran et al., 2007). Moreover, there is substantial necrotic tissue and abnormal exudate on the surface of the ulcer, often accompanied by multiple bacterial infections. Thus, treatment of the wound surface is also necessary. The Ag foam dressing absorbs a large amount of exudate, and it can be used for the prevention of infection. The dressing can be combined with compression therapy to promote wound healing. The alginate dressing absorbs large amounts of exudate and is also suitable for the treatment of VLU. As shown in **Figures 4A,B**, silver ion dressing plays a positive role in wound healing (Harding et al., 2016). Of course, debridement is inevitable. A new type of porous mesh foam dressing, cell foam dressing with through holes (ROCF-CC), was introduced into negative pressure wound therapy with instillation and dwell. As shown in **Figures 4C–E**, this dressing is highly effective on debridement (McElroy et al., 2018).

A study evaluated the effectiveness of knitted viscose and hydrocolloid dressings for venous ulceration. The results indicated that there are no significantly differences in these two dressings (Nelson et al., 2007). Maggio et al. tested the effectiveness and safety of Vulnamin® gel (Errekappa, Milan, Italy) and compressive bandages in patients with lower limb chronic venous ulcers. The results indicated that the use of Vulnamin® together with elastic compressive bandages is safe and more effective than standard dressing (Maggio et al., 2012). Another study compared the wound healing efficacy of AQUACEL® Ag dressing and Urgotul® (Laboratoires Urgo, Chenove, France) Silver dressing for the treatment of venous ulcers at risk of infection. The results showed that both silver dressings were effective in the healing of venous ulcers (Harding et al., 2012). Lammoglia et al. reported the effectiveness and safety of *M. tenuiflora* cortex extract (MTC-2G) in patients with VLU. The results indicated that there was no significant difference between hydrogel containing MTC-2G and hydrogel alone for the treatment of VLU (Lammoglia-Ordiales et al., 2012). A study evaluated LyphoDermTM (XCELLentis, Belgium) gel containing allogeneic epidermal keratinocytes in the treatment of patients with venous ulcers, which are difficult to heal. The results indicated that, in the subgroup with enlarging ulcers, there were significantly more healed ulcers in the LyphoDerm™ group vs. the control group (Harding et al., 2005). Franks et al. compared the effectiveness of ALLEVYN® Hydrocellular and Mepilex®, two commonly used foam dressings, in the treatment of chronic VLU. Although the results did not reveal significant differences in the number of patients achieving complete repair of ulcers between the two groups, both dressings reduced pain after treatment (Franks et al., 2007). Another study compared the treatment effect and cost-effectiveness of silver-containing and non-silver low-adherence dressings in the management of VLU. The results indicated that there were no significant differences between the silver-containing dressing group and the control group (Michaels et al., 2009). A study evaluated the effectiveness and safety of Contreet Foam, a dressing with sustained release of silver, in the management of chronic VLU with moderate and high exudation. The results indicated that Contreet Foam combined with silver achieved excellent exudate management in patients with hard-to-heal chronic VLU (Karlsmark et al., 2003).

Unlike the aforementioned types of wounds, VLU in the lower extremities requires treatment of lower extremity edema to promote wound healing. Tissue edema can stress the arteries and affect the blood circulation in the lower extremities, resulting in insufficient blood supply to the wound. The combination of wound dressings and multiple lamination treatments may exert the best therapeutic effect. At the meantime, a network meta-analysis show that silver-containing dressings can increase the likelihood of VLU healing, but because of the small number of related studies and high risk of bias, the most effective treatment is still not determined (Norman et al., 2018). This results of this network meta-analysis focus exclusively on complete healing, did not take other important outcomes into consideration.

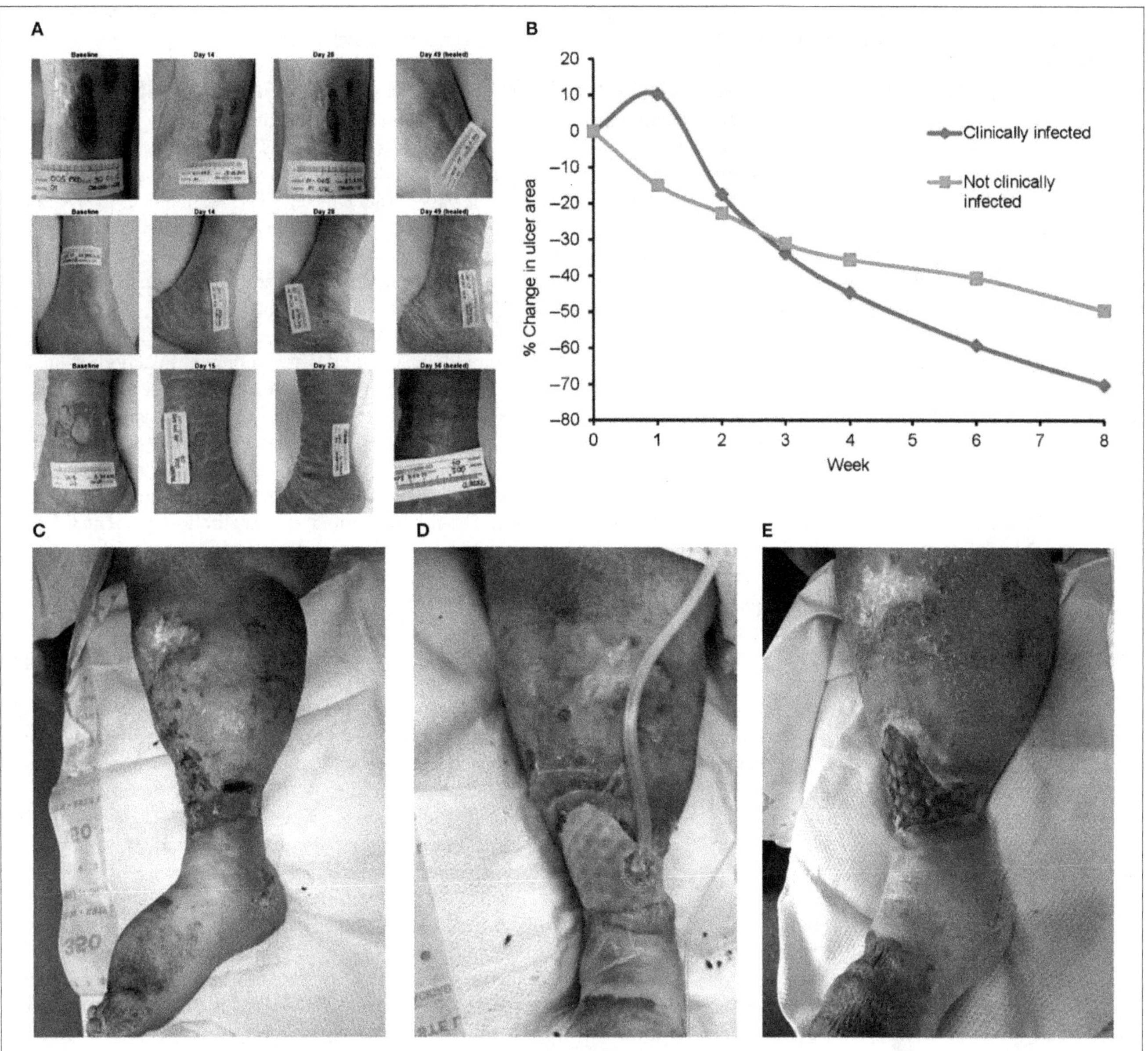

FIGURE 4 | Modern dressings promoting the healing of VLU. **(A)** Ulcer areas in patients with infected (red line) and non-infected (blue line) at different time points. **(B)** Trends in the ulcer area in different patients. **(C)** Initial state of the wound. **(D)** Dressing application of cell foam dressing with through holes (ROCF-CC). **(E)** Dressing replacement. Reproduced with permission from Harding et al. (2016) and McElroy et al. (2018).

Therefore, decision makers can appropriately draw on the results of the above studies according to the actual situation of the wound when choosing a dressing. At the same time, more high-quality research is needed in order to obtain more definitive evidence-based evidence in order to provide reliable decision-making basis for decision makers.

Radiation Dermatitis

Radiation therapy is a common method for the treatment of cancer. It is used to treat cancer that is not suitable for surgery or assist surgery (Terasawa et al., 2009). Radiation-related skin lesions are most common in radioactive local lesions and can be classified as acute radiation-induced skin injury, chronic radiation-induced skin injury, and radiation skin cancer (Kirkwood et al., 2014). Skin side effects of radiation therapy occasionally limit its application (Wickline, 2004; Hird et al., 2008). Severe adverse skin reactions may affect further treatment. At present, the prevention and management of radiation-induced skin injury remains a challenge. Modern wound dressing can be used as a prevention and management method.

Radiation increases the expression of apoptosis-related genes, retards cell proliferation, and decreases cytokine activity and collagen content, resulting in delayed wound healing (Zhang et al., 2012, 2014). A transparent film dressing can be used to protect the skin in the illuminated area. The film dressing using Airwall exhibited a satisfactory prophylactic effect (Arimura et al., 2016).

Radiation dermatitis severity was reduced in patients with breast cancer radiotherapy after prophylactic use of Hydrofilm (Paul Hartmann AG, Heidenheim, Germany) compared with control (Schmeel et al., 2019). A study examined the effect of a film dressing (Airwall) in the management of acute radiation dermatitis induced by proton beam therapy. The results indicated that the Airwall group experienced less severe acute radiation dermatitis compared with the standard management group (Arimura et al., 2016). Perea et al. evaluated the effectiveness of silver-containing Hydrofiber® dressings in minimizing or preventing radiation-induced dermatitis. They suggested that silver-containing Hydrofiber® dressings are effective in reducing radiation dermatitis and arresting its progression, consequently leading to shorter healing time (Whaley et al., 2013). A clinical study investigated the effects of film dressings 3M™ Cavilon® No Sting Barrier Film (3M, Minneapolis, MN, USA), and topical corticosteroids on skin exposed to radiotherapy and compared the effects of the two methods in preventing radiation dermatitis. The results showed that although 3M™ film dressings and corticosteroids were not significantly different vs. control in all respects, 3M™ film dressings may reduce skin itching, while corticosteroids may delay the onset of severe skin inflammation (Shaw et al., 2015). In a single-blind, randomized controlled trial for the prophylactic use of a silicone-based film forming gel dressing (StrataXRT® Stratpharma AG, Basel, Switzerland) in patients with head and neck cancer undergoing radiation therapy, the results show that it is effective for preventing, and delaying the development of grade 2 and 3 skin toxicity (Chan et al., 2019).

For skin already suffering from radiation dermatitis, the use of a suitable dressing can promote healing. Lee et al. studied the effects of a foam dressing combined with recombinant human epidermal growth factor on the treatment of seven patients with head and neck cancer experiencing radiation-induced dermatitis. The wounds of these seven patients with radiation-induced dermatitis healed within 14 days (Lee J. et al., 2016). A study compared the effects of Mepilex® Lite dressing on wound healing and the quality of life in patients with nasopharyngeal carcinoma. The results indicated that the patients in the Mepilex® group had significantly shorter wound healing time and improved sleep quality compared with those in the control group (Zhong et al., 2013).

The onset time of chronic dermatitis usually occurs after radiotherapy for a prolonged period of time (Spalek, 2016). Therefore, the application of modern dressings in radiation dermatitis is mostly focused on acute dermatitis. Although the above studies have concluded that the use of modern dressings and growth factors can improve radiation dermatitis, there is a lack of evidence-based, randomized, controlled trials comparing different types of these dressings. Importantly, future studies should examine skin-specific quality of life and cost-effectiveness. Medical staff should focus on the prevention of radiation dermatitis. They can comprehensively evaluate the skin in the radiotherapy area prior to radiotherapy and use film dressings or liquid dressings to protect the skin.

Split-Thickness Skin Grafting (SSG)

SSG is a common reconstructive technique used to repair orthopedic wounds and burns. However, the repair and regeneration of the donor site is overlooked, causing unnecessary pain to the patient (Shoemaker, 1982; Kirsner et al., 1997; Coruh and Yontar, 2012). In recent years, the application of new dressings is one of the common methods used to promote the repair of the donor site (Malakar and Malakar, 2001). Studies have shown that as many as half of donor sites show signs of infection, and patients often experience pain at these sites. Leakage of blood and fluid is also common. Infections, pain, and leakage are factors that complicate and retard the healing process, as well as cause hypertrophic scars and hypopigmentation or hyperpigmentation. Therefore, appropriate management of the donor site after the collection of SSG is essential. The application of the dressing is a key part of this process. The ideal dressing should assist rapid epithelialization, prevent infection and leakage, and feel comfortable and painless for the patients. It is also adjustable according to different parts, easy to use, and cost-effective.

The skin graft donor site is a type of surgical wound; therefore, it is less likely to be infected than the aforementioned types of wounds. Dressings used in this condition provide a good healing environment to prevent wound infection and reduce the formation of scars. Researchers have combined antimicrobial-impregnated dressing with negative-pressure wound therapy to greatly improve the survival rate of skin grafts (Wu C. C. et al., 2015). Alginate dressings, hydrocolloid dressings, and foam dressings are used in this setting. A study compared the effectiveness of two types of advanced dressings, namely polyurethane foam (ALLEVYN™) and CA (Kaltostat®), in the management of the donor site after SSG. The results indicated that, although there were no significant differences in wound healing time, pain intensity, length of stay, and staff and patient satisfaction between the ALLEVYN™ group and Kaltostat® group, the former dressing was more cost effective than the latter (Higgins et al., 2012). A study compared the effectiveness of two silver dressings, AQUACEL® Ag (Convatec) and Alginate Silver (Coloplast), in the management of donor site wounds. The results showed that Alginate Silver exhibited superior performance in terms of pain and re-epithelialization time (Ding et al., 2013). A trial compared the effectiveness of six wound dressings, including semipermeable film, alginate, hydrocolloid, gauze dressing, hydrofiber, and silicon, in the management of donor-site wounds. The results showed that the hydrocolloid group had the fastest epithelialization rate, and the wound infection rate in the gauze group was 2-fold higher than that reported in the other five groups (Brolmann et al., 2013). A study compared the effectiveness of banded dressings and not banded dressings in patients who underwent skin grafting. Studies showed that the use of polyurethane foams and elastic tape was a simpler but effective method of trimming and may be associated with a shorter operating time than conventional fixation methods using bonded pads (Yuki et al., 2017).

SSG, as a reconstructive technique, is used in burn patients with larger wound bed. The goal of donor site management is to achieve a faster healing speed without pain. Treatment of donor site wounds after SSG is an important clinical issue because patients generally report greater pain at the donor site than at the graft receiving site (Voineskos et al., 2009). Acute wound pain has been shown to increase patient stress and subsequently negatively affect quality of life and lead to delayed wound healing (Broadbent et al., 2003). An evidence-based review summarizes the current evidence that wet wound healing dressing products have clear clinical advantages over non-wet dressing products in treating SSG donor site wounds (Brown and Holloway, 2018). However, no clear trend was detected regarding the performance of each dressing type. So far, there has been limited discussion about the influence of secondary dressings as well as methods/techniques of primary dressing use on donor site wounds. Further research is clearly needed in this area. Especially should explore the role of secondary dressing use, and using more than one primary dressing product throughout the donor site wound-healing process should be taken into consideration.

PROSPECT

With the increase in the incidence of diabetes and chronic vascular diseases, wound management (especially for certain chronic wounds) has gradually attracted the attention of clinicians. The poor healing of wounds results in pain to patients and causes a heavy medical burden. For example, DFU can cause severe and persistent infections and, in extreme cases, lead to amputation. The use of dressings is a common treatment for the management of wounds. In particular, modern dressings are superior to traditional dressings in preventing infection, accelerating wound healing, and reducing pain in patients. The selection of the most appropriate modern dressing product is a challenge for clinicians. An ideal dressing should have the ability to maintain moisture balance in the wound, promote oxygen exchange, isolate proteases, stimulate growth factors, prevent infection, facilitate autolytic debridement, and promote the production of granulation tissue and re-epithelialization (Moura et al., 2013).

Although these modern dressing products are superior to traditional dressings in some respects, their cost is higher than that of traditional dressings. The use of modern dressings in countries and regions where health insurance systems are not well-established involves a significant cost, especially for those with low- or average-income levels. Therefore, dressing manufacturers improve production efficiency, optimize production processes, and reduce costs to ensure that more patients benefit from the use of these new dressings. At the same time, research on a variety of new materials for wounds has emerged, but few have been applied to the clinic in the end. Therefore, promoting the industrialization of scientific research results and providing patients with more alternative dressings is a problem that needs to be solved. Most of the studies discussed above were conducted in hospitals and the subjects were hospitalized patients. Nevertheless, chronic wounds (e.g., DFUs and PUs) were treated at home or nursing home in most cases. It is suggested that how to promote wound healing in a home and nursing home should be studied in the future. In particular, most studies have only evaluated the effect of a single dressing on the wound, but it may have better results when combined with other treatments, such as light therapy and topical drugs. It is suggested that this research direction can be considered in the future. At the same time, additional multi-center, high-quality, randomized, controlled clinical trials are warranted to prove the advantages of modern dressing products in wound healing. Last, systematic review and meta-analysis of DFU and pressure ulcers is slightly lagging, and it is recommended to include research in recent years for timely updates to provide reliable evidence for decision.

CONCLUSION

In summary, the process of wound healing is not static. It requires an appropriate environment at each stage of the healing process, and a reasonable approach to the selection of dressing for certain types of wounds should be clarified for clinical professionals. In the opinion of the author, an ideal dressing is expected to possess the capacity of moisture balance, promote oxygen exchange, isolate proteases, stimulate growth factors, prevent infection, facilitate autolytic debridement, and promote the production of granulation tissue and re-epithelialization. However, currently, there are no dressings that can achieve all these functions. Hence, the specific selection of modern wound dressings for different wounds should be based on the particular conditions, such as the patient's primary disease, the characteristics of the dressing, and especially the physiological mechanisms of wounds. This article summarized the advantages of various wound dressings and their applications in different wounds, aiming to provide a clinical guideline for the selection of suitable wound dressings for effective wound healing.

AUTHOR CONTRIBUTIONS

JW and YS conceived and coordinated this project. CS and CW wrote this paper. RL and YZ collected and summarized literatures. QL and YL edited pictures in this paper. HL revised this paper.

FUNDING

This work was supported by the National Natural Science Foundation of China (grant nos. 51861145311, 21174048, 81671804, and 81772456); Scientific Development Program of Jilin Province (grant nos. 20190304123YY, 20180623050TC, and 20180201041SF); Program of Jilin Provincial Health Department (grant nos. 2019SCZT001 and 2019SRCJ001); Cultivation Program from the Second Hospital of Jilin University for National Natural Science Foundation (grant no. KYPY2018-01); and Youth Talents Promotion Project of Jilin Province (grant no. 192004).

REFERENCES

Acosta, J. B., del Barco, D. G., Vera D. C., Savigne, W., Lopez-Saura, P., Guillen Nieto, G., et al. (2008). The pro-inflammatory environment in recalcitrant diabetic foot wounds. *Int. Wound J.* 5, 530–539. doi: 10.1111/j.1742-481X.2008.00457.x

Alvarez, O. (1988). Moist environment for healing: matching the dressing to the wound. *Ostomy Wound Manage.* 21, 64–83.

Amini-Nik, S., Yousuf, Y., and Jeschke, M., G. (2018). Scar management in burn injuries using drug delivery and molecular signaling: current treatments and future directions. *Adv. Drug Deliv. Rev.* 123, 135–154. doi: 10.1016/j.addr.2017.07.017

Arimura, T., Ogino, T., Yoshiura, T., Toi, Y., Kawabata, M., Chuman, I., et al. (2016). Effect of film dressing on acute radiation dermatitis secondary to proton beam therapy. *Int. J. Radiat. Oncol. Biol. Phys.* 95, 472–476. doi: 10.1016/j.ijrobp.2015.10.053

Ascione, F., Caserta, S., and Guido, S. (2017a). The wound healing assay revisited: a transport phenomena approach. *Chem. Eng. Sci.* 160, 200–209. doi: 10.1016/j.ces.2016.11.014

Ascione, F., Guarino, A., M., Calabro, V., Guido, S., and Caserta, S. (2017b). A novel approach to quantify the wound closure dynamic. *Exp. Cell Res.* 352, 175–183. doi: 10.1016/j.yexcr.2017.01.005

Barnea, Y., Weiss, J., and Gur, E. (2010). A review of the applications of the hydrofiber dressing with silver (Aquacel Ag) in wound care. *Ther. Clin. Risk Manage.* 6, 21–27. doi: 10.2147/TCRM.S3462

Blakytny, R., and Jude, E. B. (2009). Altered molecular mechanisms of diabetic foot ulcers. *Int. J. Low. Extrem. Wounds* 8, 95–104. doi: 10.1177/1534734609337151

Bolton, L. (2016). Evidence corner: dressings can prevent pressure injury. *Wounds* 28, 376–378.

Borda, L. J., Macquhae, F., and E., Kirsner, R. S. (2016). Wound dressings: a comprehensive review. *Curr. Dermatol. Rep.* 5, 287–297. doi: 10.1007/s13671-016-0162-5

Brennan, M. B., Hess, T. M., Bartle, B., Cooper, J. M., Kang, J., Huang, E. S. (2017). Diabetic foot ulcer severity predicts mortality among veterans with type 2 diabetes. *J. Diabetes Complicat.* 31, 556–561. doi: 10.1016/j.jdiacomp.2016.11.020

Brindle, C. T., and Wegelin, J. A. (2012). Prophylactic dressing application to reduce pressure ulcer formation in cardiac surgery patients. *J. Wound Ostomy Continence Nurs.* 39, 133–142. doi: 10.1097/WON.0b013e318247cb82

Broadbent, E., Petrie, K. J., Alley, P. G., and Booth, R. (2003). Psychological stress impairs early wound repair following surgery. *Psychosom. Med.* 65, 865–869. doi: 10.1097/01.PSY.0000088589.92699.30

Brolmann, F. E., Eskes, A. M., Goslings, J. C., Niessen, F. B., de Bree, R., Vahl, A. C., et al. (2013). Randomized clinical trial of donor-site wound dressings after split-skin grafting. *Br. J. Surg.* 100, 619–627. doi: 10.1002/bjs.9045

Broughton, G., II, Janis, J., and Attinger, C. E. (2006). A brief history of wound care. *Plast. Reconstr. Surg. 117,* 6S–11S. doi: 10.1097/01.prs.0000225429.76355.dd

Brown, J. E., and Holloway, S. L. (2018). An evidence-based review of split-thickness skin graft donor site dressings. *Int. Wound J.* 15, 1000–1009. doi: 10.1111/iwj.12967

Bugmann, P., Taylor, S., Gyger, D., Lironi, A., Genin, B., Vunda, A., et al. (1998). A silicone-coated nylon dressing reduces healing time in burned paediatric patients in comparison with standard sulfadiazine treatment: a prospective randomized trial. *Burns* 24, 609–612. doi: 10.1016/S0305-4179(98)0 0095-3

Call, E., Pedersen, J., Bill, B., Black, J., Alves, P., Brindle, C., et al. (2015). Enhancing pressure ulcer prevention using wound dressings: what are the modes of action? *Int. Wound J.* 12, 408–413. doi: 10.1111/iwj.12123

Chaiken, N. (2012). Reduction of sacral pressure ulcers in the intensive care unit using a silicone border foam dressing. *J. Wound Ostomy Continence Nurs.* 39, 143–145. doi: 10.1097/WON.0b013e318246400c

Chan, R. J., Blades, R., Jones, L., Downer, T. R., Peet, S. C., Button, E., et al. (2019). A single-blind, randomised controlled trial of StrataXRT(R) - a silicone-based film-forming gel dressing for prophylaxis and management of radiation dermatitis in patients with head and neck cancer. *Radiother. Oncol.* 139, 72–78. doi: 10.1016/j.radonc.2019.07.014

Chapman, S. (2017). Venous leg ulcers: an evidence review. *Br. J. Community Nurs.* 22, S6–S9. doi: 10.12968/bjcn.2017.22.Sup9.S6

Coruh, A., and Yontar, Y. (2012). Application of split-thickness dermal grafts in deep partial- and full-thickness burns: a new source of auto-skin grafting. *J. Burn Care Res.* 33, e94–e100. doi: 10.1097/BCR.0b013e31823499e9

Davies, P., McCarty, S., and Hamberg, K. (2017). Silver-containing foam dressings with Safetac: a review of the scientific and clinical data. *J. Wound Care* 26, S1–S32. doi: 10.12968/jowc.2017.26.Sup6a.S1

Dawkins, H. (2017). Non-healing venous leg ulcer. *Br. J. Nurs.* 26, S26–S27. doi: 10.12968/bjon.2017.26.Sup20a.S26

Demarre, L., Verhaeghe, S., Van Hecke, A., Clays, E., Grypdonck, M., and Beeckman, D. (2015). Factors predicting the development of pressure ulcers in an at-risk population who receive standardized preventive care: secondary analyses of a multicentre randomised controlled trial. *J. Adv. Nurs.* 71, 391–403. doi: 10.1111/jan.12497

Ding, X., Shi, L., Liu, C., and Sun, B. (2013). A randomized comparison study of Aquacel Ag and Alginate Silver as skin graft donor site dressings. *Burns* 39, 1547–1550. doi: 10.1016/j.burns.2013.04.017

dos Santos, M. R., Alcaraz-Espinoza, J. J., da Costa, M. M., and de Oliveira, H. (2018). Usnic acid-loaded polyaniline/polyurethane foam wound dressing: preparation and bactericidal activity. *Mater. Sci. Eng. C Mater. Biol. Appl.* 89, 33–40. doi: 10.1016/j.msec.2018.03.019

Dumville, J. C., Deshpande, S., O'Meara, S., and Speak, K. (2013a). Foam dressings for healing diabetic foot ulcers. *Cochrane Database Syst. Rev.* 6:CD009111. doi: 10.1002/14651858.CD009111.pub3

Dumville, J. C., Deshpande, S., O'Meara, S., and Speak, K. (2013b). Hydrocolloid dressings for healing diabetic foot ulcers. *Cochrane Database Syst. Rev.* 2:CD009099. doi: 10.1002/14651858.CD009099.pub3

Dumville, J. C., O'Meara, S., Deshpande, S., and Speak, K. (2013c). Alginate dressings for healing diabetic foot ulcers. *Cochrane Database Syst. Rev.* 2:CD009110. doi: 10.1002/14651858.CD009110.pub3

Dumville, J. C., O'Meara, S., Deshpande, S., and Speak, K. (2013d). Hydrogel dressings for healing diabetic foot ulcers. *Cochrane Database Syst. Rev.* 9:CD009101. doi: 10.1002/14651858.CD009101.pub3

Edmonds, M., Lazaro-Martinez, J. L., Alfayate-Garcia, J. M., and Martini, J. (2018). Sucrose octasulfate dressing versus control dressing in patients with neuroischaemic diabetic foot ulcers (Explorer): an international, multicentre, double-blind, randomised, controlled trial. *Lancet Diabetes Endocrinol.* 6, 186–196. doi: 10.1016/S2213-8587(17)30438-2

Fletcher, J. (2003). Using film dressings. *Nurs. Times* 99:57.

Francesko, A., Petkova, P., and Tzanov, T. (2017). Hydrogel dressings for advanced wound management. *Curr. Med. Chem.* 25, 5782–5797. doi: 10.2174/0929867324666170920161246.

Franks, P. J., Moody, M., Moffatt, C. J., Hiskett, G., Gatto, P., Davies, C., et al. (2007). Randomized trial of two foam dressings in the management of chronic venous ulceration. *Wound Repair Regen.* 15, 197–202. doi: 10.1111/j.1524-475X.2007.00205.x

Gianfaldoni, S., Wollina, U., Lotti, J., Gianfaldoni, R., Lotti, T., Fioranelli, M., et al. (2017). History of venous leg ulcers. *J. Biol. Regul. Homeost. Agents* 31(2 Suppl. 2), 107–120.

Gil, J., Natesan, S., Li, J., Valdes, J., Harding, A., Solis, M., et al. (2017). A PEGylated fibrin hydrogel-based antimicrobial wound dressing controls infection without impeding wound healing. *Int. Wound J.* 14, 1248–1257. doi: 10.1111/iwj.12791

Goodwin, N. S., Spinks, A., and Wasiak, J. (2016). The efficacy of hydrogel dressings as a first aid measure for burn wound management in the pre-hospital setting: a systematic review of the literature. *Int. Wound J.* 13, 519–525. doi: 10.1111/iwj.12469

Graumlich, J. F., Blough, L. S., McLaughlin, R. G., and Milbrandt, J. (2003). Healing pressure ulcers with collagen or hydrocolloid: a randomized, controlled trial. *J. Am. Geriatr. Soc.* 51, 147–154. doi: 10.1046/j.1532-5415.2003.51051.x

Guo, S., and Dipietro, L. A. (2010). Factors affecting wound healing. *J. Dent. Res.* 89, 219–229. doi: 10.1177/0022034509359125

Harding, K., Gottrup, F., Jawien, A., Mikosinski, J., Twardowska-Saucha, K., Kaczmarek, S., et al. (2012). A prospective, multi-centre, randomised, open label, parallel, comparative study to evaluate effects of AQUACEL(R) Ag and Urgotul(R) Silver dressing on healing of chronic venous leg ulcers. *Int. Wound J.* 9, 285–294. doi: 10.1111/j.1742-481X.2011.00881.x

Harding, K. G., Krieg, T., Eming, S. A., and Flour, M. L. (2005). Efficacy and safety of the freeze-dried cultured human keratinocyte lysate, LyphoDerm 0.9%, in the treatment of hard-to-heal venous leg ulcers. *Wound Repair Regen.* 13, 138–147. doi: 10.1111/j.1067-1927.2005.130204.x

Harding, K. G., Szczepkowski, M., Mikosinski, J., Twardowska-Saucha, K., Blair, S., Ivins, N., et al. (2016). Safety and performance evaluation of a next-generation antimicrobial dressing in patients with chronic venous leg ulcers. *Int. Wound J.* 13, 442–448. doi: 10.1111/iwj.12450

Harper, D., Young, A., and McNaught, C.-E. (2014). The physiology of wound healing. *Surgery* 32, 445–450. doi: 10.1016/j.mpsur.2014.06.010

Hess, C. T. (2000). When to use alginate dressings. *Adv. Skin Wound Care* 13:131.

Heyer, K., Augustin, M., Protz, K., Herberger, K., Spehr, C., Rustenbach, S., et al. (2013). Effectiveness of advanced versus conventional wound dressings on healing of chronic wounds: systematic review and meta-analysis. *Dermatology* 226, 172–184. doi: 10.1159/000348331

Higgins, L., Wasiak, J., Spinks, A., and Cleland, H. (2012). Split-thickness skin graft donor site management: a randomized controlled trial comparing polyurethane with calcium alginate dressings. *Int. Wound J.* 9, 126–131. doi: 10.1111/j.1742-481X.2011.00867.x

Hird, A. E., Wilson, J., Symons, S., Sinclair, E., Davis, M., and Chow, E. (2008). Radiation recall dermatitis: case report and review of the literature. *Curr. Oncol.* 15, 53–62. doi: 10.3747/co.2008.201

Hobot, J., Walker, M., Newman, G., and Bowler, P. (2008). Effect of hydrofiber wound dressings on bacterial ultrastructure. *J. Electron Microsc.* 57, 67–75. doi: 10.1093/jmicro/dfn002

Hopper, G. P., Deakin, A. H., Crane, E. O., and Clarke, J. (2012). Enhancing patient recovery following lower limb arthroplasty with a modern wound dressing: a prospective, comparative audit. *J. Wound Care* 21, 200–203. doi: 10.12968/jowc.2012.21.4.200

Horn, T. (2012). [Wound dressings. Overview and classification]. *Unfallchirurg* 115, 774–782. doi: 10.1007/s00113-012-2209-9

Huang, Y., Li, X., Liao, Z., Zhang, G., Liu, Q., Tang, J., et al. (2007). A randomized comparative trial between Acticoat and SD-Ag in the treatment of residual burn wounds, including safety analysis. *Burns* 33, 161–166. doi: 10.1016/j.burns.2006.06.020

Hunt, D. L. (2003). Review: debridement using hydrogel seems to be better than standard wound care for healing diabetic foot ulcer. *ACP J. Club* 139:16.

Imanishi, K., Morita, K., Matsuoka, M., Hayashi, H., Furukawa, S., Terashita, F., et al. (2006). Prevention of postoperative pressure ulcers by a polyurethane film patch. *J. Dermatol.* 33, 236–237. doi: 10.1111/j.1346-8138.2006.00057.x

Imran, D., Sassoon, E., and Lewis, D. (2004). Protection of dressings and wounds by cling film. *Plast. Reconstr. Surg.* 113, 1093–1094. doi: 10.1097/01.PRS.0000107737.67371.D7

Jeffcoate, W. J. (2012). Wound healing–a practical algorithm. *Diabetes Metab. Res. Rev.* 28(Suppl. 1), 85–88. doi: 10.1002/dmrr.2235

Jude, E. B., Apelqvist, J., Spraul, M., Martini, J., and Silver Dressing Study Group. (2007). Prospective randomized controlled study of Hydrofiber dressing containing ionic silver or calcium alginate dressings in non-ischaemic diabetic foot ulcers. *Diabet. Med.* 24, 280–288. doi: 10.1111/j.1464-5491.2007.02079.x

Kamoun, E. A., Kenawy, E. S., and Chen, X. (2017). A review on polymeric hydrogel membranes for wound dressing applications: PVA-based hydrogel dressings. *J. Adv. Res.* 8, 217–233. doi: 10.1016/j.jare.2017.01.005

Karlsmark, T., Agerslev, R. H., Bendz, S. H., and Larsen, J. (2003). Clinical performance of a new silver dressing, Contreet Foam, for chronic exuding venous leg ulcers. *J. Wound Care* 12, 351–354. doi: 10.12968/jowc.2003.12.9.26534

Kasuya, A., and Tokura, Y. (2014). Attempts to accelerate wound healing. *J. Dermatol. Sci.* 76, 169–172. doi: 10.1016/j.jdermsci.2014.11.001

Khanolkar, M. P., Bain, S. C., and Stephens, J. W. (2008). The diabetic foot. *QJM* 101, 685–695. doi: 10.1093/qjmed/hcn027

Kirkwood, M. L., Arbique, G. M., Guild, J. B., and Timaran, C. (2014). Radiation-induced skin injury after complex endovascular procedures. *J. Vasc. Surg.* 60, 742–748. doi: 10.1016/j.jvs.2014.03.236

Kirsner, R. S., Eaglstein, W. H., and Kerdel, F. A. (1997). Split-thickness skin grafting for lower extremity ulcerations. *Dermatol. Surg. 23, 85–91.* doi: 10.1111/j.1524-4725.1997.tb00666.x

Kong, L. Z., Wu, Z., Zhao, H., Cui, H., Shen, J., Chang, J., et al. (2018). Bioactive injectable hydrogels containing desferrioxamine and bioglass for diabetic wound healing. *ACS Appl. Mater. Interfaces* 10, 30103–30114. doi: 10.1021/acsami.8b09191

Kuo, C. Y., Wootten, C. T., Tylor, D. A., and Werkhaven, J. A., Huffman, K. F., and Goudy, S. L. (2013). Prevention of pressure ulcers after pediatric tracheotomy using a mepilex ag dressing. *Laryngoscope* 123, 3201–3205. doi: 10.1002/lary.24094

Lammoglia-Ordiales, L., Vega-Memije, M. E., Herrera-Arellano, A., Rivera-Arce, E., Aguero, J., Vargas-Martinez, F., et al. (2012). A randomised comparative trial on the use of a hydrogel with tepescohuite extract (Mimosa tenuiflora cortex extract-2G) in the treatment of venous leg ulcers. *Int. Wound J.* 9, 412–418. doi: 10.1111/j.1742-481X.2011.00900.x

Lee, J., Lee, S. W., Hong, J. P., Shon, M., Ryu, S. H., and Ahn, S. D. (2016). Foam dressing with epidermal growth factor for severe radiation dermatitis in head and neck cancer patients. *Int. Wound J.* 13, 390–393. doi: 10.1111/iwj.12317

Lee, M., Han, S. H., Choi, W. J., Chung, K., and Lee, J. W. (2016). Hyaluronic acid dressing (*Healoderm*) in the treatment of diabetic foot ulcer: a prospective, randomized, placebo-controlled, single-center study. *Wound Repair Regen.* 24, 581–588. doi: 10.1111/wrr.12428

Li, S., Dong, S. J., Xu, W. G., Tu, S. C., Yan, L., Zhao, C. W., et al. (2018). Antibacterial hydrogels. *Adv. Sci.* 5:1700527. doi: 10.1002/advs.201700527

Li, Z., Zhou, F., Li, Z., Lin, S., Chen, L., Liu, L., et al. (2018). Hydrogel cross-linked with dynamic covalent bonding and micellization for promoting burn wound healing. *ACS Appl. Mater. Interfaces* 10, 25194–25202. doi: 10.1021/acsami.8b08165

Lohmann, M., Thomsen, J. K., Edmonds, M. E., Harding, K. G., Apelqvist, J., Gottrup, F., et al. (2004). Safety and performance of a new non-adhesive foam dressing for the treatment of diabetic foot ulcers. *J. Wound Care* 13, 118–120. doi: 10.12968/jowc.2004.13.3.26591

Lozano Sanchez, F. S., Marinel lo Roura, J., Carrasco Carrasco, E., Gonzalez-Porras, J. R., Escudero Rodriguez, J. R., Sanchez Nevarez, I., et al. (2014). Venous leg ulcer in the context of chronic venous disease. *Phlebology* 29, 220–226. doi: 10.1177/0268355513480489

Mabrouk, A., Boughdadi, N. S., Helal, H. A., Zaki, B. M., and Maher, A. (2012). Moist occlusive dressing (Aquacel® Ag) versus moist open dressing (MEBO®) in the management of partial-thickness facial burns: a comparative study in Ain Shams University. *Burns* 38, 396–403. doi: 10.1016/j.burns.2011.09.022

Maggio, G., Armenio, A., Ruccia, F., Giglietto, D., Pascone, M., and Ribatti, D. (2012). A new protocol for the treatment of the chronic venous ulcers of the lower limb. *Clin. Exp. Med.* 12, 55–60. doi: 10.1007/s10238-011-0136-7

Malakar, S., and Malakar, R. S. (2001). Surgical pearl: composite film and graft unit for the recipient area dressing after split-thickness skin grafting in vitiligo. *J. Am. Acad. Dermatol.* 44, 856–858. doi: 10.1067/mjd.2001.111334

Marks, J., and Ribeiro, D. (1983). Silicone foam dressings. *Nurs. Times* 79, 58–60.

Matsuzaki, K., and Kishi, K. (2015). Investigating the pressure-reducing effect of wound dressings. *J. Wound Care* 24, 514–517. doi: 10.12968/jowc.2015.24.11.512

McElroy, E., Lemay, S., Reider, K., and Behnam, A. B. (2018). A case review of wound bed preparation in an infected venous leg ulcer utilizing novel reticulated open cell foam dressing with through holes during negative pressure wound therapy with instillation. *Cureus* 10:e3504. doi: 10.7759/cureus.3504

Michaels, J. A., Campbell, B., King, B., Palfreyman, S. J., Shackley, P., Stevenson, M., et al. (2009). Randomized controlled trial and cost-effectiveness analysis of silver-donating antimicrobial dressings for venous leg ulcers (VULCAN trial). *Br. J. Surg.* 96, 1147–1156. doi: 10.1002/bjs.6786

Moore, Z. E., and Webster, J. (2013). Dressings and topical agents for preventing pressure ulcers. *Cochrane Database Syst. Rev.* 8:CD009362. doi: 10.1002/14651858.CD009362.pub2

Moore, Z. E., and Webster, J. (2018). Dressings and topical agents for preventing pressure ulcers. *Cochrane Database Syst. Rev.* 12:CD009362. doi: 10.1002/14651858.CD009362.pub3

Morton, L. M., and Phillips, T. J. (2012). Wound healing update. *Semin. Cutan. Med. Surg.* 31, 33–37. doi: 10.1016/j.sder.2011.11.007

Moura, L. I., Dias, A. M., Carvalho, E., and de Sousa, H. C. (2013). Recent advances on the development of wound dressings for diabetic foot ulcer treatment–a review. *Acta Biomater.* 9, 7093–7114. doi: 10.1016/j.actbio.2013.03.033

Muangman, P., Pundee, C., Opasanon, S., and Muangman, S. (2010). A prospective, randomized trial of silver containing hydrofiber dressing versus 1% silver sulfadiazine for the treatment of partial thickness burns. *Int. Wound J.* 7, 271–276. doi: 10.1111/j.1742-481X.2010.00690.x

Murakami, K., Aoki, H., Nakamura, S., Nakamura, S., Takikawa, M., Hanzawa, M., et al. (2010). Hydrogel blends of chitin/chitosan, fucoidan and alginate as healing-impaired wound dressings. *Biomaterials* 31, 83–90. doi: 10.1016/j.biomaterials.2009.09.031

Nakagami, G., Sanada, H., Konya, C., Kitagawa, A., Tadaka, E., and Matsuyama, Y. (2007). Evaluation of a new pressure ulcer preventive dressing containing ceramide 2 with low frictional outer layer. *J. Adv. Nurs.* 59, 520–529. doi: 10.1111/j.1365-2648.2007.04334.x

Nelson, E. A., Prescott, R. J., Harper, D. R., Gibson, B., Brown, D., Ruckley, C. V., et al. (2007). A factorial, randomized trial of pentoxifylline or placebo, four-layer or single-layer compression, and knitted viscose or hydrocolloid dressings for venous ulcers. *J. Vasc. Surg.* 45, 134–141. doi: 10.1016/j.jvs.2006.09.043

Norman, G., Westby, M. J., Rithalia, A. D., Stubbs, N., Soares, M. O., and Dumville, J. C. (2018). Dressings and topical agents for treating venous leg ulcers. *Cochrane Database Syst. Rev.* 6:CD012583. doi: 10.1002/14651858.CD012583.pub2

Nuutila, K., Singh, M., Kruse, C., Philip, J., Caterson, E. J., and Eriksson, E. (2016). Titanium wound chambers for wound healing research. *Wound Repair Regen.* 24, 1097–1102. doi: 10.1111/wrr.12472

Okuma, C. H., Andrade, T. A., Caetano, G. F., Finci, L. I., Maciel, N. R., Topan, J. F., et al. (2015). Development of lamellar gel phase emulsion containing marigold oil (*Calendula officinalis*) as a potential modern wound dressing. *Eur. J. Pharm. Sci.* 71, 62–72. doi: 10.1016/j.ejps.2015.01.016

O'Meara, S., and Martyn-St James, M. (2013). Alginate dressings for venous leg ulcers. *Cochrane Database Syst. Rev.* 4:CD010182. doi: 10.1002/14651858.CD010182.pub2

Opasanon, S., Muangman, P., and Namviriyachote, N. (2010). Clinical effectiveness of alginate silver dressing in outpatient management of partial-thickness burns. *Int. Wound J.* 7, 467–471. doi: 10.1111/j.1742-481X.2010.00718.x

Palfreyman, S., King, B., and Walsh, B. (2007). A review of the treatment for venous leg ulcers. *Br. J. Nurs.* 16, S6–14. doi: 10.12968/bjon.2007.16.8.23412

Pancorbo-Hidalgo, P. L., Garcia-Fernandez, F. P., Lopez-Medina, I. M., and Alvarez-Nieto, C. (2006). Risk assessment scales for pressure ulcer prevention: a systematic review. *J. Adv. Nurs.* 54, 94–110. doi: 10.1111/j.1365-2648.2006.03794.x

Park, G. B. (1978). Burn wound coverings - a review. *Biomater. Med. Devices Artif. Organs* 6, 1–35. doi: 10.3109/10731197809118690

Pieper, B., Langemo, D., and Cuddigan, J. (2009). Pressure ulcer pain: a systematic literature review and national pressure ulcer advisory panel white paper. *Ostomy Wound Manage.* 55, 16–31.

Powers, J. G., Higham, C., Broussard, K., and Phillips, T., J. (2016). Wound healing and treating wounds: Chronic wound care and management. *J. Am. Acad. Dermatol. 74, 607–25.* doi: 10.1016/j.jaad.2015.08.070

Raffetto, J. D. (2009). Dermal pathology, cellular biology, and inflammation in chronic venous disease. *Thromb. Res.* 123(Suppl. 4), S66–S71. doi: 10.1016/S0049-3848(09)70147-1

Rajendran, S., Rigby, A. J., and Anand, S. C. (2007). Venous leg ulcer treatment and practice–Part 3: the use of compression therapy systems. *J. Wound Care* 16, 107–109. doi: 10.12968/jowc.2007.16.3.27016

Rathur, H. M., and Boulton, A. J. (2005). Recent advances in the diagnosis and management of diabetic neuropathy. *J. Bone Joint Surg. Br.* 87, 1605–1610. doi: 10.1302/0301-620X.87B12.16710

Rayman, G., Rayman, A., Baker, N., R., Jurgeviciene, N., Dargis, V., Sulcaite, R., et al. (2005). Sustained silver-releasing dressing in the treatment of diabetic foot ulcers. *Br. J. Nurs.* 14, 109–114. doi: 10.12968/bjon.2005.14.2.17441

Richard, J. L., Martini, J., Bonello Faraill, M. M., Bemba, J. M., Lepeut, M., Truchetet, F., et al. (2012). Management of diabetic foot ulcers with a TLC-NOSF wound dressing. *J. Wound Care* 21, 142–147. doi: 10.12968/jowc.2012.21.3.142

Richetta, A. G., Cantisani, C., Li, V. W., Mattozzi, C., Melis, L., De Gado, F., et al. (2011). Hydrofiber dressing and wound repair: review of the literature and new patents. *Recent Pat. Inflamm. Allergy Drug Discov.* 5, 150–154. doi: 10.2174/187221311795399264

Saco, M., Howe, N., Nathoo, R., and Cherpelis, B. (2016). Comparing the efficacies of alginate, foam, hydrocolloid, hydrofiber, and hydrogel dressings in the management of diabetic foot ulcers and venous leg ulcers: a systematic review and meta-analysis examining how to dress for success. *Dermatol. Online J.* 22, 1087–2108. doi: 10.1016/j.jaad.2016.02.1129

Salome, G. M., de Almeida, S. A., de Jesus Pereira, M. T., Massahud, M. R. Jr., de Oliveira Moreira, C. N., de Brito, M. J. et al. (2016). The impact of venous leg ulcers on body image and self-esteem. *Adv. Skin Wound Care* 29, 316–321. doi: 10.1097/01.ASW.0000484243.32091.0c

Santamaria, N., Gerdtz, M., Sage, S., McCann, J., Freeman, A., Vassiliou, T., et al. (2015). A randomised controlled trial of the effectiveness of soft silicone multi-layered foam dressings in the prevention of sacral and heel pressure ulcers in trauma and critically ill patients: the border trial. *Int. Wound J.* 12, 302–308. doi: 10.1111/iwj.12101

Scanlon, L. (2003). Review: debridement using hydrogel appears to be more effective than standard wound care for healing diabetic foot ulcers. *Evid. Based Nurs.* 6:83. doi: 10.1136/ebn.6.3.83

Schmeel, L. C., Koch, D., Schmeel, F. C., Bucheler, B., Leitzen, C., Mahlmann, B., et al. (2019). Hydrofilm polyurethane films reduce radiation dermatitis severity in hypofractionated whole-breast irradiation: an objective, intra-patient randomized dual-center assessment. *Polymers* 11:2112. doi: 10.3390/polym11122112

Schreml, S., Szeimies, R. M., Prantl, L., Karrer, S., Landthaler, M., and Babilas, P. (2010). Oxygen in acute and chronic wound healing. *Br. J. Dermatol.* 163, 257–268. doi: 10.1111/j.1365-2133.2010.09804.x

Schwartz, D., and Gefen, A. (2019). The biomechanical protective effects of a treatment dressing on the soft tissues surrounding a non-offloaded sacral pressure ulcer. *Int. Wound J.* 16, 684–695. doi: 10.1111/iwj.13082

Sebern, M. D. (1986). Pressure ulcer management in home health care: efficacy and cost effectiveness of moisture vapor permeable dressing. *Arch. Phys. Med. Rehabil.* 67, 726–729. doi: 10.1016/0003-9993(86)90004-3

Sedlarik, K. M. (1994). [Modern wound dressings. 5: foam dressings]. *Z. Arztl. Fortbild.* 88, 141–143.

Serra, R., Grande, R., Buffone, G., Molinari, V., Perri, P., Perri, A., et al. (2016). Extracellular matrix assessment of infected chronic venous leg ulcers: role of metalloproteinases and inflammatory cytokines. *Int. Wound J.* 13, 53–58. doi: 10.1111/iwj.12225

Shamloo, A., Sarmadi, M., Aghababaie, Z., and Vossoughi, M. (2018). Accelerated full-thickness wound healing via sustained bFGF delivery based on a PVA/chitosan/gelatin hydrogel incorporating PCL microspheres. *Int. J. Pharm.* 537, 278–289. doi: 10.1016/j.ijpharm.2017.12.045

Shaw, S. Z., Nien, H. H., Wu, C. J., Lui, L., Su, J. F., and Lang, C. H. (2015). 3M cavilon no-sting barrier film or topical corticosteroid (*mometasone furoate*) for protection against radiation dermatitis: a clinical trial. *J. Formos. Med. Assoc.* 114, 407–414. doi: 10.1016/j.jfma.2013.04.003

Shoemaker, P. J. (1982). Split thickness skin grafting. *Can. Fam. Physician* 28, 1145–1147.

Singh, M. R., Saraf, S., Vyas, A., Jain, V., and Singh, D. (2013). Innovative approaches in wound healing: trajectory and advances. *Artif. Cells Nanomed. Biotechnol.* 41, 202–212. doi: 10.3109/21691401.2012.716065

Skorkowska-Telichowska, K., Czemplik, M., Kulma, A., and Szopa, J. (2013). The local treatment and available dressings designed for chronic wounds. *J. Am. Acad. Dermatol.* 68, e117–e126. doi: 10.1016/j.jaad.2011.06.028

Snyder, B. J., and Waldman, B. J. (2009). Venous thromboembolism prophylaxis and wound healing in patients undergoing major orthopedic surgery. *Adv. Skin Wound Care* 22, 311–315. doi: 10.1097/01.ASW.0000305485.98734.1f

Spalek, M. (2016). Chronic radiation-induced dermatitis: challenges and solutions. *Clin. Cosmet. Investig. Dermatol.* 9, 473–482. doi: 10.2147/CCID.S94320

Stavrou, D., Weissman, O., Tessone, A., Zilinsky, I., Holloway, S., Boyd, J., et al. (2014). Health related quality of life in burn patients–a review of the literature. *Burns* 40, 788–796. doi: 10.1016/j.burns.2013.11.014

Suvarna, R., Viswanadh, K. Hanumanthappa, M. B., and Devidas Shetty, N. (2016). A comparative study between hydrofiber dressing, povidone dressing in diabetic foot ulcers. *J. Evid. Based Med. Healthc.* 3, 986–991. doi: 10.18410/jebmh/2016/226

Tarnuzzer, R. W., and Schultz, G. S. (1996). Biochemical analysis of acute and chronic wound environments. *Wound Repair Regen.* 4, 321–325. doi: 10.1046/j.1524-475X.1996.40307.x

Terasawa, T., Dvorak, T., Ip, S., Raman, G., Lau, J., Trikalinos, T., et al. (2009). Systematic review: charged-particle radiation therapy for cancer. *Ann. Intern. Med.* 151, 556–565. doi: 10.7326/0003-4819-151-8-200910200-00145

Thomas, S. (1990). Semi-permeable film dressings. *Nurs. Times* 86, 49–51.

Thu, H. E., Zulfakar, M. H., and Ng, S. F. (2012). Alginate based bilayer hydrocolloid films as potential slow-release modern wound dressing. *Int. J. Pharm.* 434, 375–383. doi: 10.1016/j.ijpharm.2012.05.044

Tirgari, B., Mirshekari, L., and Forouzi, M. A. (2018). Pressure injury prevention: knowledge and attitudes of iranian intensive care nurses. *Adv. Skin Wound Care* 31, 1–8. doi: 10.1097/01.ASW.0000530848.50085.ef

Truong, B., Grigson, E., Patel, M., and Liu, X. (2016). Pressure ulcer prevention in the hospital setting using silicone foam dressings. *Cureus* 8:e730. doi: 10.7759/cureus.730

Tsang, V. L., and Bhatia, S. N. (2004). Three-dimensional tissue fabrication. *Adv. Drug Deliv. Rev.* 56, 1635–1647. doi: 10.1016/j.addr.2004.05.001

Varas, R. P., O'Keeffe, T., Namias, N., Pizano, L. R., Quintana, O. D., Herrero Tellachea, M., et al. (2005). A prospective, randomized trial of acticoat versus silver sulfadiazine in the treatment of partial-thickness burns: which method is less painful? *J. Burn Care Rehabil.* 26, 344–347. doi: 10.1097/01.BCR.0000170119.87879.CA

Verbelen, J., Hoeksema, H., Heyneman, A., Pirayesh, A., and Monstrey, S. (2014). Aquacel((R)) ag dressing versus acticoat dressing in partial thickness burns: a prospective, randomized, controlled study in 100 patients. part 1: burn wound healing. *Burns* 40, 416–427. doi: 10.1016/j.burns.2013.07.008

Voineskos, S. H., Ayeni, O. A., McKnight, L., and Thoma, A. (2009). Systematic review of skin graft donor-site dressings. *Plast. Reconstr. Surg.* 124, 298–306. doi: 10.1097/PRS.0b013e3181a8072f

Vowden, K., and Vowden, P. (2014). Wound dressings: principles and practice. *Surgery* 32, 462–467. doi: 10.1016/j.mpsur.2014.07.001

Walsh, N. S., Blanck, A. W., Smith, L., Cross, M., Andersson, L., Polito, C. (2012). Use of a sacral silicone border foam dressing as one component of a pressure ulcer prevention program in an intensive care unit setting. *J. Wound Ostomy Continence Nurs.* 39, 146–149. doi: 10.1097/WON.0b013e3182435579

Wang, M., Wang, C., Chen, M., Xi, Y., Cheng, W., Mao, C., et al. (2019). Efficient angiogenesis-based diabetic wound healing/skin reconstruction through bioactive antibacterial adhesive ultraviolet shielding nanodressing with exosome release. *ACS Nano.* 13, 10279–10293. doi: 10.1021/acsnano.9b03656

Webb, R. (2017). Pressure ulcer over pressure injury. *Br. J. Nurs.* 26:S4. doi: 10.12968/bjon.2017.26.6.S4

Weller, C. D., Gershenzon, E. R., Evans, S. M., Team, V., McNeil, J. J. (2018). Pressure injury identification, measurement, coding, and reporting: key challenges and opportunities. *Int. Wound J.* 15, 417–423. doi: 10.1111/iwj.12879

Westby, M. J., Dumville, J. C., Soares, M. O., Stubbs, N., Norman, G. (2017). Dressings and topical agents for treating pressure ulcers. *Cochrane Database Syst. Rev.* 6:CD011947. doi: 10.1002/14651858.CD011947.pub2

Whaley, J. T., Kirk, M., Cengel, K., McDonough, J., Bekelman, J., Christodouleas, J., et al. (2013). Protective effect of transparent film dressing on proton therapy induced skin reactions. *Radiat. Oncol.* 8:19. doi: 10.1186/1748-717X-8-19

Wickline, M. M. (2004). Prevention and treatment of acute radiation dermatitis: a literature review. *Oncol. Nurs. Forum* 31, 237–247. doi: 10.1188/04.ONF.237-247

Wilhelm, K. P., Wilhelm, D., and Bielfeldt, S. (2017). Models of wound healing: an emphasis on clinical studies. *Skin Res. Technol.* 23, 3–12. doi: 10.1111/srt.12317

Williams, C. (2000). 3M tegasorb thin: a hydrocolloid dressing for chronic wounds. *Br. J. Nurs.* 9, 720–723. doi: 10.12968/bjon.2000.9.11.6263

Wu, C. C., Chew, K. Y., Chen, C. C., Kuo, Y. R. (2015a). Antimicrobial-impregnated dressing combined with negative-pressure wound therapy increases split-thickness skin graft engraftment: a simple effective technique. *Adv. Skin Wound Care* 28, 21–27. doi: 10.1097/01.ASW.0000459038.81701.fb

Wu, L., Norman, G., Dumville, J. C., O'Meara, S., Bell-Syer, S. E. (2015). Dressings for treating foot ulcers in people with diabetes: an overview of systematic reviews. *Cochrane Database Syst. Rev.* 7:CD010471. doi: 10.1002/14651858.CD010471.pub2.

Yuki, A., Takenouchi, T., Takatsuka, S., Fujikawa, H., and Abe, R. (2017). Investigating the use of tie-over dressing after skin grafting. *J. Dermatol.* 44, 1317–1319. doi: 10.1111/1346-8138.13916

Zhang, S., Song, C., Zhou, J., Xie, L., Meng, X., Liu, P., et al. (2012). Amelioration of radiation-induced skin injury by adenovirus-mediated heme oxygenase-1 (HO-1) overexpression in rats. *Radiat. Oncol.* 7:4. doi: 10.1186/1748-717X-7-4

Zhang, S., Wang, W., Gu, Q., Xue, J., Cao, H., Tang, Y., et al. (2014). Protein and miRNA profiling of radiation-induced skin injury in rats: the protective role of peroxiredoxin-6 against ionizing radiation. *Free Radic. Biol. Med.* 69, 96–107. doi: 10.1016/j.freeradbiomed.2014.01.019

Zhang, Y., and Xing, S. Z. (2014). Treatment of diabetic foot ulcers using Mepilex Lite Dressings: a pilot study. *Exp. Clin. Endocrinol. Diabetes* 122, 227–230. doi: 10.1055/s-0034-1370918

Zhong, W. H., Tang, Q. F., Hu, L. Y., and Feng, H. X. (2013). Mepilex lite dressings for managing acute radiation dermatitis in nasopharyngeal carcinoma patients: a systematic controlled clinical trial. *Med. Oncol.* 30:761. doi: 10.1007/s12032-013-0761-y

Zhu, Y. N., Zhang, J. M., Song, J. Y., Yang, J., Du, Z., Zhao, W. Q., et al. (2019). A multifunctional pro-healing zwitterionic hydrogel for simultaneous optical monitoring of pH and glucose in diabetic wound treatment. *Adv. Func. Mater.* 30:1905493. doi: 10.1002/adfm.201905493

2

The Injury Mechanism of Traumatic Amputation

*Iain A. Rankin[1], Thuy-Tien Nguyen[1], Louise McMenemy[1,2], Jonathan C. Clasper[1,3] and Spyros D. Masouros[1]**

[1] Department of Bioengineering, Imperial College London, London, United Kingdom, [2] Academic Department of Military Surgery and Trauma, Royal Centre for Defence Medicine, ICT Centre, Birmingham Research Park, Birmingham, United Kingdom, [3] Department of Trauma and Orthopaedic Surgery, Frimley Park Hospital, Surrey, United Kingdom

Traumatic amputation has been one of the most defining injuries associated with explosive devices. An understanding of the mechanism of injury is essential in order to reduce its incidence and devastating consequences to the individual and their support network. In this study, traumatic amputation is reproduced using high-velocity environmental debris in an animal cadaveric model. The study findings are combined with previous work to describe fully the mechanism of injury as follows. The shock wave impacts with the casualty, followed by energised projectiles (environmental debris or fragmentation) carried by the blast. These cause skin and soft tissue injury, followed by skeletal trauma which compounds to produce segmental and multifragmental fractures. A critical injury point is reached, whereby the underlying integrity of both skeletal and soft tissues of the limb has been compromised. The blast wind that follows these energised projectiles completes the amputation at the level of the disruption, and traumatic amputation occurs. These findings produce a shift in the understanding of traumatic amputation due to blast from a mechanism predominately thought mediated by primary and tertiary blast, to now include secondary blast mechanisms, and inform change for mitigative strategies.

Correspondence:
Spyros D. Masouros
s.masouros04@imperial.ac.uk

Keywords: biomechanics, traumatic amputation, fracture, blast injury, military, mouse, soil, sand

INTRODUCTION

Recent conflicts have seen improvised explosive devices (IEDs) rise as the insurgents' weapon of choice, where they have been the primary cause of military deaths (Clasper and Ramasamy, 2013). Outside of the military setting, use of IEDs by terrorist organisations has increased steadily over the last 40 years (Edwards et al., 2016). One of the most common and defining injuries of an IED explosion is of blast-mediated traumatic amputation (Ramasamy et al., 2009a). This injury represents a significant cause of morbidity and mortality. It is associated with fatality either directly through haemorrhage, or indirectly as a marker of other severe blast trauma (Mellor and Cooper, 1989). With regards to morbidity, a US-Army study showed only a 2.3% return-to-duty rate for soldiers who had sustained a traumatic amputation (of whom most had suffered only partial hand or foot loss) (Kishbaugh et al., 1995). The 2013 Boston Marathon bombing caused 17 lower limb traumatic amputations and a further 10 severe soft tissue extremity injuries (King et al., 2015); the morbidity in these civilian injuries is likewise extensive with reduced mobility, phantom limb pain, and an overall reduced quality of life reported (Sinha et al., 2011;

Azocar et al., 2020). To limit future morbidity and mortality through mitigative strategies, an accurate understanding of the mechanism of injury is essential.

The mechanisms of injury due to an explosion in general can be separated into five distinct categories: primary (direct effects of the shock front over-pressurisation), secondary (injury caused by energised projectiles propagated by the blast), tertiary (bodily displacement, either directly or indirectly as a result of the blast wind), quaternary (a miscellaneous category of injuries, including burns), and quinary (non-explosion related effects resulting in a hyper-inflammatory state, including through the use of biological, chemical or nuclear products). The mechanism of injury by which blast results in traumatic amputation is not clearly understood. Several mechanisms of injury have been proposed. The first proposed mechanism was hypothesised to occur due to a combination of primary and tertiary blast mechanisms, whereby the shock front over-pressurisation causes diaphyseal fracture through shear and axial stress, followed by the blast wind completing the amputation (Hull and Cooper, 1996). Other proposed mechanisms of injury include tertiary blast injury in isolation, as rapid lower limb movement propagated by the blast wind results in traumatic amputation (Singleton et al., 2014). Secondary blast injury has also been linked to traumatic amputation, where single large fragments propagated by the blast have resulted in "guillotine type" injuries (Hull and Cooper, 1996). More recently, we have shown secondary blast injury as a result of energised environmental debris to be linked to causing traumatic amputation in an animal model (Rankin et al., 2020a). Whilst we showed that high velocity environmental debris (sandy gravel soil) can cause a cohort of injuries, including traumatic amputation, the exact mechanism by which the traumatic amputation had occurred was not examined specifically.

With regards to the type of environmental debris, North Atlantic Treaty Organization (NATO) standards for testing protection against a buried explosive device defines the testing conditions as utilising a soil type which is of a sandy gravel composition (Nato/PfP Unclassified, 2006). Whilst the mechanism by which energised sandy gravel soil causes traumatic amputation is not clear, the process by which it propagates following an explosion is known. When a buried explosive is detonated, the resultant shockwave compresses this surrounding sandy gravel soil. Immediately following this, gas from the explosion is released at high velocity and acts to eject this compressed soil at supersonic speeds, which rapidly decelerate to below 600 m/s before impacting with casualties (Bowyer, 1996; Tremblay et al., 1998). The soil is carried upwards from the ground by the gas flow to project, dependent upon the soil's characteristics, at an angle of between 45 and 120 degrees, in a cone shape. With dry soil, easier venting of gaseous detonation products results in a wider spread. In contrast, water saturated soil resists gaseous venting to a greater degree; this results in a tunnelling effect and concentration of the soil in a vertical direction, which may result in increased injury at the point of impact (Grujicic et al., 2008; Ramasamy et al., 2009b). This injury mechanism has previously been referred to as "sand blast" (Webster et al., 2018).

A further variable which may affect injury risk is the size of the propagated soil. Typical sandy gravel soil granulometry has been described, with ideally distributed particle sizes ranging from 0.1 to 40 mm (Nato/PfP Unclassified, 2006). The effect that variations in soil size or moisture content may have on the injury risk of traumatic amputation is not known.

The aims of this study were (1) to replicate isolated traumatic amputation in a cadaveric small animal mouse model, caused by propagated high velocity sandy gravel soil (subsequently referred to as "sand blast"), (2) to investigate and describe the mechanism of injury of sand blast mediated traumatic amputation, through high-speed video recording and injury documentation, and (3) to investigate the effect of changes in sandy gravel soil size and moisture content on the risk for sustaining traumatic amputation.

MATERIALS AND METHODS

The experimental design and procedures were carried out in compliance with the UK Animal (Scientific Procedures) Act 1986. Testing was conducted using an established model on fresh-frozen cadaveric male MF-1 (out-bred, ex-breeder, wild type) murine specimens (8–9 weeks of age, Charles River Ltd., United Kingdom) (Rankin et al., 2019). Specimens were stored at −20°C and thawed at room temperature (21 ± 2°C) prior to testing.

Sandy gravel soil sizes were chosen based upon NATO unclassified AEP-55 recommendations for typical sandy gravel soil granulometry (Nato/PfP Unclassified, 2006). This was subsequently scaled to the murine model based upon recommended animal scaling parameters in blast, where the scale is equal to the length of a parameter of the human species divided by that of the animal species used ($\lambda_L = L_1/L_2$) (Panzer et al., 2014). The thigh circumference of each species was taken as the representative parameter for scaling, in view of traumatic amputation of the lower limb as the primary outcome. Median mouse thigh circumference was calculated as 2.7 cm (range 2.4–3.2 cm) from specimens ($n = 59$), whilst human thigh circumference was taken from literature as 55 cm (White and Churchill, 1971). From this, a downscaling of 20× for sandy gravel size was utilized ($\lambda_L = 55 / 2.7 = 20$). A minimum sandy gravel size cut-off of 0.1 mm was taken to avoid sublimation of sandy gravel particles smaller than this at high velocity.

Testing with different sandy gravel soil size and moisture content was performed to ascertain for any difference seen in injury risk. Three sandy gravel soil size ranges were tested, consisting of (1) ideally distributed, (2) minimum, and (3) maximum sandy gravel soil size range. These groups were further subdivided into dry, or saturated with water prior to testing. Sand saturated with water was formed by first submerging a sample of dry sand into a beaker of shallow water (with sufficient quantity to cover the total sand mass). The sand was then removed from the beaker by means of a laboratory micro spatula and transferred to absorbent tissue paper, to remove excess water. The sand was subsequently transferred from the tissue paper via micro spatula to the hollow polycarbonate sabot, for use immediately in an experiment.

This gave a total of six different sandy gravel soil test groups. The ideally distributed sandy gravel soil size range chosen consisted of sandy gravel as closely representative to human scaled values, ranging from the human ideal particle size median value to the 85th centile value, consisting of 60% sandy gravel sized 0.1 to 0.3 mm, 20% sized 0.3 to 0.5 mm, and 20% sized 0.5 to 1 mm. The minimum sandy gravel soil size group consisted of 100% sandy gravel sized 0.1 to 0.3 mm. The maximum sandy gravel soil size group consisted of 100% sandy gravel sized 0.5 to 1 mm. The experimental sand sizes and distribution used (scaled to human values) are shown alongside those recommended in NATO AEP-55, ideally distributed particle sizes in **Figure 1** (Nato/PfP Unclassified, 2006).

The sandy gravel was housed within a hollow polycarbonate sabot which was loaded into the firing chamber of a double-reservoir gas-gun system (Nguyen et al., 2018). Within this system, a 2-litre reservoir charged with air or helium and a Mylar® diaphragm firing mechanism was used to accelerate the sabot-sand unit down a 3-m-long, 32-mm-bore barrel. The output velocity was controlled by the thickness of the Mylar® diaphragm. The reservoir section of the gas gun was charged to a predetermined firing pressure, to accelerate the sabot-sand unit to the desired velocity. The pressure was maintained within the reservoir section by a Mylar® diaphragm of appropriate thickness (ranging from 50 to 150 μm). The system utilises a priming section, which is charged to a pressure below the rupture pressure of the diaphragm. This reduces the pressure gradient across the mylar diaphragm (containing the reservoir system) and prevents it from rupturing early, as the reservoir is filled. The pressure in the prime section is vented at the point of initiating firing of the gas gun, resulting in rupture of the diaphragm, with release of the pressurised gas. The gas-gun system accelerates the sabot-sandy-gravel unit down a barrel to exit into a target chamber, where the sabot is separated from the sandy gravel by a sabot stripper. The sabot is halted at this point, while the sandy gravel continues to travel toward the mouse specimen at the intended terminal velocity.

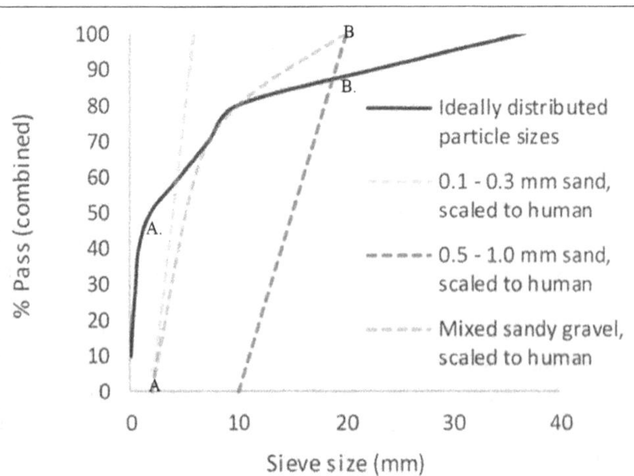

FIGURE 1 | Experimental sandy gravel sizes used, scaled to human values, shown alongside ideally distributed particle sizes. (A) = human median value. (B) = human 85th centile. (A) = lower limit of experimental sandy gravel range. (B) = upper limit of experimental sandy gravel range. % pass (combined) describes the percentage of total volume of sandy gravel passing a specific sieve size; sieve size (mm) relates to the diameter of each hole within the sieve.

Mice were secured in an upright posture on a steel mount of 10 mm diameter fixed within the target chamber, 50 mm distal to the gas-gun outlet. A single cable tie across the thorax was applied to secure the specimens in position on the mount, whilst leaving the lower limbs exposed and freely mobile (**Figure 2**). The right lower limb was centred in the midpoint of the path of the focused sand blast. Experiments were then repeated with re-positioning of the mount to target the contralateral limb.

The speed of the sandy gravel particles at the point of impact with the specimen was estimated using high-speed photography (Phantom VEO710L, AMETEK, United States) at 68,000-fps. An average velocity for the sand blast was determined based upon identifying and tracking four unique points evenly distributed across the sandy gravel. From this, the mean with standard deviation of the velocity of the sand blast as a whole was calculated.

A single control test was performed utilising the maximum gas-gun pressure used previously with the absence of any sandy gravel ejecta. This was performed in order to ascertain whether any injurious effects are caused by the pressurised air alone. This control test was performed on a single mouse specimen.

Prior to and following each test, mouse specimens underwent radiographic imaging using a mini C-arm (Fluoroscan® InSight™ FD system, United States) to identify any lower limb fractures. Following this, the specimens were reviewed to identify lower limb traumatic amputation. Where a lower limb open fracture was present with extensive soft tissue loss, the injury was classified as a traumatic amputation.

Statistical Analysis and Development of the Risk Function

The NCSS statistical software was used for statistical analysis (version 12, UT, United States). A likelihood-criteria best-fit analysis, with the aid of probability plots, was performed to choose the distribution that best fit the data for each injury type. The Weibull distribution was shown to be the best fit in the majority of cases; hence, it was chosen as the probability distribution to represent the risk for all injury types observed in this study. Weibull survival analysis was used to examine the association between sandy gravel velocity and traumatic amputation. The Weibull regression model is $P(v) = 1 - e^{-(v/\lambda)^{\kappa}}$, where P is the probability of injury, v (the average velocity of the sandy gravel) is the predictor variable, and λ and κ are the corresponding coefficients associated with the predictor variable. To derive the injury-risk curves, data were classified as left censored where injury was present and right censored where there was no injury. A *post hoc* two-sample Kolmogorov-Smirnov test was performed to assess

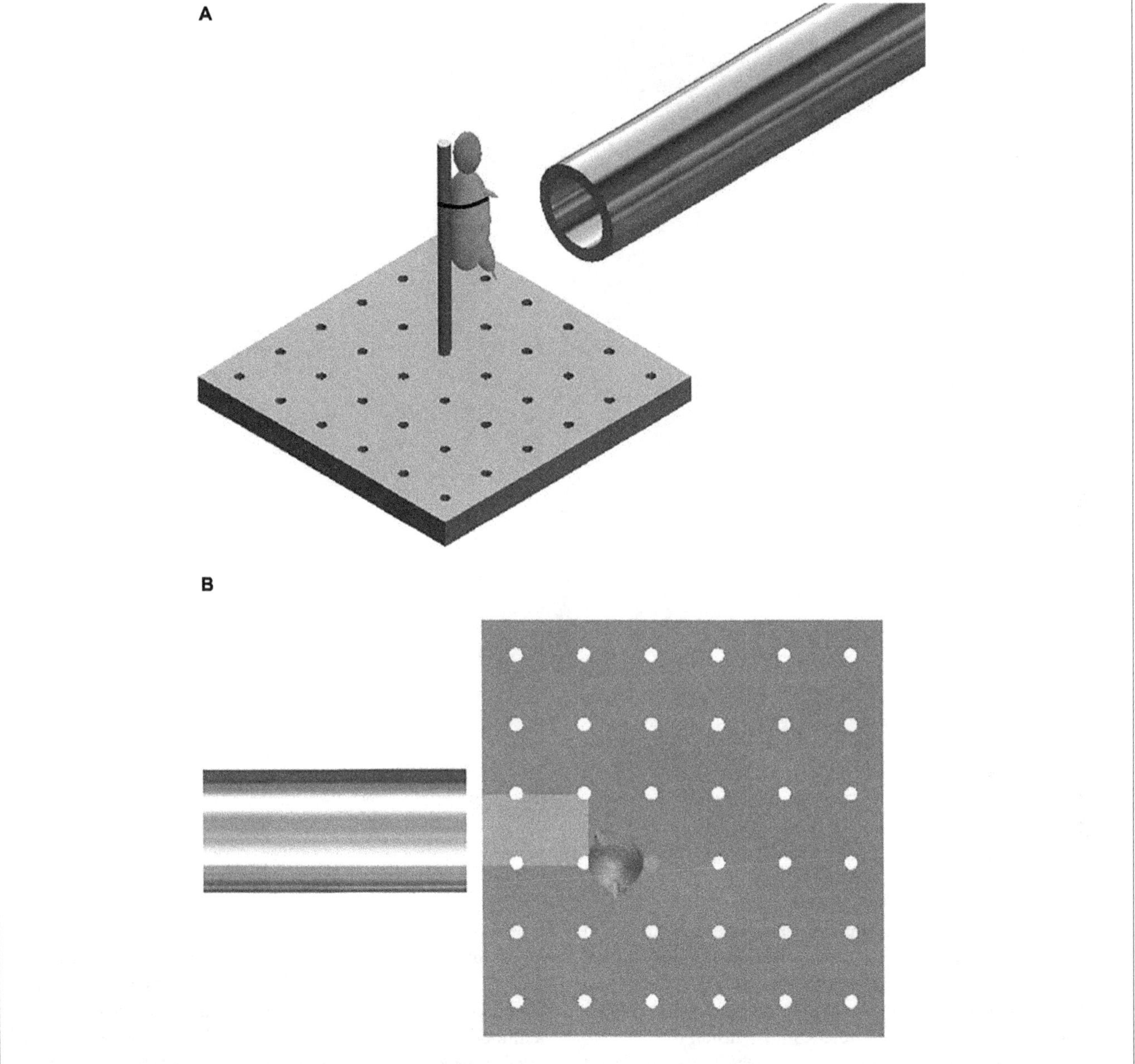

FIGURE 2 | (A) Schematic illustrating the experimental setup showing the gas-gun outlet with mounting platform and mouse. The mouse represented with a model. **(B)** Aerial view of schematic illustrating initial sandy gravel stream passing through distal outlet to impact with offset lower limb of mouse. The mouse is represented with a model.

for significant differences between the distribution of injury-risk curves across groups. A Bonferroni corrected α value of 0.0083 was used to compensate for multiple comparisons (0.0083 = 0.05/6).

RESULTS

Fifty-nine cadaveric mice were used across experiments, comprising of a total of 117 lower limbs impacted by high-velocity sandy gravel soil, and one lower limb control specimen. No injuries were seen in the control specimen. A gas-gun system was used to accelerate the sandy gravel; the average sand blast velocity at the exit of the gun's barrel ranged from 20 ± 5 to 136 ± 5 m/s. A radiograph showing a mouse which sustained a traumatic amputation due to high velocity sand blast is shown in **Figure 3**. **Supplementary Material Video 1** shows a 68,000 frames per second (fps) recorded video with an aerial viewpoint, played at 30 fps, capturing sandy gravel soil travelling at 64 m/s as it impacts a specimen. **Supplementary Material Video 2** shows a 68,000-fps recorded video with a side-on viewpoint, played at 30 fps, capturing sandy gravel impact at 130 m/s. Images from **Supplementary Material Video 2**, showing the sequential stages of sand blast impact, can be seen in **Figure 4**.

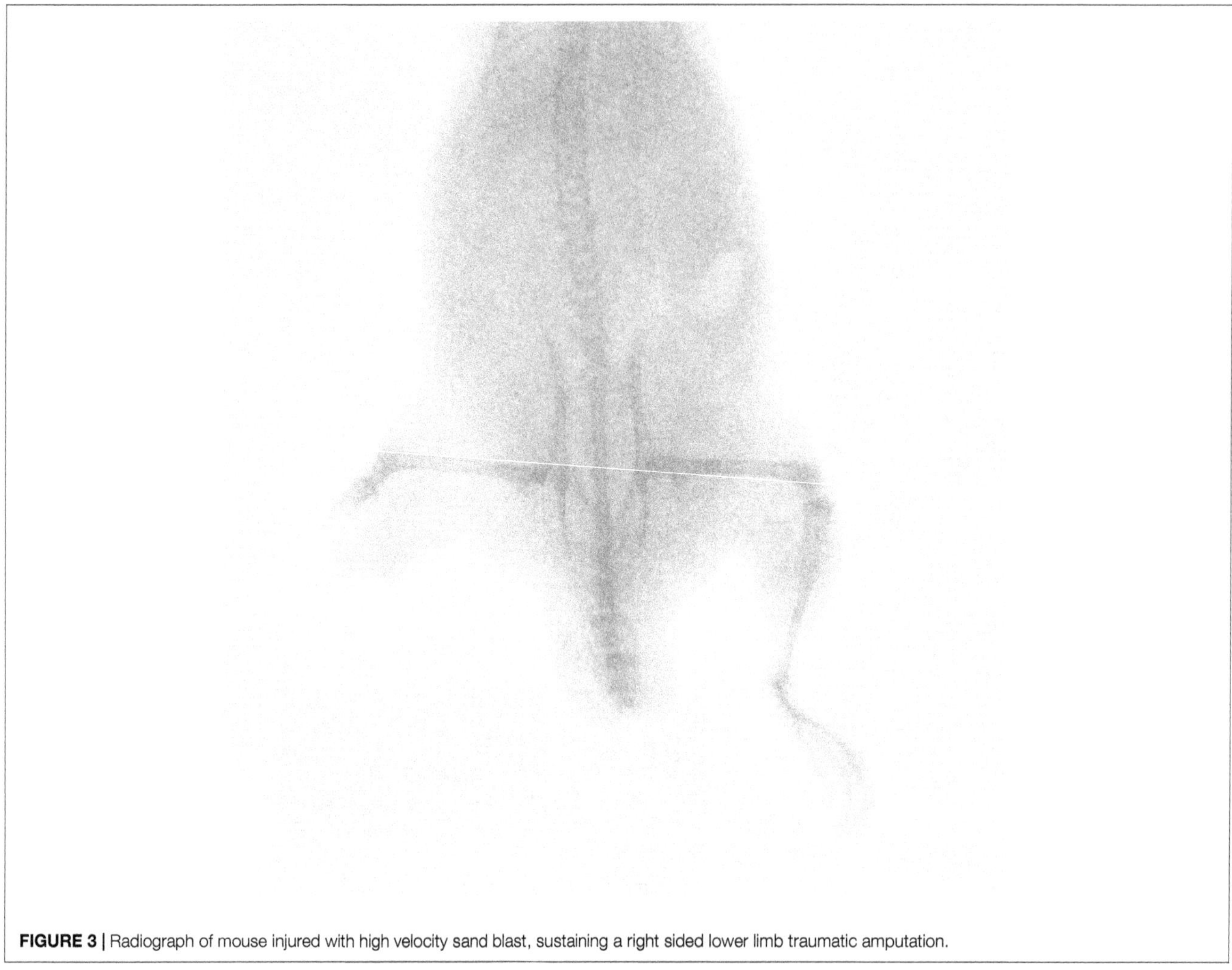

FIGURE 3 | Radiograph of mouse injured with high velocity sand blast, sustaining a right sided lower limb traumatic amputation.

Images showing exemplar injuries sustained are shown in **Figure 5**. These images show increasing severity of injury: initial skin lacerations and superficial wounding only (A), skin and underlying soft tissue injury (B), associated open fracture with extensive tissue loss (C), and complete limb avulsion (D).

Risk of traumatic amputation increased with increasing sand blast velocity across all groups. The 50% risk of traumatic amputation ranged from 70 m/s (95% CI 63–77 m/s) in the 0.1–0.3 mm wet sandy gravel group to 77 m/s (95% CI 69–86 m/s) in the 0.5–1.0 mm dry sandy gravel group. No significant differences between the distribution of injury-risk curves for sandy gravel soil groups were seen, including across size ranges and moisture content (**Table 1**). Full injury risk curves with 95% CIs are shown in **Figure 6**, with the 25, 50, and 75% risks of injury presented in **Table 2**.

DISCUSSION

The first aim of this study was to reproduce isolated traumatic amputation due to sand blast in a cadaveric mouse model, utilising a gas-gun system. We showed that high velocity sand blast is an independent mechanism of injury causing traumatic amputation, with extensive soft tissue and skeletal disruption seen at high velocities. The injury curves presented (**Figure 4**) show a clear link between increasing sandy gravel velocity and likelihood of injury. For example, ideally distributed dry sandy gravel showed a 25, 50, and 75% risk of traumatic amputation at sand blast velocities of 62, 71, and 79 m/s, respectively.

We have previously demonstrated traumatic amputation in conjunction with pelvic fractures, perineal injury and open abdominal trauma, due to impact with a widely dispersed cloud of high velocity sandy gravel, from an under-body blast position (Rankin et al., 2020a). High velocity sand blast was implicated in the mechanism of injury for traumatic amputation, however, from the injury outcome data alone a characterisation of the process was not possible. In the present study, we have utilised a focused sand blast to impact the lower limb in isolation. This has allowed us to characterise the pattern and development of injury and provide a detailed account of the underlying mechanism of injury. Based on these findings, we describe in detail and characterise the process of traumatic amputation due to high velocity sand blast: an initial bolus of compressed sandy gravel soil is propagated at high velocity toward the

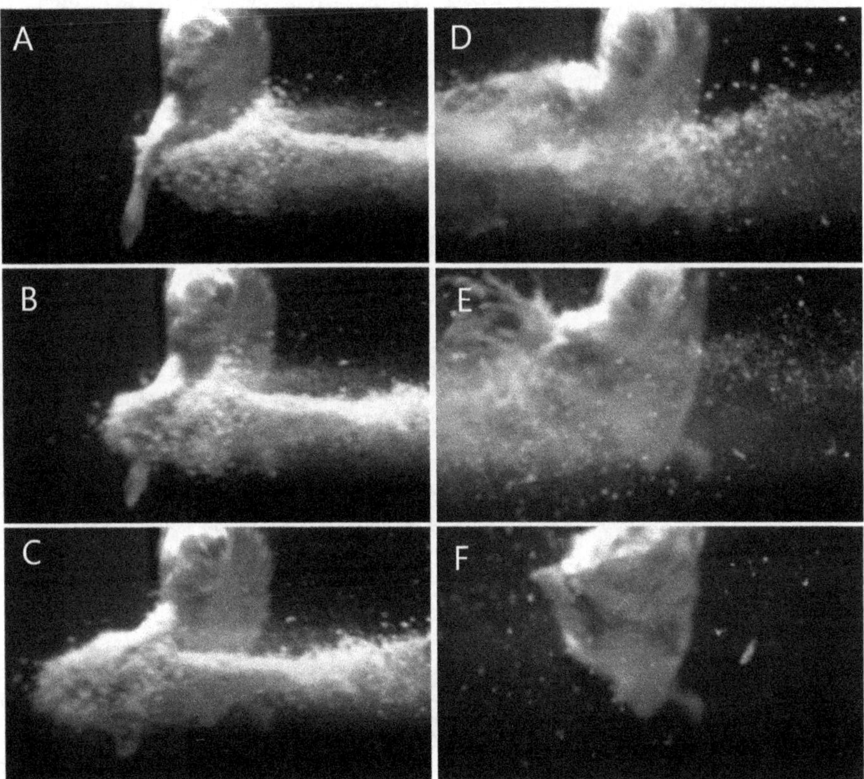

FIGURE 4 | Images illustrating the stages of traumatic amputation secondary to high velocity sand blast. **(A)** Immediately pre-impact. **(B)** Point of initial impact. The sandy gravel has begun to move through and around the tissues of the lower limb at high velocity. Due to the experimental setup the foot has evaded the trajectory of the sandy gravel, whilst the limb above has begun to fragment and displace relative to the foot below. **(C)** The foot has been pulled upward into the trajectory of the sandy gravel, whilst the skeletal and soft tissue above are now significantly fragmented and displaced. **(D)** The lower limb has now been entirely shattered and displaced, with soft tissue stripping on the periphery of the blast now evident as the muscle is seen moving outwards. **(E)** As the sand blast dissipates, the remaining surrounding soft tissues can be seen more clearly to be stripped and displaced. **(F)** Completed traumatic amputation. (A schematic to provide context of the animal's position and orientation is provided in **Figures 2A,B**).

casualty (**Figure 4A**). The initial impact results in superficial burst lacerations and tears to the skin of impacted limbs (**Figure 5A**). As the soil continues to propagate (**Figure 4B**), it progresses to infiltrate deep to the skin, spreading out both within and through tissue planes; this occurs through a series of multiple microtraumas to the underlying fascia and muscular tissue, where the sand blast damages and displaces these soft tissues (**Figure 5B**). With sufficient velocity, the soil progresses to cause a series of microfractures to the underlying skeletal structures which compound to cause segmented or multifragmentary fractures to the long bones of the lower limb; the ongoing impact of soil to the soft tissues of the limb has at this stage resulted in extensive soft tissue loss in association with long bone fractures (**Figure 5C**). The skeletal and soft tissue are now seen to be fragmented and displaced (**Figure 4C**). A critical injury point is reached, whereby the underlying integrity of both skeletal and soft tissues of the limb has been compromised (**Figure 4D**). These tissues progress to be avulsed, whilst tissues in the periphery are injured and propagated outward from the point of maximal impact (**Figure 4E**). At this stage, a completed traumatic amputation of the limb has occurred (**Figures 4F, 5D**).

Multiple mechanisms of injury for blast-related traumatic amputation have been described. The initial accepted mechanism of injury was hypothesised to be due to the initial blast shock front causing a diaphyseal fracture of the limb, with the subsequent blast wind separating and amputating the limb at the point of fracture. This theory was based on laboratory work with a goat hind limb model, which showed that a diaphyseal fracture occurred when a long bone was impacted with a shock front but shielded from the subsequent blast wind or any associated secondary blast injury (Hull and Cooper, 1996). Of note, diaphyseal fracture occurred at distances of 0.5 m proximity to the explosive, but not at 1 m, suggesting the requirement for the casualty to be in close proximity to the explosive for this mechanism of injury to occur (Hull and Cooper, 1996). Further underpinning this mechanism was the clinical association at the time of traumatic amputation to fatal traumatic blast-lung injury, and a lack of through-joint traumatic amputations (Mellor and Cooper, 1989; Hull et al., 1994). More recent military data have questioned this theory. Data from the recent conflicts in Iraq and Afghanistan showed no link between traumatic amputation and primary blast-lung injury, with a high proportion of amputees surviving their injuries;

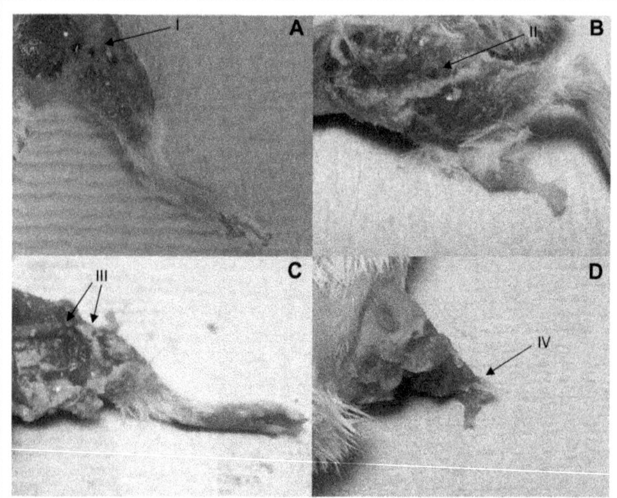

FIGURE 5 | Four separate injuries of worsening severity sustained following impact with high velocity sand blast. **(A)** Burst lacerations and skin tears seen at I. **(B)** Involvement of the underlying subcutaneous and muscular layers, with muscle tears and stripping seen at II. **(C)** Associated open segmental femoral fracture seen at III, with extensive surrounding soft tissue damage and loss. **(D)** Complete limb avulsion with traumatic amputation seen at IV.

TABLE 1 | Two sample Kolmogorov-Smirnov test to assess for significant differences between the distribution of injury risk curves.

	0.1–0.3 dry	0.5–1.0 dry	Mix dry	0.1–0.3 wet	0.5–1.0 wet
0.1–0.3 dry					
0.5–1.0 dry	0.591				
Mix dry	1.000	0.358			
0.1–0.3 wet	0.841	0.095	0.841		
0.5–1.0 wet	0.591	0.841	0.358	0.194	
Mix wet	0.591	0.841	0.358	1.000	0.194

P values shown.

furthermore, a substantially higher incidence of through-joint traumatic amputation was seen, again questioning the shockwave mediated diaphyseal fracture mechanism of injury (Singleton et al., 2014). In that study, we hypothesised that the blast wind played a far more substantial role in the mechanism of injury for traumatic amputation and could itself be a mechanism of injury independent of other factors (Singleton et al., 2014).

Our previous work investigating pelvic fracture and vascular injury due to a shock-tube mediated blast wave (consisting of both a shock front and subsequent blast wind) using a cadaveric mouse model, showed traumatic amputation rates following blast far lower than what would be expected to be present in association with the pelvic fractures and vascular injury seen, as compared to battlefield data (Rankin et al., 2019, 2020b). We subsequently showed that when an initial injuring force to the lower limb occurred prior to impact with the blast wind, traumatic amputation occurred. We concluded that the lower-than-expected traumatic amputation rates were likely due to the absence of any secondary blast injury from the experimental model, to cause this initial injury (Rankin et al., 2019). The current study has shown that high velocity sand blast (a secondary blast-injury mechanism) can be in and of itself, an independent mechanism of injury causing traumatic amputation. Both shock tube and gas-gun experimental models are surrogates of the blast environment. Both platforms provide parts of the blast injury in isolation: a shock-tube system allows focused study of the shock front and blast wind (primary and tertiary blast injury) whilst the gas-gun system allows focused study of energised environmental debris (secondary blast injury). Both platforms have produced traumatic amputation, of varying incidence rates, in a cadaveric animal model. In a blast environment, all of these mechanisms (the primary shock front, the secondary energised environmental debris, and the tertiary blast wind causing bodily displacement) occur together. As such, whilst each is possible of causing traumatic amputation in isolation, the reality likely is that traumatic amputation is caused by all three of these described mechanisms synergistically, to varying degrees of each, dependent upon the blast conditions. These mechanisms acting synergistically are thought to be the causative factors for both military and civilian blast-mediated traumatic amputation, where in the civilian setting the sand blast effect is replaced by explosive fragmentation and any surrounding environmental debris. Whilst other authors have linked energised environmental debris following blast to infection and delayed amputation, we are the first to implicate it as a causative mechanism of injury for traumatic amputation, either independently or in association with the shock front and blast wind (Khatod et al., 2003; Covey and Ficke, 2016; Rankin et al., 2020a).

The second aim of the study was to ascertain differences to the risk of injury from different loading conditions of the energised environmental debris, with reference to size and moisture content. No significant differences were seen across groups when comparing sandy gravel size (ideally distributed, small, large), moisture content (dry or saturated with water), or both. Whilst a type II error of non-significance is possible, the *P* values obtained were far from reaching significance, with values ranging from 0.194 to 1.0. As such, the data leads us to accept the null hypothesis that neither sandy gravel size nor moisture content increase the risk of traumatic amputation as occurs following high velocity sand blast in this model. Of note, the mass of sandy gravel was standardised across all experiments, irrespective of sandy gravel size. As such, it could be concluded that failure to reject the null hypothesis highlights that the total mass and dissipation of energy is the determinant factor in causing injury, as opposed to the individual size of any one piece of environmental debris.

In the present study, the 50% risk of traumatic amputation ranged from 70 m/s (95% CI 63–77 m/s) in the 0.1–0.3 mm wet sandy gravel group to 77 m/s (95% CI 69–86 m/s) in the 0.5–1.0 mm dry sandy gravel group. This compares to our previous work which showed the 50% risk of traumatic amputation in the mouse model to occur, following impact with a widely dispersed high velocity sand blast cloud, at 247 m/s (95% CI: 222–274 m/s). The same gas-gun system and standardised mass of sandy gravel was used in both experiments. In our previous work, the sandy gravel ejecta was widely dispersed to encompass a whole-body

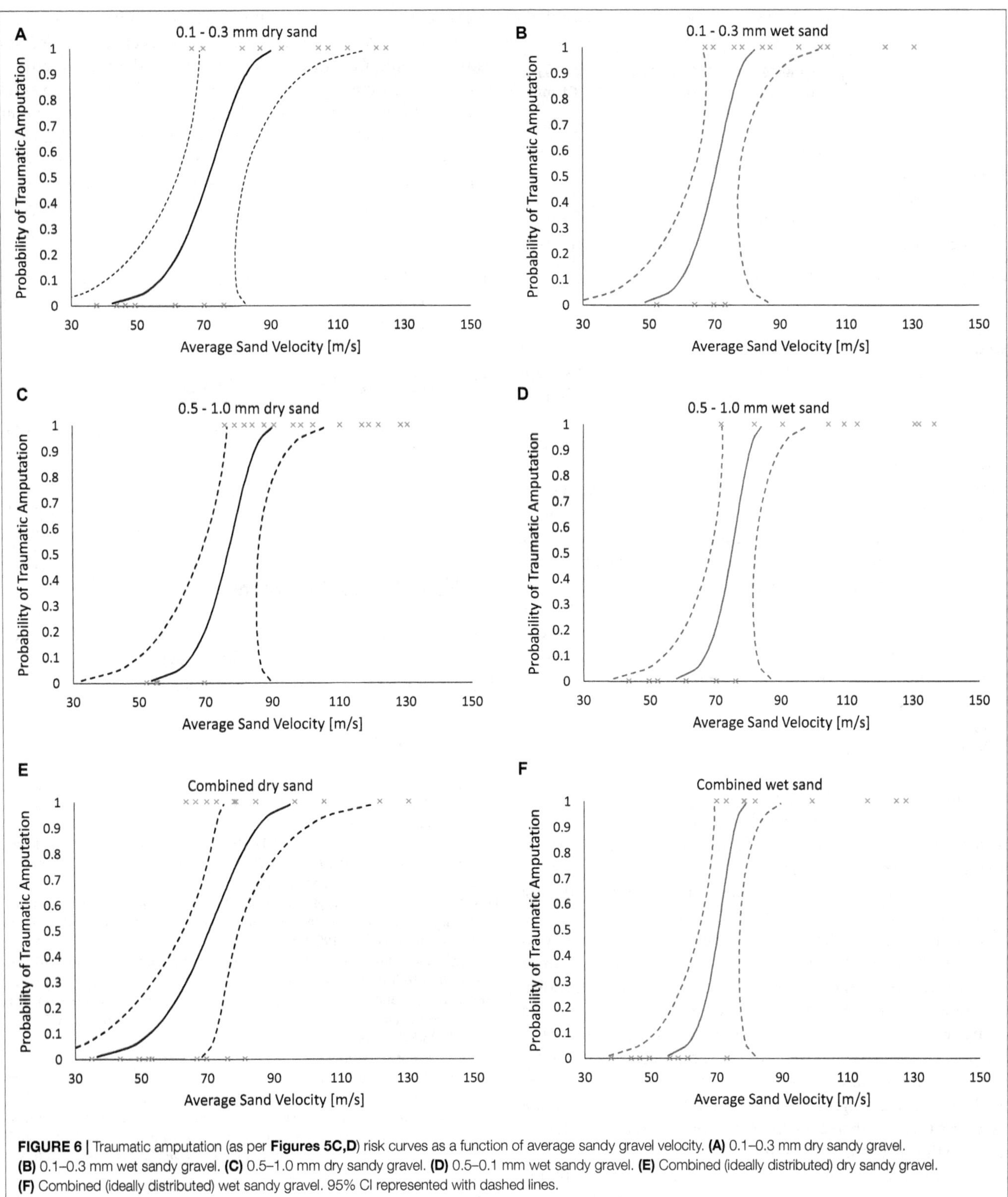

FIGURE 6 | Traumatic amputation (as per **Figures 5C,D**) risk curves as a function of average sandy gravel velocity. **(A)** 0.1–0.3 mm dry sandy gravel. **(B)** 0.1–0.3 mm wet sandy gravel. **(C)** 0.5–1.0 mm dry sandy gravel. **(D)** 0.5–0.1 mm wet sandy gravel. **(E)** Combined (ideally distributed) dry sandy gravel. **(F)** Combined (ideally distributed) wet sandy gravel. 95% CI represented with dashed lines.

field of impact, as occurs following blast, to best recreate the boundary conditions of a blast scenario. As the present work focused on traumatic amputation in isolation, a proportionately greater mass of sandy gravel impacted with the lower limb of the specimen. As such, a greater amount of kinetic energy is expected to be imparted upon the lower limb, where kinetic energy is equal to half of an object's mass multiplied by the velocity squared. It is therefore not unexpected that traumatic amputation was

TABLE 2 | The velocities (m/s) at 25, 50, and 75% risk of injury (V_{25}, V_{50}, and V_{75}, respectively) for traumatic amputation across all group.

	V_{25} (95% CI) m/s	V_{50} (95% CI) m/s	V_{75} (95% CI) m/s
0.1–0.3 mm, dry	64 (52–80)	72 (63–83)	78 (67–90)
0.5–1.0 mm, dry	71 (60–85)	77 (69–86)	81 (74–89)
Ideally distributed, dry	62 (50–75)	71 (63–80)	79 (70–89)
0.1–0.3 mm, wet	65 (55–77)	70 (63–77)	74 (67–82)
0.5–1.0, wet	71 (62–81)	75 (68–82)	78 (72–85)
Ideally distributed, wet	67 (58–77)	71 (65–77)	74 (68–79)

95% confidence intervals (CI) in parenthesis.

seen to occur at a lower velocity than our previous work, nor that any difference in injury risk curve distribution across groups was seen, where the sandy gravel mass across these experiments was standardised.

The current study used a focused sand blast impacting specimens from the front. This experimental setup was utilised as it most accurately allowed for traumatic amputation secondary to high velocity sand blast to occur in a reproducible manner and allowed for accurate characterisation of the injury process. It is more likely in the combat environment, however, that sand blast is encountered below the casualty and that the sand blast projectiles scatter outwards, rather than to focus on a specific target (the lower extremity as in this study). As such, the velocity values obtained from our previous work, utilising an under-body dispersing blast wave, are thought to more accurately represent the velocities required to cause traumatic amputation secondary to high velocity sand blast.

A limitation of the present study is that it was not possible to alter the standardised mass of sandy gravel, due to the experimental setup and customised sabots used in the delivery of the sand. Future work could address this limitation with further customised sabots, of differing sizes and geometry, to accommodate varying sand masses.

Whilst the current study's findings have shown sand blast to be a mechanism of injury for traumatic amputation, scaled animal models cannot be expected to be exact replicates of what occurs in humans (Bowen et al., 1968; Bowyer, 1996; Panzer et al., 2014). Irrespective of scaling, however, this study has shown that sand blast causes significant and progressively worsening injury at high and increasing velocities, resulting in extensive soft tissue and skeletal disruption in the mouse model, and a similar effect therefore should be expected in the human. Future work reproducing high velocity sand blast could utilise human cadaveric tissue, with a focus on protective equipment which may mitigate this mechanism of injury.

This work has now allowed us to describe in detail the complete injury mechanism of traumatic amputation. Following the energy imparted by the initial shock wave (which itself may cause skeletal trauma, if the casualty is sufficiently close to the explosive), energised projectiles (sand blast; or fragmentation and other environmental debris in an urban setting) are propagated at high velocity toward the casualty. This causes initial lacerations to the skin followed by continued progression through tissue planes, as a series of microtraumas to the underlying fascia and muscular tissue occurs. With sufficient velocity the energised projectiles cause multiple fractures to the underlying skeletal structures, which compound to cause segmental and multifragmental fractures to the long bones of the limb. A critical injury point is reached, whereby the underlying integrity of both skeletal and soft tissues of the limb has been compromised. The blast wind that follows these energised projectiles completes the amputation at the level of the disruption, and traumatic amputation occurs. In cases of through-joint amputations, the energised projectiles and subsequent blast wind results in failure of the supportive soft tissues (including the ligamentous structures, but with integrity of the skeletal structures intact) to result in limb avulsion and through-joint amputation.

AUTHOR CONTRIBUTIONS

IR, SM, and JC were involved in the conception of the study. IR and T-TN were involved in the preparation of tests, data acquisition, and in conducting the tests. IR, T-TN, and LM were involved in the data analysis. IR drafted the manuscript. All authors revised it and involved in the interpretation of the data.

ACKNOWLEDGMENTS

This study was conducted in the Royal British Legion Centre for Blast Injury Studies. We would like to thank the Royal British Legion for their ongoing funding and support.

REFERENCES

Azocar, A. F., Mooney, L. M., Duval, J. F., Simon, A. M., Hargrove, L. J., and Rouse, E. J. (2020). Design and clinical implementation of an open-source bionic leg. *Nat. Biomed. Eng.* 4, 941–953. doi: 10.1038/s41551-020-00619-3

Bowen, I., Fletcher, E., and Richmond, D. (1968). *Estimate of man's tolerance to the direct effects of air blast. TIechniCal Progress Report,. DASA-2113.* Washington, DC: Defense Atomic Support Agency.

Bowyer, G. W. (1996). Management of small fragment wounds: experience from the Afghan border. *J. Trauma Inj. Infect. Crit. Care* 40(Suppl. 3), S170–S172. doi: 10.1097/00005373-199603001-00037

Clasper, J., and Ramasamy, A. (2013). Traumatic amputations. *Br. J. Pain* 7, 67–73. doi: 10.1177/2049463713487324

Covey, D. C., and Ficke, J. (2016). "Blast and fragment injuries of the musculoskeletal system," in *Orthopedics in Disasters*, eds N. Wolfson, A. Lerner, and L. Roshal (Heidelberg: Springer), 269–280.

Edwards, D. S., McMenemy, L., Stapley, S. A., Patel, H. D. L., and Clasper, J. C. (2016). 40 years of terrorist bombings–a meta-analysis of the casualty and injury profile. *Injury* 47, 646–652. doi: 10.1016/j.injury.2015.12.021

Grujicic, M., Pandurangan, B., Qiao, R., Cheeseman, B. A., Roy, W. N., Skaggs, R. R., et al. (2008). Parameterization of the porous-material model for sand with different levels of water saturation. *Soil Dyn. Earthq. Eng.* 28, 20–35. doi: 10.1016/j.soildyn.2007.05.001

Hull, J. B., and Cooper, G. J. (1996). Pattern and mechanism of traumatic amputation by explosive blast. *J. Trauma* 40, S198–S205.

Hull, J. B., Bowyer, G. W., Cooper, G. J., and Crane, J. (1994). Pattern of injury in those dying from traumatic amputation caused by bomb blast. *Br. J. Surg.* 81, 1132–1135.

Khatod, M., Botte, M. J., Hoyt, D. B., Meyer, R. S., Smith, J. M., and Akeson, W. H. (2003). Outcomes in open tibia fractures: Relationship between delay in treatment and infection. *J. Trauma* 55, 949–954. doi: 10.1097/01.TA.0000092685.80435.63

King, D. R., Larentzakis, A., and Ramly, E. P. (2015). Tourniquet use at the Boston Marathon bombing. *J. Trauma Acute Care Surg.* 78, 594–599. doi: 10.1097/TA.0000000000000561

Kishbaugh, D., Dillingham, T. R., Howard, R. S., Sinnott, M. W., and Belandres, P. V. (1995). Amputee soldiers and their return to active duty. *Mil. Med.* 160, 82–84. doi: 10.1093/milmed/160.2.82

Mellor, S. G., and Cooper, G. J. (1989). Analysis of 828 servicemen killed or injured by explosion in Northern Ireland 1970–84: the hostile action casualty system. *Br. J. Surg.* 76, 1006–1010. doi: 10.1002/bjs.1800761006

Nato/PfP Unclassified. (2006). Procedures for Evaluating the Protection Level of Logistic and Light Armoured Vehicles Volume 2 For Mine Threat. AEP-55 2, Annex C. NATO/PfP Unclassified, Brussels.

Nguyen, T. T. N., Tear, G. R., Masouros, S. D., and Proud, W. G. (2018). Fragment penetrating injury to long bones. *AIP Conf. Proc.* 1979, 90011–90011. doi: 10.1063/1.5044868

Panzer, M. B., Wood, G. W., and Bass, C. R. (2014). Scaling in neurotrauma: how do we apply animal experiments to people? *Exp. Neurol.* 261, 120–126. doi: 10.1016/j.expneurol.2014.07.002

Ramasamy, A., Hill, A. M., and Clasper, J. C. (2009a). Improvised explosive devices: pathophysiology, injury profiles and current medical management. *J. R. Army Med. Corps* 155, 265–272. doi: 10.1136/jramc-155-04-05

Ramasamy, A., Hill, A. M., Hepper, A. E., Bull, A. M., and Clasper, J. C. (2009b). Blast mines: physics, injury mechanisms and vehicle protection. *J. R. Army Med. Corps* 155, 258–264. doi: 10.1136/jramc-155-04-06

Rankin, I. A., Nguyen, T. T., Carpanen, D., Clasper, J. C., and Masouros, S. D. (2019). Restricting lower limb flail is key to preventing fatal pelvic blast injury. *Ann. Biomed. Eng.* 47, 2232–2240. doi: 10.1007/s10439-019-02296-z

Rankin, I. A., Nguyen, T.-T., Carpanen, D., Clasper, J. C., and Masouros, S. D. (2020a). A new understanding of the mechanism of injury to the pelvis and lower limbs in blast. *Front. Bioeng. Biotechnol.* 8:960. doi: 10.3389/fbioe.2020.00960

Rankin, I. A., Webster, C. E., Gibb, I., Clasper, J. C., and Masouros, S. D. (2020b). Pelvic injury patterns in blast. *J. Trauma Acute Care Surg.* 88, 832–838. doi: 10.1097/ta.0000000000002659

Singleton, J. A. G., Gibb, I. E., Bull, A. M. J., and Clasper, J. C. (2014). Blast-mediated traumatic amputation: evidence for a revised, multiple injury mechanism theory. *J. R. Army Med. Corps* 160, 175–179. doi: 10.1136/jramc-2013-000217

Sinha, R., Van Den Heuvel, W. J. A., and Arokiasamy, P. (2011). Factors affecting quality of life in lower limb amputees. *Prosthet. Orthot. Int.* 35, 90–96. doi: 10.1177/0309364610397087

Tremblay, J., Bergeron, D., and Gonzalez, R. (1998). "KTA1-29: protection of soft-skinned vehicle occupants from landmine effects," in *Val-Belair, Canada, Defence Research Establishment*, ed. T. T. C. P. Program (Quebec: Valcartier).

Webster, C. E., Clasper, J., Stinner, D. J., Eliahoo, J., and Masouros, S. D. (2018). Characterization of lower extremity blast injury. *Mil. Med.* 183, e448–e453. doi: 10.1093/milmed/usx126

White, R., and Churchill, E. (1971). *The Body Size of Soldiers U.S. Army Anhropometry. Report Number 72-51-CE (CPLSEL-94).* Natick, MA: U.S. Army Natick Laboratories.

3

Targeting Tunable Physical Properties of Materials for Chronic Wound Care

Yuzhen Wang [1,2,3,4], *Ubaldo Armato* [5,6] *and Jun Wu* [6*]

[1] Research Center for Tissue Repair and Regeneration Affiliated to the Medical Innovation Research Department and 4th Medical Center, PLA General Hospital and PLA Medical College, Beijing, China, [2] PLA Key Laboratory of Tissue Repair and Regenerative Medicine and Beijing Key Research Laboratory of Skin Injury, Repair and Regeneration, Beijing, China, [3] Research Unit of Trauma Care, Tissue Repair and Regeneration, Chinese Academy of Medical Sciences, 2019RU051, Beijing, China, [4] Department of Burn and Plastic Surgery, Air Force Hospital of PLA Central Theater Command, Datong, China, [5] Histology and Embryology Section, Department of Surgery, Dentistry, Pediatrics and Gynecology, University of Verona Medical School Verona, Verona, Italy, [6] Department of Burn and Plastic Surgery, Second People's Hospital of Shenzhen, Shenzhen University, Shenzhen, China

Correspondence:
Jun Wu
junwupro@126.com

Chronic wounds caused by infections, diabetes, and radiation exposures are becoming a worldwide growing medical burden. Recent progress highlighted the physical signals determining stem cell fates and bacterial resistance, which holds potential to achieve a better wound regeneration *in situ*. Nanoparticles (NPs) would benefit chronic wound healing. However, the cytotoxicity of the silver NPs (AgNPs) has aroused many concerns. This review targets the tunable physical properties (i.e., mechanical-, structural-, and size-related properties) of either dermal matrixes or wound dressings for chronic wound care. Firstly, we discuss the recent discoveries about the mechanical- and structural-related regulation of stem cells. Specially, we point out the currently undocumented influence of tunable mechanical and structural properties on either the fate of each cell type or the whole wound healing process. Secondly, we highlight novel dermal matrixes based on either natural tropoelastin or synthetic elastin-like recombinamers (ELRs) for providing elastic recoil and resilience to the wounded dermis. Thirdly, we discuss the application of wound dressings in terms of size-related properties (i.e., metal NPs, lipid NPs, polymeric NPs). Moreover, we highlight the cytotoxicity of AgNPs and propose the size-, dose-, and time-dependent solutions for reducing their cytotoxicity in wound care. This review will hopefully inspire the advanced design strategies of either dermal matrixes or wound dressings and their potential therapeutic benefits for chronic wounds.

Keywords: chronic wounds, stem cells, mechanical properties, structural properties, nanotechnology

INTRODUCTION

Infections, diabetes, or radiation exposures promote chronic wounds. About 1–2% of the population in developed countries suffer from chronic wounds throughout their lifetime (Dovi et al., 2003; Satish et al., 2017). In China, the prevalence rate of chronic wounds was 1.7‰ among hospitalized patients based on the latest cross-sectional epidemiological survey (Jiang et al., 2011). The feet of diabetic patients usually suffer more as compared with other bodily parts because of further aggravations due to persistent bacterial infections, to sympathetic nerve dysfunctions, and to the continuous frictions of walking (Akash et al., 2020). Approximately one diabetic patient in six suffers from chronic foot wounds (Bakker et al., 2016). Among them, each year almost one million diabetic patients have to undergo lower limb amputation (Boulton et al., 2005). With the aging of the global population, chronic wounds are becoming a worldwide growing medical burden.

Traditional therapeutic approaches to chronic wounds are unsatisfactory because patients suffer prolonged pain as well as unavoidable upshots such as scarring and physical dysfunctions. Commonly used therapeutic approaches are chemical strategies, such as drugs, growth factors, agonists, or inhibitors of critical signaling pathways. However, recent advances in the fields of stem cells and nanotechnology highlighted some knowledge-updating discoveries of physical properties (i.e., mechanical-, structural-, and size-related properties) in directing endogenous stem cell fates (Jiang et al., 2018) and fighting bacterial resistance (Bhattacharya et al., 2019), which might play major roles in chronic wound healing.

The World Health Organization reported that about 265,000 deaths occur every year caused by burns or lack of appropriate treatments including skin substitutes or wound dressings (Das et al., 2016; Khorasani et al., 2018). Generally, skin substitutes aim at replacing missing tissues with gradually degrading dermal matrixes (Ramanathan et al., 2017), while wound dressings cover wound beds acting as temporary mechanical barriers to prevent bacterial infections and to avoid the loss of water and nutrients (Kalantari et al., 2020). Herein, we respectively discuss how the mechanical and structural properties of dermal matrixes affect stem cell behavior, as well as the application of nanoparticle-based (size-related properties) wound dressings for treating infections of chronic wounds. Moreover, we also discuss some worries about mechanical- and structure-related regulation of stem cells. We also address current biosafety concerns about nanoparticles (NPs) and examine workable solutions to reduce their cytotoxicity.

CHRONIC WOUND HEALING

Endogenous Stem Cells

Concerning acute wounds, healing processes are singled out in stages such as hemostasis, inflammation, novel tissue generation, and remodeling, which successively appear and overlap one after the other. Endogenous stem cells (i.e., endothelial progenitor cells, epidermal stem cells, etc.) can both undergo self-renewal and differentiate into one or multiple lineages to repair tissue losses (Kanji and Das, 2017). However, infection, diabetes or radiation exposure may disrupt the well-orchestrated stem cell behaviors and result in chronic wounds (**Figure 1**). Even worse, continuing pathological risks (i.e., bacterial infection, high blood glucose levels, local continuous pressure or friction, etc.) hinder the healing of wounds, which become chronic when they did not show any sign of improved healing after 30 days (Kim et al., 2018).

Endogenous endothelial progenitor cells, which are either resident in wound environments or originate from bone marrow, can promote wound healing via angiogenesis (Kanji and Das, 2017). Angiogenesis involves the sequential occurrence and overlap of various stages, i.e. the activation of endothelial cells, the degradation of the endothelial cells' basement membranes, and the sprouting and ripening of newly-formed vascular structures (Huang et al., 2019). Various alterations of oxygen, nutrients, metabolites' levels, and inflammatory events easily impact on the whole angiogenic process. For example, diabetic wounds easily suffer from hypoxia (or reduced oxygen supply) due to inadequate angiogenesis and a concurring vascular dysfunction and neuropathy. Even more worrying, diabetic wounds usually exhibit higher oxygen consumption rates causing a further lessening of available oxygen *in situ* (Hopf and Rollins, 2007). Concurrently, an inadequate angiogenesis due to an impaired function of endogenous endothelial progenitor cells restricts the proliferation of fibroblasts and their collagen deposition by affecting the hydroxylation of proline and lysine residues, which impacts on scarring's outcomes (**Figure 1**; Desmet et al., 2018).

Endogenous epidermal stem cells with different lineages inhabit the basal layers, interfollicular epidermis, sebaceous glands, eccrine sweat ducts, or hair follicles bulges. During wound healing processes, epidermal stem cells are capable of differentiating into multiple lineages and of repopulating other epidermal components (Haensel et al., 2020). In chronic wounds, most epidermal stem cells show a blunted self-renewal or have been destroyed together with the missing deep tissue. In this case, re-epithelialization typically occurs from the peripheral edges of chronic wounds, being mediated by the recruitment of mobilized stem cells from wound-adjacent stem cell sources (Vagnozzi et al., 2015). Therefore, regulating endogenous stem cells behaviors plays a vital role in chronic wound care.

Infection

Persistent infections help bring about chronic wounds, which are all susceptible to a contaminating localization of microorganisms. The proliferation coupled with toxins release of the localized microorganisms causes inflammatory reactions in the host. Microorganisms can form polymicrobic biofilms, which are one of the mechanisms underlying antibiotic resistance. If left untreated, the infected wounds do not heal (**Figure 1**).

The infecting organisms, most often bacteria, can easily attach to the wound bed and enter into the blood system because the skin barrier is no longer present. *Staphylococcus*, a genus of Gram-positive bacteria which includes more than 40 species, is the most common type of infectious agent found in burn wounds (Dhanalakshmi et al., 2016). The methicillin-resistant *Staphylococcus aureus* (MRSA) is the most common antibiotic-resistant microorganism responsible for hospital-acquired infections (Dantes et al., 2013). Other bacteria genuses found in wounds environment are *Pseudomonas aeruginosa*, *Klebsiella pneumoniae*, *Proteus mirabilis*, *Streptococcus faecalis*,

Abbreviations: AgNPs, silver nanoparticles; ARID1A, AT-rich interactive-domain 1A; ELRs, elastin-like recombinamers; MRSA, methicillin-resistant *Staphylococcus aureus*; MSCs, mesenchymal stem cells; NPs, nanoparticles; PLGA, poly(lactic-co-glycolic acid); ROS, reactive oxygen species; SWI/SNF, switch/sucrose non-fermenting; TAZ, transcriptional co-activator with PDZ-binding motif; YAP, yes-associated protein.

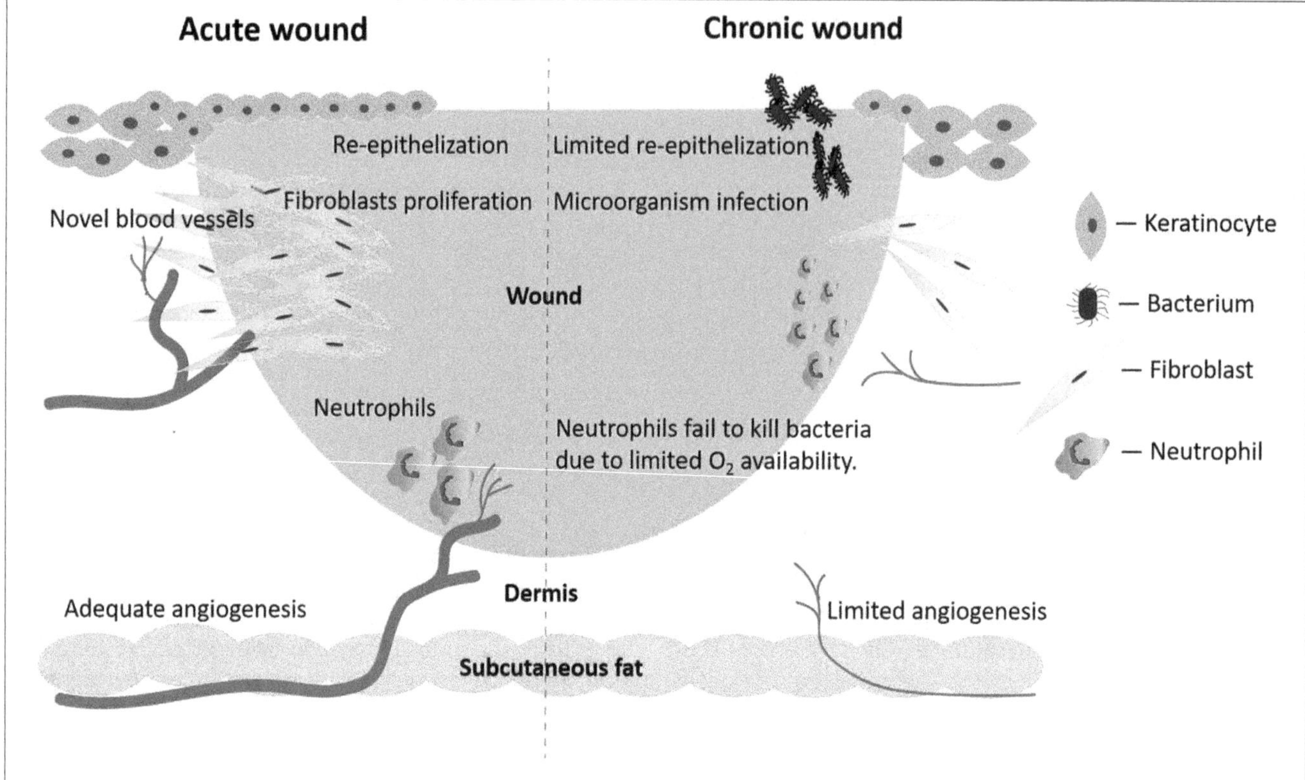

FIGURE 1 | Pathological mechanisms active in acute wounds and chronic wounds, respectively. Acute wounds **(Left Side)**: an adequate angiogenesis promotes re-epithelialization, fibroblasts' proliferation, and neutrophils' anti-infection activities. Chronic wounds **(Right Side)**: persistent local bacterial infections hinder the formation of novel blood vessels. In turn, the restricted angiogenesis hampers fibroblasts' proliferation and the neutrophils' anti-infection activities.

and others more. Besides, an alteration of intestinal flora might cause the gut bacteria to trespass into circulating blood; this has become a current research hotspot and has attracted a lot of attention (He et al., 2019).

In chronic wounds, inadequate angiogenesis due to functionally impaired endogenous endothelial progenitor cells might further reduce the innate anti-infection capabilities. When wounds have become infected, the phagocytosis of the involved pathogens by leukocytes will trigger the respiratory burst process resulting in the release of massive amounts of bactericidal reactive oxygen species (ROS). Reportedly, the respiratory burst process consumes about 98% of the oxygen in neutrophils (Bryan et al., 2012). A lack of oxygen in chronic wounds impairs the anti-infection abilities of neutrophils (**Figure 1**).

Usually, diabetic patients show high blood glucose levels due to reduced autologous insulin secretion or increased insulin resistance, which result in multiple metabolic dysfunctions. Several underlying pathological factors also contribute to the delayed healing of diabetic wounds, such as local persistent bacterial infections coupled with excessive levels of pro-inflammatory cytokines, proteases, ROS (Frykberg and Banks, 2015), and with a worsening vascular dysfunction combined with the cells' inability to respond to pro-reparative stimuli (Kim et al., 2018).

MECHANICAL PROPERTIES

Mechanical properties of dermal matrixes include stiffness, elastic modulus, tensile strength, viscoelasticity, stress stiffening effects, stress-relaxation rate, and more. Recent studies about mechanical-related regulation of stem cells and elastin-based dermal matrixes highlighted the practical solutions for chronic wound care.

Mechanical-Related Regulation During Wound Healing

Clinical practice in wound healing has shown that higher tension sutures of surgical wounds increase scar tissue formation, and that the stress and stiffness of wound fixation could also affect wound healing speed and quality. However, the underlying mechanism is still unclear.

Recently, mechanical signals have increasingly shown an overarching ability to regulate stem cell characteristics and lineages. Among mechanical signals, stiffness-related control of cell fates has been studied extensively. For example, mesenchymal stem cells (MSCs) show distinctive differentiation patterns when cultured in matrixes of tunable stiffness. MSCs changed their lineage specification into neurons, myoblasts or osteoblasts when cultured in polyacrylamide hydrogels with a tunable stiffness gradient varying from 0.1 to 25 kPa (Engler et al., 2006). In other words, MSCs "felt" matrixes stiffness and then "chose" their direction of differentiation.

Further research showed that the transcriptional co-activator with PDZ-binding motif (TAZ) and Yes-associated protein (YAP) played vital roles in the stiffness-related regulation of stem cell fates (Yang et al., 2014). YAP/TAZ are two highly related downstream readers and transcriptional regulators of mechanotransduction, serving as molecular "beacons" of cellular responses to surrounding mechanical stimuli (Brusatin et al., 2018). Reportedly, the AT-rich interactive domain-containing protein 1A (ARID1A) is located in the chromosome 1p36 region acting as a tumor suppressor gene (Guan et al., 2011). The ARID1A belongs to the switch/sucrose non-fermenting (SWI/SNF) chromatin remodeling complex, which encodes a large nuclear protein involved in chromatin remodeling (Guan et al., 2011). The full activation of YAP/TAZ activity needs to meet two requirements: i.e., both the promotion of YAP/TAZ nuclear accumulation and the inhibition of the ARID1A-containing SWI/SNF complex (Chang et al., 2018). In other words, the ARID1A-containing SWI/SNF complex works as a mechano-regulated inhibitor of YAP/TAZ. In multiple experimental organoids, YAP/TAZ activity modulates stem cells' stemness and cell fates, which are eventually dictated by the spatio-temporal balance between material stiffness and degradability (Brusatin et al., 2018). Specifically, the stiffness-sensing YAP/TAZ is gradually inactivated due to the "contact inhibition" of cell proliferation; while this happens, the stem cells lose their stemness and choose a specific direction of differentiation. At this very moment, a suitable speed of biomaterial degradation could supply extra inner spaces for cellular proliferation thus preserving cellular stemness for organoid generation. These novel discoveries have highlighted how to spatio-temporally control stem cells differentiation through mechanically related YAP/TAZ activity and biomaterials degradation for best dermal matrixes.

As regards wound healing, experimental work uncovered an interesting "mechanical memory" effect: epithelial cells primed on stiff matrixes exhibited higher capabilities of migration and adhesion even after transfer onto a softer secondary matrixes (Nasrollahi et al., 2017). These interesting results showed that migrating cells can "remember" information from past physical environments and that these "mechanical memories" may be exploited to influence cell fates. As stem cells in chronic wounds show a slow self-renewal and remain uncommitted to differentiation, the tailored control of stem cells is believed to help wound healing.

Moreover, mechanical properties can influence scar formation. Reportedly, aberrant mechanotransduction is regarded as a driver of fibrosis (Brusatin et al., 2018). For chronic wounds, the mechanical signals might either affect extracellular matrixes remodeling through the "stiffness-sensing" capability of fibroblasts (Zhou et al., 2016) or impact the delivery of bioactive agents during the fibroblasts-to-myofibroblasts transdifferentiation, a key pathological process underlying the development of hypertrophic scars (Jiang et al., 2018).

Last but not least, the mechanical signals were also reported to regulate immune responses by influencing the behavior of human monocyte-derived macrophages (Adlerz et al., 2016), which is related to bacterial resistance in chronic wounds.

Elastin-Based Dermal Matrixes

Due to the huge impact exerted by mechanical signals on the regulation of stem cell differentiation and of mechanotransduction in the course of wound healing, elastin-based dermal matrixes have recently emerged as means to provide elastic recoil and resilience to the wounded dermis and to prevent pathological scar retractions.

Generally, dermal elastic fibers and collagen fibers are responsible for Young's (elastic) modulus and the tensile strength of human dermis, respectively (Wang et al., 2015). In healthy skin, elastin monomers derive from the tropoelastin precursor and are then further crosslinked into polymeric networks. The latter enable healthy skin to recover its original shape once stretched to a great extent. In wounded skin, as compared to normal, a smaller amount of elastin monomers is produced, while most of the dermal fibers are deposited in an aberrant manner, resulting in a disorderly fibrous and poorly elastic network. Although elastin accounts for only about 2–4% of the human skin dry weight (Rodriguez-Cabello et al., 2018), its significant functional role is attracting a growing attention aimed at improving dermis mechanical properties and at regulating cellular activities during wound healing.

Currently, dermal matrixes trying to mimic the natural elastic properties of human skin are based on either natural tropoelastin or synthetic elastin-like recombinamers (ELRs) (Rodriguez-Cabello et al., 2018).

Tropoelastin-Based Dermal Matrixes

Tropoelastin, which naturally exists in all vertebrates except Cyclostomes, is a 60–72 kDa protein made of 750–800 amino acid residues constituting the dominant building block of the elastic fibers that imbue tissues with elasticity and resilience. Tropoelastin is made up of alternating hydrophilic and hydrophobic domains. The latter show elastic properties while the intercalated hydrophilic lysine-rich domains act as crosslinkers. As recently reported, the established atomic structure of human tropoelastin is an extended molecular body flanked by two protruding legs (Wang et al., 2015). The lysine residues of the hydrophilic domains show a substantial variation in their locations, which might contribute to their greater accessibility and cross-linking capacities (Tarakanova et al., 2019).

The versatile and pliable potentialities of tropoelastin have attracted interest from several biomedical fields. Tropoelastin and silk fibroin were blended to produce electrospun yarns, in which the elasticity of the former is combined with the mechanical strength of the latter. The results of the subcutaneous implantation of such yarns in mice proved their good tolerance and persistence for over 8 weeks, supporting their potential application to tissue engineering (Aghaei-Ghareh-Bolagh et al., 2019). In another study, the engineered tropoelastin-polydopamine-coated tendon scaffolds promoted the tenogenic commitment of human adipose tissue-derived stem cells which remarkably synthesized and deposited elastin in the generated elastin-rich matrixes *in vitro* (Almeida et al., 2019). Yeo et al. (2019) immobilized tropoelastin on plasma-coated polyurethane films, which significantly promoted the adhesion and proliferation of multipotent adult progenitor cells.

The first *in vivo* study focusing on the therapeutic effects of tropoelastin on full-thickness dermal wounds was recently reported by Mithieux et al. (2018). The implanted pure tropoelastin exhibited superior cell recruiting properties and significantly promoted angiogenesis, resulting in an enhanced healing of full-thickness pig skin wounds. The pure tropoelastin used for the experiments was dissolved, dried, and heated in a stepwise procedure with no addition of other chemicals. Although the regeneration included vessels, rete ridges, and a keratinizing stratified epithelium, no results were reported about the recovery of any degree of elasticity on the part of the tropoelastin-treated wounds.

Although the above discoveries highlighted the potential therapeutic values of tropoelastin as regards wound healing, we still lack *in vivo* evidences in terms of a restored elasticity of regenerated wound tissues during lengthy follow-up observations.

ELRs-Based Dermal Matrixes

ELRs are genetically engineered polypeptides having the repeated elastin sequence valine-proline-glycine-X-glycine (VPGXG), where X can be any amino acid excepting proline. The structures made of engineered ELRs are tunable and offer versatile elastic-tailored applications. Gonzalez de Torre et al. (2018) described the "clickable" properties of ELRs and used electrospinning to prepare bioactive fibers from clickable ELRs with no crosslinking agent added. In another study, Changi et al. (2018) developed thermo-sensitive ELRs which contained bioactive molecules and showed good biocompatibility and limited immunogenicity in BALB/c and C57BL/6 mouse models. Moreover, some functional sequences, such as growth factors, can be attached via chemical reactions to ELRs molecule or can be directly inserted into main sequences of ELRs through recombinant techniques (Flora et al., 2019).

To sum up, mechanical signals can regulate stem cells, scar formation, or immune responses during wound healing. Current studies have shown that both tropoelastin and ELRs exhibit a potential for chronic wound care. However, limited research has been hitherto focused on the recovered elasticity of the regenerated skin. Further experiments need to be carried out to confirm the long-term therapeutic effects of elastin- and ELRs-based dermal matrixes.

STRUCTURAL PROPERTIES

Structure-Related Regulation During Wound Healing

Structural properties of dermal matrixes include pore sizes, porosity, surface topology, organization of inner frames, etc. Among structural properties, pore sizes (Wang et al., 2016) and porosity (i.e. the ratio between the hollow space inside a scaffold and its overall volume; Xu et al., 2016) have been extensively studied. Dermal matrixes presently available in clinical settings have suitable pore sizes and high degrees of inner connections to allow cell migration as well as nutrients exchange. The Wnt/β-catenin signaling pathway was recently reported to regulate pore-size-related cell proliferation (Xu et al., 2018). The current consensus is that ideal pore sizes or porosity have yet to be ascertained for the different kinds of matrixes and seeded cells (Xu et al., 2015).

Interestingly, surface topology was found to regulate stem cells mainly via roughness and texture (Xing et al., 2019). Firstly, a rough surface can attract stem cell aggregation. In human skin, stem cells usually gather and undergo self-renewal in "niches," i.e., the interfollicular epidermis, the basal layers, and the hair follicle bulges (Alonso and Fuchs, 2006). Likewise, stem cells tend to aggregate on rough surfaces endowed with topologically "artificial niches," such as holes, canyons, grooves, or craters (Cooper et al., 2012). Secondly, surface textures with different shapes further direct stem cell fates. Kilian et al. (2010) patterned the mesenchymal stem cell individually on a substrate and each cell was patterned with a certain shape, i.e. rectangles or pentagonal symmetries (five-pointed star). The mesenchymal stem cells were found to display different adipogenesis and osteogenesis profiles once seeded onto different shapes. Furthermore, the mesenchymal stem cells were then patterned individually onto different rectangles with increasing aspect ratios as well as onto dissimilar pentagonal symmetries with varied subcellular curvatures. Their results showed that changing the cell shapes correspondingly changed the cell lineages. In other words, altering the shapes of stem cells can influence the cell lineages they generate. Therefore, manipulating the roughness and texture of surface topology could enable us to tailor the fate of the individual cell.

Recently, surface micropatterning methods (i.e., nanotechnology, 3D bio-printing, laser photolithography, microcontact transfer method, electron beam etching, etc.) can manipulate the microgeographic structures on matrix surfaces (Bui et al., 2018). Therefore, surface micropatterning methods hold potential to regulate the stem cell fates during wound healing via tailoring the surface topology. In a recent study, a crossed groove/column micropattern was constructed on the surface of bacterial cellulose matrix using low-energy CO_2 laser photolithography. Animal experiments indicated that this micropatterned shape guided a "basket-woven" organization of collagen distribution that may reduce scar formation (Hu et al., 2019).

Anyhow, natural skin environment acts as the blueprint for engineered dermal matrixes. Maximally mimicking the natural skin environment holds potential to achieve a scarless regeneration *in situ* (MacEwan et al., 2017). Traditional dermal matrixes create less biomimetic environments that do not help commit stem cells to differentiation. Consequently, higher numbers of fibroblasts transdifferentiate into myofibroblasts, which possibly leads to hypertrophic scars (**Figure 2A**; Li Y. et al., 2019). Nowadays, advanced dermal matrixes endowed with more skin-like biomimetic architectures and mechanical properties as well as with the necessary biochemical signals are believed to commit stem cells to differentiation (MacEwan et al., 2017), which further reduces scar formation while

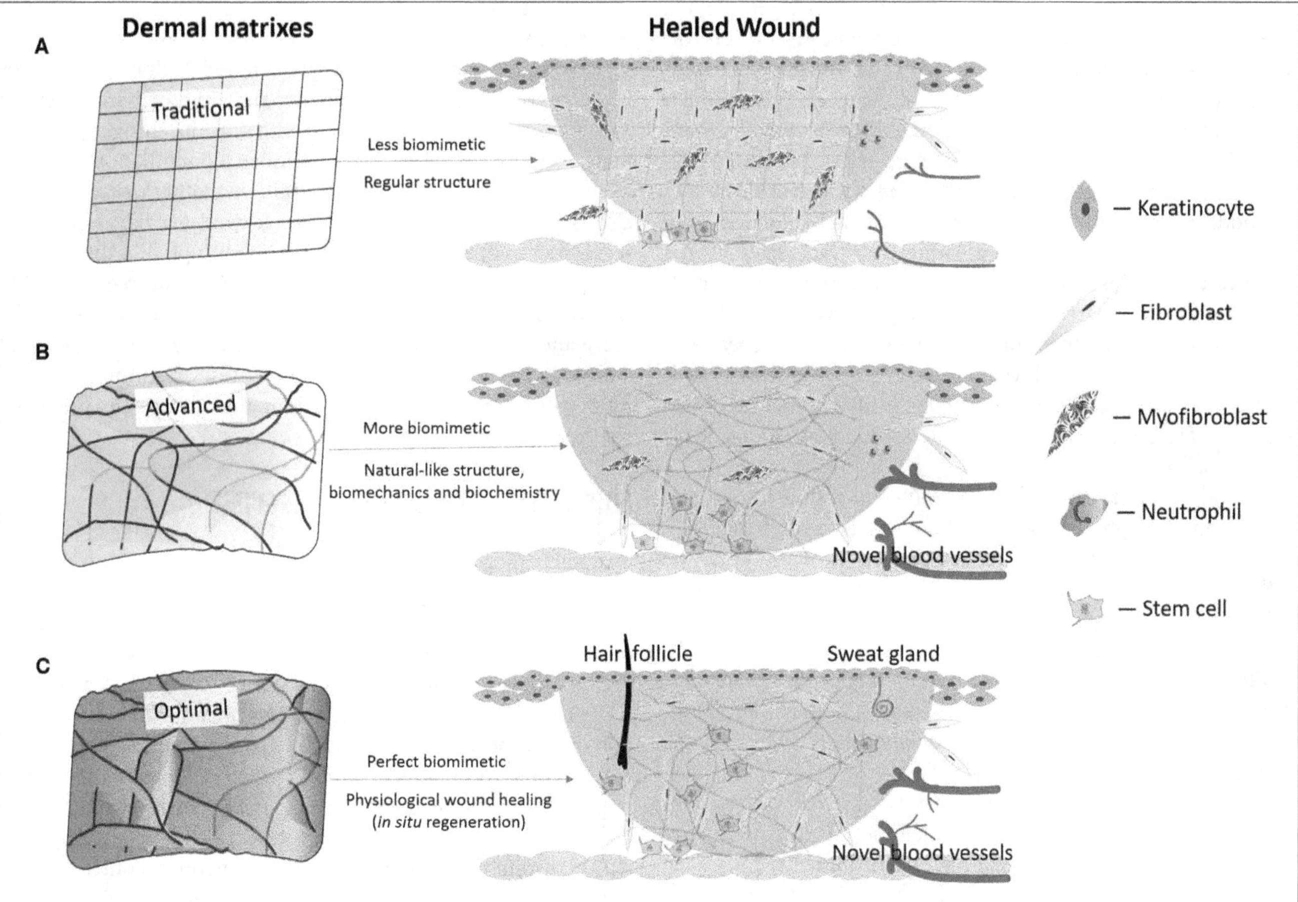

FIGURE 2 | Schematic diagram of traditional, advanced, and best dermal matrixes and their respective therapeutic outcomes. **(A)** Traditional dermal matrixes create less biomimetic environments leading to a more abundant scar formation and fewer regenerated blood vessels. **(B)** Advanced dermal matrixes mimic the natural skin environment better than traditional dermal matrixes, thereby leading to a less abundant scar formation and a more intense regeneration of blood vessels. However, the regeneration of cutaneous appendages (i.e., hair follicles, sweat, and sebaceous glands) remains difficult to achieve. **(C)** Optimal dermal matrixes enable wounds to reach a complete tissue regeneration (theoretically physiological wound healing) *in situ*.

promoting angiogenesis (**Figure 2B**). However, the regeneration of cutaneous appendages (i.e. hair follicles or sweat glands) is not yet satisfactory. Theoretically, optimal dermal matrixes should enable wounds to achieve tissue regeneration (i.e. physiological wound healing) *in situ*, which means that the healed wound has the same morpho-functional features as the natural skin, is devoid of scar tissue, and has concurrently regenerated the cutaneous appendages (i.e. hair follicles or sweat glands; **Figure 2C**). However, it is still beyond our sight what the best dermal matrixes might be and how they would regulate stem cells differentiation.

Further understanding of natural dermal structures might inspire the organization of the inner structures (e.g. random, aligned, gradient, porous, or filamentous) of dermal matrixes. Reportedly, collagen/elastin-based three-dimensional (3D) histological images indicated that the human dermis amounts to a "sandwich" structure with gradient changes in gradual terms of either interstitial spaces or architecture at different dermal depths (Wang et al., 2015). However, no solid conclusion has been hitherto reached whether dermal aligned or gradient structures are significantly better than random or homogeneous structures. The best patterns of the inner structures of dermal matrixes are yet to be assessed for the different cell types and chemical components.

Concerns Regarding Mechanical and Structural Regulation of Cells

Although mechanical and structural properties of dermal matrixes have shown crucial effects on cell behaviors, we cannot yet reach a solid conclusion concerning one or another specific parameter and its corresponding therapeutic effects. Tunable mechanical and structural properties exert a previously undocumented influence on either the fate of each cell type or the whole wound healing process.

First, it is difficult to decouple the interplay between structural and mechanical properties. When we tune one physical property and study its therapeutic effects, inevitably other properties concurrently change. For example, when we tried to fabricate a series of scaffolds with varied stiffness gradients, the other intrinsic properties (e.g., pore size, porosity, organization of inner structures, and elastic modulus) changed correspondingly. One study reported that mixtures with different proportions of collagen and hydroxyapatite could be coated on decellularized cancellous bone to vary its stiffness with no statistically significant after-coating changes in the scaffold architecture. Notwithstanding this, the chemical composition and related cell binding sites underwent concomitant changes (Chen et al., 2015). In another study, the cryoprotectant dimethyl-sulfoxide was used to control pore size by regulating ice crystal sizes in 3D freeze-dried porous scaffolds, while the stiffness was regulated by adjusting the degree of cross-linking (Jiang et al., 2019). Although using the above methods achieved an independent control of pore size and stiffness, the decoupling of structural and mechanical properties affecting cellular activities was far from being satisfactory due to variations in chemical inhomogeneity among scaffolds.

Second, it is difficult to observe cellular responses to a single tunable physical property due to the complex and changeable spatio-temporal microenvironments, because so many kinds of cells are involved in wound healing and each cell type is regulated by a specific set of multiple factors. For example, porosity and pore size are two correlated physical properties. On the one hand, smaller pores favor cell adhesion and immigration because of their higher surface area and ligand density. On the other hand, smaller pores are easily subject to clogging when cells grow on their inside, the upshot being a decreased porosity which further reduces permeability to oxygen and nutrients. It seems that we cannot find the "best choice" for a single specific parameter due to the great complexity of cellular microenvironments.

Third, cellular behaviors distinctly differ going from individual cell level to tissue/organ level. Micropatterning technologies (Brusatin et al., 2018) have been intensively used to study individual cell's behaviors with respect to various physical properties in two dimensions (2D). By this way the first evidences and groundbreaking discoveries were mostly gained about mechanical-related cellular responses. However, from what is known about 2D cultures, it is difficult to extrapolate the cellular behaviors in complex 3D environments. Moreover, precisely tuning physical properties of 3D matrixes faces insurmountable difficulties due to the concomitant changes in the other parameters, just as we mentioned above.

Fourth, the confusion about bulk stiffness and local stiffness also causes concerns. Bulk stiffness is usually measured via tensile/compression tests and refers to the scaffolds overall macroscopic features. However, local stiffness is usually measured via atomic force microscopy and is believed to be the only biophysical signal scaffolds-attached cells can sense and respond to. A study using atomic force microscopy indicated that the local stiffness of different sites within acellular fibrotic lungs was very inhomogeneous (Melo et al., 2014). Therefore, when attached cells are migrating through a scaffold, they will experience significantly heterogeneous degrees of local stiffness from their own perspective. There are worrying trends that many studies of cellular mechano-responsiveness only focus on bulk stiffness, yet unintentionally neglect local stiffness. Concerning dermal matrixes, it is still unclear how local stiffness and bulk stiffness antagonistically regulate stem cell fates during wound healing.

Hopefully, many scientists have started taking heed of this problem. In order to mimic the dynamic microenvironments, a 4D programmable culture system with self-morphing capabilities was developed to regulate the controlled differentiation of neural stem cells (Miao et al., 2020). In addition, mathematical methods also help to solve these problems. Recently, a Bayesian linear regression mathematical model was used to predict the changes of topography-induced gene expression (Cutiongco et al., 2020). In another case, a mathematical model was used to assess the correlation between local and bulk stiffness, i.e., the bulk/local stiffness ratio. The results showed that the local stiffness detected by atomic force microscopy fell within the value ranges predicted via the mathematical model (Jiang et al., 2019).

SIZE-RELATED PROPERTIES

Nanotechnology has become known as an exciting wound treatment tool. Multiple kinds of macroscopic nanobiomaterials (e.g., electrospun nanofibers, nanosheets, nanoemulsions, carbon nanotubes-based, or graphene-based nanocomposites) and nano-sized biomaterials (e.g., NPs, ions, molecules, nucleic acids, functional peptides, proteins, oligosaccharides, or polysaccharides) have exhibited great potential capabilities of modulating vascularization, bacterial resistance, and inflammation during wound healing (Chakrabarti et al., 2019).

In this regard, size-related physical properties targeting chronic wound care are anti-infection outcomes contributed by NPs. Common NPs in use are metals (e.g., Ag, TiO_2, ZnO, MgF_2, CeO_2), lipid-based vesicles (e.g., liposome, exosomes), and polymers. Compared with materials of regular sizes, NPs quite differ in regard to mechanical strengths, melting points, surface areas, optical, and magnetic properties (Das and Baker, 2016).

Metal NPs

The silver NPs (AgNPs) are the most widely used metal NPs in both laboratory and clinical applications. AgNPs ranging from 1 to 100 nm in size or silver nanoclusters with an ultrasmall size (<2 nm) have shown good antimicrobial properties. Solid evidence has been provided that AgNPs can prevent and/or fight microorganism infections and significantly enhance the healing of chronic wounds (Sandri et al., 2019).

Bacterial biofilms are associated with the resistance to an extensive range of antibiotics, contributing to chronic wounds formation. Recent studies have shown that AgNPs exert promising therapeutic effects against the biofilm-forming MRSA (Zhang et al., 2018). Another study also reported the inhibiting ability of AgNPs loaded with thymol and chitosan on the biofilm formation by MRSA with a 10.08 ± 0.06 mm zone of inhibition (ZOI) and a minimum inhibitory concentration of 100 $\mu g\ mL^{-1}$ (Manukumar et al., 2017). The AgNPs killing efficacy on biofilms of *Vibrio* species, another group of clinically multi-drug resistant bacteria, was also verified (Satish et al., 2017). Moreover, clinical data further confirmed the effectiveness of AgNPs against biofilm-forming bacteria. Thomas et al. (2014) isolated from clinical samples a series of multidrug-resistant biofilm-forming coagulase-negative staphylococci, e.g. *S. epidermidis* strains, *S. aureus*, *Salmonella typhi*, and *Salmonella paratyphi*. Surprisingly, AgNPs exerted their antibacterial activity against all the tested strains. A randomized and double-blind pilot clinical trial study also revealed that Nano Silver Fluoride particles can inhibit the formation of *Streptococcus* mutants' biofilms (Freire et al., 2017).

The likely underlying mechanisms of AgNPs' antibacterial properties lie in structurally damaging the cell membranes and in deeply altering the intracellular metabolic activities of the bacteria (Eckhardt et al., 2013). AgNPs also inhibit the activities of bacterial respiratory enzymes (Franci et al., 2015). In addition, other evidences demonstrated that AgNPs control inflammatory processes and modulate cytokines' activities (Rigo et al., 2013), which might be additional mechanisms benefiting chronic wound healing.

Lipid NPs

Liposomes, also known as phospholipid vesicles, are the most widely used lipid NPs for wound dressings (Nasab et al., 2019). In contact with an aqueous solution liposomes can be automatically assembled into enclosed phospholipid bilayers containing a watery core surrounded by a hydrophobic membrane (Ahmed et al., 2019). Reportedly, vancomycin-loaded nanoliposomes coupled with an anti-staphylococcal protein (lysostaphin) can serve as potential antimicrobial formulations for wound infections caused by MRSA, which is resistant to several conventional antibiotics (Hajiahmadi et al., 2019).

The lipid-based NPs versatile capabilities due to their nanoscales, biocompatibility, and high permeability might change our classical views on drugs pharmacokinetics. For example, egg lecithin and soy lecithin liposomes showed superior antioxidant activity *in vitro* and significantly accelerated wound-healing *in vivo* (Nasab et al., 2019). Reportedly, farnesyl-encapsulated liposomes promoted wound healing in a rat model with third-degree burns (Wu et al., 2019). More interestingly, liposomes encapsulating propolis, a natural bee product, showed both antimicrobial and antioxidant activities (Aytekin et al., 2019), which indicated the multiplicity of potential applications of liposomes in pharmacotherapy.

Besides discovering the potential therapeutic effects of new drugs, lipid-based NPs might also enable us to amplify the applications of traditional drugs regarding chronic wound care. Insulin administered by injection is a drug used to regulate blood sugar levels in Internal Medicine. Recently, the promising therapeutic effects of insulin's external administration on chronic wounds were noted, probably because insulin regulates nutrients' metabolism further helping cellular activities during wound healing. However, insulin's external administration is a great technical challenge due to its limited transdermal absorption and its rapid degradation in the wound's bed. To solve this problem, Dawoud et al. (2019) formulated insulin-loaded chitosan NPs liposomes which successfully prolonged the release of insulin.

Moreover, the use of liposomes for intracellular drug delivery is a promising approach to reduce scarring, promote vascularization of ischemic wounds or regulate inflammation in cases of diabetic ulcers and other types of chronic wounds (Choi et al., 2017). Reportedly, glucocorticoid-loaded liposomes did induce a pro-resolution phenotype in human primary macrophages, which significantly promoted the healing of chronic wounds (Gauthier et al., 2018). Similarly, fibroblast growth factor-encapsulating liposomes advanced wound healing in rats (Xiang et al., 2011). Nunes et al. (2016) developed an usnic acid/liposomes-embedded gelatin-based membrane which is capable of transdermal absorption by skin layers and of controlled drug release. Another intracellular delivery use of liposomes aimed at upregulating growth factor co-receptors in diabetic wounds, which usually heal with difficulty to due to growth factor resistance (Das et al., 2014).

Other widely used lipid NPs are exosomes (Chen et al., 2019), solid lipid NPs, and more. Exosomes have diameter sizes ranging from 30 to 100 nm, and are usually released from cells when multivesicular bodies fuse with the plasma membrane (Zarrintaj et al., 2017). Reports indicated that exosomes derived from gene-modified microRNA-126-overexpressing synovium MSCs significantly promoted the proliferation of human dermal microvascular endothelial cells and of human dermal fibroblasts in a dose-dependent manner (Tao et al., 2017). Besides, solid lipid NPs (Eskiler et al., 2019) also exhibited superior capabilities of controlling drugs delivery for potential wound care applications. Moreover, lipid-based NPs partake in emerging applications in relation to several fields, such as cancer therapy, vaccines, dermatological treatments, ocular delivery (Li N. et al., 2019), and post-surgery pain control (Cohen et al., 2019).

Polymeric NPs

Polymeric NPs are usually used to encapsulate drugs, nucleic acids, proteins, macromolecules, and growth factors in order to extend their half-life and improve their bioavailability by physically isolating them from the wound's bed environment, in which multiple kinds of proteases are present. Moreover, the sustained release of drugs at therapeutic concentrations not only can reduce the frequency of drug deliveries but also achieves optimized pharmacokinetics profiles (Kim et al., 2018). Therefore, wound dressings with polymeric NPs have drawn increasing attention due to their intracellular delivery capabilities.

Among them, poly (lactic-co-glycolic acid) (PLGA)-based NPs are widely used for controlled drug releasing due to their versatile degradation kinetics. PLGA biodegradation can also release lactate byproducts further advancing wound healing processes. An endogenous human host defense peptide, LL37, was encapsulated into PLGA NPs to prevent infection and accelerate wound healing (Chereddy et al., 2014). Karimi Dehkordi et al. (2019) formulated a nanocrystalline cellulose-hyaluronic acid composite embedded with granulocyte-macrophage-colony-stimulating-factor-loaded chitosan NPs to promote wound healing. In the last composite, nanocrystalline cellulose acts as a strengthening agent boosting the mechanical properties of hyaluronic acid.

As biological macromolecular compounds, polymeric NPs exhibit bioactivities that are easily affected by several physical properties, such as sizes, components, surface charges, shapes, etc. Hasan et al. (2019) developed positively- and negatively-charged, respectively, PLGA NPs containing the antibiotic

Clindamycin. Although both kinds of nanoparticles did no detectable harm to healthy fibroblasts, the positively charged NPs elicited significantly better therapeutic outcomes of wound healing in a MRSA-infected mouse model. The different effectiveness in antibacterial activity exhibited by the positively charged *vs.* the negatively charged polymeric NPs was probably due to their dissimilar capability of adhering to bacteria. To systematically compare the effects of NPs surface charges and shapes on wound healing, Mahmoud et al. (2019) synthesized a series of polymeric hydrogels loaded with gold NPs of differing shapes (rods and spheres) and introduced various surface modifications (neutral, cationic, and anionic charged polymers). Both the inherent parameters (e.g., colloidal stability and release behavior) and therapeutic outcomes (e.g., wound healing, skin re-epithelialization, collagen deposition, inflammation level, and antibacterial activity) were assessed in an animal wound model. Their results showed that hydrogels of gold nanorods constitute a promising nano-platform for wound healing.

Like lipid-based NPs, polymeric NPs might also affect drugs' pharmacokinetics in wound environments, thus enabling us to explore potential off-label uses of current drugs. Jia et al. (2018) developed nanofibrous PLGA incorporating andrographolide-loaded mesoporous silica NPs. Their results showed that the sustained releasing of andrographolide, which is extracted from a Chinese herb, surprisingly reduced inflammation intensity while promoting epidermal cells adhesion. Another kind of Chinese herb, *Aloe vera*, was reported to enhance wound healing when encapsulated inside PLGA NPs to be used in wound dressings (Garcia-Orue et al., 2019). A further recent example comes from the interesting works of Farghaly Aly et al. (2019) who showed that hydrogels containing polymeric NPs loaded with Simvastatin, a cardiovascular drug commonly used to treat serum hyperlipidemia, can benefit wound healing processes. Once encapsulated in chitosan NPs, Phenytoin, an antiepileptic drug, also exhibits a potential capability to accelerate wound healing, a suggestion inspired by recently reported clinical cases of gingival hyperplasia after Phenytoin's oral administration (Cardoso et al., 2019).

Biosafety Concerns of NPs

The biosafety and cytotoxicity of AgNPs have already aroused many concerns. AgNPs seem to be cytotoxic for many species including human beings (Shavandi et al., 2011; Pratsinis et al., 2013). Newly published research showed the toxicity of AgNPs on marine microalgae (Hazeem et al., 2019) and the yeast *Saccharomyces cerevisiae* BY4741 (Kasemets et al., 2019). As regards human beings, prolonged exposures to AgNPs can cause argyria (Richter et al., 2015), whose symptoms include blue gray skin color changes and multiple alterations of bodily functions such as gastrointestinal disorders, spasms, and even death (Rice, 2009). Importantly, AgNPs have produced genotoxicity in the testicles of Sprague Dawley rats (Elsharkawy et al., 2019) and in the embryos of Zebrafish (Chakraborty et al., 2016). As regards human beings, AgNPs have showed genotoxicity in human liver HepG2 and colon Caco2 cells (Sahu et al., 2016). These results revealed a possible reproductive genotoxicity of AgNPs on human offspring especially when AgNPs are used at high doses and for lengthy periods in patients with large area burns or chronic wounds. Moreover, AgNPs can possibly induce neurotoxicity by crossing the brain blood barrier and penetrating the central nervous system of human beings (Khan et al., 2019).

To test the toxicity when AgNPs are applied on wounds, Pang et al. (2020) applied AgNPs onto the wounds of Zebrafish after the amputation of fins. AgNPs were found to impair epithelialization and blastema formation especially during the first few days, showing that the cytotoxicity of AgNPs is time-dependent and is more obvious at the initial stages of wound healing. Konop et al. (2019) used micellar electro kinetic chromatography to detect the releasing profile of AgNPs from wound dressings. AgNPs at concentration higher than 10 ppm exerted significant ($p < 0.05$) toxicity on the fibroblasts isolated from diabetic mice vs. a murine fibroblasts cell line and a human fibroblasts cell line. Our team also found that an exposure to high concentrations of AgNPs significantly inhibited the proliferation of mice fibroblasts (Liu et al., 2018b). Specially, we noticed that the antibacterial efficiency stopped growing and entered a plateau stage as the AgNPs doses increased, which indicated that an optimized dose range does exist for AgNPs (Liu et al., 2017).

Also, attentions have already been paid to the biosafety and toxicity of other metal NPs, such as TiO_2, ZnO, magnesium fluoride (MgF_2), cerium oxide (CeO_2), copper, iron oxide, gold, etc. Wang et al. (2018) compared the toxicity of Ag, TiO_2, and ZnO NPs to human smooth-muscle cells. Their results showed that all the three kinds of metal NPs could induce inflammatory responses. More importantly, ZnO NPs significantly increased intracellular ROS showing a stronger cellular cytotoxicity than that of Ag and TiO_2 NPs. In another case, Filipova et al. (2018) reported a "three-in-one" screening assay to test the toxicity of three kinds of NPs for human umbilical vein endothelial cells. The three NPs are silica NPs (7–14 nm), superparamagnetic iron oxide NPs (8 nm), and carboxylated multiwall carbon nanotubes (60 nm), all of which were tested at the same concentration of 100 μg/ml. Surprisingly, all the NPs types tested exhibited a gradual toxic effect which decreased cell viability.

Solutions to Reduce Cytotoxicity of AgNPs in Wound Care

Reportedly, a general mechanism for AgNPs-mediated intracellular toxicity is that AgNPs can enter human cells either by endosomal uptake or by diffusion (Frohlich and Frohlich, 2016). The cytotoxicity of AgNPs is a size-, dose-, and time-dependent, which means that it is closely related to nanoparticle size, shape, surface charge, oxidation state, agglomeration condition, administration route, and dosage (Liao et al., 2019). Correspondingly, potential solutions to reducing cytotoxicity of AgNPs are focused on the tunable size-, dose-, or time-dependent features of AgNPs.

First, increasing the size of AgNPs can reduce their cytotoxicity, but the antibacterial efficacy is concurrently reduced. Reportedly, AgNPs with sizes below 10 nm exhibited both a higher antibacterial efficiency and cytotoxicity (Gahlawat et al., 2016). Zille et al. (2015) tested the antibacterial efficacy of AgNPs with 10, 20, 40, 60, and 100 nm particle sizes. The antibacterial inhibition values against *S. aureus* were 19% for the 100 nm-AgNPs and 95% for the 10 nm-AgNPs, showing that antibacterial effectiveness increases with decreasing nanoparticle size. On the other hand, AgNPs of sizes below 10 nm showed to be more cytotoxic than those of other sizes (Recordati et al., 2016). AgNPs of sizes below 3 nm can be deposited within multiple organs of male mice, such as liver, spleen, kidney, heart, lungs, testicles, stomach, and intestine (Yang et al., 2017). Therefore, a balance needs to be achieved between antimicrobial efficiency and biosafety due to the size-dependent cytotoxicity of AgNPs.

Second, combining AgNPs with other antibacterial strategies can reduce the administered doses to lessen the dose-dependent cytotoxicity. For example, antimicrobial peptides (AMPs), which are integral compounds secreted by natural organisms and act as natural immune defenses (Kokel and Torok, 2018), can possibly reinforce AgNPs in terms of killing antibiotic-resistant bacteria. In a recent study, AMPs were included at the peripheral hydrophilic region of polymersomes, while AgNPs were included inside the hydrophobic corona. *In vitro* tests indicated that the AMP/AgNPs polymersomes exhibited a satisfactory bacteriostatic activity as well as a low cytotoxicity toward human dermal fibroblasts (Bassous and Webster, 2019). In other cases, AgNPs-coated zwitterionic hydrogels, which confer superhydrophilic properties to resist bacterial attachment, were reported to promote wound healing (GhavamiNejad et al., 2016). Our team recently used N,N-dimethylformamide-treated poly(vinylidene fluoride), in which the Ag^{+} ions were reduced to elemental silver. The impregnated AgNPs were then generated *in situ* and the surface hydrophobicity was significantly increased. Then, we tried different concentrations of ingredient materials and eventually reduced the cytotoxicity and achieved optimized anti-bacterial capacities against *A. baumannii* and *E. coli* (Menglong Liu et al., 2018).

Third, novel drug delivery system can release AgNPs in a spatio-temporally controlled or stimuli-responsive profile to reduce dosing frequency and amounts. As regards chronic wounds, the stimuli which trigger the release of AgNPs can be pH levels, lactic acid, glucose, proteases, and matrix metalloproteinases, etc. Among all the peculiar stimuli, pH changes play a vital role by revealing pathophysiological alterations occurring during the transformation of acute wounds into chronic wounds due to infection, ischemia, or inflammation. Recently, our team reported the pH-responsive releasing of AgNPs reinforced via a chemo-photothermal therapy targeting chronic wounds with bacterial infections. The infectious wound environment (pH $\sim$ 6.3) can trigger the release of AgNPs, which contributes to lower their cytotoxicity (Liu et al., 2018a).

OVERVIEW

Obviously, stem cell fates are spatio-temporally modulated by concurrent signals from both physical and chemical stimuli. Surface micropatterning methods, especially the nanotechnology, 3D bio-printing, and laser photolithography enable us to precisely tailor the surface topology and biomechanical features to study the behaviors of individual cells. These discoveries highlighted that in some cases physical properties can be the predominating and independent factors that direct stem cell fates (Kilian et al., 2010).

Earlier strategies for the regeneration of cutaneous appendages (i.e., sweat glands and hair follicles) were focused on chemical approaches, which entailed insurmountable difficulties. The physical property-based regulation of stem cells has been tracking down potential solutions. For example, 3D bio-printed dermal matrixes served as "artificial niches" to direct epidermal progenitors (Liu et al., 2016) and MSCs (Yao et al., 2020) into sweat gland differentiation.

Traditional fabrication techniques do not tailor spatial structures or control modeling for the regenerations of human cutaneous appendages. Recently, a microfluidic device, which can manipulate fluids at the submillimeter scale (Sackmann et al., 2014), was ingeniously designed to recapitulate the development of human epiblast and amniotic ectoderm using human pluripotent stem cells (Zheng et al., 2019). This study showed that the guides of biomimetic spatial structures and physical cues play key roles during the regeneration of organoids with complex microstructures and microfluidics technology holds potential for the regenerations of human cutaneous appendages.

AUTHOR CONTRIBUTIONS

YW provided the main concept for this review and wrote the manuscript. UA and JW prepared the figures and improved the language of the manuscript.

ACKNOWLEDGMENTS

We would like to thank the kind aid and the inspiring ideas about regenerating cutaneous appendages from Dr. Sha Huang in the Medical Innovation Research Department, PLA General Hospital and PLA Medical College, Beijing, China.

REFERENCES

Adlerz, K. M., Aranda-Espinoza, H., and Hayenga, H. N. (2016). Substrate elasticity regulates the behavior of human monocyte-derived macrophages. *Eur. Biophys. J.* 45, 301–309. doi: 10.1007/s00249-015-1096-8

Aghaei-Ghareh-Bolagh, B., Mithieux, S. M., Hiob, M. A., Wang, Y., Chong, A., and Weiss, A. S. (2019). Fabricated tropoelastin-silk yarns and woven textiles for diverse tissue engineering applications. *Acta Biomater.* 91, 112–122. doi: 10.1016/j.actbio.2019.04.029

Ahmed, K. S., Hussein, S. A., Ali, A. H., Korma, S. A., Lipeng, Q., and Jinghua, C. (2019). Liposome: composition, characterisation, preparation, and recent innovation in clinical applications. *J. Drug Target.* 27, 742–761. doi: 10.1080/1061186X.2018.1527337

Akash, M. S. H., Rehman, K., Fiayyaz, F., Sabir, S., and Khurshid, M. (2020). Diabetes-associated infections: development of antimicrobial resistance and possible treatment strategies. *Arch. Microbiol.* doi: 10.1007/s00203-020-01818-x. [Epub ahead of print].

Almeida, H., Domingues, R. M. A., Mithieux, S. M., Pires, R. A., Goncalves, A. I., Gomez-Florit, M., et al. (2019). Tropoelastin-coated tendon biomimetic scaffolds promote stem cell tenogenic commitment and deposition of elastin-rich matrix. *ACS Appl. Mater. Interfaces* 11, 19830–19840. doi: 10.1021/acsami.9b04616

Alonso, L., and Fuchs, E. (2006). The hair cycle. *J. Cell Sci.* 119, 391–393. doi: 10.1242/jcs.02793

Aytekin, A. A., Tuncay Tanriverdi, S., Aydin Kose, F., Kart, D., Eroglu, I., and Ozer, O. (2019). Propolis loaded liposomes: evaluation of antimicrobial and antioxidant activities. *J. Liposome Res.* 30, 107–116. doi: 10.1080/08982104.2019.1599012

Bakker, K., Apelqvist, J., Lipsky, B. A., Van Netten, J. J., and International Working Group on the Diabetic (2016). The 2015 IWGDF guidance documents on prevention and management of foot problems in diabetes: development of an evidence-based global consensus. *Diabetes Metab. Res. Rev.* 32(Suppl. 1), 2–6. doi: 10.1002/dmrr.2694

Bassous, N. J., and Webster, T. J. (2019). The binary effect on methicillin-resistant *Staphylococcus aureus* of polymeric nanovesicles appended by proline-rich amino acid sequences and inorganic nanoparticles. *Small* 15:e1804247. doi: 10.1002/smll.201804247

Bhattacharya, D., Ghosh, B., and Mukhopadhyay, M. (2019). Development of nanotechnology for advancement and application in wound healing: a review. *IET Nanobiotechnol.* 13, 778–785. doi: 10.1049/iet-nbt.2018.5312

Boulton, A. J., Vileikyte, L., Ragnarson-Tennvall, G., and Apelqvist, J. (2005). The global burden of diabetic foot disease. *Lancet* 366, 1719–1724. doi: 10.1016/S0140-6736(05)67698-2

Brusatin, G., Panciera, T., Gandin, A., Citron, A., and Piccolo, S. (2018). Biomaterials and engineered microenvironments to control YAP/TAZ-dependent cell behaviour. *Nat. Mater.* 17, 1063–1075. doi: 10.1038/s41563-018-0180-8

Bryan, N., Ahswin, H., Smart, N., Bayon, Y., Wohlert, S., and Hunt, J. A. (2012). Reactive oxygen species (ROS)–a family of fate deciding molecules pivotal in constructive inflammation and wound healing. *Eur. Cell. Mater.* 24, 249–265. doi: 10.22203/eCM.v024a18

Bui, V. T., Thi Thuy, L., Choi, J. S., and Choi, H. S. (2018). Ordered cylindrical micropatterned Petri dishes used as scaffolds for cell growth. *J. Colloid Interface Sci.* 513, 161–169. doi: 10.1016/j.jcis.2017.11.024

Cardoso, A. M., de Oliveira, E. G., Coradini, K., Bruinsmann, F. A., Aguirre, T., Lorenzoni, R., et al. (2019). Chitosan hydrogels containing nanoencapsulated phenytoin for cutaneous use: skin permeation/penetration and efficacy in wound healing. *Mater. Sci. Eng. C Mater. Biol. Appl.* 96, 205–217. doi: 10.1016/j.msec.2018.11.013

Chakrabarti, S., Chattopadhyay, P., Islam, J., Ray, S., Raju, P. S., and Mazumder, B. (2019). Aspects of nanomaterials in wound healing. *Curr. Drug Deliv.* 16, 26–41. doi: 10.2174/1567201815666180918110134

Chakraborty, C., Sharma, A. R., Sharma, G., and Lee, S. S. (2016). Zebrafish: a complete animal model to enumerate the nanoparticle toxicity. *J. Nanobiotechnol.* 14:65. doi: 10.1186/s12951-016-0217-6

Chang, L., Azzolin, L., Di Biagio, D., Zanconato, F., Battilana, G., Lucon Xiccato, R., et al. (2018). The SWI/SNF complex is a mechanoregulated inhibitor of YAP and TAZ. *Nature* 563, 265–269. doi: 10.1038/s41586-018-0658-1

Changi, K., Bosnjak, B., Gonzalez-Obeso, C., Kluger, R., Rodriguez-Cabello, J. C., Hoffmann, O., et al. (2018). Biocompatibility and immunogenicity of elastin-like recombinamer biomaterials in mouse models. *J. Biomed. Mater. Res. A* 106, 924–934. doi: 10.1002/jbm.a.36290

Chen, B., Sun, Y., Zhang, J., Zhu, Q., Yang, Y., Niu, X., et al. (2019). Human embryonic stem cell-derived exosomes promote pressure ulcer healing in aged mice by rejuvenating senescent endothelial cells. *Stem Cell Res. Ther.* 10:142. doi: 10.1186/s13287-019-1253-6

Chen, G., Dong, C., Yang, L., and Lv, Y. (2015). 3D scaffolds with different stiffness but the same microstructure for bone tissue engineering. *ACS Appl. Mater Interfaces* 7, 15790–15802. doi: 10.1021/acsami.5b02662

Chereddy, K. K., Her, C. H., Comune, M., Moia, C., Lopes, A., Porporato, P. E., et al. (2014). PLGA nanoparticles loaded with host defense peptide LL37 promote wound healing. *J. Control. Release* 194, 138–147. doi: 10.1016/j.jconrel.2014.08.016

Choi, J. U., Lee, S. W., Pangeni, R., Byun, Y., Yoon, I. S., and Park, J. W. (2017). Preparation and in vivo evaluation of cationic elastic liposomes comprising highly skin-permeable growth factors combined with hyaluronic acid for enhanced diabetic wound-healing therapy. *Acta Biomater.* 57, 197–215. doi: 10.1016/j.actbio.2017.04.034

Cohen, B., Glosser, L., Saab, R., Walters, M., Salih, A., Zafeer-Khan, M., et al. (2019). Incidence of adverse events attributable to bupivacaine liposome injectable suspension or plain bupivacaine for postoperative pain in pediatric surgical patients: a retrospective matched cohort analysis. *Paediatr. Anaesth.* 29, 169–174. doi: 10.1111/pan.13561

Cooper, A., Leung, M., and Zhang, M. (2012). Polymeric fibrous matrices for substrate-mediated human embryonic stem cell lineage differentiation. *Macromol. Biosci.* 12, 882–892. doi: 10.1002/mabi.201100269

Cutiongco, M. F. A., Jensen, B. S., Reynolds, P. M., and Gadegaard, N. (2020). Predicting gene expression using morphological cell responses to nanotopography. *Nat. Commun.* 11:1384. doi: 10.1038/s41467-020-15114-1

Dantes, R., Mu, Y., Belflower, R., Aragon, D., Dumyati, G., Harrison, L. H., et al. (2013). National burden of invasive methicillin-resistant *Staphylococcus aureus* infections, United States. *JAMA Intern. Med.* 173, 1970–8. doi: 10.1001/jamainternmed.2013.10423

Das, S., and Baker, A. B. (2016). Biomaterials and nanotherapeutics for enhancing skin wound healing. *Front. Bioeng. Biotechnol.* 4:82. doi: 10.3389/fbioe.2016.00082

Das, S., Singh, G., and Baker, A. B. (2014). Overcoming disease-induced growth factor resistance in therapeutic angiogenesis using recombinant co-receptors delivered by a liposomal system. *Biomaterials* 35, 196–205. doi: 10.1016/j.biomaterials.2013.09.105

Das, U., Behera, S. S., Singh, S., Rizvi, S. I., and Singh, A. K. (2016). Progress in the development and applicability of potential medicinal plant extract-conjugated polymeric constructs for wound healing and tissue regeneration. *Phytother. Res.* 30, 1895–1904. doi: 10.1002/ptr.5700

Dawoud, M. H. S., Yassin, G. E., Ghorab, D. M., and Morsi, N. M. (2019). Insulin mucoadhesive liposomal gel for wound healing: a formulation with sustained release and extended stability using quality by design approach. *AAPS Pharm.* 20:158. doi: 10.1208/s12249-019-1363-6

Desmet, C. M., Preat, V., and Gallez, B. (2018). Nanomedicines and gene therapy for the delivery of growth factors to improve perfusion and oxygenation in wound healing. *Adv. Drug Deliv. Rev.* 129, 262–284. doi: 10.1016/j.addr.2018.02.001

Dhanalakshmi, V., Nimal, T. R., Sabitha, M., Biswas, R., and Jayakumar, R. (2016). Skin and muscle permeating antibacterial nanoparticles for treating Staphylococcus aureus infected wounds. *J. Biomed. Mater. Res. Part B Appl. Biomater* 104, 797–807. doi: 10.1002/jbm.b.33635

Dovi, J. V., He, L. K., and DiPietro, L. A. (2003). Accelerated wound closure in neutrophil-depleted mice. *J. Leukoc. Biol.* 73, 448–455. doi: 10.1189/jlb.0802406

Eckhardt, S., Brunetto, P. S., Gagnon, J., Priebe, M., Giese, B., and Fromm, K. M. (2013). Nanobio silver: its interactions with peptides and bacteria, and its uses in medicine. *Chem. Rev.* 113, 4708–4754. doi: 10.1021/cr300288v

Elsharkawy, E. E., Abd El-Nasser, M., and Kamaly, H. F. (2019). Silver nanoparticles testicular toxicity in rat. *Environ. Toxicol. Pharmacol.* 70:103194. doi: 10.1016/j.etap.2019.103194

Engler, A. J., Sen, S., Sweeney, H. L., and Discher, D. E. (2006). Matrix elasticity directs stem cell lineage specification. *Cell* 126, 677–689. doi: 10.1016/j.cell.2006.06.044

Eskiler, G. G., Cecener, G., Dikmen, G., Egeli, U., and Tunca, B. (2019). Talazoparib loaded solid lipid nanoparticles: preparation, characterization and evaluation of the therapeutic efficacy *in vitro*. *Curr. Drug Deliv.* 16, 511–529. doi: 10.2174/1567201816666190515105532

Farghaly Aly, U., Abou-Taleb, H. A., Abdellatif, A. A., and Sameh Tolba, N. (2019). Formulation and evaluation of simvastatin polymeric nanoparticles loaded in hydrogel for optimum wound healing purpose. *Drug Des. Devel. Ther.* 13, 1567–1580. doi: 10.2147/DDDT.S198413

Filipova, M., Elhelu, O. K., De Paoli, S. H., Fremuntova, Z., Mosko, T., Cmarko, D., et al. (2018). An effective "three-in-one" screening assay for testing drug and nanoparticle toxicity in human endothelial cells. *PLoS ONE* 13:e0206557. doi: 10.1371/journal.pone.0206557

Flora, T., de Torre, I. G., Alonso, M., and Rodriguez-Cabello, J. C. (2019). Tethering QK peptide to enhance angiogenesis in elastin-like recombinamer (ELR) hydrogels. *J. Mater. Sci. Mater. Med* 30:30. doi: 10.1007/s10856-019-6232-z

Franci, G., Falanga, A., Galdiero, S., Palomba, L., Rai, M., Morelli, G., et al. (2015). Silver nanoparticles as potential antibacterial agents. *Molecules* 20, 8856–8874. doi: 10.3390/molecules20058856

Freire, P. L. L., Albuquerque, A. J. R., Sampaio, F. C., Galembeck, A., Flores, M. A. P., Stamford, T. C. M., et al. (2017). AgNPs: the new allies against *S. mutans* biofilm - a pilot clinical trial and microbiological assay. *Braz. Dent. J.* 28, 417–422. doi: 10.1590/0103-6440201600994

Frohlich, E. E., and Frohlich, E. (2016). Cytotoxicity of nanoparticles contained in food on intestinal cells and the gut microbiota. *Int. J. Mol. Sci.* 17:509. doi: 10.3390/ijms17040509

Frykberg, R. G., and Banks, J. (2015). Challenges in the treatment of chronic wounds. *Adv Wound Care* 4, 560–582. doi: 10.1089/wound.2015.0635

Gahlawat, G., Shikha, S., Chaddha, B. S., Chaudhuri, S. R., Mayilraj, S., and Choudhury, A. R. (2016). Microbial glycolipoprotein-capped silver nanoparticles as emerging antibacterial agents against cholera. *Microb. Cell Fact.* 15:25. doi: 10.1186/s12934-016-0422-x

Garcia-Orue, I., Gainza, G., Garcia-Garcia, P., Gutierrez, F. B., Aguirre, J. J., Hernandez, R. M., et al. (2019). Composite nanofibrous membranes of PLGA/Aloe vera containing lipid nanoparticles for wound dressing applications. *Int. J. Pharm.* 556, 320–329. doi: 10.1016/j.ijpharm.2018.12.010

Gauthier, A., Fisch, A., Seuwen, K., Baumgarten, B., Ruffner, H., Aebi, A., et al. (2018). Glucocorticoid-loaded liposomes induce a pro-resolution phenotype in human primary macrophages to support chronic wound healing. *Biomaterials* 178, 481–495. doi: 10.1016/j.biomaterials.2018.04.006

GhavamiNejad, A., Park, C. H., and Kim, C. S. (2016). *In situ* synthesis of antimicrobial silver nanoparticles within antifouling zwitterionic hydrogels by catecholic redox chemistry for wound healing application. *Biomacromolecules* 17, 1213–1223. doi: 10.1021/acs.biomac.6b00039

Gonzalez de Torre, I., Ibanez-Fonseca, A., Quintanilla, L., Alonso, M., and Rodriguez-Cabello, J. C. (2018). Random and oriented electrospun fibers based on a multicomponent, in situ clickable elastin-like recombinamer system for dermal tissue engineering. *Acta Biomater.* 72, 137–149. doi: 10.1016/j.actbio.2018.03.027

Guan, B., Mao, T. L., Panuganti, P. K., Kuhn, E., Kurman, R. J., and Maeda, D., et al. (2011). Mutation and loss of expression of ARID1A in uterine low-grade endometrioid carcinoma. *Am. J. Surg. Pathol.* 35, 625–632. doi: 10.1097/PAS.0b013e318212782a

Haensel, D., Jin, S., Sun, P., Cinco, R., Dragan, M., Nguyen, Q., et al. (2020). Defining epidermal basal cell states during skin homeostasis and wound healing using single-cell transcriptomics. *Cell Rep.* 30, 3932–3947.e6. doi: 10.1016/j.celrep.2020.02.091

Hajiahmadi, F., Alikhani, M. Y., Shariatifar, H., Arabestani, M. R., and Ahmadvand, D. (2019). The bactericidal effect of lysostaphin coupled with liposomal vancomycin as a dual combating system applied directly on methicillin-resistant *Staphylococcus aureus* infected skin wounds in mice. *Int. J. Nanomedicine* 14, 5943–5955. doi: 10.2147/IJN.S214521

Hasan, N., Cao, J., Lee, J., Hlaing, S. P., Oshi, M. A., Naeem, M., et al. (2019). Bacteria-targeted clindamycin loaded polymeric nanoparticles: effect of surface charge on nanoparticle adhesion to MRSA, antibacterial activity, wound healing. *Pharmaceutics* 11:236. doi: 10.3390/pharmaceutics11050236

Hazeem, L. J., Kuku, G., Dewailly, E., Slomianny, C., Barras, A., Hamdi, A., et al. (2019). Toxicity effect of silver nanoparticles on photosynthetic pigment content, growth, ROS production and ultrastructural changes of microalgae *Chlorella vulgaris*. *Nanomaterials* 9:914. doi: 10.3390/nano9070914

He, W., Wang, Y., Wang, P., and Wang, F. (2019). Intestinal barrier dysfunction in severe burn injury. *Burns Trauma* 7:24. doi: 10.1186/s41038-019-0162-3

Hopf, H. W., and Rollins, M. D. (2007). Wounds: an overview of the role of oxygen. *Antioxid. Redox Signal.* 9, 1183–1192. doi: 10.1089/ars.2007.1641

Hu, Y., Liu, H., Zhou, X., Pan, H., Wu, X., Abidi, N., et al. (2019). Surface engineering of spongy bacterial cellulose via constructing crossed groove/column micropattern by low-energy CO_2 laser photolithography toward scar-free wound healing. *Mater. Sci. Eng. C Mater. Biol. Appl.* 99, 333–343. doi: 10.1016/j.msec.2019.01.116

Huang, X., Sun, J., Chen, G., Niu, C., Wang, Y., Zhao, C., et al. (2019). Resveratrol promotes diabetic wound healing via SIRT1-FOXO1-c-Myc signaling pathway-mediated angiogenesis. *Front. Pharmacol.* 10:421. doi: 10.3389/fphar.2019.00421

Jia, Y., Zhang, H., Yang, S., Xi, Z., Tang, T., Yin, R., et al. (2018). Electrospun PLGA membrane incorporated with andrographolide-loaded mesoporous silica nanoparticles for sustained antibacterial wound dressing. *Nanomedicine* 13, 2881–2899. doi: 10.2217/nnm-2018-0099

Jiang, S., Li, S. C., Huang, C., Chan, B. P., and Du, Y. (2018). Physical properties of implanted porous bioscaffolds regulate skin repair: focusing on mechanical and structural features. *Adv. Healthc. Mater.* 7: E1700894. doi: 10.1002/adhm.201700894

Jiang, S., Lyu, C., Zhao, P., Li, W., Kong, W., Huang, C., et al. (2019). Cryoprotectant enables structural control of porous scaffolds for exploration of cellular mechano-responsiveness in 3D. *Nat. Commun.* 10:3491. doi: 10.1038/s41467-019-11397-1

Jiang, Y., Huang, S., Fu, X., Liu, H., Ran, X., Lu, S., et al. (2011). Epidemiology of chronic cutaneous wounds in China. *Wound Repair Regen.* 19, 181–188. doi: 10.1111/j.1524-475X.2010.00666.x

Kalantari, K., Mostafavi, E., Afifi, A. M., Izadiyan, Z., Jahangirian, H., Rafiee-Moghaddam, R., et al. (2020). Wound dressings functionalized with silver nanoparticles: promises and pitfalls. *Nanoscale* 12, 2268–2291. doi: 10.1039/C9NR08234D

Kanji, S., and Das, H. (2017). Advances of Stem Cell Therapeutics in Cutaneous Wound Healing and Regeneration. *Mediators Inflamm.* 2017:5217967. doi: 10.1155/2017/5217967

Karimi Dehkordi, N., Minaiyan, M., Talebi, A., Akbari, V., and Taheri, A. (2019). Nanocrystalline cellulose-hyaluronic acid composite enriched with GM-CSF loaded chitosan nanoparticles for enhanced wound healing. *Biomed. Mater.* 14:035003. doi: 10.1088/1748-605X/ab026c

Kasemets, K., Kaosaar, S., Vija, H., Fascio, U., and Mantecca, P. (2019). Toxicity of differently sized and charged silver nanoparticles to yeast *Saccharomyces cerevisiae* BY4741: a nano-biointeraction perspective. *Nanotoxicology* 13, 1041–1059. doi: 10.1080/17435390.2019.1621401

Khan, A. M., Korzeniowska, B., Gorshkov, V., Tahir, M., Schroder, H., Skytte, L., et al. (2019). Silver nanoparticle-induced expression of proteins related to oxidative stress and neurodegeneration in an *in vitro* human blood-brain barrier model. *Nanotoxicology* 13, 221–239. doi: 10.1080/17435390.2018.1540728

Khorasani, M. T., Joorabloo, A., Moghaddam, A., Shamsi, H., and MansooriMoghadam, Z. (2018). Incorporation of ZnO nanoparticles into heparinised polyvinyl alcohol/chitosan hydrogels for wound dressing application. *Int. J. Biol. Macromol.* 114, 1203–1215. doi: 10.1016/j.ijbiomac.2018.04.010

Kilian, K. A., Bugarija, B., Lahn, B. T., and Mrksich, M. (2010). Geometric cues for directing the differentiation of mesenchymal stem cells. *Proc. Natl. Acad. Sci. U.S.A* 107, 4872–4877. doi: 10.1073/pnas.0903269107

Kim, H. S., Sun, X., Lee, J. H., Kim, H. W., Fu, X., and Leong, K. W. (2018). Advanced drug delivery systems and artificial skin grafts for skin wound healing. *Adv. Drug Deliv. Rev.* 146, 209–239. doi: 10.1016/j.addr.2018.12.014

Kokel, A., and Torok, M. (2018). Recent advances in the development of antimicrobial peptides (AMPs): attempts for sustainable medicine? *Curr. Med. Chem.* 25, 2503–2519. doi: 10.2174/0929867325666180117142142

Konop, M., Klodzinska, E., Borowiec, J., Laskowska, A. K., Czuwara, J., Konieczka, P., et al. (2019). Application of micellar electrokinetic chromatography for detection of silver nanoparticles released from wound dressing. *Electrophoresis* 40, 1565–1572. doi: 10.1002/elps.201900020

Li, N., Xie, X., Hu, Y., He, H., Fu, X., Fang, T., et al. (2019). Herceptin-conjugated liposomes co-loaded with doxorubicin and simvastatin in targeted prostate cancer therapy. *Am. J. Transl. Res.* 11, 1255–1269.

Li, Y., Zhang, J., Zhou, Q., Wang, H., Xie, S., Yang, X., et al. (2019). Linagliptin inhibits high glucose-induced transdifferentiation of hypertrophic scar-derived fibroblasts to myofibroblasts via IGF/Akt/mTOR signalling pathway. *Exp. Dermatol* 28, 19–27. doi: 10.1111/exd.13800

Liao, C., Li, Y., and Tjong, S. C. (2019). Bactericidal and cytotoxic properties of silver nanoparticles. *Int. J. Mol. Sci.* 20:449. doi: 10.3390/ijms20020449

Liu, M., He, D., Yang, T., Liu, W., Mao, L., Zhu, Y., et al. (2018a). An efficient antimicrobial depot for infectious site-targeted chemo-photothermal therapy. *J. Nanobiotechnol.* 16:23. doi: 10.1186/s12951-018-0348-z

Liu, M., Liu, T., Chen, X., Yang, J., Deng, J., He, W., et al. (2018b). Nano-silver-incorporated biomimetic polydopamine coating on a thermoplastic polyurethane porous nanocomposite as an efficient antibacterial wound dressing. *J. Nanobiotechnol.* 16:89. doi: 10.1186/s12951-018-0416-4

Liu, M., Luo, G., Wang, Y., He, W., Liu, T., Zhou, D., et al. (2017). Optimization and integration of nanosilver on polycaprolactone nanofibrous mesh for bacterial inhibition and wound healing in vitro and in vivo. *Int. J. Nanomedicine* 12, 6827–6840. doi: 10.2147/IJN.S140648

Liu, N., Huang, S., Yao, B., Xie, J., Wu, X., and Fu, X. (2016). 3D bioprinting matrices with controlled pore structure and release function guide in vitro self-organization of sweat gland. *Sci. Rep.* 6:34410. doi: 10.1038/srep34410

MacEwan, M. R., MacEwan, S., Kovacs, T. R., and Batts, J. (2017). What makes the optimal wound healing material? A review of current science, and introduction of a synthetic nanofabricated wound care scaffold. *Cureus* 9:e1736. doi: 10.7759/cureus.1736

Mahmoud, N. N., Hikmat, S., Abu Ghith, D., Hajeer, M., Hamadneh, L., Qattan, D., et al. (2019). Gold nanoparticles loaded into polymeric hydrogel for wound healing in rats: Effect of nanoparticles' shape and surface modification. *Int. J. Pharm.* 565, 174–186. doi: 10.1016/j.ijpharm.2019.04.079

Manukumar, H. M., Chandrasekhar, B., Rakesh, K. P., Ananda, A. P., Nandhini, M., Lalitha, P., et al. (2017). Novel T-C@AgNPs mediated biocidal mechanism against biofilm associated methicillin-resistant *Staphylococcus aureus* (Bap-MRSA) 090, cytotoxicity and its molecular docking studies. *Medchemcomm* 8, 2181–2194. doi: 10.1039/C7MD00486A

Melo, E., Cardenes, N., Garreta, E., Luque, T., Rojas, M., Navajas, D., et al. (2014). Inhomogeneity of local stiffness in the extracellular matrix scaffold of fibrotic mouse lungs. *J. Mech. Behav. Biomed. Mater.* 37, 186–195. doi: 10.1016/j.jmbbm.2014.05.019

Menglong Liu, Y. W., Xiaodong, H., Weifeng, H., Yali, G., Xiaohong, H., Meixi, L., et al. (2018). Janus N-dimethylformamide as a solvent for a gradient porous wound dressing of poly(vinylidene fluoride) and as a reducer for *in situ* nano-silver production: anti-permeation, antibacterial and antifouling activities against multi-drug-resistant bacteria both *in vitro* and *in vivo*. *RSC Adv.* 8, 26626–26639. doi: 10.1039/C8RA03234C

Miao, S., Cui, H., Esworthy, T., Mahadik, B., Lee, S. J., Zhou, X., et al. (2020). 4D self-morphing culture substrate for modulating cell differentiation. *Adv. Sci.* 7:1902403. doi: 10.1002/advs.201902403

Mithieux, S. M., Aghaei-Ghareh-Bolagh, B., Yan, L., Kuppan, K. V., Wang, Y., Garces-Suarez, F., et al. (2018). Tropoelastin implants that accelerate wound repair. *Adv. Healthc. Mater.* 7 e1701206. doi: 10.1002/adhm.201701206

Nasab, M. E., Takzaree, N., Saffaria, P. M., and Partoazar, A. (2019). *In vitro* antioxidant activity and *in vivo* wound-healing effect of lecithin liposomes: a comparative study. *J. Comp. Eff. Res.* 8, 633–643. doi: 10.2217/cer-2018-0128

Nasrollahi, S., Walter, C., Loza, A. J., Schimizzi, G. V., Longmore, G. D., and Pathak, A. (2017). Past matrix stiffness primes epithelial cells and regulates their future collective migration through a mechanical memory. *Biomaterials* 146, 146–155. doi: 10.1016/j.biomaterials.2017.09.012

Nunes, P. S., Rabelo, A. S., Souza, J. C., Santana, B. V., da Silva, T. M., Serafini, M. R., et al. (2016). Gelatin-based membrane containing usnic acid-loaded liposome improves dermal burn healing in a porcine model. *Int. J. Pharm.* 513, 473–482. doi: 10.1016/j.ijpharm.2016.09.040

Pang, S., Gao, Y., Wang, F., Wang, Y., Cao, M., Zhang, W., et al. (2020). Toxicity of silver nanoparticles on wound healing: a case study of zebrafish fin regeneration model. *Sci. Total Environ.* 717:137178. doi: 10.1016/j.scitotenv.2020.137178

Pratsinis, A., Hervella, P., Leroux, J. C., Pratsinis, S. E., and Sotiriou, G. A. (2013). Toxicity of silver nanoparticles in macrophages. *Small* 9, 2576–2584. doi: 10.1002/smll.201202120

Ramanathan, G., Singaravelu, S., Muthukumar, T., Thyagarajan, S., Perumal, P. T., and Sivagnanam, U. T. (2017). Design and characterization of 3D hybrid collagen matrixes as a dermal substitute in skin tissue engineering. *Mater. Sci. Eng. C Mater. Biol. Appl.* 72, 359–370. doi: 10.1016/j.msec.2016.11.095

Recordati, C., De Maglie, M., Bianchessi, S., Argentiere, S., Cella, C., Mattiello, S., et al. (2016). Tissue distribution and acute toxicity of silver after single intravenous administration in mice: nano-specific and size-dependent effects. *Part. Fibre Toxicol* 13:12. doi: 10.1186/s12989-016-0124-x

Rice, L. B. (2009). The clinical consequences of antimicrobial resistance. *Curr. Opin. Microbiol* 12, 476–481. doi: 10.1016/j.mib.2009.08.001

Richter, A. P., Brown, J. S., Bharti, B., Wang, A., Gangwal, S., Houck, K., et al. (2015). An environmentally benign antimicrobial nanoparticle based on a silver-infused lignin core. *Nat. Nanotechnol.* 10, 817–823. doi: 10.1038/nnano.2015.141

Rigo, C., Ferroni, L., Tocco, I., Roman, M., Munivrana, I., Gardin, C., et al. (2013). Active silver nanoparticles for wound healing. *Int. J. Mol. Sci.* 14, 4817–4840. doi: 10.3390/ijms14034817

Rodriguez-Cabello, J. C., Gonzalez de Torre, I., Ibanez-Fonseca, A., and Alonso, M. (2018). Bioactive scaffolds based on elastin-like materials for wound healing. *Adv. Drug Deliv. Rev.* 129, 118–133. doi: 10.1016/j.addr.2018.03.003

Sackmann, E. K., Fulton, A. L., and Beebe, D. J. (2014). The present and future role of microfluidics in biomedical research. *Nature* 507, 181–189. doi: 10.1038/nature13118

Sahu, S. C., Njoroge, J., Bryce, S. M., Zheng, J., and Ihrie, J. (2016). Flow cytometric evaluation of the contribution of ionic silver to genotoxic potential of nanosilver in human liver HepG2 and colon Caco2 cells. *J. Appl. Toxicol.* 36, 521–531. doi: 10.1002/jat.3276

Sandri, G., Miele, D., Faccendini, A., Bonferoni, M. C., Rossi, S., Grisoli, P., et al. (2019). Chitosan/glycosaminoglycan scaffolds: the role of silver nanoparticles to control microbial infections in wound healing. *Polymers* 11:1207. doi: 10.3390/polym11071207

Satish, L., Santhakumari, S., Gowrishankar, S., Pandian, S. K., Ravi, A. V., and Ramesh, M. (2017). Rapid biosynthesized AgNPs from Gelidiella acerosa aqueous extract mitigates quorum sensing mediated biofilm formation of Vibrio species-an in vitro and in vivo approach. *Environ. Sci. Pollut. Res. Int.* 24, 27254–27268. doi: 10.1007/s11356-017-0296-4

Shavandi, Z., Ghazanfari, T., and Moghaddam, K. N. (2011). In vitro toxicity of silver nanoparticles on murine peritoneal macrophages. *Immunopharmacol. Immunotoxicol.* 33, 135–140. doi: 10.3109/08923973.2010.487489

Tao, S. C., Guo, S. C., Li, M., Ke, Q. F., Guo, Y. P., and Zhang, C. Q. (2017). Chitosan wound dressings incorporating exosomes derived from MicroRNA-126-overexpressing synovium mesenchymal stem cells provide sustained release of exosomes and heal full-thickness skin defects in a diabetic rat model. *Stem Cells Transl. Med.* 6, 736–747. doi: 10.5966/sctm.2016-0275

Tarakanova, A., Yeo, G. C., Baldock, C., Weiss, A. S., and Buehler, M. J. (2019). Tropoelastin is a flexible molecule that retains its canonical shape. *Macromol Biosci.* 19:e1800250. doi: 10.1002/mabi.201800250

Thomas, R., Nair, A. P., Kr, S., Mathew, J., and Ek, R. (2014). Antibacterial activity and synergistic effect of biosynthesized AgNPs with antibiotics against multidrug-resistant biofilm-forming coagulase-negative staphylococci isolated from clinical samples. *Appl. Biochem. Biotechnol.* 173, 449–460. doi: 10.1007/s12010-014-0852-z

Vagnozzi, A. N., Reiter, J. F., and Wong, S. Y. (2015). Hair follicle and interfollicular epidermal stem cells make varying contributions to wound regeneration. *Cell Cycle* 14, 3408–3417. doi: 10.1080/15384101.2015.1090062

Wang, M., Yang, Q., Long, J., Ding, Y., Zou, X., Liao, G., et al. (2018). A comparative study of toxicity of TiO2, ZnO, and Ag nanoparticles to human aortic smooth-muscle cells. *Int. J. Nanomedicine* 13, 8037–8049. doi: 10.2147/IJN.S188175

Wang, Y., Xu, R., He, W., Yao, Z., Li, H., Zhou, J., et al. (2015). Three-dimensional histological structures of the human dermis. *Tissue Eng. Part C Methods* 21, 932–944. doi: 10.1089/ten.tec.2014.0578

Wang, Y., Xu, R., Luo, G., Lei, Q., Shu, Q., Yao, Z., et al. (2016). Biomimetic fibroblast-loaded artificial dermis with "sandwich" structure and designed gradient pore sizes promotes wound healing by favoring granulation tissue formation and wound re-epithelialization. *Acta Biomater.* 30, 246–257. doi: 10.1016/j.actbio.2015.11.035

Wu, Y. C., Wu, G. X., Huang, H. H., and Kuo, S. M. (2019). Liposome-encapsulated farnesol accelerated tissue repair in third-degree burns on a rat model. *Burns* 45, 1139–1151. doi: 10.1016/j.burns.2019.01.010

Xiang, Q., Xiao, J., Zhang, H., Zhang, X., Lu, M., Zhang, H., et al. (2011). Preparation and characterisation of bFGF-encapsulated liposomes and evaluation of wound-healing activities in the rat. *Burns* 37, 886–895. doi: 10.1016/j.burns.2011.01.018

Xing, F., Li, L., Zhou, C., Long, C., Wu, L., Lei, H., et al. (2019). Regulation and directing stem cell fate by tissue engineering functional microenvironments: scaffold physical and chemical cues. *Stem Cells Int.* 2019:2180925. doi: 10.1155/2019/2180925

Xu, R., Bai, Y., Zhao, J., Xia, H., Kong, Y., Yao, Z., et al. (2018). Silicone rubber membrane with specific pore size enhances wound regeneration. *J. Tissue Eng. Regen. Med.* 12, e905–e917. doi: 10.1002/term.2414

Xu, R., Luo, G., Xia, H., He, W., Zhao, J., Liu, B., et al. (2015). Novel bilayer wound dressing composed of silicone rubber with particular micropores enhanced wound re-epithelialization and contraction. *Biomaterials* 40, 1–11. doi: 10.1016/j.biomaterials.2014.10.077

Xu, R., Xia, H., He, W., Li, Z., Zhao, J., Liu, B., et al. (2016). Controlled water vapor transmission rate promotes wound-healing via wound re-epithelialization and contraction enhancement. *Sci. Rep.* 6:24596. doi: 10.1038/srep24596

Yang, C., Tibbitt, M. W., Basta, L., and Anseth, K. S. (2014). Mechanical memory and dosing influence stem cell fate. *Nat. Mater.* 13, 645–652. doi: 10.1038/nmat3889

Yang, L., Kuang, H., Zhang, W., Aguilar, Z. P., Wei, H., and Xu, H. (2017). Comparisons of the biodistribution and toxicological examinations after repeated intravenous administration of silver and gold nanoparticles in mice. *Sci. Rep.* 7:3303. doi: 10.1038/s41598-017-03015-1

Yao, B., Wang, R., Wang, Y., Zhang, Y., Hu, T., Song, W., et al. (2020). Biochemical and structural cues of 3D-printed matrix synergistically direct MSC differentiation for functional sweat gland regeneration. *Sci. Adv.* 6:eaaz1094. doi: 10.1126/sciadv.aaz1094

Yeo, G. C., Kosobrodova, E., Kondyurin, A., McKenzie, D. R., Bilek, M. M., and Weiss, A. S. (2019). Plasma-activated substrate with a tropoelastin anchor for the maintenance and delivery of multipotent adult progenitor cells. *Macromol Biosci.* 19:e1800233. doi: 10.1002/mabi.201800233

Zarrintaj, P., Moghaddam, A. S., Manouchehri, S., Atoufi, Z., Amiri, A., Amirkhani, M. A., et al. (2017). Can regenerative medicine and nanotechnology combine to heal wounds? The search for the ideal wound dressing. *Nanomedicine* 12, 2403–2422. doi: 10.2217/nnm-2017-0173

Zhang, X., Manukumar, H. M., Rakesh, K. P., Karthik, C. S., Nagendra Prasad, H. S., Swamy, S. N., et al. (2018). Role of BP*C@AgNPs in Bap-dependent multicellular behavior of clinically important methicillin-resistant Staphylococcus aureus (MRSA) biofilm adherence: A key virulence study. *Microb. Pathog.* 123, 275–284. doi: 10.1016/j.micpath.2018.07.025

Zheng, Y., Xue, X., Shao, Y., Wang, S., Esfahani, S. N., Li, Z., et al. (2019). Controlled modelling of human epiblast and amnion development using stem cells. *Nature* 573, 421–425. doi: 10.1038/s41586-019-1535-2

Zhou, C., Jin, S., and Willing, R. (2016). Simulation of extracellular matrix remodeling by fibroblast cells in soft three-dimensional bioresorbable scaffolds. *Biomech. Model. Mechanobiol.* 15, 1685–1698. doi: 10.1007/s10237-016-0791-4

Zille, A., Fernandes, M. M., Francesko, A., Tzanov, T., Fernandes, M., Oliveira, F. R., et al. (2015). Size and aging effects on antimicrobial efficiency of silver nanoparticles coated on polyamide fabrics activated by atmospheric DBD plasma. *ACS Appl. Mater. Interfaces* 7, 13731–13744. doi: 10.1021/acsami.5b04340

4

Indentation Stiffness Measurement by an Optical Coherence Tomography-Based Air-Jet Indentation System can Reflect Type I Collagen Abundance and Organisation in Diabetic Wounds

*Harry Ming Chun Choi[1], Alex Kwok-Kuen Cheung[1], Michelle Chun Har Ng[1], Yongping Zheng[2], Yih-Kuen Jan[3] and Gladys Lai Ying Cheing[1]**

[1] Department of Rehabilitation Sciences, The Hong Kong Polytechnic University, Kowloon, Hong Kong, [2] Department of Biomedical Engineering, The Hong Kong Polytechnic University, Kowloon, Hong Kong, [3] Department of Kinesiology and Community Health, University of Illinois at Urbana-Champaign, Urbana, IL, United States

***Correspondence:**
Gladys Lai Ying Cheing
Gladys.cheing@polyu.edu.hk

There is a lack of quantitative and non-invasive clinical biomechanical assessment tools for diabetic foot ulcers. Our previous study reported that the indentation stiffness measured by an optical coherence tomography-based air-jet indentation system in a non-contact and non-invasive manner may reflect the tensile properties of diabetic wounds. As the tensile properties are known to be contributed by type I collagen, this study was aimed to establish the correlations between the indentation stiffness, and type I collagen abundance and organisation, in order to further justify and characterise the *in vivo* indentation stiffness measurement in diabetic wounds. In a male streptozotocin-induced diabetic rat model, indentation stiffness, and type I collagen abundance and organisation of excisional wounds were quantified and examined using the optical coherence tomography-based air-jet indentation system and picrosirius red polarised light microscopy, respectively, on post-wounding days 3, 5, 7, 10, 14, and 21. The results showed significant negative correlations between indentation stiffness at the wound centre, and the collagen abundance and organisation. The correlations between the indentation stiffness, as well as collagen abundance and organisation of diabetic wounds suggest that the optical coherence tomography-based air-jet indentation system can potentially be used to quantitatively and non-invasively monitor diabetic wound healing in clinical settings, clinical research or preclinical research.

Keywords: biomechanical properties, collagen, diabetic wounds, non-invasive measurement, diagnostic device

INTRODUCTION

Diabetes mellitus is a metabolic disease characterised by hyperglycaemia. Peripheral polyneuropathy, regional ischaemia in the limbs and foot ulceration are common diabetes-related complications. Due to impaired sensation and circulation, people with diabetes are susceptible to repeated cutaneous injuries and possible wound infection, which may result in delayed healing and chronic foot ulcers (Jeffcoate and Harding, 2003; Bjarnsholt et al., 2008).

Chronic diabetic foot ulcers may subsequently result in lower limb amputation and thus require prompt medical attention.

Precise, objective, reliable, and quantitative measurements of wounds are needed to determine prognosis and ensure best strategies adopted in treating and preventing the development of ulcers. Common clinical assessments for diabetic ulcers include gross observation of wound size, colour, and depth (tendon/capsule/bone involvements), as well as the presence of gangrene, infection, and/or ischaemia (Oyibo et al., 2001; Gul et al., 2006). However, these assessments rely only on the observation of the wound appearance, which are not shown to reflect the underlying histology and the biomechanical strength. During wound healing, collagen, which is a major protein in the cutaneous extracellular matrix, is deposited, organised, and contributing to the biomechanical properties as well as the integrity of the skin. The biomechanical properties can thus be a potential quantitative measurement for chronic wounds such as diabetic ulcers to reflect the functional histological integrity of the wounds. Conventional tensile testing is a common strategy to measure the tensile biomechanical properties which are dependent on the abundance, alignment and orientation of collagen, in particular type I collagen (Silver et al., 1992). Therefore, tensile testing is useful in assessing wound healing and recovery of collagen histology in the literature (Howes et al., 1929; Dogan et al., 2009; Dadpay et al., 2012; Minossi et al., 2014; Lau et al., 2015). Preclinical studies have consistently concluded that impaired wound healing in diabetic condition is characterised by decreased tensile strength, as well as reduced collagen abundance and organisation (Yue et al., 1987; Davidson et al., 1997; Schäffer et al., 1997; Reddy et al., 2001; Immonen et al., 2013; Minossi et al., 2014; Zhang et al., 2016). Nevertheless, both tensile testing and histological examination are not feasible in clinical settings because the excision of tissue samples from the subject is required. Optical coherence tomography (OCT) has been applied to assess *in vivo* skin in real time and non-invasively. Advanced OCT systems were also developed to even image the skin in human at high resolution but only required brief contact (Monnier et al., 2020). Recently, our research team conducted a pilot study utilising an OCT-based air-jet indentation system to assess the indentation stiffness of diabetic wounds in a non-contact manner (Choi et al., 2015). By using the air-jet as an indenter, deformation of the wounds can be achieved by a small force in a non-contact manner, which minimises the risk of contamination or damage due to direct contact. We have demonstrated that the OCT-based air-jet indentation system can accurately and reliably measure the indentation force and deformation in the plantar tissues of patients with diabetes (Chao et al., 2011). Unlike tensile testing that involves the extraction and rupture of specimens, the OCT-based air-jet indentation system reversibly deforms the wounds inward to measure their indentation stiffness at low load and strain (i.e., it does not disrupt the wound tissue). The load of indentation is mainly absorbed by the cutaneous proteoglycans in the extracellular matrix (Silver et al., 1992), which participate in regulating collagen deposition and maturation (Raghow, 1994; Reed and Iozzo, 2002) as well as in the whole wound healing process (Werner and Grose, 2003; Schultz and Wysocki, 2009). Together with our earlier study that demonstrated the negative correlations between the tensile strength and indentation stiffness of a diabetic rat wound model (Choi et al., 2015), we hypothesised that the indentation stiffness is also associated with the recovery of type I collagen histology during wound healing.

The objective of the present study was therefore to establish the correlations between indentation stiffness, and type I collagen abundance and organisation in a diabetic rat wound model.

MATERIALS AND METHODS

Animal Handling and Diabetes Induction

The protocol of this study was approved by the Animal Subjects Ethics Sub-Committee of the Hong Kong Polytechnic University. All the rats received humane care and the protocols were in compliance with the guidelines and regulations from the Animal Subjects Ethics Sub-Committee and Institutional Animal Care and Use Committee[1]. Ten-week-old male (300–400 g) Sprague-Dawley rats used in this study were obtained from the Centralised Animal Facilities of The Hong Kong Polytechnic University. The rats were kept at 21°C and 60% relative humidity under a 12-h light-dark cycle. They were fed with a standard laboratory diet and sterile water *ad libitum*. Before diabetes induction, the rats were fasted for 12 h and their blood glucose level was measured to exclude any abnormally hyper- or hypoglycaemic animals from the study. Intra-peritoneal injection of streptozotocin (50 mg/kg; Sigma-Aldrich, St. Louis, MO, United States) in sterile citrate buffer (pH 4.4) was given to induce diabetes in the rats. After 7 days, the blood glucose level of the rats was measured and monitored once a week throughout the experiment to ensure diabetes was successfully induced and sustained in these rats. Any rats with a blood glucose level lower than 16.7 mM were excluded from the study (King, 2012; Lei et al., 2020).

Wound Induction

Prior to wound induction, the rats were anaesthetised by an intra-peritoneal injection of a mixture of ketamine (100 mg/kg) and xylazine (3.33 mg/kg). After shaving and cleansing the skin, wounds were induced with a 6 mm biopsy punch on the lateral side of each hind limb (about 3 mm distal to the fibular head). The wounds were left opened without dressing. The rats were then housed individually to prevent cannibalism. At the time points of harvest, photos of the wounds were taken and the wound area was estimated by Fiji software (Schindelin et al., 2012). Percentage of wound area was defined as the area of the wound at a particular time point divided by the initial wound area (post-wounding day 0).

OCT-Based Air-Jet Indentation Assessment

Wounds were randomly selected for assessment using the OCT-based air-jet indentation system (Choi et al., 2015) on post-wounding days 3, 5, 7, 10, 14, and 21 so that data from various

[1] http://www.polyu.edu.hk/ro/forms/Attachment%202_Guidelines%20for%20the%20assessment%20&%20mgmt%20of%20pain.pdf

phases of wound healing could be collected. Immediately before the assessment, the rats were anaesthetised by ketamine and xylazine injection as mentioned. The technical details of the OCT-based air-jet indentation system have been documented in our previous studies (Huang et al., 2009; Choi et al., 2015). The schematic diagram is shown in **Figure 1**.

Briefly, the probe of the OCT device consisted of a 1-mm air-jet bubbler together with a super-luminescent diode light source (Dense Light, DL-CS3055A, Singapore) operating at a central wavelength of 1,310 nm, a nominal −3 dB spectral bandwidth of 50 nm, and a nominal output power of 5 mW. The OCT unit provided an axial resolution of 18 μm and an imaging depth of approximately 2 to 3 mm in highly scattered materials. An electronic proportional valve with pressure feedback (ITV 1030-311L-Q, SMC Corporation, Tokyo, Japan) at a measurement range of 0.5 MPa was installed. In-house OCT software was used to collect the signals and to control the air valve with a step motor.

The system was used to measure the indentation stiffness of the wounds *in vivo*. There were five measurement sites including one at the centre of the wound with reference to the wound margin, and four at the periphery (proximal, distal, medial, and lateral to the wound with reference to the fibula, 3 mm from the centre of the wound). Two measurements were made at each site with a 5 min resting interval between each measurement; a total of ten measurements were taken for each wound. Three cycles of loading and unloading at an indentation rate of around 0.13 mm/s were applied and recorded, which lasted for approximately 30 s in total. The maximum indentation force was approximately 0.012 N. The deformation was measured by the OCT probe as the inward displacement of the surface of the wound, in accordance with the shift of the OCT signal corresponding to the tissue surface. The stiffness coefficient presented as force/deformation ratio (N/mm) was calculated to represent indentation stiffness. The first loading and unloading cycle was the preconditioning cycle. The indentation stiffness measurements calculated in the loading phases of the second and third cycles were averaged. The typical load-deformation curve including both loading and unloading phases in each cycle is illustrated in **Supplementary Figure 1**.

Histological Analysis of Collagen

The full-thickness wounds of randomly selected rats were harvested on post-wounding days 3, 5, 7, 10, 14, and 21 with 8 mm biopsy punches. The wound tissues were then fixed, processed, embedded in paraffin wax, and then sectioned into 5 μm thickness. The sections of the wound centre, which is defined by the sections with the largest wound gap between morphologically mature epidermis and dermis amongst the series of consecutive sections, were deparaffinised and stained with picrosirius red (Sigma-Aldrich, St. Louis, MO, United States) according to the standard procedures (Kiernan, 2002). Type I collagen is the only type of collagen to appear red upon the staining and examination under a polarised light microscope (Nikon Eclipse 80i, Nikon Corporation, Tokyo, Japan) (Kiernan, 2002). Images of the wound centre were captured using a digital camera (Spot Flex 15.2 64 Mp Shifting Pixel, Diagnostic Instruments Inc., Sterling Heights, MI, United States). The quantification of collagen was executed by Fiji software. The red channel of the images was converted to 8-bit colour depth for analysis. The amount of collagen was quantified as area. The percentage of collagen abundance was represented by the amount of collagen normalised by the area of dermis, where collagen is normally present. The intensity of the staining was measured to represent the alignment of collagen fibrils as better aligned collagen fibrils have a higher degree of birefringence and thus generate brighter image under polarised light microscope (Montes and Junqueira, 1991). Greater Feret length indicates greater continuation of a collagen fibre and also reflects greater degrees of orientation and anisotropy (Melis et al., 2002; Noorlander et al., 2002). The average Feret length of the top ten longest collagen fibres of the wound was calculated to represent the orientation of the collagen fibres (Melis et al., 2002; Noorlander et al., 2002). By selecting six representative regions of interest in the dermis, the energy and coherency values from the Fiji plug-in, OrientationJ, were also obtained as parameters of orientation and anisotropy of collagen fibres by structure tensor evaluation (Rezakhaniha et al., 2012). Briefly, the coherency value ranges from 0 to 1, where a coherency value that is close to 1 indicates coherently oriented fibres of the same direction (Fonck et al., 2009); the energy value, consistent to the coherency value, reflects the directionality of the fibres, but is also a function of the area of fibres (Rezakhaniha et al., 2012).

Statistical Analysis

Intraclass correlation (ICC) [3, 2] analysis was performed to assess the test-retest reliability. Two-way analysis of variance with *post hoc* Tukey's tests was conducted to examine differences between indentation stiffness measured at the wound centre and periphery over time. Spearman's Rho was conducted to explore the correlations between the indentation stiffness, and collagen abundance and organisation. The two-sided significance level was set at 0.05. The ICC coefficient was generated by IBM SPSS Statistics for Windows version 21.0 (Armonk, NY, United States: IBM Corp.). The other statistics were performed by GraphPad Prism version 6.00 for Windows (GraphPad Software, La Jolla, CA, United States)[2]. Data were displayed as individual data points and mean ± standard error of mean.

RESULTS

The diabetic rat model was induced using streptozotocin injection. The streptozotocin injection led to 21.8% mortality. Among the surviving rats, 4.4% did not develop hyperglycaemia.

Wound Size, Indentation Stiffness, and Type I Collagen Deposition

Excisional wounds were inflicted on the hind limbs of the rats for the assessment of indentation stiffness, and collagen abundance and organisation. By 14 days, all wounds were grossly closed without notable infection (**Figure 2**).

[2]www.graphpad.com

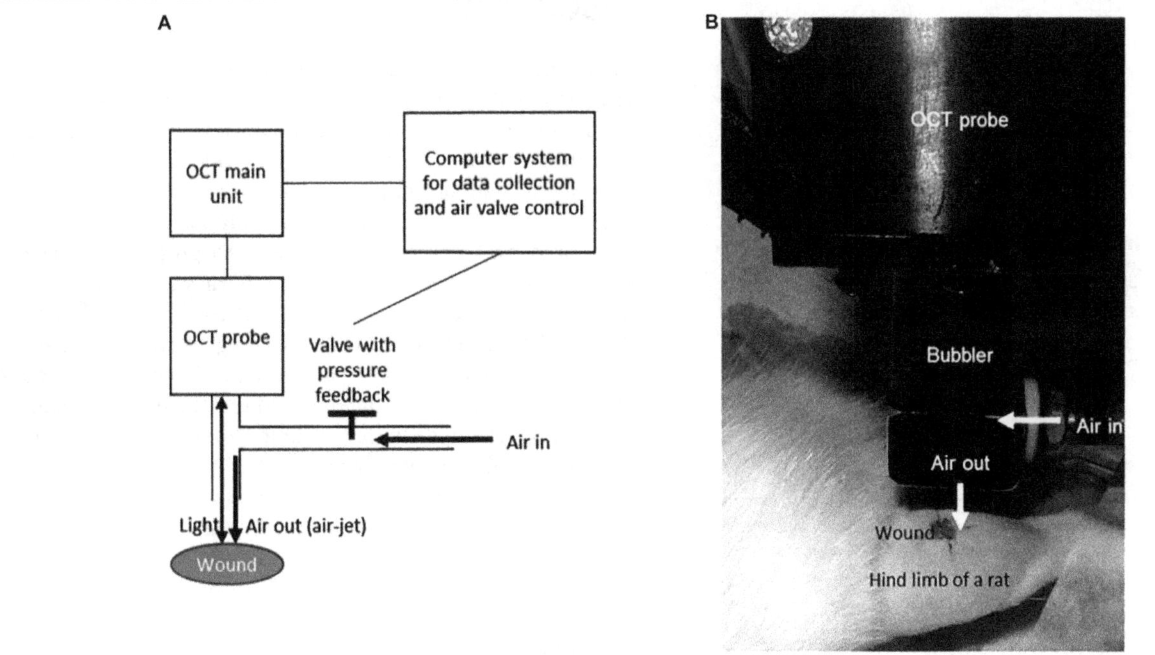

FIGURE 1 | The design of the OCT-based air-jet indentation system used for measuring indentation stiffness of wounds. **(A)** Schematic diagram showing that air-jet whose pressure or flow was controlled by a valve with pressure feedback and a computer system. The air-jet was used as an indenter while the reflected light signal is captured by the OCT probe so that the displacement was detected by the computer system. **(B)** A wound on a hind limb of a diabetic rat was assessed by the OCT-based air-jet indentation system.

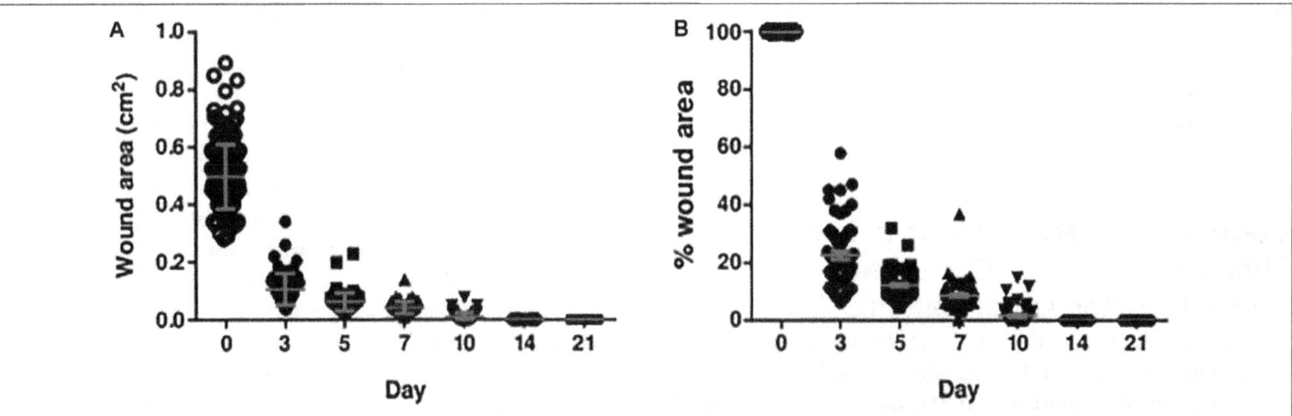

FIGURE 2 | The **(A)** area and **(B)** percentage of area of the diabetic wounds measured over 3 weeks. The area and percentage of area of the diabetic wounds decreased over time. All wounds were closed by post-wounding day 14. The percentage of wound area was the wound area on the specific day divided by the initial wound area (day 0). Data are expressed as individual data points as well as mean ± standard error of mean. Day 0: n = 191 wounds, 96 rats; day 3: n = 68 wounds, 34 rats; day 5: n = 68 wounds, 34 rats; day 7: n = 64 wounds, 32 rats; day 10: n = 56 wounds, 28 rats; day 14: n = 56 wounds, 28 rats; and day 21: n = 56 wounds, 28 rats.

Intraclass correlation [3, 2] analysis indicated an excellent test-retest reliability of the indentation stiffness measurement at both the centre and periphery of 46 randomly selected wounds at different time points [ICC (3, 2) = 0.92]. This finding shows that the measurement made in current experimental setting was reliable.

At the wound centre, the indentation stiffness was comparable in the early phase (days 3, 5, and 7; **Figure 3**). However, it significantly dropped in the later phase (days 10, 14, and 21; $P < 0.0001$). In contrast, the indentation stiffness at the wound periphery demonstrated negligible change over time and was consistently smaller as compared to the wound centre.

Picrosirius red staining was performed to visualise type I collagen fibres (appear in red under polarised light), which is the main contributor to the tensile strength of the wounds and the skin. Images taken at the centre of the wounds harvested on post-wounding days 3, 5, 7, 10, 14, and 21 revealed that the majority of the staining appeared red indicating type I

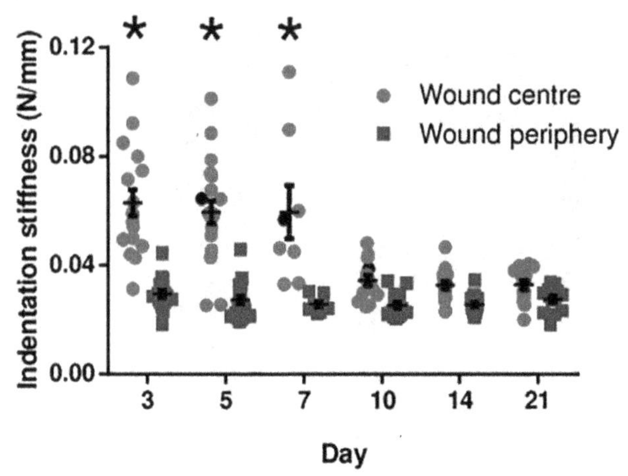

FIGURE 3 | The indentation stiffness measured at the centre and periphery of the diabetic wounds over 3 weeks. The indentation stiffness measurements at the wound centre on days 3, 5, and 7 were significantly greater than those measured on days 10, 14, and 21 (*$P < 0.0001$). Data are expressed as individual data points as well as mean ± standard error of mean. Day 3: $n = 17$ wounds, 9 rats; day 5: $n = 20$ wounds, 11 rats; day 7: $n = 8$ wounds, 4 rats; day 10: $n = 14$ wounds, 7 rats; day 14: $n = 16$ wounds, 9 rats; and day 21: $n = 14$ wounds, 8 rats.

collagen fibres. However, green signals, which indicates thinner and less aligned collagen fibres, such as type III, were negligible in abundance. Type I collagen fibres were quantified in terms of collagen abundance, fibril alignment and fibre orientation (**Figure 4**). The collagen abundance showed an notable increase from day 7 to day 21. However, there were no substantial changes in collagen organisation (i.e., fibril alignment, fibre orientation, and anisotropy) throughout the study period.

Correlations Between Indentation Stiffness, and Type I Collagen Abundance and Organisation

As type I collagen is the major structural protein in the extracellular matrix underlying biomechanical properties, correlations were established between the indentation stiffness and the abundance and organisation of type I collagen. The indentation stiffness at the wound centre was significantly negatively correlated with the collagen abundance (absolute abundance and percentage abundance) and organisation (fibril alignment, fibre orientation, energy of anisotropy, and coherency of anisotropy; **Figure 5**). As a negative control, the indentation stiffness at the wound periphery was not correlated with the collagen abundance and organisation at the wound centre. These findings confirm that the correlations are region specific (i.e., only indentation stiffness measured at the wound centre, but not periphery, reflects the collagen at the wound centre). Interestingly, such negative correlations between the indentation stiffness at the wound centre (but not the wound periphery) and collagen abundance and organisation were also found significant in non-diabetic wounds of strain-, sex-, and age-matched rats (**Supplementary Figure 2**).

DISCUSSION

This study is the first one to show that the abundance and organisation of collagen in wounds could be reflected by an *in vivo*, non-contact and non-invasive biomechanical measurement. This provides further evidence to support the use of indentation stiffness as a biomechanical assessment of diabetic wounds. As our previous study have shown that the indentation stiffness could reflect the tensile properties of diabetic wounds, we postulated that collagen fibril alignment and fibre orientation should also be factors in the correlation (Choi et al., 2015). The current study demonstrating negative correlations between indentation stiffness, and type I collagen abundance and organisation in diabetic wounds may therefore further explain the negative correlations between the indentation stiffness and tensile properties, which are mainly contributed by type I collagen fibres.

Proteoglycans may absorb compressive stress and resist tissue deformation upon compression, thus contributing to the compressive/indenting property of the skin (Silver et al., 1992). Correlation between indentation stiffness and collagen shown in the current study suggests interesting relationships between indenting property, proteoglycans and collagen in wound healing. Proteoglycans, which is a component of the ground substance, have roles in collagen deposition and maturation. Decorin, regarded as one of the small-sized proteoglycans found in the skin, interacts with various types of collagen (Vogel et al., 1984; Brown and Vogel, 1989; Tenni et al., 2002). It plays an important role in regulating collagen deposition (Reed and Iozzo, 2002) and also the recovery of collagen organisation upon injury (Dunkman et al., 2014). Hence, it potentially affects the tensile properties of the skin wounds (Carrino et al., 2000). It should be noted that the abundance of decorin increases following wound closure (Yeo et al., 1991). In contrast, other proteoglycans such as chondroitin sulphate proteoglycans of large molecular size remain dominant during the wound healing process, when the wound is not completely closed (Yeo et al., 1991). Proteoglycans of large size (e.g., chondroitin sulphate proteoglycans) are interlaced with thin collagen fibrils, vice versa, the smaller-sized (e.g., decorin) are distributed among thicker collagen (Kuwaba et al., 2002). Owing to such characteristic, we speculate that the dynamic changes in molecular size of proteoglycans do not only contribute to the organisation and maturation of collagen fibres, but also the indentation stiffness during wound healing. The predominance of large-sized proteoglycans may contribute to an increased indentation stiffness in the early phase (day 3 to day 7), prior to wound closure. They are then replaced by the smaller-sized proteoglycans following wound closure, which may account for the reduced indentation stiffness in the later phase (day 10 to day 21). This may not only justify the negative correlations between the indentation stiffness and collagen abundance and organisation found in the current study, but also explain the consistently smaller indentation stiffness at the wound periphery, which is presumably uninjured skin, with proteoglycans of smaller size (Kuwaba et al., 2002). Future study is warranted to confirm the relationships between the indentation stiffness, proteoglycans, and collagen deposition and organisation of

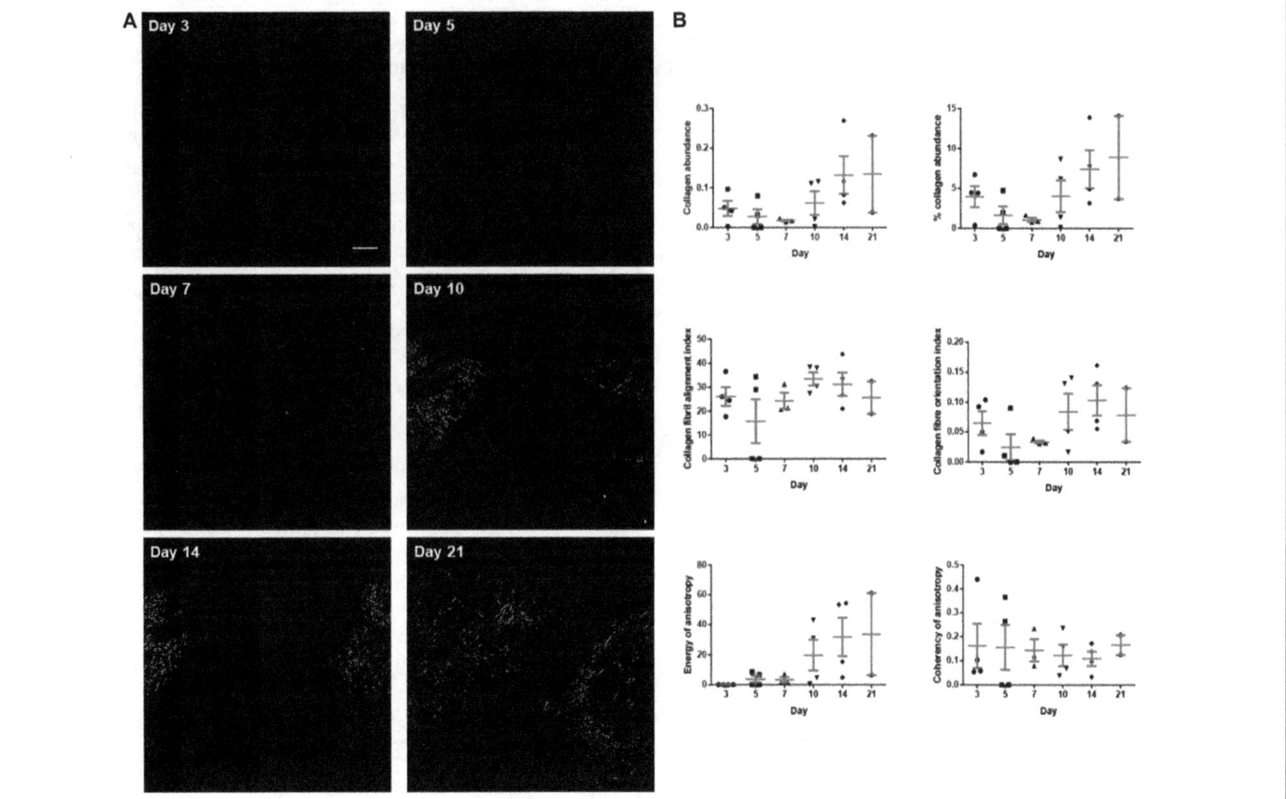

FIGURE 4 | The collagen histology of the diabetic wounds examined over 3 weeks. **(A)** Representative picrosirius red stained sections at the centre of the diabetic wounds examined under polarised light microscope on post-wounding day 3, day 5, day 7, day 10, day 14, and day 21. Type I collagen fibres appear red under polarised light. No collagen was observed to be deposited on days 3 and 5. Very limited collagen was observed on day 7. The abundance of collagen increased as the wounds healed on days 10, 14, and 21. Scale bar = 150 μm. **(B)** The collagen histology including collagen abundance, percentage collagen abundance, collagen fibril alignment, collagen fibre orientation, energy of anisotropy and coherency of anisotropy quantified over 3 weeks. Both abundance of collagen and energy of anisotropy showed obvious increasing trend from post-wounding day 7 to day 21. Data are expressed as individual data points as well as mean ± standard error of mean. Day 3: $n = 4$ wounds, 4 rats; day 5: $n = 4$ wounds, 4 rats; day 7: $n = 3$ wounds, 3 rats; day 10: $n = 4$ wounds, 4 rats; day 14: $n = 4$ wounds, 4 rats; and day 21: $n = 2$ wounds, 2 rats.

diabetic wounds, in order to provide concrete support on the clinical use of the indentation stiffness measurement.

Although the present study focuses on the dermal layer of the skin/wound, wound healing does involve re-epithelialisation. Particularly in the early phase where the dermal layer is still very thin or even absent, the epidermal layer may probably be the main structure contributing to the biomechanical properties of the wound. Indeed, our data show that the thicker epidermal layer in the early phase (**Supplementary Figure 3**) coincides with the greater indentation stiffness in the early phase of diabetic wound healing (days 3, 5, and 7; **Figure 3**). The epidermal thickness at different time points has a significant positive correlation with the indentation stiffness at the wound centre (**Supplementary Figure 3**). Keratinocyte is the major cell type in the epidermal layer, which synthesises protein fibre keratin that can potentially contribute to compressive/indenting biomechanical properties (Wang et al., 2016). The presence of epidermal layer in the early phase of wound centre in the current study suggests the presence of keratin and keratinocytes at the wound centre in the early phase. Other studies conducted with excisional wounds in rats (Sabol et al., 2012) and humans (Usui et al., 2005) have also found the presence of keratin and keratinocytes in the early phase of wound healing. During wound healing, keratinocytes proliferate, migrate, differentiate into different stages and express distinct types of keratins such as K16 in activated proliferating keratinocytes and K10 in terminally differentiated keratinocytes (Freedberg et al., 2001; Santos et al., 2002; Usui et al., 2008). It has been suggested that different types of keratins with different structures and molecular weights could have different biomechanical properties (Bragulla and Homberger, 2009). Therefore, in different phases of wound healing, different compositions and abundance of various types of keratins may possibly contribute to the different indentation stiffness. This may also explain why the indentation stiffness at the wound centre is significantly different from that at the periphery as the compositions of keratins at these sites are probably different. At the wound centre, it is expected that keratinocytes are more activated and proliferative expressing high level of K16. Conversely, keratinocytes in the uninjured area at the wound periphery express less K16 but more K10. Interestingly, keratinocytes expressing different types of keratins release different signalling molecules such as cytokines (e.g.,

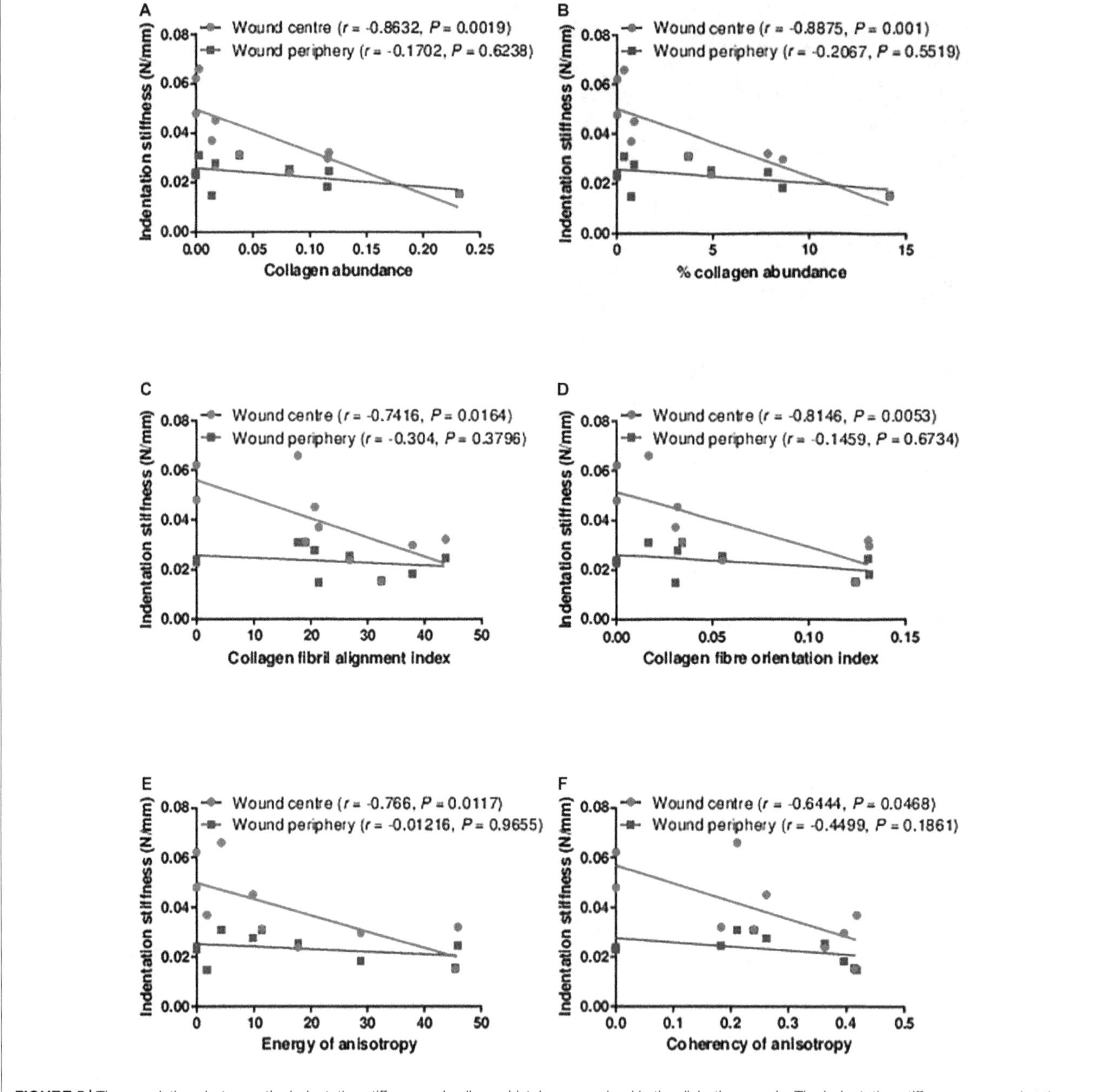

FIGURE 5 | The correlations between the indentation stiffness and collagen histology examined in the diabetic wounds. The indentation stiffness measured at the wound centre was significantly negatively correlated to the **(A,B)** collagen abundance, **(C)** alignment, **(D)** orientation, and **(E,F)** anisotropy on post-wounding day 3 (n = 1 wound, 1 rat), 5 (n = 2 wounds, 2 rats), 7 (n = 2 wounds, 2 rats), 10 (n = 1 wound, 1 rat), 14 (n = 2 wounds, 2 rats), and 21 (n = 2 wounds, 2 rats). Data at different time points were pooled together.

TNF-α) and growth factors (TGF-β) to regulate the signalling and differentiation of fibroblasts. The release of various signalling molecules has potential effects on the collagen deposition and maturation in dermis (Werner et al., 2007; Pastar et al., 2014). Future studies are needed to clarify the indentation stiffness of specific types, compositions and abundance of keratins in *in vivo* wound models and, in addition, to examine the regulation of collagen deposition and maturation in dermal layer by keratinocytes expressing distinct types of keratins in wound healing process. This series of studies will hopefully be able to further elucidate the biomechanical and molecular characteristics of the wounds reflected by the indentation stiffness in different phases of wound healing.

Apart from the possible contribution by proteoglycans and keratins, the consistently high indentation stiffness in the early phase of wound healing could be related to wound oedema. The histological finding in the present study suggests that oedema was present in the wounds on days 3, 5, and 7 but not on days 10, 14, and 21 (**Supplementary Figure 3**). This observation is consistent with the report by Vexler et al. (1999) who reported skin oedema to be associated with increased stiffness. In addition, it is generally agreed that oedema increases the stiffness of the tissue due to hydrostatic pressure in a confined space. The hypothesis that the high indentation stiffness is related to wound oedema is also partly supported by the present finding that the indentation stiffness at the wound periphery, where no wound oedema was found, was substantially smaller than that at the wound centre.

The main focus of the current study is to evaluate the correlations between the indentation stiffness, and type I collagen abundance and organisation in diabetic wounds. Nevertheless, to the best of our knowledge, this study is the first study to illustrate the quantitative changes in collagen abundance and organisation of diabetic wounds, over a period of time from the early phase (post-wounding day 3) to the later phase (day 21). Existing literature on the collagen histology is lacking the presentation of changes at various time points. Therefore, the present findings may provide insights to the research on optimal time points for specific interventions to diabetic wounds in different phases of wound healing. For the collagen abundance, our data show a non-significant decreasing trend from post-wounding day 3 to day 7 and an increasing trend thereafter. Majority of the studies which investigated the time course changes in collagen using either diabetic (Ponrasu and Suguna, 2012; Ram et al., 2015; Zhang et al., 2016) or non-diabetic wound models (Oxlund et al., 1996; Ponrasu and Suguna, 2012; Almeida et al., 2014) demonstrated an increase in collagen abundance over time and plateau or slightly decreases in the very late phase, which is consistent with the rising trend from day 7 to day 21 concluded in the current study. Therefore, the non-significant decrease from day 3 to day 7 in the collagen abundance shown in the present study could be attributed to individual variation. However, since limited study has focussed on the time course changes of collagen abundance between day 3, or earlier, and day 7 in diabetic wound models, we are unable to rule out the possibility that the decreasing trend of collagen abundance on post-wounding day 7 is as a result of diabetes-related complications in wound healing.

For collagen fibril alignment and fibre orientation indices, as well as the coherency of anisotropy which is also a measurement of collagen fibre orientation estimated by tensor analysis, there was no obvious increase or decrease across the time points. On the other hand, the energy of anisotropy is a function of both area and orientation of fibres. The rising trend of the energy of anisotropy corresponds to the increasing trend of the collagen abundance. In agreement with the unchanged collagen fibril alignment and fibre orientation in the current study, our previous study have also found no significant difference in the collagen fibril alignment and fibre orientation between post-wounding day 7 and day 14 in a diabetic rat excisional wound model (Choi et al., 2016). Broadley et al. (1989) demonstrated that even though the collagen concentration in diabetic wounds approached to the non-diabetic wound level over time, the tensile strength of the diabetic wounds remained impaired. Since tensile strength is contributed by all collagen abundance, alignment and orientation, they extrapolated that wounds in diabetic rat model might have deficits in the recovery of collagen alignment and orientation (Broadley et al., 1989). To date, no other published studies have quantitatively assessed the collagen fibril alignment and fibre orientation in wounds over a period of time. We therefore believe that the recovery of collagen alignment and orientation may not be significant in the current diabetic wound model within the experimental period, which is in agreement with the literature.

In conclusion, we established correlations between the indentation stiffness, type I collagen abundance and organisation of diabetic wounds in a rat model. Our findings provide evidence supporting the potential clinical use of the OCT-based air-jet indentation system for biomechanical assessment of diabetic wounds. In the future, we anticipate investigations using a more clinically relevant wound model involving repetitive stress and chronic inflammation resembling foot ulcers in patients to explore the correlations between the indentation stiffness and more clinically oriented parameters such as the prognosis of the wounds, risk of infections and severity of diabetes.

AUTHOR CONTRIBUTIONS

HC, AC, and GC: conceptualisation. HC: data curation, formal analysis, visualisation, and writing – original draft. GC: funding acquisition and project administration. HC and MN: investigation. YZ: methodology. AC and GC: supervision. HC, AC, YZ, Y-KJ, and GC: writing – review and editing. All authors contributed to the article and approved the submitted version.

REFERENCES

Almeida, B. M., Nascimento, M. F., Pereira-Filho, R. N., Melo, G. C., Santos, J. C., Oliveira, C. R., et al. (2014). Immunohistochemical profile of stromal constituents and lymphoid cells over the course of wound healing in murine model. *Acta Cir. Bras.* 29, 596–602.

Bjarnsholt, T., Kirketerp-Møller, K., Jensen, P. Ø, Madsen, K. G., Phipps, R., Krogfelt, K., et al. (2008). Why chronic wounds will not heal: a novel hypothesis. *Wound Repair Regen.* 16, 2–10. doi: 10.1111/j.1524-475X.2007.00283.x

Bragulla, H. H., and Homberger, D. G. (2009). Structure and functions of keratin proteins in simple, stratified, keratinized and cornified epithelia. *J. Anat.* 214, 516–559. doi: 10.1111/j.1469-7580.2009.01066.x

Broadley, K. N., Aquino, A. M., Hicks, B., Ditesheim, J. A., McGee, G. S., Demetriou, A. A., et al. (1989). The diabetic rat as an impaired wound healing model: stimulatory effects of transforming growth factor-beta and basic fibroblast growth factor. *Biotechnol. ther.* 1, 55–68.

Brown, D. C., and Vogel, K. G. (1989). Characteristics of the in vitro interaction of a small proteoglycan (PG II) of bovine tendon with type I collagen. *Matrix* 9, 468–478.

Carrino, D. A., Sorrell, J. M., and Caplan, A. I. (2000). Age-related changes in the proteoglycans of human skin. *Arch. Biochem. Biophys.* 373, 91–101. doi: 10.1006/abbi.1999.1545

Chao, C. Y. L., Zheng, Y. P., and Cheing, G. L. Y. (2011). A novel noncontact method to assess the biomechanical properties of wound tissue. *Wound Repair Regen.* 19, 324–329. doi: 10.1111/j.1524-475X.2011.00694.x

Choi, M. C., Cheung, K. K., Li, X., and Cheing, G. L. (2016). Pulsed electromagnetic field (PEMF) promotes collagen fibre deposition associated with increased myofibroblast population in the early healing phase of diabetic wound. *Arch. Dermatol. Res.* 308, 21–29. doi: 10.1007/s00403-015-1604-9

Choi, M. C., Cheung, K. K., Ng, G. Y., Zheng, Y. P., and Cheing, G. L. (2015). Measurement of diabetic wounds with optical coherence tomography-based air-jet indentation system and a material testing system. *J. Wound Care* 24, 519–528. doi: 10.12968/jowc.2015.24.11.519

Dadpay, M., Sharifian, Z., Bayat, M., Bayat, M., and Dabbagh, A. (2012). Effects of pulsed infra-red low level-laser irradiation on open skin wound healing of healthy and streptozotocin-induced diabetic rats by biomechanical evaluation. *J. Photochem. Photobiol. B* 111(Suppl. C), 1–8. doi: 10.1016/j.jphotobiol.2012.03.001

Davidson, J. M., Broadley, K. N., and Quaglino, D. (1997). Reversal of the wound healing deficit in diabetic rats by combined basic fibroblast growth factor and transforming growth factor-β1 therapy. *Wound Repair Regen.* 5, 77–88. doi: 10.1046/j.1524-475X.1997.50115.x

Dogan, S., Demirer, S., Kepenekci, I., Erkek, B., Kiziltay, A., Hasirci, N., et al. (2009). Epidermal growth factor-containing wound closure enhances wound healing in non-diabetic and diabetic rats. *Int. Wound J.* 6, 107–115. doi: 10.1111/j.1742-481X.2009.00584.x

Dunkman, A. A., Buckley, M. R., Mienaltowski, M. J., Adams, S. M., Thomas, S. J., Satchell, L., et al. (2014). The tendon injury response is influenced by decorin and biglycan. *Ann. Biomed. Eng.* 42, 619–630. doi: 10.1007/s10439-013-0915-2

Fonck, E., Feigl, G. G., Fasel, J., Sage, D., Unser, M., Rüfenacht, D. A., et al. (2009). Effect of aging on elastin functionality in human cerebral arteries. *Stroke* 40, 2552–2556. doi: 10.1161/strokeaha.108.528091

Freedberg, I. M., Tomic-Canic, M., Komine, M., and Blumenberg, M. (2001). Keratins and the keratinocyte activation cycle. *J. Invest. Dermatol.* 116, 633–640. doi: 10.1046/j.1523-1747.2001.01327.x

Gul, A., Basit, A., Ali, S. M., Ahmadani, M. Y., and Miyan, Z. (2006). Role of wound classification in predicting the outcome of diabetic foot ulcer. *J. Pak. Med. Assoc.* 56, 444–447.

Howes, E. L., Sooy, J. W., and Harvey, S. C. (1929). The healing of wounds as determined by their tensile strength. *J. Am. Med. Assoc.* 92, 42–45. doi: 10.1001/jama.1929.02700270046011

Huang, Y. P., Zheng, Y. P., Wang, S. Z., Chen, Z. P., Huang, Q. H., and He, Y. H. (2009). An optical coherence tomography (OCT)-based air jet indentation system for measuring the mechanical properties of soft tissues. *Meas. Sci. Technol.* 20, 1–11.

Immonen, J. A., Zagon, I. S., Lewis, G. S., and McLaughlin, P. J. (2013). Topical treatment with the opioid antagonist naltrexone accelerates the remodeling phase of full-thickness wound healing in type 1 diabetic rats. *Exp. Biol. Med.* 238, 1127–1135. doi: 10.1177/1535370213502632

Jeffcoate, W. J., and Harding, K. G. (2003). Diabetic foot ulcers. *Lancet* 361, 1545–1551.

Kiernan, J. A. (2002). Collagen type I staining. *Biotech. Histochem.* 77:31.

King, A. J. (2012). The use of animal models in diabetes research. *Br. J. Pharmacol.* 166, 877–894. doi: 10.1111/j.1476-5381.2012.01911.x

Kuwaba, K., Kobayashi, M., Nomura, Y., Irie, S., and Koyama, Y. (2002). Size control of decorin dermatan sulfate during remodeling of collagen fibrils in healing skin. *J. Dermatol. Sci.* 29, 185–194.

Lau, P. S., Bidin, N., Krishnan, G., Nassir, Z., and Bahktiar, H. (2015). Biophotonic effect of diode laser irradiance on tensile strength of diabetic rats. *J. Cosmet. Laser Ther.* 17, 86–89. doi: 10.3109/14764172.2014.968587

Lei, X., Huo, P., Wang, Y., Xie, Y., Shi, Q., Tu, H., et al. (2020). Lycium barbarum polysaccharides improve testicular spermatogenic function in streptozotocin-induced diabetic rats. *Front. Endocrinol.* 11:164. doi: 10.3389/fendo.2020.00164

Melis, P., Noorlander, M. L., van der Horst, C. M., and van Noorden, C. J. (2002). Rapid alignment of collagen fibers in the dermis of undermined and not undermined skin stretched with a skin-stretching device. *Plast. Reconstr. Surg.* 109, 674–680.

Minossi, J. G., Lima, F. D. O., Caramori, C. A., Hasimoto, C. N., Ortolan, ÉV. P., Rodrigues, P. A., et al. (2014). Alloxan diabetes alters the tensile strength, morphological and morphometric parameters of abdominal wall healing in rats. *Acta Cir. Bras.* 29, 118–124.

Monnier, J., Tognetti, L., Miyamoto, M., Suppa, M., Cinotti, E., Fontaine, M., et al. (2020). In vivo characterization of healthy human skin with a novel, non-invasive imaging technique: line-field confocal optical coherence tomography. *J. Eur. Acad. Dermatol. Venereol.* 34, 2914–2921. doi: 10.1111/jdv.16857

Montes, G., and Junqueira, L. (1991). The use of the Picrosirius-polarization method for the study of the biopathology of collagen. *Mem. Inst. Oswaldo Cruz* 86, 1–11.

Noorlander, M. L., Melis, P., Jonker, A., and Van Noorden, C. J. (2002). A quantitative method to determine the orientation of collagen fibers in the dermis. *J..Histochem. Cytochem.* 50, 1469–1474.

Oxlund, H., Christensen, H., Seyer-Hansen, M., and Andreassen, T. T. (1996). Collagen deposition and mechanical strength of colon anastomoses and skin incisional wounds of rats. *J. Surg. Res.* 66, 25–30. doi: 10.1006/jsre.1996.0367

Oyibo, S. O., Jude, E. B., Tarawneh, I., Nguyen, H. C., Harkless, L. B., and Boulton, A. J. (2001). A comparison of two diabetic foot ulcer classification systems: the Wagner and the University of Texas wound classification systems. *Diabetes Care* 24, 84–88.

Pastar, I., Stojadinovic, O., Yin, N. C., Ramirez, H., Nusbaum, A. G., Sawaya, A., et al. (2014). Epithelialization in wound healing: a comprehensive review. *Adv. wound care* 3, 445–464. doi: 10.1089/wound.2013.0473

Ponrasu, T., and Suguna, L. (2012). Efficacy of *Annona squamosa* on wound healing in streptozotocin-induced diabetic rats. *Int. Wound J.* 9, 613–623. doi: 10.1111/j.1742-481X.2011.00924.x

Raghow, R. (1994). The role of extracellular matrix in postinflammatory wound healing and fibrosis. *FASEB J.* 8, 823–831.

Ram, M., Singh, V., Kumawat, S., Kumar, D., Lingaraju, M. C., Uttam Singh, T., et al. (2015). Deferoxamine modulates cytokines and growth factors to accelerate cutaneous wound healing in diabetic rats. *Eur. J. Pharmacol.* 764, 9–21. doi: 10.1016/j.ejphar.2015.06.029

Reddy, G. K., Stehno-Bittel, L., and Enwemeka, C. S. (2001). Laser photostimulation accelerates wound healing in diabetic rats. *Wound Repair Regen.* 9, 248–255.

Reed, C. C., and Iozzo, R. V. (2002). The role of decorin in collagen fibrillogenesis and skin homeostasis. *Glycoconj. J.* 19, 249–255. doi: 10.1023/a:1025383913444

Rezakhaniha, R., Agianniotis, A., Schrauwen, J. T., Griffa, A., Sage, D., Bouten, C. V., et al. (2012). Experimental investigation of collagen waviness and orientation in the arterial adventitia using confocal laser scanning microscopy. *Biomech. Model. Mechanobiol.* 11, 461–473. doi: 10.1007/s10237-011-0325-z

Sabol, F., Dancakova, L., Gal, P., Vasilenko, T., Novotny, M., Smetana, K., et al. (2012). Immunohistological changes in skin wounds during the early periods of healing in a rat model. *Vet. Med.* 57, 77–82. doi: 10.17221/5253-vetmed

Santos, M., Paramio, J. M., Bravo, A., Ramirez, A., and Jorcano, J. L. (2002). The expression of keratin K10 in the basal layer of the epidermis inhibits cell proliferation and prevents skin tumorigenesis. *J. Biol. Chem.* 277, 19122–19130. doi: 10.1074/jbc.M201001200

Schäffer, M. R., Tantry, U., Efron, P. A., Ahrendt, G. M., Thornton, F. J., and Barbul, A. (1997). Diabetes-impaired healing and reduced wound nitric oxide synthesis: a possible pathophysiologic correlation. *Surgery* 121, 513–519. doi: 10.1016/S0039-6060(97)90105-7

Schindelin, J., Arganda-Carreras, I., Frise, E., Kaynig, V., Longair, M., Pietzsch, T., et al. (2012). Fiji: an open-source platform for biological-image analysis. *Nat. Methods* 9, 676–682. doi: 10.1038/nmeth.2019

Schultz, G. S., and Wysocki, A. (2009). Interactions between extracellular matrix and growth factors in wound healing. *Wound Repair Regen.* 17, 153–162. doi: 10.1111/j.1524-475X.2009.00466.x

Silver, F. H., Kato, Y. P., Ohno, M., and Wasserman, A. J. (1992). Analysis of mammalian connective tissue: relationship between hierarchical structures and mechanical properties. *J. Long Term Eff. Med. Implants* 2, 165–198.

Tenni, R., Viola, M., Welser, F., Sini, P., Giudici, C., Rossi, A., et al. (2002). Interaction of decorin with CNBr peptides from collagens I and II. evidence for multiple binding sites and essential lysyl residues in collagen. *Eur. J. Biochem.* 269, 1428–1437.

Usui, M. L., Mansbridge, J. N., Carter, W. G., Fujita, M., and Olerud, J. E. (2008). Keratinocyte migration, proliferation, and differentiation in chronic ulcers from patients with diabetes and normal wounds. *J. Histochem. Cytochem.* 56, 687–696. doi: 10.1369/jhc.2008.951194

Usui, M. L., Underwood, R. A., Mansbridge, J. N., Muffley, L. A., Carter, W. G., and Olerud, J. E. (2005). Morphological evidence for the role of suprabasal keratinocytes in wound reepithelialization. *Wound Repair Regen.* 13, 468–479. doi: 10.1111/j.1067-1927.2005.00067.x

Vexler, A., Polyansky, I., and Gorodetsky, R. (1999). Evaluation of skin viscoelasticity and anisotropy by measurement of speed of shear wave propagation with viscoelasticity skin analyzer. *J. Invest. Dermatol.* 113, 732–739. doi: 10.1046/j.1523-1747.1999.00751.x

Vogel, K. G., Paulsson, M., and Heinegård, D. (1984). Specific inhibition of type I and type II collagen fibrillogenesis by the small proteoglycan of tendon. *Biochem. J.* 223, 587–597.

Wang, B., Yang, W., McKittrick, J., and Meyers, M. A. (2016). Keratin: structure, mechanical properties, occurrence in biological organisms, and efforts at bioinspiration. *Prog. Mat. Sci.* 76, 229–318. doi: 10.1016/j.pmatsci.2015.06.001

Werner, S., and Grose, R. (2003). Regulation of wound healing by growth factors and cytokines. *Physiol. Rev.* 83, 835–870.

Werner, S., Krieg, T., and Smola, H. (2007). Keratinocyte–fibroblast interactions in wound healing. *J. Investig. Dermatol.* 127, 998–1008. doi: 10.1038/sj.jid.5700786

Yeo, T. K., Brown, L., and Dvorak, H. F. (1991). Alterations in proteoglycan synthesis common to healing wounds and tumors. *Am. J. Pathol.* 138, 1437–1450.

Yue, D. K., McLennan, S., Marsh, M., Mai, Y. W., Spaliviero, J., Delbridge, L., et al. (1987). Effects of experimental diabetes, uremia, and malnutrition on wound healing. *Diabetes* 36, 295–299. doi: 10.2337/diab.36.3.295

Zhang, Y., McClain, S. A., Lee, H.-M., Elburki, M. S., Yu, H., Gu, Y., et al. (2016). A novel chemically modified curcumin "normalizes" wound-healing in rats with experimentally induced type I diabetes: initial studies. *J. Diabetes Res.* 2016:5782904. doi: 10.1155/2016/5782904

5

Three-Layered Silk Fibroin Tubular Scaffold for the Repair and Regeneration of Small Caliber Blood Vessels: From Design to *in vivo* Pilot Tests

Antonio Alessandrino[1], Anna Chiarini[2], Marco Biagiotti[1], Ilaria Dal Prà[2], Giulia A. Bassani[1], Valentina Vincoli[1], Piergiorgio Settembrini[3], Pasquale Pierimarchi[4], Giuliano Freddi[1] and Ubaldo Armato[2]*

[1] Silk Biomaterials Srl, Lomazzo, Italy, [2] Human Histology & Embryology Section, Department of Surgery, Dentistry, Pediatrics & Gynecology, University of Verona Medical School, Verona, Italy, [3] Department of Vascular Surgery, San Carlo Borromeo Hospital, Milan, Italy, [4] Institute of Translational Pharmacology, National Research Council, Rome, Italy

***Correspondence:**
Giuliano Freddi
giuliano@silkbiomaterials.com

Silk fibroin (SF) is an eligible biomaterial for the development of small caliber vascular grafts for substitution, repair, and regeneration of blood vessels. This study presents the properties of a newly designed multi-layered SF tubular scaffold for vascular grafting (SilkGraf). The wall architecture consists of two electrospun layers (inner and outer) and an intermediate textile layer. The latter was designed to confer high mechanical performance and resistance on the device, while electrospun layers allow enhancing its biomimicry properties and host's tissues integration. *In vitro* cell interaction studies performed with adult Human Coronary Artery Endothelial Cells (HCAECs), Human Aortic Smooth Muscle Cells (HASMCs), and Human Aortic Adventitial Fibroblasts (HAAFs) demonstrated that the electrospun layers favor cell adhesion, survival, and growth. Once cultured *in vitro* on the SF scaffold the three cell types showed an active metabolism (consumption of glucose and glutamine, release of lactate), and proliferation for up to 20 days. HAAF cells grown on SF showed a significantly lower synthesis of type I procollagen than on polystyrene, meaning a lower fibrotic effect of the SF substrate. The cytokine and chemokine expression patterns were investigated to evaluate the cells' proliferative and pro-inflammatory attitude. Interestingly, no significant amounts of truly pro-inflammatory cytokines were secreted by any of the three cell types which exhibited a clearly proliferative profile. Good hemocompatibility was observed by complement activation, hemolysis, and hematology assays. Finally, the results of an *in vivo* preliminary pilot trial on minipig and sheep to assess the functional behavior of implanted SF-based vascular graft identified the sheep as the more apt animal model for next medium-to-long term preclinical trials.

Keywords: silk fibroin, small caliber vascular graft, morphological structure, mechanical performance, *in vitro* biocompatibility, *in vivo* pilot test

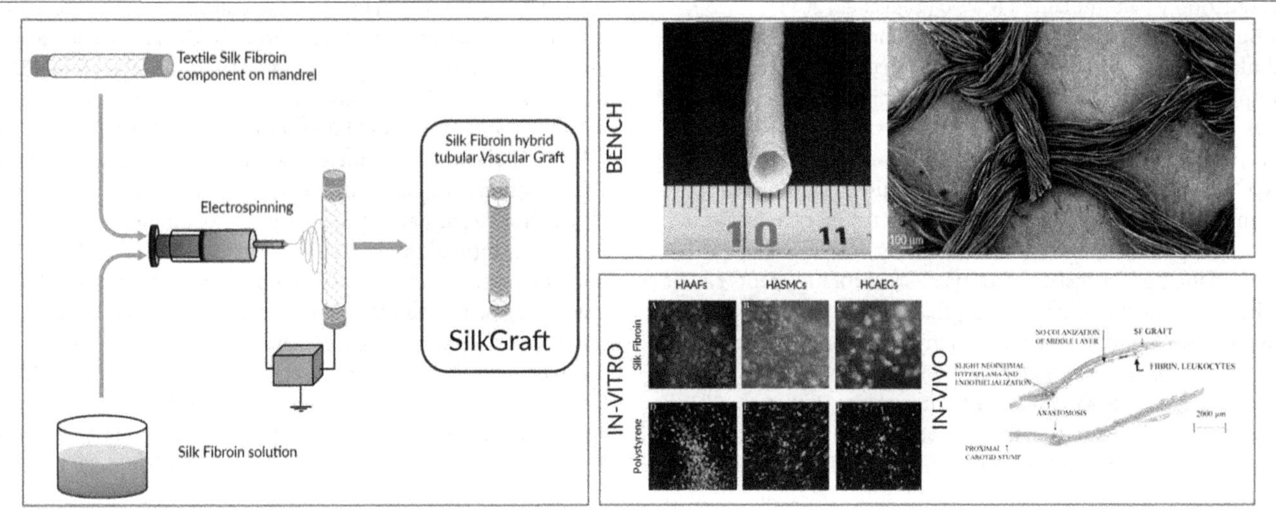

GRAPHICAL ABSTRACT | Novel hybrid textile-electrospun tubular architecture for vascular grafting, highly biocompatible, preventing fibrotic tissue responses, promising off-the-shelf solution for treating vascular diseases.

INTRODUCTION

Cardiovascular pathologies are the leading cause of death worldwide (World Health Organization, 2012), with very high overall incidence on health expenditures. As the vascular diseases progress with age, the related burden is likely to increase with the global rise in life expectancy. Thus, the availability of grafts for the treatment of vascular diseases becomes a real and urgent need. In the vascular surgery field of either coronary or peripheral bypass procedures, there is a crucial necessity of novel viable solutions, which might complement or even replace current surgical approaches, based on autografts, or synthetic grafts (Catto et al., 2014; Hiob et al., 2017; Sugiura et al., 2017). Autografts (using native vessels such as superficial veins or rarely umbilical veins) still remain the standard clinical approach for the replacement of small diameter blood vessels. However, there are some factors which may strongly curb the use of autografts: absence of a usable graft, significative atherosclerosis of the arteries, previous usage of an autograft for surgical procedures, or angiographic approaches (Catto et al., 2014).

Nowadays, small caliber synthetic grafts are made of polyethylene terephthalate (PET) or expanded polytetrafluoroethylene (ePTFE). Their use leads to possible multiple complications like aneurysm, intimal hyperplasia, calcification, thrombosis, infection, and lack of growth potential for pediatric applications. These drawbacks are mainly correlated to the regeneration of a non-functional endothelium and a mismatch between the mechanical properties of grafts and native blood vessels leading to the development of an intimal hyperplasia with subsequent reduction of the patency rate (Catto et al., 2014 and references therein cited).

As a biodegradable and biocompatible natural polymer Silk Fibroin (SF) has the potential to become the biomaterial of choice for the development of a range of medical applications, including small caliber blood vessel grafts (Altman et al., 2003; Thurber et al., 2015; Wang et al., 2017). The starting material can be easily purified and processed in different 2D/3D shapes. It is not immunogenic in humans (preliminary proteomic data revealed that several human proteins expressed by both epithelial and connective tissue cells exhibit homology sequences with SF Armato et al., 2011) and favors angiogenesis, an essential feature for tissue repair/regeneration (Dal Prà et al., 2005).

Manufacturing technologies of SF-based small caliber tubular grafts span from filament winding (Enomoto et al., 2010; Nakazawa et al., 2011), braiding (Ding et al., 2016; Zamani et al., 2017), and knitting (Yagi et al., 2011; Yamamoto et al., 2016), which are textile techniques making use of native microfiber yarns as starting material, to electrospinning (Wang et al., 2010; Liu et al., 2011; Xiang et al., 2011), and gel spinning (Lovett et al., 2008, 2010), which lead to various formats of regenerated SF tubular scaffolds. A recent research trend is to simulate in the scaffold the three-layered structure of the native blood vessel. Thus, designing multi-layered tubular scaffolds is seen as an effective way to mimic not only the native architecture but also to approach functional features of the artery. In particular, the aim is to create regionally selective environments in favor of the infiltration, adhesion, and spreading of cells conducive to the regeneration of neo-tissues with biological features and mechanical behaviors similar to the native ones.

The simplest technical approach to create at least an additional layer is to coat the textile tubular scaffold with a film-forming biocompatible polymer (SF or gelatin) (Fukayama et al., 2015; Yamamoto et al., 2016). The use of SF microfibers as scaffold material and of SF aqueous solution as coating showed advantages in terms of enhanced *in vivo* endothelialization, which corresponded to improved graft performance (e.g., medium-to-long term patency). Addition of crosslinking agents, like poly(ethylene glycol diglycidyl ether), to aqueous SF enhanced stability, and protected the scaffold from rapid degradation when implanted *in vivo* (Yagi et al., 2011).

Building a 3D sponge-like layer on one or both sides of the tubular braided/knitted textile core may represent a step forward in approaching more complex scaffold architectures (Aytemiz et al., 2013; Liu et al., 2013, 2018; Ding et al., 2016; Zamani et al., 2017; Tanaka et al., 2018). The manufacturing techniques used by various authors, albeit with minor variations, share common steps: immersion of the tubular textile core in a mold, pouring a polymer solution, freeze-drying, and possible solvent consolidation of the just created layer. Crosslinking agents can be added to modulate porosity, strength, elasticity, and degradation rate; functional molecules, most often anti-thrombogenic agents, can also be loaded into the sponge. *In vivo* implantation up to 1 year in dogs (Aytemiz et al., 2013) and rabbits (Liu et al., 2018), and up to 3 months in rats (Tanaka et al., 2018) resulted in high patency rate, absence of thrombus, aneurysm, or infection, and a physiological level of endothelialization of the internal lumen of the graft with no signs of intimal hyperplasia.

The three-layered concept for the wall structure of the graft was approached by Enomoto et al. (2010), who fabricated a tubular scaffold by combining two kinds of native SF microfibers, i.e., a thin silk thread and cocoon filaments, which were successively arranged around a cylindrical core. The final consolidation step consisted in dipping the scaffold into a SF solution. The scaffold implanted into the abdominal aorta of male Sprague-Dawley rats showed very good patency at 1 year, organization of endothelial and medial layers, formation of *vasa-vasorum* in the adventitia, regenerating a vascular-like structure. These findings highlighted the importance of SF as a promising material to develop vascular grafts for smaller caliber blood vessels.

Wu et al. (2018) and McClure et al. (2012) engineered three-layered tubular scaffolds using only electrospinning as the manufacturing technology. Combinations of natural (SF, collagen, elastin) and biodegradable synthetic polymers [polycaprolactone, poly(L-lactide-co-caprolactone), and poly(lactide-co-glycolide)], alone or as blends, were used to build layers with finely tuned morphological and mechanical properties. The devices were fully characterized from the mechanical point of view, but the authors reported no *in vivo* functional tests. One of the devices was subcutaneously implanted for 10 weeks in rats (Wu et al., 2018) showing a propensity to promote cell infiltration from the outside environment into the interior of the graft.

Electrospinning has the ability to mimic the nanoscale properties of fibrous components (collagen and elastin fibrils) of the extracellular matrix and to realize a range of biochemical, topographical, and mechanical properties conducive to improved cell interactions (Babitha et al., 2017). Our previous studies focused on the development of small caliber vascular grafts made of electrospun SF (Marelli et al., 2009, 2010, 2012; Cattaneo et al., 2013; Catto et al., 2015). SF tubular matrices with inner diameter of about 5 mm had a pressurized burst strength of 576 ± 17 mmHg, higher than physiological and pathological pressure thresholds, but still lower than that of human arteries (~5,000 mmHg for carotids). The compliance value of about 3.5 (radial deformation/mmHg10^{-2}) was considered very interesting since it is higher than synthetic grafts (<2) and closer to the physiological values for saphenous (4.4) and umbilical vein (3.7), the gold standard for autologous replacement of small caliber arteries. *In vitro* studies (Marelli et al., 2009, 2010, 2012; Catto et al., 2015) showed good integration of cells with the SF matrix, while functional implants in the abdominal aorta of Lewis rats proved short term patency of the grafts (Cattaneo et al., 2013). The cellular intimal thickening showed a structure similar to the tunica of native arterial vessel, with elastin and intimal layers reminiscent of the native inner vascular structure. Small blood vessels with the morphology of *vasa-vasorum* were found in the thin layer of tissue grown on the outer surface of the graft. Taken together, all these results showed that small caliber SF vascular grafts produced by electrospinning may be promising matrices for vascular tissue replacement, without requiring cell seeding before implantation.

This study reports the chemical, morphological, physical, and mechanical properties of a novel multi-layered SF tubular scaffold (SilkGraft). The hybrid architecture was designed to optimize not only production and pre-surgery manipulation of the device, but also stitching at the site of implantation, biological integration with host's tissues, and biomechanical performance (compliance, resistance to radial stresses, biodegradation rate, etc.). A wide range of *in vitro* cell interaction studies with human adult fibroblasts, endothelial cells, and smooth muscle cells were performed to investigate the biological response to the device. The cytokine and chemokine expression patterns were investigated to evaluate the cells' proliferative and/or pro-inflammatory attitude. The SilkGraft interaction with blood components was studied by means of the complement cascade activation assay, the change of the leucocyte and erythrocyte counts, and the hemolysis assay. Additionally, the results of *in vivo* preliminary pilot tests on large animals aimed at evaluating the handling of the device during the surgical procedure and identifying the more apt animal model for next medium-to-long term preclinical trials will be presented and discussed.

MATERIALS AND METHODS

Fabrication of the Three-Layered Tubular Scaffold

The vascular graft is a hybrid three-layered tubular device comprising inner and outer electrospun layers (ES), and an intermediate textile layer (TEX). The TEX layer was manufactured by warp needle braiding technology using degummed SF yarn. The ES nanofibrous layers were produced via electrospinning using pupae-free silk cocoons as starting material. Cocoons were degummed in autoclave at 120°C for 30 min and extensively washed with warm water. Pure SF microfibers thus obtained were dissolved with an aqueous solution of 9.3 M lithium bromide at 60°C for 3 h. The salt was removed by dialysis and aqueous SF was cast in Petri dishes at 35°C in a ventilated oven until complete evaporation of water to produce SF films, which were then dissolved in Formic Acid

(8% w_{SF}/v_{FA}) to prepare the spinning dope. Electrospinning was performed as previously reported (Marelli et al., 2010) using the following experimental parameters: voltage 25 kV, flow rate 0.8 ml/h, spinneret-collector distance 15 mm. Coupling of TEX and ES layers was made during electrospinning, according to a patented process (Alessandrino, 2016), with the use of an ionic liquid (1-ethyl-3-methylimidazolium acetate, Sigma Aldrich) as welding agent. Hybrid ES-TEX-ES tubular devices were finally purified by extraction with ethanol under microwave heating at 50°C for 60 min to remove processing aids, immersed in distilled water overnight, dried, packaged under laminar flow cabinet, and sterilized with ethylene oxide (EtO). Henceforth, the final three-layered SF-based ES-TEX-ES vascular graft is identified by the name "SilkGraft."

Materials and Scaffolds Characterization

Morphological and Geometrical Properties

Morphological analyses were performed with a scanning electron microscope (SEM; Zeiss EVO MA10) on Au/Pd sputter-coated samples (Desk IV, Denton Vacuum, LLC), at 10 kV acceleration voltage, 100 μA beam current, and 15 mm working distance.

Geometrical properties of SilkGraft were characterized by determining the weight per unit length, the wall thickness, and the inner diameter. Wall thickness was measured according to the ISO 7198:2016 standard method. The tubular device was cut longitudinally, flattened and measured with a thickness tester MarCator 1075R (Mahr) equipped with a constant load thickness gauge of 1 cm^2 foot area that exerts a pressure of 1 kPa. Dry state inner diameter was determined from SEM images of tubular cross-sections mounted on stubs, using the SEM software measuring tools.

Amino Acid Analysis

The amino acid composition was performed after hydrolysis with HCl 6 N, under vacuum, for 24 h. Free amino acids were quantitatively determined by Ion Exchange Chromatography using external standard calibration. Samples were analyzed in duplicate.

Attenuated Total Reflectance Fourier Transform Infrared Spectroscopy (ATR-FTIR)

ATR-FTIR spectra were made with an ALPHA FTIR spectrometer equipped with an ATR Platinum Diamond accessory, at a resolution of 4 cm^{-1}, in the infrared range of 4,000–400 cm^{-1}. Spectra were corrected with a linear baseline and normalized to the CH_2 bending peak at about 1,445 cm^{-1}. This peak was selected because it's not sensitive to SF molecular conformation.

Differential Scanning Calorimetry (DSC)

Thermal analyses were performed with a DSC 3500 Sirius (Netzsch). Samples (3–5 mg) were closed in Aluminum pans and subjected to a heating cycle from 50 to 400°C, at a heating rate of 10°C/min, under N_2 atmosphere (flow rate: 20 ml/min).

Circumferential Tensile Tests

Tests were performed according to ISO 7198:2016 using an All Electric Dynamic Test Instrument ElectroPuls E3000 (Instron), equipped with a load cell of 250 N, a thermostatic bath (BioPuls), and appropriate grips fabricated *ad hoc*. Samples (length = 10 mm, $n = 3$) were cut carefully, mounted on the grips, conditioned in water at 37°C for 5 min, and tested while submerged at a crosshead speed of 50 mm/min. Due to the difficulty in determining the correct size of the resistant cross-sectional area, the results are expressed in terms of load and not of the usual stress values.

Pressurized Burst Strength

The test was carried out according to ISO 7198:2016. A balloon was placed inside the tubular graft (length = 100 mm; $n = 3$) and filled with test fluid at a measured rate of pressure change until the sample burst or test was discontinued. Before testing, samples were conditioned in the test fluid (distilled water) at 37°C for 20 min. No sample pre-stretching was applied, but axial displacement (axial elongation of the sample) was allowed. The test was performed with the sample submerged in the testing fluid. A gear pump provided a flow through the sample and pressure was measured just upstream the sample. The rise in pressure and the pressure at which sample burst or test was discontinued were measured and recorded.

In vitro Cellular Studies

Preparation of Substrates for *in vitro* Cell Cultures

SilkGraft samples were washed, transversally cut into 1.5 cm long pieces, and opened lengthwise in order to obtain small squares with an apparent surface area of about 300 mm^2. After autoclave sterilization (121°C for 30 min), they were aseptically transferred to 2.2 cm-diameter culture plates (Falcon-Becton Dickinson). Heat-sterilized stainless-steel rings were applied onto the upper surface of the pieces to keep them flat at the bottom of the plates.

Pre-culture Intravital Cell Staining

Cells were stained with fluorescent lipophilic membrane dyes (tracers) such as the red-orange fluorescent $DilC_{18}(3)$ (1,1'-Dioctadecyl-3,3,3',3'-tetramethyl-indocarbocyanine perchlorate; maximum fluorescence excitation 549 nm and emission 565 nm; Thermo Fisher Scientific, USA) or the green fluorescent $DiOC_{18}(3)$ (3,3′-Dioctadecyl oxacarbocyanine perchlorate; maximum fluorescence excitation 484 nm and emission 590 nm; Thermo Fisher Scientific, USA) dissolved in DMSO according to seller's instructions. At intervals of 3 days, cultured specimens were observed under an inverted fluorescence microscope (IM 35, Zeiss) equipped with proper excitation and emission filters according to the intravital stain used, and digitally photographed with a DP10 Camera (Olympus, Japan).

Cell Cultures

Adult Human Coronary Artery Endothelial Cells (HCAECs), Human Aortic Smooth Muscle Cells (HASMCs), and Human Aortic Adventitial Fibroblasts (HAAFs) were provided by ScienCell Research Laboratories (Carlsbad, CA, USA). The supplier company guaranteed the cells characteristics we required via Cell Applications Inc. (San Diego, CA, USA).

For the adhesion studies, 2 × 10^4 human intravitally pre-stained cells were separately seeded onto SilkGraft samples.

HCAECs were seeded onto the inner ES layer, whereas HASMCs or HAAFs were seeded onto the outer ES layer. In parallel, the three cell types were separately seeded on 2D polystyrene plates as controls. All the tests were performed in triplicate and repeated in three separate experiments. Cell cultures were kept in an incubator at 37°C in 95 vol% air plus 5 vol% CO_2. The growth media used were: HCAECs, ready to use Endothelial Cell Medium; HAAFs, Fibroblast Medium; HASMCs, Smooth Muscle Cell Medium (all from ScienCell Research Laboratories, USA). Every 3 days the growth media were changed with fresh ones and the cell-conditioned media collected and stored at −80°C to be subsequently analyzed. The cultures were kept going for at least 20 consecutive days.

Cells Counts

Cells counts on polystyrene plates were first performed using an inverted light microscope (IM35, Zeiss) (Armato et al., 1986). On the same samples, cell number was determined by means of the Cell Titer-Blue® Cell Viability Assay (Promega, USA) fluorescence assay based on the ability of living cells to convert a redox dye (resazurin) into a final fluorescent product (resorufin). Correlating microscopic findings with resorufin Promega assay data allowed to construct cell type-specific standard curves to be used to determine total cell numbers on SilkGrafts.

Assays of Cell Metabolites

Three metabolites (D-glucose, L-glutamine, lactate) were assayed in the cell-conditioned growth medium samples from each of the three types of cells separately cultured on SilkGraft or on polystyrene surfaces. The data corrected for actual cell numbers were expressed as means ± SE of the respective time-related cumulative curves.

Cell D-glucose consumption was assessed by means of a glucose oxidase assay using the Amplex® Red Glucose/Glucose Oxidase Assay Kit (Invitrogen-USA). L-glutamine uptake/consumption was determined using the L-glutamine assay kit developed by Megazyme (Ireland). The lactic acid release was assessed via the colorimetric enzymatic Lactate Assay Kit (Sigma Aldrich).

Assay of the Extracellular C-Telopeptide of Procollagen Type I

The extracellular release (and subsequent assembly of fibers) of type I collagen was assessed by evaluating the amount of the C-telopeptide, which is released into the cell-conditioned growth medium in stoichiometrically equal amounts from precursor procollagen type I molecules. The samples were assayed using the EIA kit developed by Takara Bio Inc. (Shiga, Japan). The sensitivity of this assay is 10 ng/ml.

Human Proinflammatory Cytokines and Chemokines Antibody Array

The secretion of various cytokines/chemokines into the growth medium was assessed by using the Human Inflammation Antibody Array, C-Series (RayBiotech-USA) in three distinct experiments. In detail, 1.0 ml medium sampled between day 18th and 20th, was used. After a treatment for 60 min with blocking solution (Odissey Blocking Buffer™ (LI-COR) with 0.05% Tween 20), the cytokines and chemokines antibody array membranes were incubated with the medium samples overnight at 4°C. Next, the membranes were washed and incubated at room temperature for 2 h with 1.0 ml of primary biotin-conjugated antibody diluted 1:250 in blocking solution. This was followed by an incubation at room temperature for 1 h with 2 ml of DyLight800-Labeled streptavidin (KPL, USA) diluted 1:7,500 in blocking solution. The immunofluorescent signals were acquired by means of an Odissey Imager™ (LI-COR) scanner and quantified using the Image Studio™ software. The resulting intensity values from each array were normalized per 1,000 cells grown on either substrate. The array kit sensitivity is 4–25 pg/ml and the coefficient of variation of the intensity of the spots is 5–10%.

Hemocompatibility

The interaction between SilkGraft and blood components, i.e., the activation of the complement cascade and the alteration of the leucocyte count, the changes on erythrocyte count, and the presence of hemolysis, was studied according to the ISO 10993-4:2017 standard. As suggested by the regulation, the induction of thrombosis was assessed during the *in vivo* pilot trials. The tests reported below were performed in compliance with Good Laboratory Practices.

Activation of the Complement System

SilkGraft was incubated in human serum at 37 ± 1°C for 90 min with a surface/volume ratio of 3 cm²/ml. Zymosan A from *Saccharomyces cerevisiae* served as positive control, human serum alone as negative control and polypropylene material as negative reference material. Serum Complement Membrane Attack Complex (Sc5b-9) and Complement Component 3 (C3a) concentrations were determined with a commercial ELISA (MicroVue™ SC5b-9 Plus EIA and MicroVue™ C3a Plus EIA, Quidel Corporation).

Hemolysis

The blood was collected from three adult rabbits in test tube with anti-coagulant Sodium Citrate 3.2% (ratio 1+9 v/v Sodium Citrate/Blood). Equal quantities of blood from each rabbit were pooled and diluted with Mg- and Ca-free PBS to obtain a final hemoglobin concentration of 1,000 mg/dl.

For indirect contact assay, SilkGraft samples were dipped in Mg- and Ca-free PBS in order to reach a surface/volume ratio of 3 cm²/ml and incubated for 72 h at 50 ± 2°C. Seven milliliter of extract were added to 1 ml of diluted rabbit blood. For direct contact assay, SilkGraft samples were dipped in diluted rabbit blood and in Mg- and Ca-free PBS in order to reach a surface/volume ratio of 3 cm²/ml for SilkGraft/PBS and 0.14 ml/ml for diluted blood/PBS. Negative control (USP reference standard high-density polyethylene), positive control (water for injection) and blank (PBS) were tested.

All the samples (direct and indirect contact) were incubated in a water bath for 3 h at 37 ± 1°C and agitation was inverted twice every 30 min. After centrifugation at 800 G for 15 min, the concentration of hemoglobin in the supernatant was determined with the automatic chemistry analyzer Konelab 20 (DASIT).

Hematology

The effect of SilkGraft on red blood and white blood cells counts was evaluated after immersion in human whole blood in order to reach a surface/volume ratio of 3 cm^2/ml and incubation for 15 min at 37 ± 1°C under dynamic conditions. An automatic counter Sysmex KX-21N (DASIT) was used. As control, the remaining part of the blood that did not come in contact with SilkGraft was used.

In vivo Animal Pilot Studies

Animal Care

Pilot animal experiments were performed at NAMSA (Lyon, France), an AAALAC internationally accredited firm. The study protocol was approved by the NAMSA Ethical Committee and the French Ministry of Education, Higher Education, and Research. The study conditions conformed to the guidelines of the European Union's Directive EU/2010/63 for animal experiments. One sheep (Blanche du Massif Central) and one minipig (Göttingen) were used. Animals were kept under controlled conditions. The animal housing room temperature and relative humidity were recorded daily. Staff involved was properly qualified and trained. Standard veterinary medical care was also provided.

Pharmacological Treatment

Starting 3 days prior to the operation, the animals received daily antiaggregant treatment (sheep: oral acetylsalicylic acid, Bayer; minipig: Clopidogrel, Sanofi) to prevent thrombosis. Twenty hours before surgery the animals were weighed and Enrofloxacin (5% Baytril®, Bayer) and/or Amoxicillin (Duphamox® LA, Zoetis) were administered. After anesthesia was induced, heparin (Heparin Choay®, Sanofi) was injected into the femoral artery via an introducer sheath and Activated Clotted Time (ACT) was evaluated using a Hemochron Junior 2 (International Technidyne Corp., USA) instrument. Analgesic, anti-inflammatory drugs and antibiotic treatments were administered during surgery and the follow up period. Animals were also maintained under prophylactic anticoagulant/antiaggregant therapy for the 4 weeks of observation until termination.

Surgical Grafting Procedure and Follow-Up

A 2.5 cm (minipig) or 8.0 cm (sheep) segment of the carotid artery was excised and replaced by end-to-end anastomosis with a piece of sterilized SilkGraft (nominal 5 mm inner diameter) of corresponding length. Surgery was unilateral in the minipig and bilateral in the sheep. Angiography and doppler ultrasound controls were performed before and after the grafting procedure and just prior to sacrifice using Iomeron 400 (Bracco Imaging, France) as contrast medium.

After surgery, the animals were transferred to a recovery area and monitored for 1 h prior to be brought back to their housing. The supply of water and food was reinstalled. Animals were monitored for 4 weeks and then euthanized.

Histopathology

At autopsy, the grafts, their connected carotid stumps, and surrounding tissues were excised, endoluminal blood was removed from the carotids by gently flushing it out first with heparinized saline and then with 10% neutral buffered formalin (NBS). To complete fixation explanted samples were dipped into 10% NBS. The fixed tissues were dehydrated in ethanol solutions of increasing strength, cleared in xylene, and embedded in paraffin. Microtome sections (4–7 μm thick) were cut from each paraffin block for histopathological analysis. After removing the paraffin and rehydrating, the sections were stained with Safranin-Hematoxylin-Eosin (SHE). Histopathology analysis concerned graft endothelialization, intimal hyperplasia, thrombi, graft recellularization, potential occlusion and the presence and type of inflammatory cells.

Statistical Analysis

Data were expressed as mean values ± SE and their level of statistical significance assessed by means of one-way ANOVA followed by Holm-Sidak's *post hoc* test. A $P < 0.05$ was taken as significant.

RESULTS

Morphological, Chemical, Physical, and Mechanical Characterization

The SilkGraft device (**Figure 1A**) is a hybrid tubular structure consisting of two electrospun (ES) layers (inner and outer) and an intermediate textile (TEX) layer (**Figures 1B,C**). It is made of pure SF, present in the final device in form of native microfibers (TEX) with an average diameter of 12–14 μm (**Figure 1D**), and electrospun nanofibers (ES), whose diameter falls in the 400–600 nm range (**Figure 1E**) (Marelli et al., 2009).

To verify whether the processing steps, including the sterilization with EtO, altered the chemical structure and properties of the constituent biopolymer, the amino acid composition of the sterilized SilkGraft device, as well as that of two constituent materials, i.e., TEX microfibers, and ES nanofibers, was determined and compared to that of native SF microfibers. The results demonstrated that there were no differences in the amino acid composition, indicating that neither processing conditions nor sterilization with EtO (Zhao et al., 2011) altered the intrinsic properties of SF materials (**Table S1**).

Structural properties of SilkGraft were characterized by ATR-FTIR. The spectra of TEX microfibers and ES nanofibers (**Figure 1F**) display the typical profile of β-sheet crystalline materials (Marelli et al., 2010; Chiarini et al., 2016), as indicated by the position, shape, and intensity of the Amide bands (Amide I at 1,620 cm^{-1}, with shoulder at 1,691 cm^{-1}; Amide II at 1,512 cm^{-1}; Amide III at 1,227 cm^{-1}, and 1,262 cm^{-1}). The crystallinity index of ES nanofibers, expressed as intensity ratio between the two Amide III components at 1,227 and 1,262 cm^{-1} ($CI = I_{1227}/I_{1262}$), was 0.58 ± 0.03, close to that determined on native SF microfibers (CI ≅ 0.60) (Chiarini et al., 2016), thus confirming the completion of the conformational transition from a prevalently random coil structure of as-spun nanofibers to a fully crystallized SF material.

Thermal properties of SilkGraft were investigated by DSC analysis. Thermograms of TEX microfibers, ES nanofibers, and final tubular device are shown in **Figure 1G**. TEX

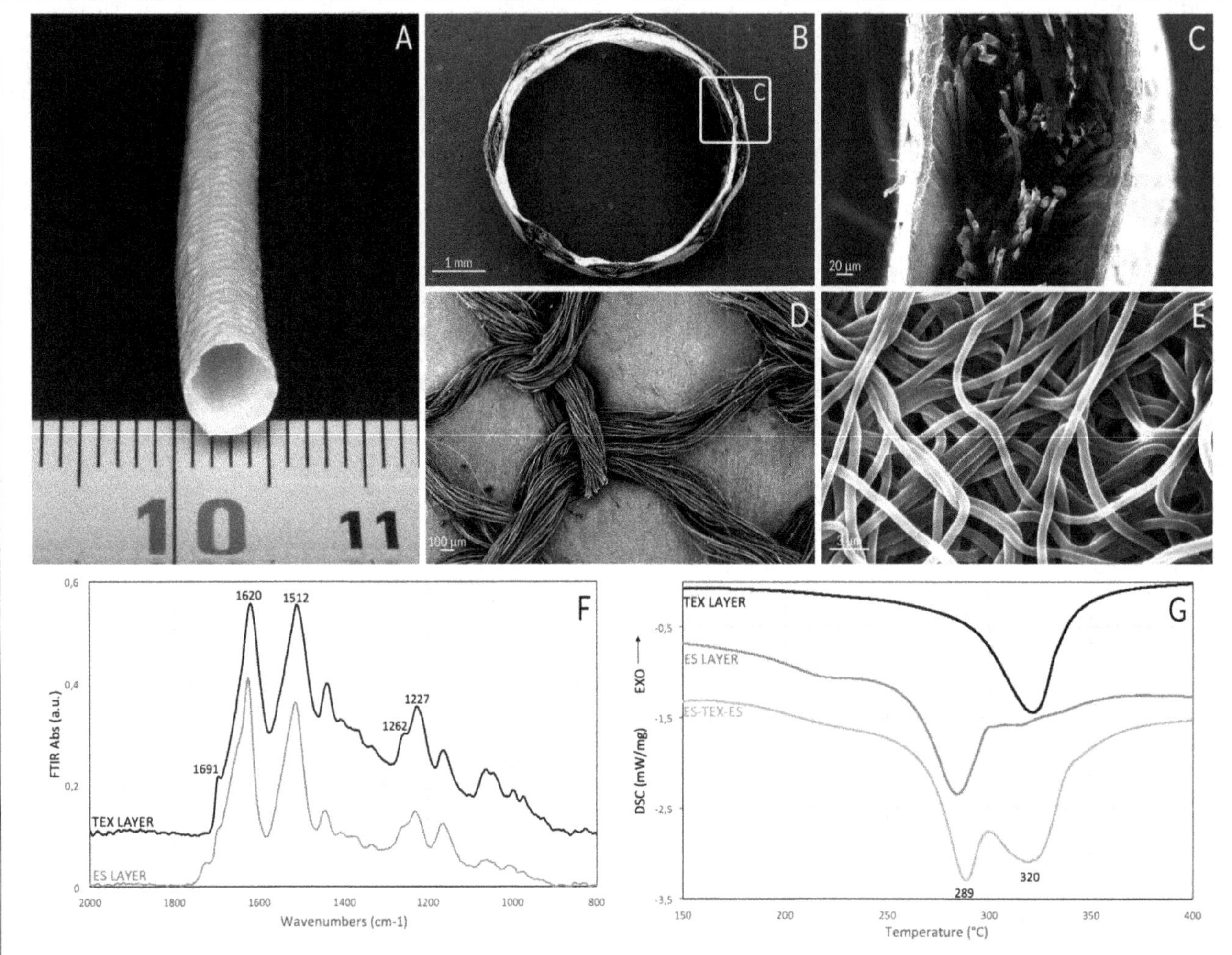

FIGURE 1 | Morphological and physico-chemical structure of SilkGraft. **(A)** Picture of a SilkGraft device with 5 mm nominal inner diameter (ruler in mm). **(B)** SEM cross-section of the graft showing the two inner and outer ES layers that enclose the intermediate TEX layer (scale bar, 1 mm). **(C)** Detail of **(B)** showing a magnification of the wall structure (scale bar 20 μm). **(D)** TEX layer coupled to an ES layer, visible in the background. The texture of the braided mesh is characterized by the presence of voids (scale bar 100 μm). **(E)** SEM detail of SF nanofibers of the ES layer (scale bar, 3 μm). **(F)** ATR-FTIR spectra of TEX and ES layers in the 2,000–800 cm^{-1} range. **(G)** DSC thermograms of TEX layer, ES layer, and SilkGraft finished device (marked ES-TEX-ES) in the 150–400°C temperature range.

TABLE 1 | Geometrical and mechanical properties of SilkGraft (nominal $\varnothing_{inner}$ = 5 mm).

Wall thickness (mm)	Unit weight (mg cm^{-1})	Weight (%)		Circumferential tensile tests		Burst pressure (mmHg)
		ES layers	TEX layer	Breaking Load (*N*)	Strain at break (mm/mm)	
0.59 ± 0.03	11.9 ± 0.5	61 ± 2	39 ± 2	29.5 ± 1.0	1.60 ± 0.05	2,308 ± 88

microfibers displayed a high thermal stability, with a main endothermic transition peaking at about 320°C, attributed to melting/degradation of highly crystalline and oriented SF microfibers (Chiarini et al., 2016). ES nanofibers, as many other regenerated SF materials, showed a marked low-temperature shift of the same transition, with a peak at about 289°C (Marelli et al., 2010). The DSC profile of the SilkGraft device was the sum of the individual components, with two discrete peaks corresponding to the thermal transitions of ES and TEX layers. The enthalpy associated with the thermal degradation of TEX ($\Delta H = -402 \pm 41$ J/g) and ES ($\Delta H = -307 \pm 32$ J/g) was used to estimate the weight contribution of each component in the final device. ES nanofibers account for about 60% by weight, while the remaining 40% is represented by the TEX layer (**Table 1**).

Geometrical parameters and mechanical properties of SilkGraft with a nominal inner diameter of 5 mm are listed in **Table 1**. The weight per unit length of the device is very low, about 5 times lower than that of a commercial ePTFE vascular

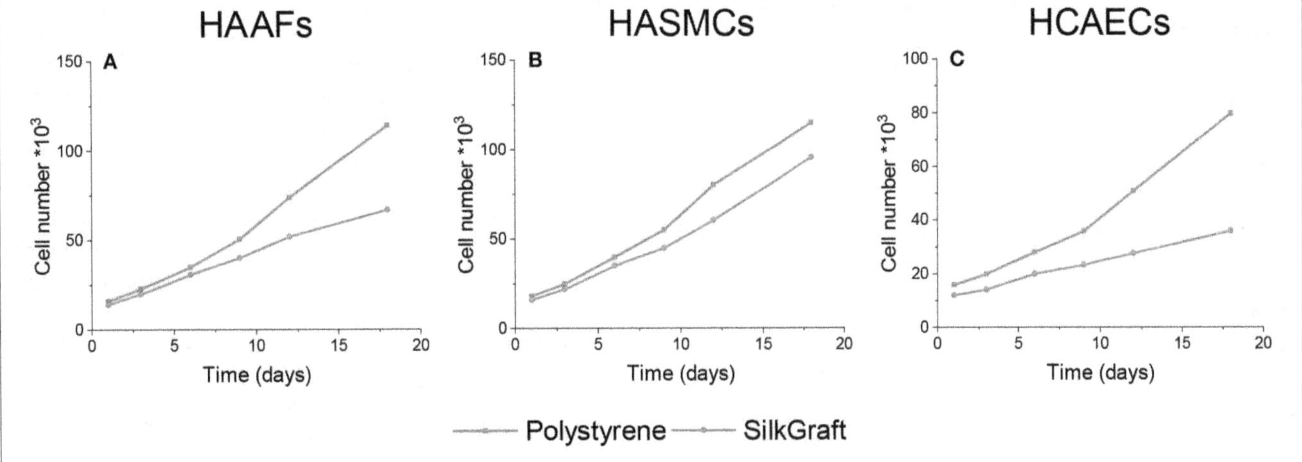

FIGURE 2 | Time dependence of the absolute cell numbers of HAAF **(A)**, HASMC **(B)**, and HCAEC **(C)** cells cultured on SilkGraft and on polystyrene. Absolute cell numbers were lower on SilkGraft than on polystyrene because the available surface area was reduced due to the use of the steel ring which kept the silk substrate under water. Total cell growth differences between cells cultured on SilkGraft or on polystyrene are expressed by the areas under the corresponding curves, the statistical levels of significance of which are: for HAAFs, $P < 0.001$; for HASMCs, $P < 0.01$; and for HCAECs, $P < 0.001$.

graft with similar inner diameter and wall thickness. While the ePTFE graft has a full thickness wall, the middle TEX layer of SilkGraft shows the typical structure of a braided mesh, with many voids that contribute to make the structure lighter (**Figure 1D**). The values of breaking load, which are about 30 times higher than those of similar grafts made only of electrospun SF nanofibers (Marelli et al., 2010), confirm that the TEX layer is the load bearing component of the graft. The contribution of the ES layers, which are solidly attached to the TEX layer through numerous welding points, is negligible. The results of burst pressure further confirm the significant contribution of the TEX layer to the mechanical performance of the multi-layered graft. The value of 2,308 mmHg is significantly larger than that of electrospun SF tubes with the same diameter (Marelli et al., 2010) and of the same order of magnitude of the values reported for internal mammary artery (3,196 ± 1,264 mmHg) and saphenous vein (1,599 ± 877 mmHg) (Konig et al., 2009).

In vitro Biocompatibility Studies

The biocompatibility of SilkGraft was tested using the three most representative cell types of human peripheral arteries, namely endothelial cells (HCAECs), smooth muscle cells (HASMCs), and adventitial fibroblasts (HAAFs). To assure the full significance and relevance of the results, we chose and applied a stringent set of selective criteria. To be eligible, the human cells had to originate from disease-free human subjects, to be of recent isolation (i.e., within the second passage *in vitro*), to be free from contaminating cells of other types, to be diploid and unprocessed, to be free from viral infections (particularly HIV-1, HHVB, HHVC), and to express cell type-specific markers.

Cell Adhesion, Survival and Proliferation Studies

$DilC_{18}(3)$ or $DiOC_{18}(3)$ intravitally stained cells were carefully seeded on the internal (HCAECs) or external (HASMCs or HAAFs) surfaces of SilkGraft and, in parallel, onto polystyrene. Next, the fluorescent cells were observed daily under an inverted microscope for up to 3 weeks of staying *in vitro*. Examples of the three types of cells grown on SilkGraft and on polystyrene substrates are shown in **Figure S1**. An adhesion fraction of 61 ± 5% for each cell type was detected 3 h after seeding, which was 2.1-fold ($P < 0.001$) the fraction of the same cells adhering to polystyrene surfaces at the same time point. Morphological indicators of apoptosis (e.g., cells with a shrunk or blebbing cytoplasm and substrate-adhering or free-floating spherical apoptotic bodies) were very rarely observed. Alike data were reported previously in the case of human dermal fibroblasts isolated from adult subjects and grown on SF-covered poly(carbonate)-urethane *vs.* polystyrene (Chiarini et al., 2003). Our present findings show that with respect to a polystyrene surface, SilkGraft neatly favors the adhesion of isolated human cells. As is well-known, adhesion to a substrate favors the survival and growth of untransformed (normal) cells.

The absolute numbers of each cell type grown on either substrate are shown and compared in **Figure 2**. Throughout 20 days HAAFs seeded onto SilkGraft increased their number by 4-fold, HCAECs by 3-fold, and HASMCs by 6.5-fold ($P < 0.001$ vs. 0 time in all instances). On polystyrene, the increases in numbers of the same cell types were greater, i.e., 7.5-fold for HAAFs, 5-fold for HCAECs, and nearly 7-fold for HASMCs ($P < 0.001$ vs. 0 time in all instances). However, if data are normalized to the apparent surface area available for growth (lower on SilkGraft due to the steel ring applied onto its surface), after 20 days HAAFs and HASMCs reached significantly ($P < 0.001$) greater cell densities on SilkGraft than on polystyrene, whereas HCAECs densities were similar between the two substrates ($P > 0.05$) (**Table 2**).

Evaluation of Cell Metabolism

The results concerning the studies on glucose and glutamine consumption, and the extracellular release of lactate were normalized per 1,000 cells and are reported in **Figure 3** and **Table 3**. Cumulative HAAFs consumption of glucose on SilkGraft was greater than on polystyrene, the difference being much more remarkable during the first 12 days of culture *in vitro* (**Figure 3A**). Conversely, the cumulative HAAFs consumption of glutamine on polystyrene was greater than on SilkGraft (**Figure 3D**), the difference becoming remarkable only after the first 12 days. On the other hand, the release of lactate into the medium was the same whichever the substrate considered (**Figure 3G**).

TABLE 2 | Living cells density/mm^2 of apparent surface area after 21 days of *in vitro* culture.

Cell type	Polystyrene (PS) plate	SilkGraft (SF)	Ratio SF/PS
HAAFs	363 ± 31	692 ± 63*	1.9 ± 0.1*
HASMCs	366 ± 28	1222 ± 106*	3.3 ± 0.2*
HCAECs	254 ± 23	232 ± 19^{ns}	0.91 ± 0.1^{ns}

*Data are normalized to the apparent surface area available for growth. Levels of statistical significance of the differences between the values on SilkGraft and on polystyrene: *P < 0.001; ns, P > 0.05.*

HASMCs cumulative consumption of glucose (**Figure 3B**) and glutamine (**Figure 3E**) and the release of lactic acid into the medium (**Figure 3H**) were not significantly affected by their attachment to either substrate.

Glutamine oxidation is the main source of energy for HCAECs. On SilkGraft the cumulative consumption of glutamine was typically much higher than on polystyrene (**Figure 3F**). The cumulative consumption of glucose was

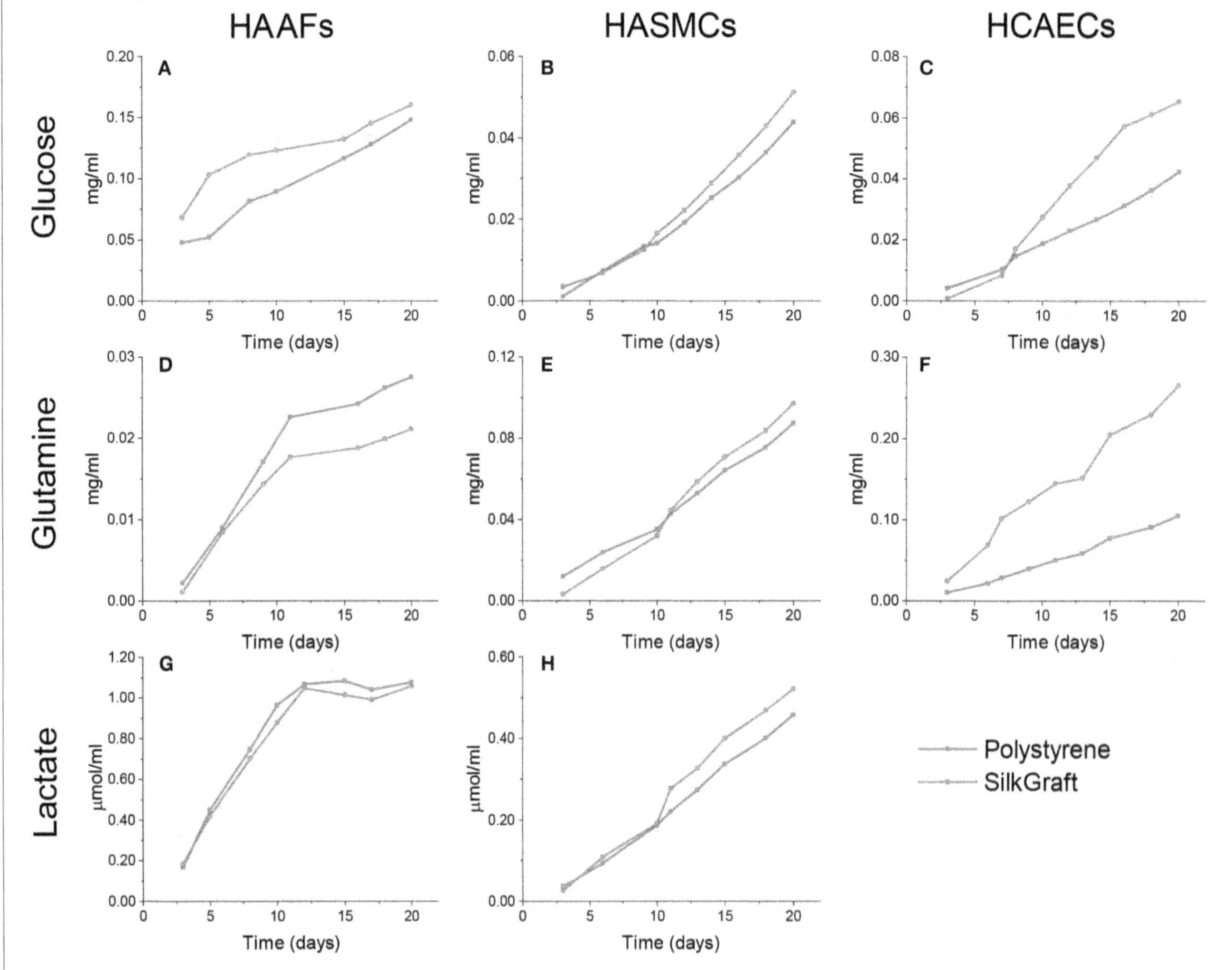

FIGURE 3 | Cumulative consumption of glucose and glutamine and release of lactate. Results were normalized per 10^3 cells. **(A–C)** The cumulative glucose consumption was higher for HAAFs ($P < 0.05$) and HCAECs ($P < 0.001$) seeded on SilkGraft, whereas it showed only marginal differences between the two substrates for HASMCs ($P > 0.05$). **(D–F)** Glutamine consumption was lower for HAAFs ($P < 0.05$) seeded on SilkGraft, similar for HASMCs ($P > 0.05$) cultured on the two substrates, and significantly larger for HCAECs ($P < 0.001$) grown on the silk substrate. **(G,H)** The cumulative amount of lactate released by HAAFs and HASMCs was the same whichever the substrate ($P > 0.05$). Lactate release could not be assessed for HCAECs because the released lactate was re-uptaken and used for metabolic purposes. The statistical analysis of these data is shown in **Table 3**.

TABLE 3 | Comparison of metabolic parameters* of the different cell types cultured on SilkGraft and polystyrene.

	Polystyrene	SilkGraft	Δ%	P
HAAFs				
Glucose uptake	1.642 ± 0.098	2.122 ± 0.150	+29.2	0.021
Glutamine uptake	0.316 ± 0.013	0.251 ± 0.012	−20.6	0.003
Lactate release	14.664 ± 0.783	13.947 ± 0.545	−4.9	0.465
Procollagen C-Telopeptide	1.500 ± 0.078	0.993 ± 0.072	−33.8	<0.001
HCAECs				
Glucose uptake	0.368 ± 0.026	0.572 ± 0.039	+55.4	<0.001
Glutamine uptake	0.919 ± 0.083	2.504 ± 0.198	+172.4	<0.001
HASMCs				
Glucose uptake	0.336 ± 0.030	0.385 ± 0.032	+14.6	0.276
Glutamine uptake	0.794 ± 0.042	0.807 ± 0.041	+1.6	0.827
Lactate release	4.016 ± 0.311	4.652 ± 0.328	+15.8	0.181

*The parameters are the areas under the respective cumulative curves shown in **Figures 3, 4**.

also greater than on polystyrene (**Figure 3C**). Undetectable levels of lactate were released into the medium by HCAECs, whichever the substrate considered, due to the known fact that endothelial cells can uptake and use lactate as an additional source of energy (Krützfeldt et al., 1990; Vegran et al., 2011).

Synthesis of Type I Collagen by HAAFs

Type I procollagen synthesis is a specific biomarker of HAAFs (Dal Prà et al., 2006). The release of the C-telopeptide of the procollagen is a stoichiometric index of the amount of collagen type I secreted, which subsequently undergoes fiber assembly. Thus, when HAAFs were grown on SilkGraft their cumulative release of C-telopeptide significantly decreased vs. that on polystyrene (**Figure 4**). A quantitative comparison of type I collagen synthesis on the two substrates is listed in **Table 3**.

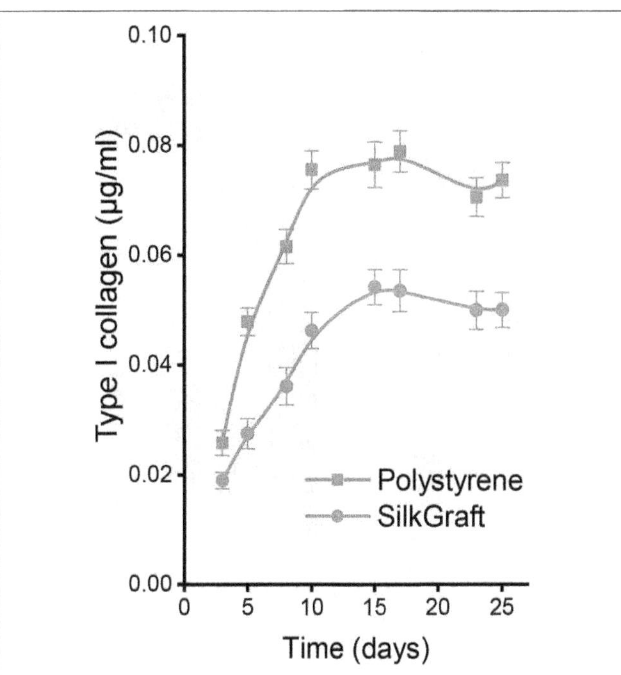

FIGURE 4 | The cumulative assembly of collagen type I (indirectly measured as the stoichiometrically released C-telopeptide of procollagen) was significantly ($P < 0.001$) lower for HAAFs cultured on SilkGraft than on polystyrene surfaces. Results were normalized per 10^3 cells. The statistical analysis of these data is shown in **Table 3**.

Cytokine and Chemokine Expression

After 20 days of staying *in vitro*, each cell type exhibited its own specific pattern of secreted cytokines and chemokines (**Figure 5**). No substantial qualitative differences emerged when comparing the expression patterns of each cell type in relation to the culture substrate. However, substrate-related significant differences in the quantitative secretion of some cytokines and chemokines could be detected.

HAAFs seeded on SilkGraft exhibited a higher secretion of IL-6 (+22%), MCP-1 (+13%), and TIMP-2 (+19%), whereas IP-10 (−26%), MCP-2 (−50%), Eotaxin-1 (−41%), and RANTES (−72%) were released at lesser extent than on polystyrene.

HCAECs grown on SilkGraft released higher amounts of IP-10 (+43%), MCP-1 (+27%), and TNF-β (+84%) as compared to polystyrene. RANTES and IL-6 were released to a lesser extent, while TIMP-2 and MIP-1β did not change significantly between the two substrates.

Finally, HASMCs discretely secreted a wider set of cytokines/chemokines. Interestingly, GM-CSF (+766%), MCP-2 (+557%), IL-1α (+561%), IL-1β (+390%), and Eotaxin-1 (+315%) were secreted at much higher levels on SilkGraft than on polystyrene, the secretion of ICAM-1 and RANTES only raised by +30%, whereas the release of IL-6, MIP-1β, TIMP-2, MCP-1, and IP-10 fell by −10/30% vs. the corresponding levels on polystyrene.

Hemocompatibility

Regarding the complement activation, a statistically significant increase ($p < 0.05$) in Sc5b-9 was noted (**Table S2**). However, the Sc5b-9 values of SilkGraft were still inside the range of the control data of a normal standard population (334–1,672 ng/ml). Based on this, the increase was regarded as not biologically relevant. The C3a concentration was comparable to that of the negative control (**Table S2**). In conclusion, it can be stated that SilkGraft did not induce a biologically relevant activation of the complement system. Both indirect and direct contact hemolysis assays showed that SilkGraft exerted no hemolytic activity (hemolytic indexes < 2%) (**Table S3**). SilkGraft did not cause any alteration of red and white blood cells counts because the difference with the respective controls was <4 and <7%, respectively (**Table S4**).

Pilot Animal Studies

The purposes of the pilot studies were first to assess which animal model would be better to use for future medium-to-long term trials, and then to establish the suitability of the surgical

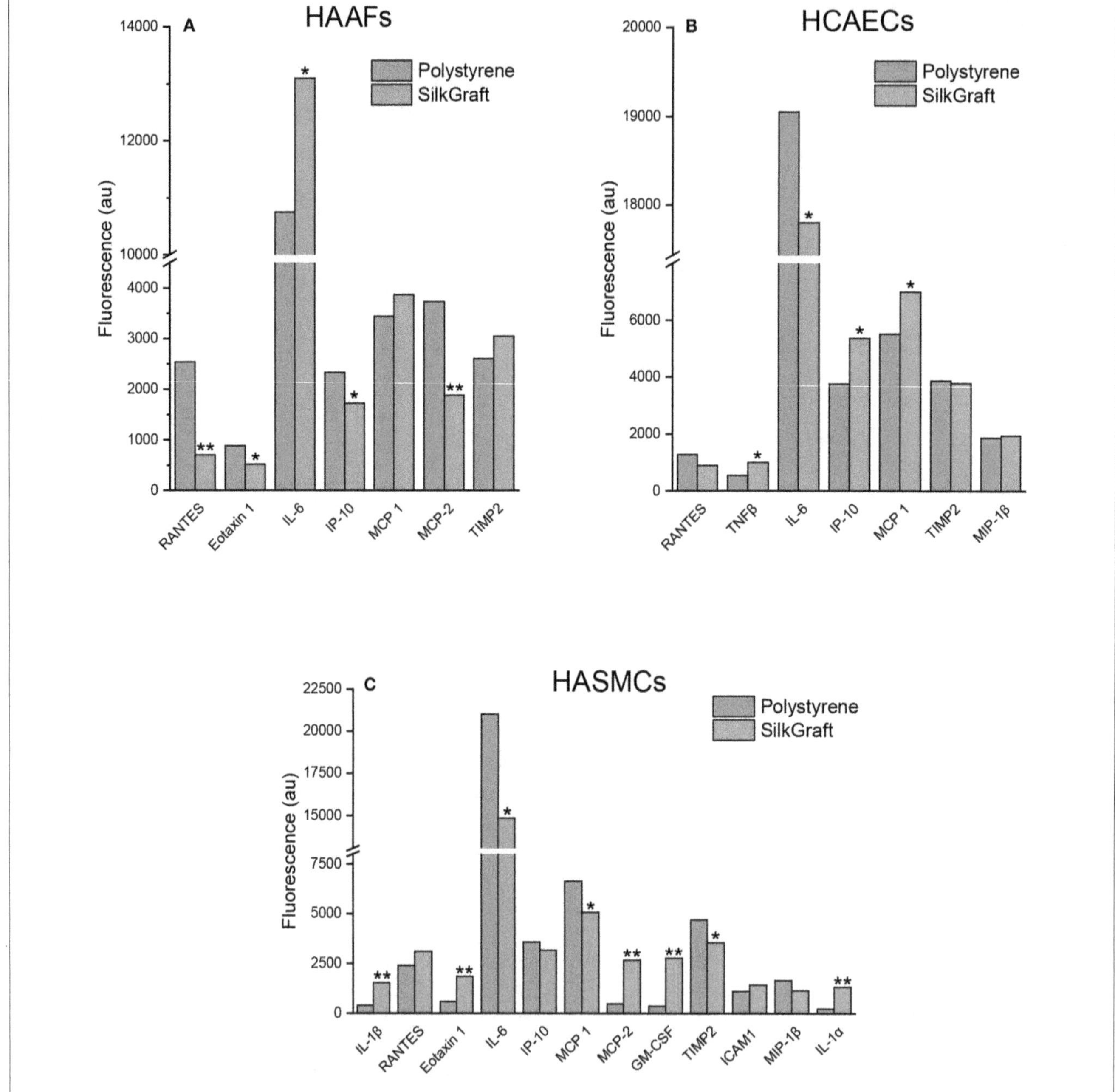

FIGURE 5 | Relevant cytokines and chemokines secreted by each cell type cultured between 18 and 20 days on SilkGraft and polystyrene: HAFFs **(A)**, HCAECs **(B)**, and HASMCs **(C)**. Results of immunofluorescence intensities were normalized to 10^3 cells. IL-6: Interleukin-6; MCP-1: Monocyte chemoattractant protein-1; TIMP-2: Tissue inhibitor of metal proteinases-2; IP-10: Interferon gamma-induced protein-10; MCP-2: Monocyte chemoattractant protein-2; Eotaxin-1; RANTES: Regulated on activation normal T cell expressed and secreted; MIP-1β: Macrophage inflammatory protein-1β; TNF-β: Tumor necrosis factor-β; GM-CSF: Granulocyte-macrophage colony stimulating factor; IL-1α: Interleukin-1α; IL-1β: Interleukin-1β; ICAM-1: Intercellular adhesion molecule-1. The bars are the mean values of three independent experiments corrected for cell numbers. $^*P < 0.01$; $^{**}P < 0.001$. SEMs, not shown, ranged between 5 and 10% of corresponding mean values.

model, to evaluate handling characteristics, aptness to stitching, patency, formation of thrombi, first signs of degradation, local tissue effects, and the general performance of SilkGraft. Resected portions of the carotid arteries of one minipig (unilateral) and one sheep (bilateral) were replaced with SilkGraft, the animals were sacrificed 4 weeks later, and histopathology of explants was examined.

Surgery was done without major difficulty on both minipig and sheep. SilkGraft preparation, handling, stitching suitability, and anastomosis capacity were overall considered as good. Moderate bleeding at the suture holes was observed. The animals survived for 4 weeks with no unwanted side effects prior to be euthanized. No graft-related clinical or macroscopic abnormalities were noted at the site of implantation or

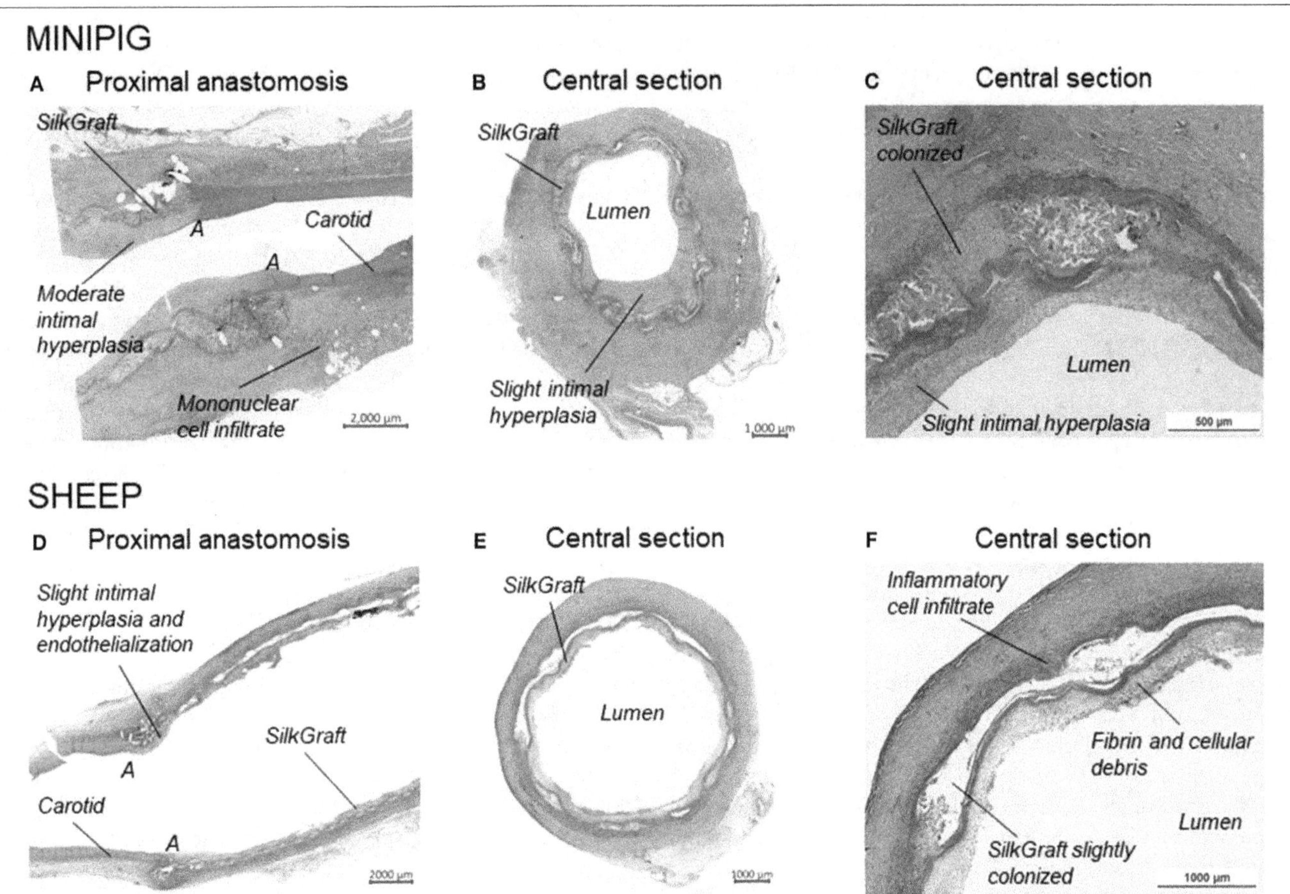

FIGURE 6 | Histopathogical analysis of a SilkGraft stitched end-to-end on the carotid artery of minipig and sheep 4 weeks after grafting. Staining: Safranin-Hematoxylin-Eosin. Minipig: **(A)** Longitudinal cut in correspondence of the proximal anastomosis showing a pervious lumen (A, anastomotic line). **(B)** Representative cross-sectional cut of the central part of the graft. The lumen is pervious, though moderately reduced by an intimal hyperplasia. **(C)** Detail of the graft wall: perivascular cell infiltrates are visible; the inner and outer ES layers appear compact, whereas the TEX layer is penetrated by growing vessels and collagen-producing fibroblasts; endothelialization is visible at the inner graft surface. Sheep: **(D)** Typical longitudinal sections of the proximal end-to-end anastomotic sites (A, anastomotic line); the lumen is pervious and devoid of any stenosis. Endothelization is restricted to a 3 mm-wide area beyond the anastomosis. **(E)** Representative cross-section of the central part of the graft; the lumen is pervious while endothelization, neointimal hyperplasia, and stenosis are absent. **(F)** Detail of the graft wall: an inflammatory infiltrate envelops the graft; a newly-formed vascularized connective tissue only partly colonizes the middle TEX layer.

in distant organs during the test period. Ultrasound and angiographic examination at day 13 and 24 after surgery showed patent carotids, no aneurysm, dilation, dissection, blood collection or signs of infection. No stenosis was identified for the sheep, whereas a slight stenosis near the proximal anastomosis was identified for the minipig. Normal blood flow was also noted at termination. The external surface of the grafts explanted from the sheep was covered by a moderate amount of thin and soft tissue, while that recovered from the minipig was surrounded by a thicker layer of soft tissue.

The histopathological analysis of the minipig explant showed that inside the graft and its attached carotid stumps the lumen was still pervious and totally devoid of thrombi (**Figure 6A**). Histopathology also confirmed the presence of a slight yet diffuse stenosis of the graft's lumen (**Figure 6B**). Endothelial-like cells lined the whole surface of the newly-formed graft's intima (**Figure 6C**). Collagen fibers, fibroblasts, macrophages, and multinucleated giant cells together with a lesser number of lymphocytes, plasma cells, and neutrophils filled the voids of the middle TEX layer. Colonizing cells circumferentially infiltrated the graft's outer nanofibrous ES layer. Moreover, the abundant periarterial tissue was infiltrated by lymphocytes and plasma cells. Altogether, these features suggested an ongoing foreign body response (FBR), as reported for other SF-based scaffolds (Dal Prà et al., 2005; Chiarini et al., 2016).

Grafted sheep carotids were pervious to blood flow and did not show any luminal stenosis (**Figures 6D,E**). Endothelization was restricted to a 3 mm-wide area beyond the end-to-end anastomotic sites. Only a thin fibrin layer and marginated leukocytes adhered to the remaining inner nanofibrous surfaces of the grafts. Also, differently from the minipig, in the long portion of the graft intervening between the anastomotic sites no newly-formed neointimal connective tissue was present. The middle TEX layer was only partially colonized by newly-formed vascularized connective tissue (**Figure 6F**). A thick infiltrate made up by lymphocytes, mononuclear macrophages, polynucleated giant cells, and neutrophils enveloped the graft's external nanofibrous layer, being less crowded around the proximal and distal arterial stumps. This picture indicated an ongoing FBR, but with no concurring subendothelial hyperplasia and no damage to neighboring tissues.

DISCUSSION

Electrospun scaffolds may suffer from some limitations when biomimicry must be coupled with a high level of mechanical performance, such as in the case of vascular grafts. An affordable solution is therefore to couple electrospinning and textile technologies (like weaving, knitting, braiding, etc.), with the aim to take advantage of both of them for realizing biomimetic scaffolds able to withstand mechanical stresses in tensile, compression, and bending modes. Zhang et al. (2017) reported the fabrication of a three-layered vascular graft where the intima and media layers were obtained by sequentially electrospinning SF and poly(L-lactide-co-ε-caprolactone), while the outer adventitia-like layer was built up by braiding SF yarns. In another study (Mi et al., 2015), a polyurethane (PU)/SF three-layered small diameter tubular scaffold was fabricated by combining electrospinning (inner PU layer) and braiding (middle SF layer) technologies. In addition, a spongy PU layer was built as third outer layer by molding and freeze drying. Both scaffolds underwent extensive mechanical and *in vitro* cytocompatibility characterization, but no *in vivo* functional tests were reported.

Coupling electrospun and textile SF matrices for the production of multi-layered tubular scaffolds is recognized as a valid approach to overcome bottlenecks due to lack of mechanical attributes of the electrospun SF scaffolds. However, the achievement of a strong adhesion between electrospun and textile layers might be a challenge, because textile surfaces onto which electrospun fibers are deposited are not homogenously flat, but present microscopic rough or sunken sites that prevent a continuous contact between the two surfaces. This results in poor adhesion strength, as demonstrated by the fact that the electrospun layer can be easily peeled off by applying a mild strength. Risks associated with poor adhesion between electrospun and textile layers may have very serious consequences on the performance of an implantable device, such as creation of morphological and mechanical discontinuities between layers, yielding and/or collapse of weaker layers, loss of geometric characteristics, thus leading to ultimate failure, especially under the stressing working conditions experienced *in vivo*.

To overcome these problems, we have developed an advanced manufacturing technology aimed at achieving an effective hybridization between electrospun and textile matrices (Alessandrino, 2016). Coating of the TEX surface with the ionic liquid before electrospinning ensures perfect welding between the electrospun and textile matrices. In fact, as soon as the first electrospun fibers reach the TEX surface, the still plastic fibers melt in contact with the ionic liquid. A dense network of strong welding points between the growing electrospun layer and the textile substrate is created. Adhesion tests showed that a force of 0.5–1 N is needed to peel off one layer from the other (Alessandrino, 2016). Therefore, the multi-layered wall of the tubular scaffold behaves as if it were made of a single piece, while harmonizing the high resistance to mechanical stresses of native SF microfibers with the enhanced biomimicking attitude of regenerated SF nanofibers. The load bearing component is the TEX layer, which confers a high mechanical resistance on the device. When stressed under wet conditions the inner and outer ES layers become very elastic. Under increasing load, they undergo extensive stretching deformation without fracturing or breaking. Interestingly, ES and TEX layers remain strongly attached to each other until the ultimate breaking point is reached, thus confirming the effectiveness of the patented coupling technology, which allows the formation of a dense network of welding points between the ES layers and the meshes of the TEX layer.

The production technology allows the fabrication of SilkGraft in a wide range of inner diameters, overlapping those of currently marketed small caliber synthetic vascular grafts. Compared to available ePTFE and PET vascular devices, SilkGraft is characterized by a design which results in a light but mechanically resistant structure. The light weight is likely to bring biological advantages because the burden of foreign material at the site of implantation is significantly reduced, thus avoiding excessive stresses to surrounding tissues during remodeling. This feature doesn't seem to negatively impact on the mechanical performance, as demonstrated by the values of circumferential breaking load and burst strength. In fact, if the breaking load reported in **Table 1** is normalized to the cross-section surface, a stress value of about 3 MPa is obtained, which underestimates the real value due to the open texture of the wall of the device (see: **Figure 1D**). The stress value is significantly larger than that reported for the human descending mid-thoracic aorta with roughly similar inner diameter (1.72 ± 0.89 MPa) (Mohan and Melvin, 1982). Interestingly, the value of strain falls in the same range of that reported for human aorta (1.53 ± 0.28) (Mohan and Melvin, 1982).

The manufacturing protocol of SilkGraft includes various washing treatments with hydro-alcoholic solutions, which are aimed not only at achieving the complete removal of processing aids, but also at consolidating as-spun SF nanofibers that are still prevalently amorphous and more sensitive to physical, (bio)chemical, and mechanical stresses. The IR crystallinity index confirmed that nanofibers in the final device are fully crystallized. Actually, this structural feature is very important for the functionality of the device because, according to unanimous consensus, the degree of crystallinity of regenerated SF scaffolds strongly impacts on the rate of *in vivo* biodegradation (Thurber et al., 2015). In our case, the nanofibers are expected to undergo remodeling in the medium term, while in the meantime supporting neo-vascular tissue formation. To this purpose, fully crystalline ES nanofibers are more favorable to ensure a slow degradation rate in the biological environment.

The results of the *in vitro* studies on SilkGraft showed a high biocompatibility of the device, which was evaluated by seeding the three main types of cells inhabiting the arterial wall (HCAECs, HASMCs, and HAAFs). Cell adhesion to SilkGraft was in all instance superior to polystyrene, in keeping with previous observations (Chiarini et al., 2003; Dal Prà et al., 2006). The preferential energy source for both HASMCs and HCAECs was glutamine, while it was glucose for HAAFs (Wu et al., 2000; Eelen et al., 2013). HAAFs and HASMCs also secreted large amounts of lactic acid into the medium, whereas HCAECs released none. This occurred because HCAECs have the metabolic capability to convert lactate into pyruvate and to use it for oxidative metabolism, thus saving glucose which they cede to the surrounding tissues (Dal Prà et al., 2005; Chiarini et al., 2016). It should be noted that the cumulative curves of consumed glucose and glutamine and of released lactate proper of HAAFs and HASMCs exhibited similar patterns, matching the metabolic activities and the expansion of the respective cell populations.

Notably, addition of serum suppresses the contact inhibition of growth in HASMCs (Krützfeldt et al., 1990; Viñals and Pouysségur, 1999). This may explain why they reached the highest density when seeded on SilkGraft, which did not happen for HCAECs. Moreover, the observed behavioral differences could be due to unlike cell sizes (endothelial cells > fibroblasts > smooth muscle cells), morphological features, and regulatory mechanisms intrinsic to each cell type. In addition, the different characteristics of SilkGraft and polystyrene surfaces, including the adhesiveness for cells and the somewhat broader surface area offered by the nanofibers, also had an impact. Having larger sizes, the HCAECs seeded on the inner nanofibrous surface reached the confluence and the contact inhibition of growth at an earlier time and more permanently than the other two cell types. This could be beneficial because *in vivo* HCAECs, once they had reached confluence on the surface of the graft, would stop proliferating and thus keep the lumen pervious to the flowing blood. Moreover, according to our previous observations concerning HAAFs grown on SF microfibers (Chiarini et al., 2003), the present results strengthen the view that HAAFs growing on an SF substrate significantly curtail their *de novo* production of type I collagen, which translates into a remarkable antifibrogenic upshot and could be significantly relevant in the clinical settings. In other words, it can be concluded that the SF substrate in a nanofibrous format exerts a neat antifibrotic effect on HAAFs.

Some cytokines and/or chemokines are cell type-specific biomarkers. The pattern of cytokines and chemokines secreted into the growth medium under the conditions examined would reveal the proliferative and/or pro-inflammatory proclivities of the cells. In particular, released chemokines may attract circulating leukocytes. Moreover, cytokines and chemokines play important roles in several cellular processes like growth, differentiation, apoptosis, angiogenesis, inflammation, and innate immunity. Among the identified cytokines and chemokines, IL-6 stands out, being the most intensely secreted one by each of the three cell types both on SilkGraft and on polystyrene. IL-6 is considered a biomarker of cell proliferation, differentiation and survival (Morimoto et al., 1991; Krishnaswamy et al., 1998; Kyurkchiev et al., 2014). Similarly, the basal secretion of MCP-1 and/or MCP-2 is indicative of a cell proliferation capacity. MCP-1 promotes the arteriogenesis associated with the induction of Vascular Endothelial Growth Factor (VEGF)-A expression (Keeley et al., 2008). Among the other important chemokines secreted by the three cell types, we mention here IP-10, known for its antifibrotic and angiostatic properties, and RANTES protein, known for its ability to regulate leucocyte diapedesis, angiogenesis and some scarring processes (Bujak et al., 2009; Lin et al., 2018). In human aorta-derived SMCs, RANTES increased the expression of cell cycle regulatory proteins and of markers of their synthetic phenotype (Lin et al., 2018). GM-CSF is constitutively expressed by HASMCs and an elevation in GM-CSF expression associates with the HASMCs synthetic phenotype (Plenz et al., 1997). As well, the cellular adhesion molecule ICAM-1 and the HASMCs basal secretion of cytokines IL-1α and IL-1β can influence and potentiate cellular proliferation by playing an autocrine role (Braun et al., 1999; Schultz et al., 2007; Bonin et al., 2009). The low secretion of TNF-β from HCAECs on polystyrene surged significantly when the cells were grown on SilkGraft. Notably, TNF-β signals control the proper development and maintenance of endothelial cells (Zindl et al., 2009).

All the three cell types, once cultured on either SilkGraft or polystyrene, exhibited similarly low basal levels of TIMP-2, a metalloprotease blocker which regulates extracellular matrix (ECM) remodeling processes and interactions between cells and ECM, as well as cell proliferation by an autocrine mechanism (Hayakawa et al., 1994). On the other hand, it is important to note that no significant amounts of truly pro-inflammatory cytokines, such as Tumor Necrosis Factor-α (TNF-α), or of profibrotic cytokines, such as Transforming growth factor-β (TGF-β) were secreted by any of the three cell types grown on either substrate. Therefore, the patterns of cytokines and chemokines secreted by the three cell types cultured on SilkGraft suggest a proliferative attitude while neatly excluding a pro-inflammatory and/or pro-fibrogenic proclivity.

The complement system is part of the innate immune system and may be involved in promoting and accelerating hemolysis, platelet and leukocyte activation and thrombosis on device material surfaces, while hemolysis is the liberation of hemoglobin following disruption of the erythrocytes. The hemocompatibility assays demonstrated that SilkGraft did not activate the Sc5b-9 and C3a components of the complement system, did not result in hemolytic effects, and did not alter the counts of red and white blood cells. Moreover, no thrombi formation was observed during the *in vivo* pilot trials. The latter parameter will be further controlled during the on-going long-term studies (up to 1 year).

Finally, the pilot animal study showed the feasibility of using SilkGraft as small caliber vessel graft *in vivo*. Due to the size of the graft, a large animal model with vessels similar in size to human's was needed to allow appropriate placement and evaluation in view of future clinical use. Both minipig and sheep are used as appropriate animal models to evaluate performance, and local tissue effects after vascular implantation (Byrom et al., 2010).

Carotid implantation was chosen to mimic clinical use and to avoid anatomical limitations (carotids are straighter and with less branches than femoral arteries). Advantages associated with using sheep as the animal model are: (i) blood vessels easily accessible and more superficial; (ii) slower endothelialization, more similar to human; (iii) ability to perform blood tests and eco-doppler with animals awake, which translates into the possibility to perform more exams with less stress for the animal; and last but not least (iv) the sheep model allows to evaluate a longer graft, up to 10 cm. Therefore, long-term studies (up to 1 year) aimed at assessing the patency and wall restructuration ability of the graft are already under course in sheep, to demonstrate the feasibility of testing SilkGraft in human clinical settings.

CONCLUSIONS

SilkGraft is a small caliber vascular graft entirely made of pure silk fibroin. The fabrication technology was progressively refined through recursive testing and optimization procedures which led to a standardized production protocol. Particular attention was devoted to the careful selection of starting materials and processing aids (e.g., size of the SF yarn, texture and mechanical performance of the TEX layer, chemical properties and efficacy of the welding medium, etc.), as well as to fine-tuning key processing parameters (e.g., electrospinning, strategy of coupling TEX and ES layers, consolidation of the hybrid structure, final purification before sterilization, etc.). The process development led to a tubular device where the inner and outer ES layers and the middle TEX layer are perfectly integrated at the structural and functional level and respond as a single body to mechanical stresses, without showing any mutual slipping or separation. In fact, the main target was to manufacture a multi-layered scaffold characterized by an easy handling during surgery and, when implanted, able to achieve top level biomimicking performance with the surrounding living tissues while avoiding the onset of any biomechanical mismatch with the native artery.

In vitro studies with three main types of cells inhabiting the arterial wall, i.e., HCAECs, HASMCs, and HAAFs, showed that SilkGraft exhibited a high degree of biocompatibility and a level of cell adhesion superior to polystyrene. The trends of specific metabolic markers, like consumption of glucose and glutamine and release of acid lactic into the medium, confirmed the intense metabolic activities and the expansion of the cell populations cultured on SilkGraft coupled with a curtailed production of collagen and with no secretion of pro-inflammatory or pro-fibrotic cytokines and chemokines. Furthermore, blood hemocompatibility was corroborated by the lack of complement activation, hemolysis, and alteration of cell counts assays.

The results of pilot animal studies indicated the sheep as the model of choice to carry out the preclinical *in vivo* tests before the clinical trials in humans and confirmed that the device is easy to handle and surgically stitch. Finally, it is important to highlight that in our setting, thanks to its promising biological responses, SilkGraft is intended as an "off-the-shelf" device, no longer requiring pre-seeding with cells, thus eliminating related time delays and costs and minimizing the steps for graft preparation before implantation.

AUTHOR CONTRIBUTIONS

This is a multi-disciplinary project that has been conducted by three groups coordinated by GF. Biomaterial development group: AA and GF led the conception and design of the project. MB, GB, and VV contributed to designing, planning, and executing all the experimental activities. Data interpretation responsibility was collectively shared by the entire group. *In vitro* preclinical study group: UA, AC, and ID were responsible for the design and planning of the *in vitro* tests. The experimental execution was performed by AC and ID, who also acquired and validated the results under the supervision of UA. *In vivo* preclinical/clinical study group: PS and PP designed the experimental approach for the *in vivo* pilot study. They shared the responsibility of selecting models, addressing surgical techniques, and evaluating the histological results. GF was responsible for drafting the text of the biomaterial development part of the work, as well as for collecting and critically revising the text contributions drafted by the other two participating groups and gathering the final approval of all authors for the publishable version. All authors ensure that questions related to the accuracy or integrity of any part of the work are appropriately investigated and resolved.

FUNDING

This study was entirely funded by Silk Biomaterials Srl, whose stock owners and employees were deeply involved in study design, data collection and analysis, decision to publish, preparation of the manuscript, and decision about submission.

ACKNOWLEDGMENTS

The authors express their deep gratitude to Dr. Hu Peng (from the First Affiliated Hospital of Zunyi Medical University, China and currently Ph.D. Student in Verona's Laboratory, Italy) for his skillful handling of human cell lines. The authors would like to address heartfelt thanks to Dr. Alberto Settembrini (Department of Vascular Surgery, Fondazione Ca' Granda Ospedale Maggiore, Milan) for his fruitful contribution to the development of the device and to the execution of the *in vivo* tests. This research did not receive any specific grant from funding agencies in the public, commercial, or not-for-profit sectors.

REFERENCES

Alessandrino, A. (2016). *Process for the Production of a Hybrid Structure Consisting of Coupled Silk Fibroin Microfibers and Nanofibers, Hybrid Structure Thus Obtained and Its Use as Implantable Medical Device*. WIPO/PCT Patent No. WO 2016/067189 A1. World Intellectual Property Organization.

Altman, G. H., Diaz, F., Jakuba, C., Calabro, T., Horan, R. L., Chen, J., et al. (2003). Silk-based biomaterials. *Biomaterials*. 24, 401–416. doi: 10.1016/S0142-9612(02)00353-8

Armato, U., Dal Prà, I., Chiarini, A., and Freddi, G. (2011). Will silk fibroin nanofiber scaffolds ever hold a useful place in translational regenerative medicine? *Int. J. Burn Trauma*. 1, 27–33.

Armato, U., Romano, F., Andreis, P. G., Paccagnella, L., and Marchesini, C. (1986). Growth stimulation and apoptosis induced in cultures of neonatal rat liver cells by repeated exposures to epidermal growth factor/urogastrone with or without associated pancreatic hormones. *Cell Tissue Res*. 245, 471–480. doi: 10.1007/BF00218546

Aytemiz, D., Sakiyama, W., Suzuki, Y., Nakaizumi, N., Tanaka, R., Ogawa, Y., et al. (2013). Small-diameter silk vascular grafts (3 mm diameter) with a double-raschel knitted silk tube coated with silk fibroin sponge. *Adv. Health. Mater.* 2, 361–368. doi: 10.1002/adhm.2012 00227

Babitha, S., Rachita, L., Karthikeyan, K., Shoba, E., Janani, I., Poornima, B., et al. (2017). Electrospun protein nanofibers in healthcare: a review. *Int. J. Pharm.* 523, 52–90. doi: 10.1016/j.ijpharm.2017.03.013

Bonin, P. D., Fic, G. J., and Singh, P. (2009). Interleukin-1 promotes proliferation of vascular smooth muscle cells in coordination with PDGF or a monocyte derived growth factor. *Exp. Cell Res.* 181, 475–482. doi: 10.1016/0014-4827(89)90104-3

Braun, M., Pietsch, P., Schrör, K., Baumann, G., and Felix, S. B. (1999). Cellular adhesion molecules on vascular smooth muscle cells. *Cardiovasc. Res.* 41, 395–401. doi: 10.1016/S0008-6363(98)00302-2

Bujak, M., Dobaczewski, M., Gonzalez-Quesada, C., Xia, Y., Leucker, T., Zymek, P., et al. (2009). Induction of the CXC chemokine interferon-gamma-inducible protein 10 regulates the reparative response following myocardial infarction. *Circ. Res.* 105, 973–983. doi: 10.1161/CIRCRESAHA.109.199471

Byrom, M. J., Bannon, P. G., and White, G. H., Ng, M.K.C. (2010). Animal models for the assessment of novel vascular conduits. *J. Vasc. Surg.* 52, 176–195. doi: 10.1016/j.jvs.2009.10.080

Cattaneo, I., Figliuzzi, M., Azzollini, N., Catto, V., Farè, S., Tanzi, M. C., et al. (2013). *In vivo* regeneration of elastic lamina on fibroin biodegradable vascular scaffold. *Int. J. Artif. Organs*. 36, 166–174. doi: 10.5301/ijao.5000185

Catto, V., Farè, S., Cattaneo, I., Figliuzzi, M., Alessandrino, A., Freddi, G., et al. (2015). Small diameter electrospun silk fibroin vascular grafts: mechanical properties, *in vitro* biodegradability, and *in vivo* biocompatibility. *Mater. Sci. Eng. C*. 54, 101–111. doi: 10.1016/j.msec.2015.05.003

Catto, V., Farè, S., Freddi, G., and Tanzi, M. C. (2014). Vascular tissue engineering: recent advances in small diameter blood vessel regeneration. *ISRN Vasc. Med.* 923030. doi: 10.1155/2014/923030

Chiarini, A., Freddi, G., Liu, D., Armato, U., and Dal Prà, I. (2016). Biocompatible silk noil-based three-dimensional carded-needled nonwoven scaffolds guide the engineering o novel skin connective tissue. *Tissue Eng. Part A*. 22, 1047–1060. doi: 10.1089/ten.tea.2016.0124

Chiarini, A., Petrini, P., Bozzini, S., Dal Prà, I., and Armato, U. (2003). Silk fibroin/poly(carbonate)-urethane as a substrate for cell growth: *in vitro* interactions with human cells. *Biomaterials* 24, 789–799. doi: 10.1016/S0142-9612(02)00417-9

Dal Prà, I., Chiarini, A., Boschi, A., Freddi, G., and Armato, U. (2006). Novel dermo-epidermal equivalents on silk fibroin-based formic acid-crosslinked three-dimensional nonwoven devices with prospective applications in human tissue engineering/regeneration/repair. *Int. J. Mol. Med.* 18, 241–247. doi: 10.3892/ijmm.18.2.241

Dal Prà, I., Freddi, G., Minic, J., Chiarini, A., and Armato, U. (2005). *De novo* engineering of reticular connective tissue *in vivo* by silk fibroin nonwoven materials. *Biomaterials*. 26, 1987–1999. doi: 10.1016/j.biomaterials.2004.06.036

Ding, X., Zou, T., Gong, X., Ren, C., Kang, H., Xu, P., et al. (2016). Trilayered sulfated silk fibroin vascular grafts enhanced with braided silk tube. *J. Bioact. Compat. Polym.* 31, 613–623. doi: 10.1177/08839115166 43107

Eelen, G., Cruys, B., Welti, J., De Bock, K., and Carmeliet, P. (2013). Control of vessel sprouting by genetic and metabolic determinants. *Trends Endocrinol. Metab.* 24, 589–596. doi: 10.1016/j.tem.2013.08.006

Enomoto, S., Sumi, M., Kajimoto, K., Nakazawa, Y., Takahashi, R., Takabayashi, C., et al. (2010). Long-term patency of small-diameter vascular graft made from fibroin, a silk-based biodegradable material. *J. Vasc. Surg.* 51, 155–164. doi: 10.1016/j.jvs.2009.09.005

Fukayama, T., Ozai, Y., Shimokawadoko, H., Aytemiz, D., Tanaka, R., Machida, N., et al. (2015). Effect of fibroin sponge coating on *in vivo* performance of knitted silk small diameter vascular grafts. *Organogenesis* 11, 137–151. doi: 10.1080/15476278.2015.1093268

Hayakawa, T., Yamashita, K., Ohuchi, E., and Shinagawa, A. (1994). Cell growth-promoting activity of tissue inhibitor of metalloproteinases-2 (TIMP-2). *J. Cell Sci.* 107, 2373–2379.

Hiob, M. A., She, S., Muiznieks, L. D., and Weiss, A. S. (2017). Biomaterials and modifications in the development of small-diameter vascular grafts. *ACS Biomater. Sci. Eng.* 3, 712–723. doi: 10.1021/acsbiomaterials.6b 00220

Keeley, E. C., Mehrad, B., and Strieter, R. M. (2008). Chemokines as mediators of neovascularization. *Arterioscler. Thromb. Vasc. Biol.* 28, 1928–1936. doi: 10.1161/ATVBAHA.108.162925

Konig, G., McAllister, T. N., Dusserre, N., Garrido, S. A., Iyican, C., Marini, A. (2009). Mechanical properties of completely autologous human tissue engineered blood vessels compared to human saphenous vein and mammary artery. *Biomaterials* 30, 1542–1550. doi: 10.1016/j.biomaterials.2008.11.011

Krishnaswamy, G., Smith, J. K., Mukkamala, R., Hall, K., Joyner, W., Yerra, L., et al. (1998). Multifunctional cytokine expression by human coronary endothelium and regulation by monokines and glucocorticoids. *Microvasc. Res.* 55, 189–200. doi: 10.1006/mvre.1998.2079

Krützfeldt, A., Spahr, R., Mertens, S., Siegmund, B., and Piper, H. M. (1990). Metabolism of exogenous substrates by coronary endothelial cells in culture. *J. Mol. Cell. Cardiol.* 22, 1393–1404. doi: 10.1016/0022-2828(90) 90984-A

Kyurkchiev, D., Bochev, I., Ivanova-Todorova, E., Mourdjeva, M., Oreshkova, T., Belemezova, K., et al. (2014). Secretion of immunoregulatory cytokines by mesenchymal stem cells. *World J. Stem Cells*. 6, 552–570. doi: 10.4252/wjsc.v6.i5.552

Lin, C. S., Hsieh, P. S., Hwang, L. L., Lee, Y. H., Tsai, S. H., Tu, Y. C., et al. (2018). The CCL5/CCR5 axis promotes vascular smooth muscle cell proliferation and atherogenic phenotype switching. *Cell. Physiol. Biochem.* 47, 707–720. doi: 10.1159/000490024

Liu, H., Li, X., Zhou, G., Fan, H., and Fan, Y. (2011). Electrospun sulfated silk fibroin nanofibrous scaffolds for vascular tissue engineering. *Biomaterials* 32, 3784–3793. doi: 10.1016/j.biomaterials.2011.02.002

Liu, S., Dong, C., Lu, G., Lu, Q., Li, Z., Kaplan, D. L., et al. (2013). Bilayered vascular grafts based on silk proteins. *Acta Biomater.* 9, 8991–9003. doi: 10.1016/j.actbio.2013.06.045

Liu, Y., Tu, F., Li, H., Shi, P., Yin, Y., Dong, F., et al. (2018). Preparation, characterization and *in vivo* graft patency of a silk fibroin tubular scaffold. *Mater. Technology.* 33, 227–234. doi: 10.1080/10667857.2017.1405889

Lovett, M. L., Cannizzaro, C. M., Vunjak-Novakovic, G., and Kaplan, D. L. (2008). Gel spinning of silk tubes for tissue engineering, *Biomaterials* 29, 4650–4657. doi: 10.1016/j.biomaterials.2008.08.025

Lovett, M. L., Eng, G., Kluge, J. A., Cannizzaro, C. M., Vunjak-Novakovic, G., and Kaplan, D. L. (2010). Tubular silk scaffolds for small diameter vascular grafts, *Organogenesis* 6, 217–224. doi: 10.4161/org.6.4.13407

Marelli, B., Achilli, M., Alessandrino, A., Freddi, G., Tanzi, M. C., Farè, S., et al. (2012). Collagen-reinforced electrospun silk fibroin tubular construct as small calibre vascular graft. *Macromol. Biosci.* 12, 1566–1574. doi: 10.1002/mabi.201200195

Marelli, B., Alessandrino, A., Farè, S., Freddi, G., Mantovani, D., and Tanzi, M. C. (2010). Compliant electrospun silk fibroin tubes for small vessel bypass grafting. *Acta Biomater.* 6, 4019–4026. doi: 10.1016/j.actbio.2010.05.008

Marelli, B., Alessandrino, A., Farè, S., Tanzi, M. C., and Freddi, G. (2009). Electrospun silk fibroin tubular matrixes for small vessel bypass grafting. *Mater. Technol.* 24, 52–57. doi: 10.1179/175355509X417945

McClure, M. J., Simpson, D. G., and Bowlin, G. L. (2012). Tri-layered vascular grafts composed of polycaprolactone, elastin, collagen, and silk: optimization of graft properties. *J. Mech. Behav. Biomed. Mater.* 10, 48–61. doi: 10.1016/j.jmbbm.2012.02.026

Mi, H.-Y., Jing, X., Yu, E., McNulty, J., Peng, X.-F., and Turng, L.-S. (2015). Fabrication of triple-layered vascular scaffolds by combining electrospinning, braiding, and thermally induced phase separation. *Mater. Lett.* 161, 305–308. doi: 10.1016/j.matlet.2015.08.119

Mohan, D., and Melvin, J. W. (1982). Failure properties of passive human aortic tissue. I–Uniaxial tension tests. *J.* Biomech. 15, 887–902. doi: 10.1016/0021-9290(82)90055-0

Morimoto, S., Nabata, T., Koh, E., Shiraishi, T., Fukuo, K., Imanaka, S., et al. (1991). Interleukin-6 stimulates proliferation of cultured vascular smooth muscle cells independently of interleukin-1 beta. *J. Cardiovasc. Pharmacol.* 17 (Suppl. 2), S117–118. doi: 10.1097/00005344-199117002-00026

Nakazawa, Y., Sato, M., Takahashi, R., Aytemiz, D., Takabayashi, C., Tamura, T., et al. (2011). Development of small-diameter vascular grafts based on silk fibroin fibers from *Bombyx mori* for vascular regeneration. *J. Biomater. Sci. Polym. Ed.* 22, 195–206. doi: 10.1163/092050609X125863816 56530

Plenz, G., Koenig, C., Severs, N. J., and Robenek, H. (1997). Smooth muscle cells express Granulocyte-Macrophage Colony-Stimulating Factor in the undiseased and atherosclerotic human coronary artery. *Arterioscl. Thromb. Vasc. Biol.* 17, 2489–2499. doi: 10.1161/01.ATV.17.11.2489

Schultz, K., Murthy, V., Tatro, J. B., and Beasley, D. (2007). Endogenous interleukin-1 alpha promotes a proliferative and proinflammatory phenotype in human vascular smooth muscle cells. *Am. J. Physiol. Heart. Circ. Physiol.* 292, H2927–H2934. doi: 10.1152/ajpheart.007 00.2006

Sugiura, T., Lee, A. Y., and Shinoka, T. (2017). "Tissue engineering in vascular medicine," in *Frontiers in Stem Cell and Regenerative Medicine Research*, Vol 4, eds A.-U. Rahman and S. Anjum (Sharjah: Bentham Science Publisher), 3–35. doi: 10.2174/9781681084756117050003

Tanaka, T., Uemura, A., Tanaka, R., Tasei, Y., and Asakura, T. (2018). Comparison of the knitted silk vascular grafts coated with fibroin sponges prepared using glycerin, poly(ethylene glycol diglycidyl ether) and poly(ethylene glycol) as porogens. *J. Biomater. Appl.* 32, 1239–1252. doi: 10.1177/0885328218758276

Thurber, A. E., Omenetto, F. G., and Kaplan, D. L. (2015). *In vivo* bio responses to silk proteins. *Biomaterials.* 71, 145–157. doi: 10.1016/j.biomaterials.2015.08.039

Vegran, F., Boidot, R., Michiels, C., Sonveaux, P., and Feron, O., and (2011). Lactateinflux through the endothelial cell monocarboxylate transporter MCT1 supports an NF-kappaB/IL-8 pathway that drives tumor angiogenesis. *Cancer Res.* 71, 2550–2560. doi: 10.1158/0008-5472.CAN-10-2828

Viñals, F., and Pouysségur, J. (1999). Confluence of vascular endothelial cells induces cell cycle exit by inhibiting p42/p44 mitogen-activated protein kinase activity. *Mol Cell Biol.* 19, 2763–2772. doi: 10.1128/MCB.19.4.2763

Wang, D., Liu, H., and Fan, Y. (2017). Silk fibroin for vascular regeneration. *Microsc. Res. Tech.* 80, 280–290. doi: 10.1002/jemt.22532

Wang, S.-D., Zhang, Y.-Z., Yin, G.-B., Wang,. H. W., and Dong, Z.-H. (2010). Fabrication of a composite vascular scaffold using electrospinning technology. *Mater. Sci. Eng. C.* 30, 670–676. doi: 10.1016/j.msec.2010.02.021

World Health Organization (2012). *Cardiovascular Diseases.* Fact Sheet No, 317.

Wu, G., Haynes, T. E., Li, H., and Meininger, C. J. (2000). Glutamine metabolism in endothelial cells: ornithine synthesis from glutamine via pyrroline-5-carboxylate synthase. *Comp. Biochem. Physiol. A Mol. Integr. Physiol.* 126, 115–123. doi: 10.1016/S1095-6433(00) 00196-3

Wu, T., Zhang, J., Wang, Y., Li, D., Sun, B., El-Hamshary, H., et al. (2018). Fabrication and preliminary study of a biomimetic tri-layer tubular graft based on fibers and fiber yarns for vascular tissue engineering. *Mater. Sci. Eng C.* 82, 121–129. doi: 10.1016/j.msec.2017.08.072

Xiang, P., Li, M., Zhang, C.-Y., Chen, D.-L., and Zhou, Z.-H. (2011). Cytocompatibility of electrospun nanofiber tubular scaffolds for small diameter tissue engineering blood vessels. *Int. J. Biol. Macromol.* 49, 281–288. doi: 10.1016/j.ijbiomac.2011.05.004

Yagi, T., Sato, M., Nakazawa, Y., Tanaka, K., Sata, M., Itoh, K., et al. (2011). Preparation of double-raschel knitted silk vascular grafts and evaluation of short-term function in a rat abdominal aorta. *J. Artif. Organs.* 14, 89–99. doi: 10.1007/s10047-011-0554-z

Yamamoto, S., Okamoto, H., Haga, M., Shigematsu, K., Miyata, T., Watanabe, T., et al. (2016). Rapid endothelialization and thin luminal layers in vascular grafts using silk fibroin. *J. Mater. Chem. B.* 4, 938–946. doi,: 10.1039/C.5T. B.02528A.

Zamani, M., Khafaji, M., Naji, M., Vossoughi, M., Alemzadeh, I., and Haghighipour, N. (2017). A biomimetic heparinized composite silk-based vascular scaffold with sustained antithrombogenicity. *Sci. Rep.* 7:4455. doi: 10.1038/s41598-017-04510-1

Zhang, J., Huang, H., Ju, R., Chen, K., Li, S., Wang, W., et al. (2017). *In vivo* biocompatibility and hemocompatibility of a polytetrafluoroethylene small diameter vascular graft modified with sulfonated silk fibroin. *Am. J. Surg.* 213, 87–93. doi: 10.1016/j.amjsurg,0.2016.04.005

Zhao, Y., Yan, X., Ding, F., Yang, Y., and Gu, X. (2011). The effects of different sterilization methods on silk fibroin. *Biomed. Sci. J. Eng.* 4, 397–402. doi: 10.4236/jbise.2011.45050

Zindl, C. L., Kim, T. H., Zeng, M., Archambault, A. S., Grayson, M. H., Choi, K., et al. (2009). The lymphotoxin LTalpha(1)beta(2) controls postnatal and adult spleen marginal sinus vascular structure and function. *Immunity* 30, 408–420. doi: 10.1016/j.immuni.2009.01.010

6

Relationship between Plantar Tissue Hardness and Plantar Pressure Distributions in People with Diabetic Peripheral Neuropathy

Yijie Duan[1†], Weiyan Ren[2†], Wei Liu[1], Jianchao Li[1], Fang Pu[1] and Yih-Kuen Jan[3*]*

[1]Key Laboratory of Biomechanics and Mechanobiology, Ministry of Education, Beijing Advanced Innovation Center for Biomedical Engineering, School of Biological Science and Medical Engineering, Beihang University, Beijing, China, [2]Key Laboratory of Rehabilitation Technical Aids for Old-Age Disability, Key Laboratory of Human Motion Analysis and Rehabilitation Technology of the Ministry of Civil Affairs, National Research Center for Rehabilitation Technical Aids, Beijing, China, [3]Department of Kinesiology and Community Health, University of Illinois at Urbana-Champaign, Champaign, IL, United States

***Correspondence:**
Fang Pu
pufangbme@buaa.edu.cn
Yih-Kuen Jan
yjan@illinois.edu

[†]These authors have contributed equally to this work and share first authorship

Objective: People with diabetic peripheral neuropathy (DPN) are usually accompanied with increased plantar pressure. Such high plantar loading during daily activities may cause changes in the biomechanical properties of plantar soft tissue, whose viability is critical to the development of foot ulcers. This study aimed to investigate the relationship between plantar tissue hardness and plantar pressure in people with and without DPN, and preliminarily explore the influence of plantar loading patterns on the plantar pressure and tissue hardness.

Methods: The study was conducted on 14 people with DPN and 14 diabetic people without DPN. The Shore durometer and MatScan System were used to measure the plantar tissue hardness and plantar pressure, respectively. The plantar loading level was evaluated by the duration of daily weight-bearing activity and was used to group diabetic participants with and without DPN into two subgroups (lower loading group and higher loading group).

Results: The plantar tissue hardness was significantly correlated with static peak plantar pressure (PPP, $p < 0.05$) and dynamic pressure-time integral (PTI, $p < 0.05$) in the forefoot region in people with DPN. Results of variance analysis showed a significant interaction effect between peripheral neuropathy and plantar loading on tissue hardness ($p < 0.05$), but not plantar pressure. For people with DPN, significant differences in tissue hardness between the higher loading group and lower loading group were observed in the forefoot, midfoot and hindfoot regions. In the higher loading group, people with DPN had significantly greater tissue hardness than that in people without DPN in the toes, forefoot, midfoot and hindfoot regions ($p < 0.05$).

Conclusions: There is a significant correlation between tissue hardness and PPP, and between tissue hardness and PTI in people with DPN. Plantar loading associated with daily activities plays a significant role on the plantar tissue hardness in people with DPN. The findings of this study contribute to further understand the relationship between increased plantar tissue hardness and high plantar pressure in people with diabetic peripheral neuropathy.

Keywords: diabetic peripheral neuropathy, foot ulcers, plantar soft tissue hardness, plantar pressure, plantar loading

INTRODUCTION

Diabetic foot ulcers (DFUs) are one of the most serious complications of diabetes, with a global prevalence of 6.3% (Zhang et al., 2017). Studies have shown that the amputation rate in diabetics is much higher than non-diabetics (Ahmad et al., 2016; Claessen et al., 2018; Gurney et al., 2018), which seriously affects the physical health and imposes additional financial burden for people with diabetes.

Peripheral neuropathy is an important risk factor for DFUs (Monteiro-Soares et al., 2012; Armstrong et al., 2017), which may lead to foot deformities, biomechanical abnormalities, and the loss of protective sensation (Volmer-Thole and Lobmann, 2016). Several studies demonstrated that people with diabetic peripheral neuropathy (DPN) have a higher peak plantar pressure (Sacco et al., 2014; Halawa et al., 2018) and show an imbalance in plantar pressure distribution (Caselli et al., 2002; Kernozek et al., 2013; Al-Angari et al., 2017), compared with people without DPN. The loss of protective sensation caused by neuropathy also prevents people with DPN from responding promptly to abnormal mechanical stress during daily activities (Armstrong et al., 2017). These factors may affect their ambulatory function.

Plantar soft tissue is the first contact with the ground during daily activities, such as standing and walking, and plays a key role in shock-absorbing and protecting foot from external mechanical damage. The accumulation of advanced glycation end-products in people with diabetes can lead to histological changes in plantar soft tissue (Ramasamy et al., 2005). Abnormal microvascular function and dysfunctional secretion of sweat caused by peripheral neuropathy may further aggravate histological changes (Volmer-Thole and Lobmann, 2016). Several studies have found that plantar soft tissue of people with DPN was thinner and stiffer than healthy people (Klaesner et al., 2002; Chao et al., 2011; Sun et al., 2011; Jan et al., 2013). Periyasamy et al. further reported significant differences in plantar tissue hardness between diabetic people with and without DPN using a shore durometer (Periyasamy et al., 2012a; Periyasamy et al., 2012b). Increased tissue hardness in people with DPN may be accompanied by stress concentration during daily activities (Klaesner et al., 2002; Chatzistergos et al., 2014). Over time, the dry skin and abnormal plantar pressure may cause hyperkeratosis under repeated and elevated plantar pressure loading (Volmer-Thole and Lobmann, 2016), which may affect the biomechanical properties of the soft tissue, and increase the vulnerability of plantar tissue to trauma and ulceration.

Several studies have shown the potential link between plantar pressure and the biomechanical properties of soft tissue (Gefen, 2003; Jan et al., 2013; Helili et al., 2021). Jan et al.'s study demonstrated a correlation between the soft tissue biomechanical properties and plantar pressure gradient in the first metatarsal region in people with DPN (Jan et al., 2013). Helili et al. also reported a correlation between plantar soft tissue hardness and average dynamic pressure in healthy people (Helili et al., 2021). However, the whole plantar regions and more plantar pressure characteristics (both peak plantar pressure and pressure-time integral (Duckworth et al., 1985; Patry et al., 2013; Chatwin et al., 2020) in static and dynamic conditions) need to be considered, in order to better understand the relationship between the biomechanical properties of soft tissue and plantar pressure distribution in people with DPN.

In daily activities, plantar loading may be an important factor affecting the plantar pressure and tissue hardness of people with DPN. Limited joint mobility, muscular alterations and foot deformities associated with peripheral neuropathy may altered the postural control and balance function during gait (Simoneau et al., 1994; Periyasamy et al., 2012a; Volmer-Thole and Lobmann, 2016), which results in an insecure gait. Such deficit of balance and posture may exacerbate their plantar biomechanical abnormalities under the excessive mechanical stress stimulus. In addition, studies showed that different levels of plantar loading have an effect on microvascular regulation (Wu et al., 2020; Duan et al., 2021). Excessive plantar pressure load may increase the degree of compression of plantar tissue and the occlusion duration of microvessels, which leads to an insufficient blood perfusion and a lack of nutrients in soft tissue. These factors may jointly influence the biomechanical properties of plantar soft tissue. It is of great significance to explore the effects of plantar loading on plantar pressure and tissue hardness for understanding the changes of soft tissue biomechanical properties on the development of ulceration in people with DPN.

Therefore, this study aimed to investigate the relationship between plantar tissue hardness and plantar pressure in people with and without DPN, and preliminarily explore the influence of plantar loading on plantar pressure and tissue hardness. This study hypothesized that the increased plantar tissue hardness was related to plantar pressure, and the plantar loading associated with daily activities has an effect on the plantar pressure and tissue hardness.

MATERIALS AND METHODS

Participants

People with type 2 diabetes were recruited from nearby hospitals and communities. The inclusion criteria were: 1) diagnosed type 2 diabetes mellitus, 2) no symptoms such as redness, inflammation, or wounds on the skin of the feet or legs, 3) no history of amputation, and 4) performed regular moderate-intensity physical activities at least 150 min/week over the course of one year on the basis of self-report (American Diabetes Association, 2021). Moderate-intensity physical activity was defined as a metabolic equivalent (MET) of 3–5.9 Mets, according to the compendium of physical activities (Ainsworth et al., 2011).

The 10 g Semmes-Weinstein monofilament was used to identify peripheral neuropathy in people with diabetes. Participants who were unable to sense the touch of the 10 g monofilament at all four areas on the plantar surface (1st, 3rd and 5th metatarsal heads and distal hallux) were assigned to the diabetic peripheral neuropathy group (DPN group) (Boulton et al., 2008), otherwise, the participant was assigned to the non-diabetic peripheral neuropathy group (Non-DPN group).

The criterion of physical activities is the minimum weekly physical activity level recommended by ADA guidelines for

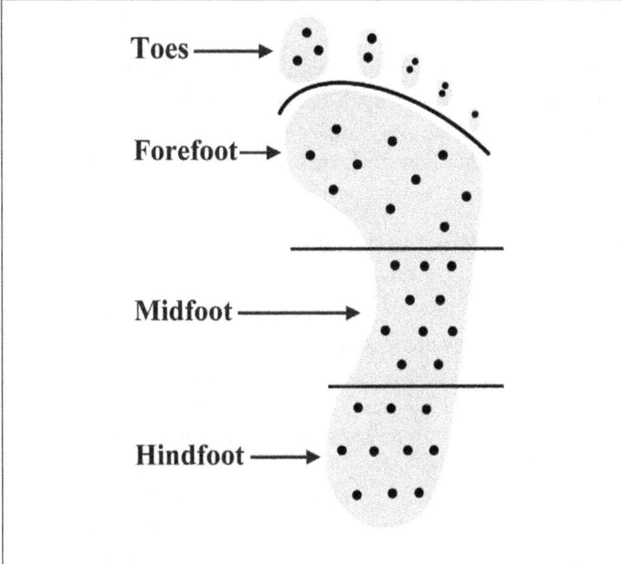

FIGURE 1 | Measurement of plantar soft tissue hardness by using the Shore (OO) durometer. The black dots indicate the measurement site of plantar tissue hardness.

people with diabetes (American Diabetes Association, 2021). The type, frequency and duration of daily physical activities of each participant were firstly recorded using the International Physical Activity Questionnaire (IPAQ) (Mynarski et al., 2012), which has been proven to be a validated tool for physical activity assessment. The median duration of weight-bearing physical activity per day of all participants (LeMaster et al., 2003) was used to divided participants of each group into two subgroups (lower loading group and higher loading group).

This study was conducted in accordance with clinical protocols approved by the institutional review board of Affiliated Hospital of National Research Center for Rehabilitation Technical Aids (20190101) and the Declaration of Helsinki (2013 revision). All participants were briefed on the study purposes and procedures and gave written informed consent prior to participation.

Measurement of Plantar Tissue Hardness and Plantar Pressure

All tests were performed in a climate-controlled room at 24°C.

A Shore durometer (Model 1600, Type OO, Rex Co., Buffalo Grove, USA) was used to measure the plantar tissue hardness, which has been used in several studies (Periyasamy et al., 2012b; Helili et al., 2021). During measurement, the durometer was pressed perpendicular to the plantar skin surface and expresses the hardness in degrees of Shore (unit: °Shore). A lower Shore value indicates a softer material. The plantar surface was divided into four regions: toes, forefoot, midfoot and hindfoot. Ten sites were selected for each of four regions of interest. Plantar tissue hardness over these sites were measured and mean values of tissue hardness were calculated for comparisons to investigate the relationship between plantar tissue hardness and plantar pressure. All measurements were performed by one skilled experimenter. **Figure 1** shows the measurement sites of plantar tissue hardness by using the Shore (OO) durometer. The locations and area of callus were special recorded.

A MatScan System (HR Mat, Tekscan, Inc., Boston, USA) was used to measure plantar pressure. It has a spatial resolution of 4 Sensels™/cm^2 (25 Sensels/in^2) with 8,448 individual pressure sensing locations. After calibration based on the manufacturer recommendations, the pressure was recorded at static conditions (standing) and dynamic conditions (taking one step on the MatScan) (Sacco et al., 2014). Recordings were made at 50 Hz for 30 s, and the analysis was made using the FootMat Research software. Plantar pressure parameters included static peak plantar pressure (PPP), dynamic peak plantar pressure (PPP) and dynamic pressure-time integral (PTI).

Data and Statistical Analyses

The plantar foot was divided into four regions, including toes, forefoot, midfoot, and hindfoot. The plantar tissue hardness of the whole foot was the average value of the tissue hardness in the regions of toes, forefoot, midfoot and hindfoot. Static PPP, dynamic PPP and PTI of corresponding area (toes, forefoot, midfoot, hindfoot, and whole foot) were calculated to assess plantar pressure distribution. The average values of tissue hardness and plantar pressure in the corresponding regions of the left and right feet were calculated and compared.

The correlations between tissue hardness and plantar pressure in each plantar region were determined using Pearson correlation analysis. When taking the plantar loading into consideration, two-way analysis of variance (ANOVA) was used to compare the plantar tissue hardness and plantar pressure between four subgroups to investigate the effect of plantar loading and neuropathy on tissue hardness and plantar pressure in people with diabetes. If there was a significant interaction between neuropathy and plantar loading, the simple effect (examined through univariate ANOVA) was used to assess the effect of neuropathy with restricted levels of plantar loading and vice versa. If no interaction was found, the main effects of neuropathy and plantar loading on tissue hardness and plantar pressure were assessed, respectively. The main effect is defined as an integrated effect of neuropathy, which disregard the levels of plantar loading, and vice versa.

The significant level was set as 0.05. All statistical analyses were performed in SPSS (Version 26.0, IBM, Armonk, NY, USA).

RESULTS

A total of 28 people with diabetes volunteered in this study, including 14 people with DPN (DPN group) and 14 people without DPN (Non-DPN group). Participants' characteristics are shown in **Table 1**. The median duration of daily weight-bearing activities of all participants was 2 h per day. In the DPN group, nine participants were divided into the higher loading group, and five participants were divided into the lower loading group. In the Non-DPN group, eight

TABLE 1 | Demographic and physiological information of participants in DPN group and Non-DPN group (Mean ± SD).

Variables	DPN Group	Non-DPN Group
Gender (Male/Female)	5/9	7/7
Age (years)	67.93 ± 5.72	67.86 ± 6.20
BMI (kg/m^2)	25.95 ± 2.77	25.91 ± 2.77
Systolic blood pressure (mmHg)	136.92 ± 11.54	132.43 ± 11.88
Diastolic blood pressure (mmHg)	71.38 ± 6.47	69.29 ± 7.39
Heart rate (bpm)	71.15 ± 7.94	73.36 ± 7.69
Duration of diabetes (years)	17.64 ± 11.88	14.82 ± 6.52
Fasting blood glucose (mmol/L)	7.90 ± 1.79	8.09 ± 1.65
ABI (left)	1.08 ± 0.12	1.03 ± 0.08
ABI (right)	1.00 ± 0.13	1.08 ± 0.06

There was no significant difference in all parameters between the DPN group and Non-DPN group (p > 0.05). BMI: body mass index; ABI: Ankle-brachial index. DPN: people with diabetic peripheral neuropathy; Non-DPN: people without diabetic peripheral neuropathy.

participants were divided into the higher loading group, and six participants were divided into the lower loading group. Except for one participant in the Non-DPN group engaged in square dancing and walking, the other participants only performed walking during daily activities. The daily weight-bearing physical activities duration of DPN group and Non-DPN group was 1.93 ± 0.92 h/day and 1.75 ± 0.80 h/day, respectively.

In DPN group, three participants had callus over the forefoot region, two participants had callus over the big toe, and one participant had callus over both forefoot region and big toe. In the Non-DPN group, none of them had callus in their feet.

Relationships Between Soft Tissue Hardness and Plantar Pressure

For all participants, tissue hardness in the forefoot region was significantly correlated with static PPP and dynamic PTI (Static PPP: r = 0.556, p = 0.002, and Dynamic PTI: r = 0.447, p = 0.017). No significant correlations between tissue hardness and plantar pressure in other plantar regions were observed (p > 0.05).

Figure 2 shows the correlations between the soft tissue hardness and plantar pressure in each plantar region of people with DPN. The tissue hardness of the forefoot region was significantly correlated with static PPP and dynamic PTI (tissue hardness and static PPP: r = 0.599, p = 0.024, tissue hardness and Dynamic PTI: r = 0.573, p = 0.032). No significant correlations between the soft tissue hardness and

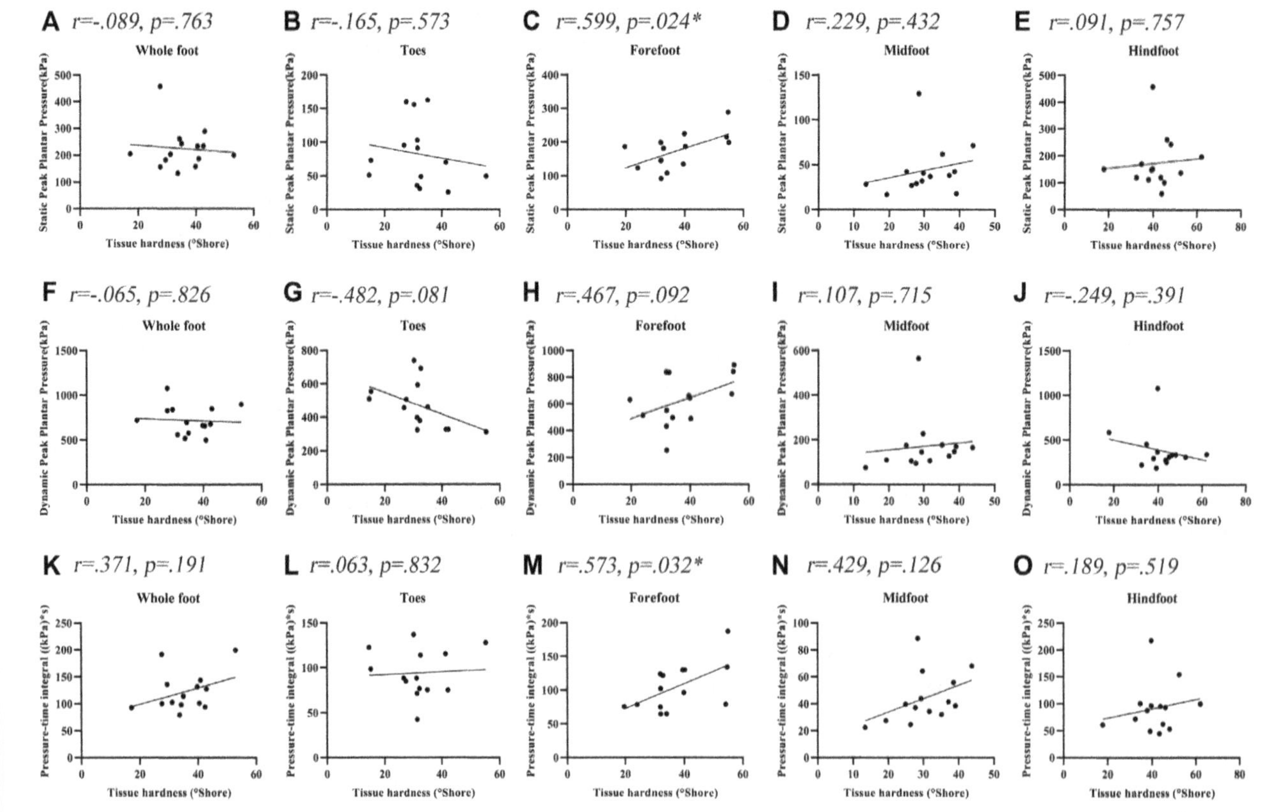

FIGURE 2 | Correlation coefficients between plantar tissue hardness and plantar pressure in people with DPN. * indicates a significant correlation (p < 0.05). **(A-E)** represent the correlation coefficients between plantar tissue hardness and static peak plantar pressure in the whole foot, toes region, forefoot region, midfoot region and hindfoot region, respectively. **(F-J)** represent the correlation coefficients between plantar tissue hardness and dynamic peak plantar pressure in the whole foot, toes region, forefoot region, midfoot region and hindfoot region, respectively. **(K-O)** represent the correlation coefficients between plantar tissue hardness and pressure-time integral in the whole foot, toes region, forefoot region, midfoot region and hindfoot region, respectively.

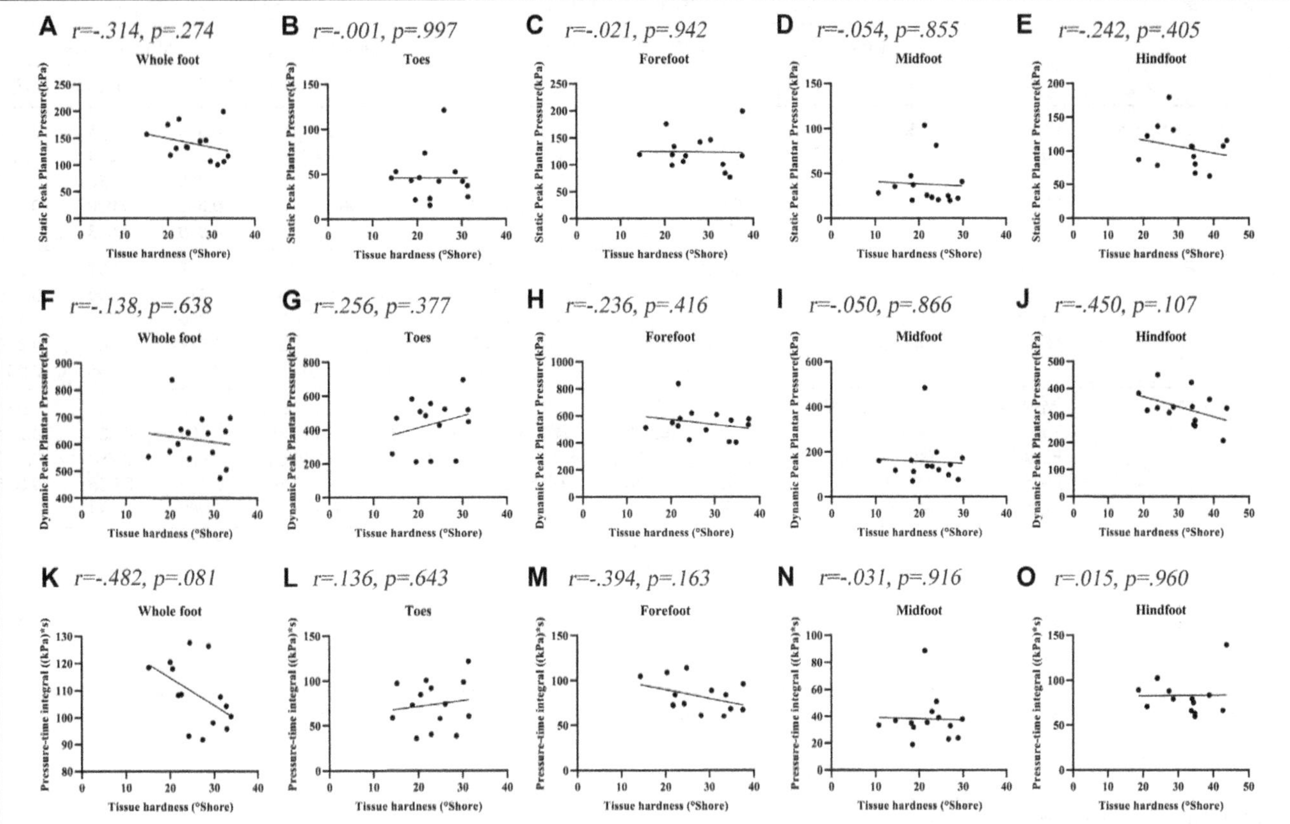

FIGURE 3 | Correlation coefficients between plantar tissue hardness and plantar pressure in people without DPN. **(A-E)** represent the correlation coefficients between plantar tissue hardness and static peak plantar pressure in the whole foot, toes region, forefoot region, midfoot region and hindfoot region, respectively. **(F-J)** represent the correlation coefficients between plantar tissue hardness and dynamic peak plantar pressure in the whole foot, toes region, forefoot region, midfoot region and hindfoot region, respectively. **(K-O)** represent the correlation coefficients between plantar tissue hardness and pressure-time integral in the whole foot, toes region, forefoot region, midfoot region and hindfoot region, respectively.

plantar pressure in other plantar regions were observed ($p > 0.05$).

Figure 3 shows the correlations between the soft tissue hardness and plantar pressure in each plantar region of people without DPN. The correlations between the soft tissue hardness and plantar pressure both did not reach statistical significance in each plantar region ($p > 0.05$).

Effect of Plantar Loading and Neuropathy on Tissue Hardness and Plantar Pressure

The interaction and main effect of peripheral neuropathy and plantar loading on tissue hardness and plantar pressure was showed in **Table 2.**

There was an interaction between the peripheral neuropathy and plantar loading on tissue hardness, with a statistical significance over the whole foot, forefoot, midfoot, and hindfoot region ($p < 0.05$). The results of simple effect on tissue hardness showed that people with DPN and higher loading had significantly higher tissue hardness, compared with people without DPN and higher loading ($p < 0.05$, **Table3**). Similarly, significant differences were also found between people with DPN and higher loading and people with DPN and lower loading, and between people with DPN and higher loading people and people without DPN and lower loading ($p < 0.05$). No significant differences in tissue hardness were observed among other subgroups ($p > 0.05$).

There was no significant interaction between the peripheral neuropathy and plantar loading on plantar pressure ($p > 0.05$). Peripheral neuropathy and plantar loading caused a significant main effect on plantar pressure, respectively (**Table 2**). The static PPP of participants in the DPN group was higher than Non-DPN group, with a significant difference over the whole foot, toes, forefoot, and hindfoot region ($p < 0.05$). The PTI of participants in the DPN group was significantly higher than Non-DPN group over the toes region ($p < 0.05$). In comparison to participants in lower loading group, people with higher loading showed significantly higher static PPP, dynamic PPP and PTI over the midfoot region and lower dynamic PPP over the toes region ($p < 0.05$).

In addition, people with callus over the forefoot region had significantly greater values of tissue hardness compared people without callus in the DPN group (50.94 ± 7.37 vs. 31.87 ± 6.19 Shore, $p < 0.05$). Their plantar pressure also higher than people without callus (static PPP: 232.18 ± 39.33 *vs.* 149.99 ± 36.69 kPa, $p < 0.05$, dynamic PPP: 764.69 ± 123.29 *vs.* 569.73 ± 179.61 kPa,

TABLE 2 | The interaction and main effects of peripheral neuropathy and plantar loading patterns on plantar tissue hardness and plantar pressure (Mean ± SD).

		DPN	Non-DPN	Lower Loading	Higher Loading	ANOVA p Value		
						P_I	P_N	P_L
Tissue hardness (°Shore)	Whole foot	35.39 ± 8.81	26.12 ± 5.72	27.24 ± 5.61	33.03 ± 9.67	**0.019**	**0.006**	**0.043**
	Toes	31.94 ± 10.29	23.44 ± 5.61	24.39 ± 6.17	29.82 ± 10.35	0.261	**0.026**	0.127
	Forefoot	37.32 ± 10.91	27.51 ± 7.24	28.25 ± 6.05	35.11 ± 11.78	**0.019**	**0.022**	0.053
	Midfoot	30.34 ± 8.14	21.94 ± 5.44	23.31 ± 6.21	27.97 ± 8.7	**0.045**	**0.009**	0.099
	Hindfoot	41.58 ± 10.19	31.5 ± 7.74	33.86 ± 8.99	38.27 ± 10.9	**0.016**	**0.018**	0.225
Static PPP (kPa)	Whole foot	224.15 ± 79.87	139.61 ± 30.56	177.22 ± 41.92	184.9 ± 89.14	0.170	**0.003**	0.918
	Toes	82.49 ± 48.01	45.68 ± 26.56	78.55 ± 49.51	54.72 ± 35.64	0.473	**0.009**	0.075
	Forefoot	173.47 ± 52.67	123.79 ± 33.64	140.16 ± 41.24	154.11 ± 55.76	0.060	**0.018**	0.497
	Midfoot	43.75 ± 28.75	37.79 ± 24.92	28.03 ± 6.77	49.01 ± 31.29	0.777	0.703	**0.049**
	Hindfoot	173.98 ± 97.63	105.15 ± 31.32	137.65 ± 51.78	140.79 ± 94.52	0.541	**0.035**	0.961
Dynamic PPP (kPa)	Whole foot	716.27 ± 162.5	616.08 ± 92.34	658.84 ± 109.2	670.92 ± 158.93	0.712	0.062	0.941
	Toes	471.09 ± 138.3	437.01 ± 153.78	547.55 ± 95.13	393.54 ± 140.38	0.568	0.306	**0.004**
	Forefoot	625.43 ± 184.92	546.46 ± 108.96	521.65 ± 151.07	627.55 ± 145.65	0.472	0.283	0.087
	Midfoot	170.56 ± 120.44	154.94 ± 100.86	107.66 ± 21.81	198.39 ± 128.16	0.809	0.865	**0.037**
	Hindfoot	380.85 ± 222.22	327.43 ± 63.78	331.2 ± 106.24	368.98 ± 192.42	0.686	0.394	0.618
Dynamic PTI (kPa*s)	Whole foot	122.24 ± 36.23	108.36 ± 12.07	107.02 ± 14.73	120.65 ± 32.49	0.243	0.326	0.217
	Toes	94.08 ± 26.41	74.09 ± 26.46	92.87 ± 20.78	78.41 ± 30.88	0.993	**0.048**	0.127
	Forefoot	104.3 ± 35.16	82.67 ± 17.69	85.16 ± 21.19	98.88 ± 33.22	0.053	0.121	0.218
	Midfoot	44.09 ± 18.72	37.77 ± 16.82	32.17 ± 7.16	46.6 ± 20.32	0.645	0.484	**0.042**
	Hindfoot	92.2 ± 46.09	82.86 ± 20.97	83.68 ± 22.44	90.02 ± 42.31	0.573	0.621	0.683

P_I, is the interaction between plantar loading and peripheral neuropathy; P_N, is the main effect of peripheral neuropathy; P_L, is the main effect of plantar loading. P value in bold text indicate the significant interaction or main effect. DPN: people with diabetic peripheral neuropathy; Non-DPN: people without diabetic peripheral neuropathy.

TABLE 3 | The effect of peripheral neuropathy and plantar loading patterns on plantar tissue hardness (Mean ± SD).

	DPN Group		Non-DPN Group		ANOVA p Value		
	Lower Loading	Higher Loading	Lower Loading	Higher Loading	P_{LH}	P_{HH}	P_{HL}
Whole foot	27.92 ± 6.47	39.54 ± 7.13[a,b,c]	26.68 ± 5.35	25.7 ± 6.31	**0.011**	**0.001**	**0.002**
Toes	26.46 ± 6.72	34.98 ± 10.96[b,c]	22.67 ± 5.67	24.01 ± 5.89	0.144	**0.024**	**0.026**
Forefoot	28.15 ± 5.96	42.41 ± 9.69[a,b,c]	28.34 ± 6.68	26.89 ± 8.02	**0.012**	**0.003**	**0.009**
Midfoot	24.31 ± 7.7	33.69 ± 6.53[a,b,c]	22.48 ± 5.27	21.54 ± 5.9	**0.032**	**0.001**	**0.004**
Hindfoot	33.76 ± 10.35	45.92 ± 7.46[a,b,c]	33.95 ± 8.72	29.66 ± 6.92	**0.025**	**<0.001**	**0.014**

P_{LH}, is the significance test between people with DPN and lower loading, and people with DPN and higher loading; P_{HH}, is the significance test between people with DPN and higher loading, and people without DPN and higher loading; P_{HL}, is the significance test between people with DPN and higher loading, and people without DPN and lower loading.
[a]Indicates a significant difference between people with DPN and lower loading, and people with DPN and higher loading (p< 0.05).
[b]Indicates a significant difference between people with DPN and higher loading, and people without DPN and higher loading (p< 0.05).
[c]Indicates a significant difference between people with DPN and higher loading, and people without DPN and lower loading (p< 0.05). P value in bold text indicate the significant difference. DPN: people with diabetic peripheral neuropathy; Non-DPN: people without diabetic peripheral neuropathy.

$p < 0.05$, dynamic PTI: 124.25 ± 48.15 *vs*. 96.32 ± 27.66 kPa*s, p = 0.188).

DISCUSSION

This study investigated the relationship between plantar tissue hardness and plantar pressure in people with and without DPN, and preliminarily explored the influence of plantar loading associated with daily activities on plantar pressure and tissue hardness. The results showed significant correlations between tissue hardness and static PPP, and between tissue hardness and dynamic PTI in the forefoot region in people with DPN. Peripheral neuropathy and plantar loading caused a significant interaction effect on tissue hardness, but not plantar pressure. The plantar pressure distribution was independently associated with peripheral neuropathy and plantar loading. In comparison to people without DPN, significant differences in tissue hardness were only found in people with DPN and higher loading.

The results of this study showed that plantar tissue hardness of people with DPN was significantly correlated to static PPP and dynamic PTI over the forefoot region. This suggested the potential relationship between increased plantar tissue hardness and high plantar pressure. This study is an important supplement to Jan et al.'s study (Jan et al., 2013) that did not pay attention to the static plantar pressure. Static plantar pressure, reflecting the contact force of the foot with the ground during standing, is as important as dynamic plantar pressure in assessing the risk of DFUs (Duckworth et al., 1985; Patry et al., 2013). Thus, both static plantar pressure (during standing) and dynamic plantar pressure (during walking) were measured in this study. However, except the forefoot region, no significant correlation was observed between tissue hardness and plantar pressure in other plantar regions, which may be due to the fact that the forefoot is the main load-bearing area during daily activities. There was no significant correlation in the heel region may be related to the imbalanced plantar pressure distribution (Caselli et al., 2002; Kernozek et al., 2013; Al-Angari et al., 2017), which may lead to change of plantar load-bearing position. Besides, the different correlation trend between plantar pressure and tissue hardness in different plantar regions may be related to different injury thresholds, which should be explored in future studies. It should also be mentioned that no significant correlation between plantar pressure and tissue hardness was observed in people without DPN. This may be due to their relatively normal plantar pressure distribution and postural control during walking. The changes of the soft tissue biomechanical properties in diabetic people without DPN may be more influenced by the accumulation of advanced glycation end-products. Therefore, foot deformities, postural control and balance function may be considered in future studies. In this study, a significant correlation between increased plantar tissue hardness and plantar pressure could contribute to understand the changes of soft tissue biomechanical properties in people with DPN.

The findings of this study also found that increased plantar tissue hardness associated with peripheral neuropathy was affected by plantar loading level. People with DPN and higher loading had higher tissue hardness compared with people with DPN and lower loading in the forefoot, midfoot and hindfoot regions. It indicated a low shock-absorbing capacity to distribute mechanical stress during daily activities, especially weight-bearing activities (e.g. walking) in people with DPN. Excessive and repetitive plantar pressure loading may aggravate the stiffness of plantar soft tissue due to their weak ability to evenly distribute abnormal plantar pressure (Chatzistergos et al., 2014) during daily activities. Klaesner et al. demonstrated that the plantar soft tissue of people with DPN over the metatarsal heads was stiffer than healthy people using an indentor system (Klaesner et al., 2002). Several studies have also reported consistent findings using ultrasound palpation system (Sun et al., 2011). However, none of these studies involved diabetic people without DPN, which makes it difficult to determine the changes in biomechanical properties of plantar soft tissue associated with pure neuropathy. Only one study reported a significant difference in tissue hardness between diabetic people with and without DPN (Periyasamy et al., 2012b), which was consistent with the results in this study. Increased plantar tissue hardness in people with DPN and higher loading indicated a warning that excessive plantar loading during weight-bearing activities may increase the burden of fragile soft tissue caused by peripheral neuropathy (Sun et al., 2011) and make a negative effect on plantar soft tissue.

However, no significant difference was observed in plantar tissue hardness between people without DPN and lower loading and people without DPN and higher loading, which indicated the specificity and importance of the safe threshold for plantar loading during daily activities. The Physical Stress Theory (PST) proposed by Muller and his group assumes a window of "increased tolerance" between function maintenance threshold and injury threshold of plantar soft tissue. Physical stress within this window may be beneficial to enhance the adaptability of plantar soft tissue to external stress stimulus (Mueller and Maluf, 2002; Kluding et al., 2017) for people with DPN. The most important and challenging thing, however, is how to determine this safe threshold. In addition, Chao et al. showed that the stiffness of plantar soft tissue was increased in all diabetic people (diabetics with foot ulceration group, diabetics with neuropathy group, and pure diabetics group) compared healthy people, but no significant difference was reported between people with neuropathy and pure diabetics (Chao et al., 2011). This may be due to a lack of consideration of various plantar loading levels on soft tissue. In this study, no significant differences in tissue hardness were found between people with DPN and lower loading and people without DPN and lower loading. It indicated that appropriate plantar loading (e.g. performing weight-bearing physical activities) may be useful to improve the soft tissue biomechanical properties in people with DPN (Otterman et al., 2011; Mueller et al., 2013). Otterman et al. demonstrated the benefits of a 12-weeks exercise programme, consisting 30 min of aerobic exercise (e.g. cycling, walking, etc.) per day for people with DPN (Otterman et al., 2011). Mueller et al.'s study conducted a 12-weeks exercise programme for 1-h exercise sessions with 3 times per week (Mueller et al., 2013), and demonstrated the benefits of weight-bearing exercise in ambulatory function. Future studies may need to clarify the effects of different levels of plantar loading on plantar soft tissue, in order to seek the safety thresholds in people with and without DPN and guide physicians to develop exercise program for people with diabetes.

In addition, the static PPP of people with DPN were significantly higher than people without DPN, which was consistent with previous studies (Sacco et al., 2014; Halawa et al., 2018). However, no significant difference in dynamic PPP between people with and without DPN was observed in this study. Such differences may be influenced by different patient characteristics such as severity stages of diabetic peripheral neuropathy (Sacco et al., 2014) and skin health characteristics (i.e. callus presence). Because Sacco et al. found that plantar pressure gradually increased with the aggravation of neuropathy (Sacco et al., 2014). People with higher loading had higher plantar pressure in the midfoot region and lower plantar pressure in the toes region, suggesting changes of plantar pressure distribution under repeated mechanical stress stimulus. Therefore, the influence of such changes of plantar pressure distribution on diabetic foot ulcers still needs to be further studied.

In people with DPN, the forefoot region with callus had higher peak plantar pressure compared with people without callus. Studies suggested high shear stress near callus could cause abnormal peak plantar pressure and plantar pressure gradient in plantar soft tissues (Chao et al., 2011). Plantar soft tissue in callus area has impaired shock-absorbing function, which may result in tissue inflammation, skin breakdown and ulceration (Sun et al., 2011). Therefore, callus presence should be noticed immediately for people with DPN. It is necessary to ensure proper footwear and perform weight-bearing physical activities selectively.

The power analysis was performed to validate the statistical results of comparisons. There are large different effects for the comparisons of plantar tissue hardness in the whole foot and forefoot region between people with DPN and higher loading and people without DPN and higher loading (whole foot: 97.91%, forefoot region: 92.49%). In addition, the power of the difference in plantar tissue hardness in the whole foot and forefoot region between people with DPN and lower loading and people with DPN and higher loading was 80.77 and 88.55%, respectively. This may suggest an important influence of plantar loading level (i.e. weight-bearing physical activity duration) on the biomechanical properties of plantar soft tissue in people with DPN.

This study has some limitations. Firstly, plantar loading caused by exercise may result in different plantar pressures between people with and without DPN. It is necessary to examine the relationship between plantar loading and plantar pressure in a larger cohort of participants with DPN. Besides, plantar loading patterns were only divided into two levels based on the duration of daily weight-bearing activities, due to the limited sample size. More groups of plantar loading levels should be explored in the future. Secondly, this study explored the influence of plantar loading caused by exercise on plantar tissue hardness and plantar pressure in people with DPN. Future research should perform longitudinal studies to further explore the changes in the soft tissue biomechanical properties under long-term physical activities. Thirdly, walking was the main type of weight-bearing activities among the participants enrolled in this study. Other types of physical activities should be considered in future studies. Fourthly, the shore durometer has limitations in characterizing nonlinear viscoelastic behavior and tissue thickness of soft tissue. Ultrasound imaging may provide additional information on the biomechanical properties of plantar soft tissue (e.g. skin thickness). In addition, body weight and duration of diabetes may affect the results observed in our study (Abouaesha et al., 2001; Pirozzi et al., 2014; Jeong et al., 2021). Thus, our finding may not be generalized to people with DM who have different durations of diabetes and BMI. The influence of other covariates on plantar pressure and tissue hardness should be investigated in the future, such as body weight and skin quality on different regions of foot. Fifthly, the plantar surface was divided into four regions in order to explore the potential relationship between tissue hardness and plantar pressure in the whole plantar region in people with diabetes. Subdivision of plantar regions (e.g. the five metatarsal regions of the forefoot, big toe and little toes) should be considered in future studies.

CONCLUSION

In conclusion, this study found that the plantar tissue hardness was correlated to plantar pressure in people with DPN. Peripheral neuropathy and plantar loading patterns associated with various physical activities are important factors affecting the biomechanical properties of plantar soft tissue. The findings of this study contribute to further understand the relationship between increased plantar tissue hardness and high plantar pressure in people with diabetic peripheral neuropathy.

AUTHOR CONTRIBUTIONS

Methodology, FP and Y-KJ; formal analysis, YD and WR; investigation, YD, WL, and JL; data curation, YD, WL, and WR; writing—original draft preparation, YD and WR; writing—review and editing, FP and Y-KJ; funding acquisition, FP and WR. All authors have read and agreed to the published version of the manuscript.

ACKNOWLEDGMENTS

The authors thank all subjects who participated in this study.

REFERENCES

Abouaesha, F., van Schie, C. H. M., Griffths, G. D., Young, R. J., and Boulton, A. J. M. (2001). Plantar Tissue Thickness is related to Peak Plantar Pressure in the High-Risk Diabetic Foot. *Diabetes Care* 24 (7), 1270–1274. doi:10.2337/diacare.24.7.1270

Ahmad, N., Thomas, G. N., Gill, P., and Torella, F. (2016). The Prevalence of Major Lower Limb Amputation in the Diabetic and Non-diabetic Population of England 2003-2013. *Diabetes Vasc. Dis. Res.* 13 (5), 348–353. doi:10.1177/1479164116651390

Ainsworth, B. E., Haskell, W. L., Herrmann, S. D., Meckes, N., Bassett, D. R., Tudor-Locke, C., et al. (2011). 2011 Compendium of Physical Activities. *Med. Sci. Sports Exerc.* 43 (8), 1575–1581. doi:10.1249/MSS.0b013e31821ece12

Al-Angari, H. M., Khandoker, A. H., Lee, S., Almahmeed, W., Al Safar, H. S., Jelinek, H. F., et al. (2017). Novel Dynamic Peak and Distribution Plantar Pressure Measures on Diabetic Patients during Walking. *Gait & Posture* 51, 261–267. doi:10.1016/j.gaitpost.2016.11.006

American Diabetes Association (2021). 5. Facilitating Behavior Change and Well-Being to Improve Health Outcomes: Standards of Medical Care in Diabetes-2021. *Diabetes Care* 44 (Suppl. ment_1), S53–S72. doi:10.2337/dc21-S005

Armstrong, D. G., Boulton, A. J. M., and Bus, S. A. (2017). Diabetic Foot Ulcers and Their Recurrence. *N. Engl. J. Med.* 376 (24), 2367–2375. doi:10.1056/NEJMra1615439

Boulton, A. J. M., Armstrong, D. G., Albert, S. F., Frykberg, R. G., Hellman, R., Kirkman, M. S., et al. (2008). Comprehensive Foot Examination and Risk Assessment. *Endocr. Pract.* 14 (5), 576–583. doi:10.4158/ep.14.5.576

Caselli, A., Pham, H., Giurini, J. M., Armstrong, D. G., and Veves, A. (2002). The Forefoot-To-Rearfoot Plantar Pressure Ratio is increased in Severe Diabetic Neuropathy and Can Predict Foot Ulceration. *Diabetes Care* 25 (6), 1066–1071. doi:10.2337/diacare.25.6.1066

Chao, C. Y. L., Zheng, Y.-P., and Cheing, G. L. Y. (2011). Epidermal Thickness and Biomechanical Properties of Plantar Tissues in Diabetic Foot. *Ultrasound Med. Biol.* 37 (7), 1029–1038. doi:10.1016/j.ultrasmedbio.2011.04.004

Chatwin, K. E., Abbott, C. A., Boulton, A. J. M., Bowling, F. L., and Reeves, N. D. (2020). The Role of Foot Pressure Measurement in the Prediction and Prevention of Diabetic Foot Ulceration-A Comprehensive Review. *Diabetes Metab. Res. Rev.* 36 (4)e3258. doi:10.1002/dmrr.3258

Chatzistergos, P. E., Naemi, R., Sundar, L., Ramachandran, A., and Chockalingam, N. (2014). The Relationship between the Mechanical Properties of Heel-Pad and Common Clinical Measures Associated with Foot Ulcers in Patients with Diabetes. *J. Diabetes Its Complications* 28 (4), 488–493. doi:10.1016/j.jdiacomp.2014.03.011

Claessen, H., Narres, M., Haastert, B., Arend, W., Hoffmann, F., Morbach, S., et al. (2018). Lower-extremity Amputations in People with and without Diabetes in Germany, 2008–2012 - an Analysis of More Than 30 Million inhabitants. *Clep* 10, 475–488. doi:10.2147/clep.S146484

Duan, Y., Ren, W., Xu, L., Ye, W., Jan, Y.-K., and Pu, F. (2021). The Effects of Different Accumulated Pressure-Time Integral Stimuli on Plantar Blood Flow in People with Diabetes Mellitus. *BMC Musculoskelet. Disord.* 22 (1)554. doi:10.1186/s12891-021-04437-9

Duckworth, T., Boulton, A., Betts, R., Franks, C., and Ward, J. (1985). Plantar Pressure Measurements and the Prevention of Ulceration in the Diabetic Foot. *The J. Bone Jt. Surg. Br. volume* 67 (1), 79–85. doi:10.1302/0301-620x.67b1.3968150

Gefen, A. (2003). Plantar Soft Tissue Loading under the Medial Metatarsals in the Standing Diabetic Foot. *Med. Eng. Phys.* 25 (6), 491–499. doi:10.1016/s1350-4533(03)00029-8

Gurney, J. K., Stanley, J., York, S., Rosenbaum, D., and Sarfati, D. (2018). Risk of Lower Limb Amputation in a National Prevalent Cohort of Patients with Diabetes. *Diabetologia* 61 (3), 626–635. doi:10.1007/s00125-017-4488-8

Halawa, M. R., Eid, Y. M., El-Hilaly, R. A., Abdelsalam, M. M., and Amer, A. H. (2018). Relationship of Planter Pressure and Glycemic Control in Type 2 Diabetic Patients with and without Neuropathy. *Diabetes Metab. Syndr. Clin. Res. Rev.* 12 (2), 99–104. doi:10.1016/j.dsx.2017.09.010

Helili, M., Geng, X., Ma, X., Chen, W., Zhang, C., Huang, J., et al. (2021). An Investigation of Regional Plantar Soft Tissue Hardness and its Potential Correlation with Plantar Pressure Distribution in Healthy Adults. *Appl. Bionics Biomech.* 2021, 1–9. doi:10.1155/2021/5566036

Jan, Y.-K., Lung, C.-W., Cuaderes, E., Rong, D., and Boyce, K. (2013). Effect of Viscoelastic Properties of Plantar Soft Tissues on Plantar Pressures at the First Metatarsal head in Diabetics with Peripheral Neuropathy. *Physiol. Meas.* 34 (1), 53–66. doi:10.1088/0967-3334/34/1/53

Jeong, H., Johnson, A. W., Feland, J. B., Petersen, S. R., Staten, J. M., and Bruening, D. A. (2021). Added Body Mass Alters Plantar Shear Stresses, Postural Control, and Gait Kinetics: Implications for Obesity. *Plos One* 16 (2), e0246605. doi:10.1371/journal.pone.0246605

Kernozek, T. W., Greany, J. F., and Heizler, C. (2013). Plantar Loading Asymmetry in American Indians with Diabetes and Peripheral Neuropathy, with Diabetes Only, and without Diabetes. *J. Am. Podiatr Med. Assoc.* 103 (2), 106–112. doi:10.7547/1030106

Klaesner, J. W., Hastings, M. K., Zou, D., Lewis, C., and Mueller, M. J. (2002). Plantar Tissue Stiffness in Patients with Diabetes Mellitus and Peripheral Neuropathy. *Arch. Phys. Med. Rehabil.* 83 (12), 1796–1801. doi:10.1053/apmr.2002.35661

Kluding, P. M., Bareiss, S. K., Hastings, M., Marcus, R. L., Sinacore, D. R., and Mueller, M. J. (2017). Physical Training and Activity in People with Diabetic Peripheral Neuropathy: Paradigm Shift. *Phys. Ther.* 97 (1), 31–43. doi:10.2522/ptj.20160124

LeMaster, J. W., Reiber, G. E., Smith, D. G., Heagerty, P. J., and Wallace, C. (2003). Daily Weight-Bearing Activity Does Not Increase the Risk of Diabetic Foot Ulcers. *Med. Sci. Sports Exerc.* 35 (7), 1093–1099. doi:10.1249/01.Mss.0000074459.41029.75

Monteiro-Soares, M., Boyko, E. J., Ribeiro, J., Ribeiro, I., and Dinis-Ribeiro, M. (2012). Predictive Factors for Diabetic Foot Ulceration: a Systematic Review. *Diabetes Metab. Res. Rev.* 28 (7), 574–600. doi:10.1002/dmrr.2319

Mueller, M. J., and Maluf, K. S. (2002). Tissue Adaptation to Physical Stress: A Proposed "physical Stress Theory" to Guide Physical Therapist Practice, Education, and Research. *Phys. Ther.* 82 (4), 383–403. doi:10.1093/ptj/82.4.383

Mueller, M. J., Tuttle, L. J., LeMaster, J. W., Strube, M. J., McGill, J. B., Hastings, M. K., et al. (2013). Weight-Bearing versus Nonweight-Bearing Exercise for Persons with Diabetes and Peripheral Neuropathy: A Randomized Controlled Trial. *Arch. Phys. Med. Rehabil.* 94 (5), 829–838. doi:10.1016/j.apmr.2012.12.015

Mynarski, W., Psurek, A., Borek, Z., Rozpara, M., Grabara, M., and Strojek, K. (2012). Declared and Real Physical Activity in Patients with Type 2 Diabetes Mellitus as Assessed by the International Physical Activity Questionnaire and Caltrac Accelerometer Monitor: A Potential Tool for Physical Activity Assessment in Patients with Type 2 Diabetes Mellitus. *Diabetes Res. Clin. Pract.* 98 (1), 46–50. doi:10.1016/j.diabres.2012.05.024

Otterman, N. M., van Schie, C. H. M., van der Schaaf, M., van Bon, A. C., Busch-Westbroek, T. E., and Nollet, F. (2011). An Exercise Programme for Patients with Diabetic Complications: a Study on Feasibility and Preliminary Effectiveness. *Diabetic Med.* 28 (2), 212–217. doi:10.1111/j.1464-5491.2010.03128.x

Patry, J., Belley, R., Cote, M., and Chateau-Degat, M.-L. (2013). Plantar Pressures, Plantar Forces, and Their Influence on the Pathogenesis of Diabetic Foot Ulcers. *J. Am. Podiatr Med. Assoc.* 103 (4), 322–332. doi:10.7547/1030322

Periyasamy, R., Anand, S., and Ammini, A. (2012a). Association of Limited Joint Mobility and Increased Plantar Hardness in Diabetic Foot Ulceration in north Asian Indian: A Preliminary Study. *Proc. Inst. Mech. Eng. H* 226 (4), 305–311. doi:10.1177/0954411911435613

Periyasamy, R., Anand, S., and Ammini, A. C. (2012b). Investigation of Shore Meter in Assessing Foot Sole Hardness in Patients with Diabetes Mellitus - a Pilot Study. *Int. J. Diabetes Dev. Ctries* 32 (3), 169–175. doi:10.1007/s13410-012-0085-z

Pirozzi, K., McGuire, J., and Meyr, A. J. (2014). Effect of Variable Body Mass on Plantar Foot Pressure and Off-Loading Device Efficacy. *J. Foot Ankle Surg.* 53 (5), 588–597. doi:10.1053/j.jfas.2014.02.005

Ramasamy, R., Vannucci, S. J., Yan, S. S. D., Herold, K., Yan, S. F., and Schmidt, A. M. (2005). Advanced Glycation End Products and RAGE: a Common Thread in Aging, Diabetes, Neurodegeneration, and Inflammation. *Glycobiology* 15 (7), 16R–28R. doi:10.1093/glycob/cwi053

Sacco, I. C. N., Hamamoto, A. N., Tonicelli, L. M. G., Watari, R., Ortega, N. R. S., and Sartor, C. D. (2014). Abnormalities of Plantar Pressure Distribution in Early, Intermediate, and Late Stages of Diabetic Neuropathy. *Gait & Posture* 40 (4), 570–574. doi:10.1016/j.gaitpost.2014.06.018

Simoneau, G. G., Ulbrecht, J. S., Derr, J. A., Becker, M. B., and Cavanagh, P. R. (1994). Postural Instability in Patients with Diabetic Sensory Neuropathy. *Diabetes care* 17 (12), 1411–1421. doi:10.2337/diacare.17.12.1411

Sun, J.-H., Cheng, B. K., Zheng, Y.-P., Huang, Y.-P., Leung, J. Y., and Cheing, G. L. (2011). Changes in the Thickness and Stiffness of Plantar Soft Tissues in People with Diabetic Peripheral Neuropathy. *Arch. Phys. Med. Rehabil.* 92 (9), 1484–1489. doi:10.1016/j.apmr.2011.03.015

Volmer-Thole, M., and Lobmann, R. (2016). Neuropathy and Diabetic Foot Syndrome. *Ijms* 17 (6), 917. doi:10.3390/ijms17060917

Wu, F.-L., Wang, W. T.-J., Liao, F., Elliott, J., Jain, S., and Jan, Y.-K. (2020). Effects of Walking Speeds and Durations on Plantar Skin Blood Flow Responses. *Microvasc. Res.* 128, 103936. doi:10.1016/j.mvr.2019.103936

Zhang, P., Lu, J., Jing, Y., Tang, S., Zhu, D., and Bi, Y. (2017). Global Epidemiology of Diabetic Foot Ulceration: a Systematic Review and Meta-Analysis. *Ann. Med.* 49 (2), 106–116. doi:10.1080/07853890.2016.1231932

7

A Systematic Review and Meta-Analysis of Clinical Effectiveness and Safety of Hydrogel Dressings in the Management of Skin Wounds

Lijun Zhang[1†], Hanxiao Yin[1†], Xun Lei[2], Johnson N. Y. Lau[3], Mingzhou Yuan[1], Xiaoyan Wang[1], Fangyingnan Zhang[1], Fei Zhou[1], Shaohai Qi[1], Bin Shu[1] and Jun Wu[1*]*

[1] Department of Burns, The First Affiliated Hospital, Sun Yat-sen University, Guangzhou, China, [2] School of Public Health and Management, Chongqing Medical University, Chongqing, China, [3] University of Hong Kong, Hong Kong Polytechnic University, Kowloon, China

***Correspondence:**
Bin Shu
shubin29@sina.com
Jun Wu
junwupro@126.com

† These authors have contributed equally to this work

The purpose of this systematic review and meta-analysis is to assess the clinical effectiveness and safety of the medical hydrogel dressings used in skin wounds and therefore to weight the evidence for their clinical application. PubMed/Medline (1980–2019), Cochrane Library (1980–2019), ClinicalTrials.gov, Cochrane CENTRAL, Chinese Journal Full-text Database (CNKI, 1994–2019), and China Biomedy Medicine disc (CBM, 1978–2019), Chinese Scientific Journal Database (VIP, 1989–2019), and Wanfang Database (WFDATA, 1980–2019) were searched to identify relevant clinical trials and studies. Forty-three studies that assessed hydrogel vs. non-hydrogel dressings were identified. Compared to the latter, hydrogel dressings associated with a significantly shortened healing time of degree II burn (superficial and deep) wounds, diabetic foot ulcers, traumatic skin injuries, radioactive skin injuries, dog bites, and body surface ulcers. In addition, hydrogel dressing obviously increased the cure rate of diabetic foot ulcers, surgical wounds, dog bites, and body surface ulcers. Moreover, hydrogel dressing significantly relieved pain in degree II burn (superficial and deep) wounds, traumatic skin injuries, and laser treatment-induced wounds. However, no significant differences obtained between hydrogel and non-hydrogel dressings in the healing time of surgical wounds, the cure rate of inpatients' pressure ulcers, and phlebitis ulcers. This comprehensive systematic review and meta-analysis of the available evidence reveals that the application of hydrogel dressings advances the healing of various wound types and effectively alleviates the pain with no severe adverse reactions. These results strongly indicate that hydrogel products are effective and safe in wound management.

Keywords: hydrogel, wound dressing, wound healing, pain relief, meta-analysis, systematic review

INTRODUCTION

Skin is the largest human organ as it reaches almost 10% of the total body mass (Grice et al., 2009) and acts as a key protective barrier against the outside environment. Normally, the human body heal skin injuries via a set of complex and interactive processes that include hemostasis, inflammation, proliferation, and remodeling. However, this healing process can be impaired by various local and systemic factors causing more severe complications and a lower quality of life (Nourian Dehkordi et al., 2019). Plenty of wound care products have been created and developed in the latest decades aimed at promoting wound healing and improving the life quality of the patients afflicted by skin wounds (Metcalfe and Ferguson, 2007; Gil et al., 2013; Chattopadhyay and Raines, 2014; Garg et al., 2015; Xu et al., 2015; Das and Baker, 2016). Therefore, surgeons must specifically select wound treatment products according to the factors impeding wounds healing.

Since the 1960s, wound dressing was considered to play a positive role in wound healing. Wound dressing could establish and maintain an environment apt for wound repair. Winter (1962) were the pioneers of this field by initiating the concept of functional active dressings. According to them, the ideal advanced wound dressing should provide and maintain a moist environment, adequate gaseous exchange, and thermal insulation in the absence of toxic contaminants; it should protect against secondary infections, induce tissue regeneration, relieve wound pain, and promote wound healing quality; finally, it should be elastic, non-antigenic, and allow to manage wound exudate (Purna and Babu, 2000). Considering all the just mentioned factors, hydrogel products have the capacity to act as promising candidates as wound dressings for applications in clinical settings (Qu et al., 2018).

In 1960, Wichterle and Lim prepared the first hydrogels by cross-linking 2-hydroxyethyl methacrylate, thus initiating the application and practice of hydrogels in the biomedical field (Wichterle and Lím, 1960). Hydrogels are extremely hydrophilic. Advanced hydrogel materials are environment-sensitive or stimuli-sensitive, as they start swelling under certain conditions and respond to definite stimuli (Qiu and Park, 2001). They can absorb exudate from the wound surface and promote fibroblast proliferation and cell migration and keratinization. In addition, hydrogels' dense meshes can prevent bacteria from invading the wound while effectively transporting bioactive molecules (such as antibacterial agents and drugs) to the wound surface (Mohan et al., 2007; Tsao et al., 2010; Schwartz et al., 2012; Mao et al., 2017). At the same time, the unique mechanical properties of hydrogels i.e., elasticity and flexibility, allow for their adaptation to different parts of the wound, making them suitable for both wound care and tissue engineering (Huang et al., 2015).

Being a novel category of wet dressings, hydrogel products have been gradually perfected in recent years. Their clinical application has become rather extensive, ranging from dry scab wounds to multiple treatments of skin ulcers, burn wounds, animal bites, bed sores, etc. (Sood et al., 2014). Medicinal hydrogel dressings are endowed with a three-dimensional (3D) crosslinked network structure, which contains three main components, a high-molecular weight compound, propylene glycol, and water. High-molecular weight compounds such as Carboxy Methyl Cellulose (CMC) can double the absorption of wound exudate and necrotic tissue fluid (Roy et al., 2010). Propylene glycol can kill bacteria and prevent bacterial proliferation. In turn, the water in hydrogel dressings can create a relatively moist environment that prevents the wound from drying up (Fan et al., 2014). Therefore, although necrotic tissues in the making go through a slow hydration, the hydrogel dressing ensures a strong absorption of wound exudate. Concurrently, it promotes the debridement of water-soluble materials and absorbs wound carrion to provide a localized moist environment advancing wound healing (Qu et al., 2018). Besides, hydrogels' micro-acidic and hypoxic environment can attract cells involved in wound repair, help inhibit bacterial growth, and promote neoangiogenesis at the wound site (Dong et al., 2016).

Managing wounds through the use of hydrogels has been an accepted practice for decades. At present, many forms of hydrogel and non-hydrogel products are available aimed at managing wounds caused by various injuries. However, the benefits of multiple options also entail many challenges to the clinicians. The purpose of this systematic review and meta-analysis is to assess the clinical effectiveness and safety of the medicinal hydrogel dressings in treating multiple skin wounds compared to non-hydrogel dressings in terms of wound healing time, wound cure rate, pain reduction, and incidence of adverse reactions.

METHODS

Systematic Review Eligibility Criteria

A systematic review was conducted according to the Preferred Reporting Items for Systematic Reviews and Meta-analyses (PRISMA) guidelines (Shamseer et al., 2015). It was based on the planned Participants, Intervention, Control, Outcome, and Study design (PICOS) elements outlined in **Table 1**.

Search Strategy

We sought to identify suitable studies by searching the following online databases: PubMed/Medline (1980–2019), Cochrane Library (1980–2019), ClinicalTrials.gov, Cochrane CENTRAL, Chinese Journal Full-text Database (CNKI, 1994–2019), and China Biomedy Medicine disc (CBM, 1978–2019), Chinese Scientific Journal Database (VIP, 1989–2019), and Wanfang Database (WFDATA, 1980–2019). With the combination of subject words and free words, the search terms included two categories: (1) "hydrogel," "polymeric hydrophilic compound," "guar gum," "guar bean," and "polyvinylpyrrolidone (PVP);" (2) "wound," "wound surface," and "burn." The logical relationship was created with "OR" and "AND," and the search formula was thereafter developed according to the characteristics of the different databases. The search strategy was improved through a pre-retrieval process. Meanwhile, unpublished studies and conference materials were manually searched, and references of the included literature were also tracked. No language limits were applied.

Abbreviations: GRADE, Grading of Recommendations Assessment, Development and Evaluation; PRISMA, Preferred Reporting Items for Systematic Reviews and Meta-Analyses; RCT, Randomized Controlled Trial; PICOS, Participants, Intervention, Control, Outcome and Study design; PVP, Polyvinylpyrrolidone; CMC, Carboxy Methyl Cellulose; EPOC, Effective Practice and Organization of Care Group; WMD, Weighted Mean Difference; SSD, Silver Sulphadiazine; VAS, Visual Analog Scale; SMSDAR, State Monitoring System of Drug Adverse Reactions; JW scale, Jun Wu scale.

TABLE 1 | Inclusion and exclusion criteria.

Criteria	Inclusion	Exclusion
Type of study	RCTs, quasi-RCTs, CCTs	Review, case study, mechanism study, research and development, preparation and storage of materials, animal experiment, marketing strategy, editorials, news, and registered clinical trials with unfinished/unreported results.
Participants	Patients with skin wounds provoked by various causes (e.g., burns, surgery, body surface ulcers, etc.).	Patients with deep burns (degrees III and IV), treatment for bone wounds, pre-operation preparation, patients using biological tissue synthesis substitutes, and patients with autologous skin cultured transplants.
Interventions	Various types of hydrogel dressings [polymeric hydrophilic compounds such as guar gum and Lengningkang[a] (Wound Caring)].	The hydrogel is used as a non-wound dressing such as an *in vivo* drug release carrier, contact lens, tissue filling material, medical sensor, etc.
Control	Any other dressing, treatment, placebo, or blank control.	Comparison of functions before and after using hydrogel dressings or comparison between different hydrogels.
Outcomes	Effective indicators including wound healing time, wound healing rate, pain score, pain level, etc. Safety indicators referring to the incidence rate of adverse reactions including skin allergy, skin dryness, tight skin, pruritus, and fever.	Long-term follow-up results such as quality of life.

[a] *The commercial name of a hydrogel dressing.*

Study Selection

Two reviewers carried out the preliminary screening by independently reading titles and abstracts to exclude literature that obviously did not conform with the inclusion criteria. As a further screening they read the full texts of the literature that might meet the inclusion criteria. When the two researchers' opinions differed, they consulted and discussed with a third researcher to reach a final decision. During the full-text screening, the information below would be extracted: authors, date of publication, study type, subject characteristics, sample number, loss to or withdrawal from follow-up, intervention measures, and measuring indicators, etc. In case of multiple studies in a single published work, data based on study contents would be extracted as needed. With regard to repeatedly reported studies, only the latest or the most comprehensive one was included.

Quality Evaluation

The quality of the methodology employed by the included studies was evaluated according to the Effective Practice and Organization of Care Group (EPOC) improved scoring standard recommended by The Cochrane Collaboration. The evaluation package included randomization methods, allocation concealment, blinding use, control of loss to follow-up, baseline information, outcome data, etc. Scores of 5–6 were classified as grade A, 2–4 as grade B, and 0–1 as grade C.

Meta-Analysis

Meta-analysis was carried out by using the RevMan5.0 software recommended by The Cochrane Collaboration. Subgroups were divided according to patient (wound) types and types of outcome variables. The relative risk (RR) was taken as the combined effect size for categorical data, while the weighted mean difference (WMD) as the combined effect size for measuring data. Each effect size was shown as 95% CI. The heterogeneity of the study results was tested by χ^2 test. When studies showed a statistical homogeneity ($P > 0.1$, $I^2 < 50\%$), a fixed-effect model would be used; otherwise, a random effect model was adopted. For subgroups containing a single study, description, and comparative analysis would be conducted on their results.

RESULTS

Study Selection and Characteristics

One thousand four hundred and seventy three studies were selected by the preliminary screening. Only 43 studies were kept after screening titles, abstracts, and full-texts (**Figure 1**), including 29 randomized controlled trials (RCTs) and 14 clinical controlled trials (CCTs) with a total of 3,521 patients. The basic characteristics of the included studies and the results of methodological quality evaluations are shown in **Table 2**. In all studies, patients' basic situations were comparable between intervention groups and control groups ($P > 0.05$).

Data Synthesis

Healing Times Comparison of Degree-II Superficial and Deep Burn Wounds

Eleven studies, reported by Cui et al. (2007), Jiang et al. (2008), Gong et al. (2009), Jin et al. (2009), Wang et al. (2011), Diao et al. (2012), Liu and Ye (2014), Liu (2015), Jin et al. (2017), Li and Wu (2018), Lin et al. (2018), compared the healing times of degree-II superficial burn wounds treated with hydrogel dressings or other treatments. There existed a statistical heterogeneity among the study results ($P < 0.0001$, $I^2 = 76\%$). Therefore, the random effect model was applied for meta-synthesis (**Figure 2A**). The results showed that on average the wound healing time of the hydrogel dressings group was shortened by 2.87 days as compared with the control group and that the difference had a high statistical significance (MD = −2.87, 95% CI: −3.35 to −2.38, $P < 0.00001$).

Twelve studies, reported by Cui et al. (2007), Jiang et al. (2008), Gong et al. (2009), Jin et al. (2009), Cai et al. (2010), Wang

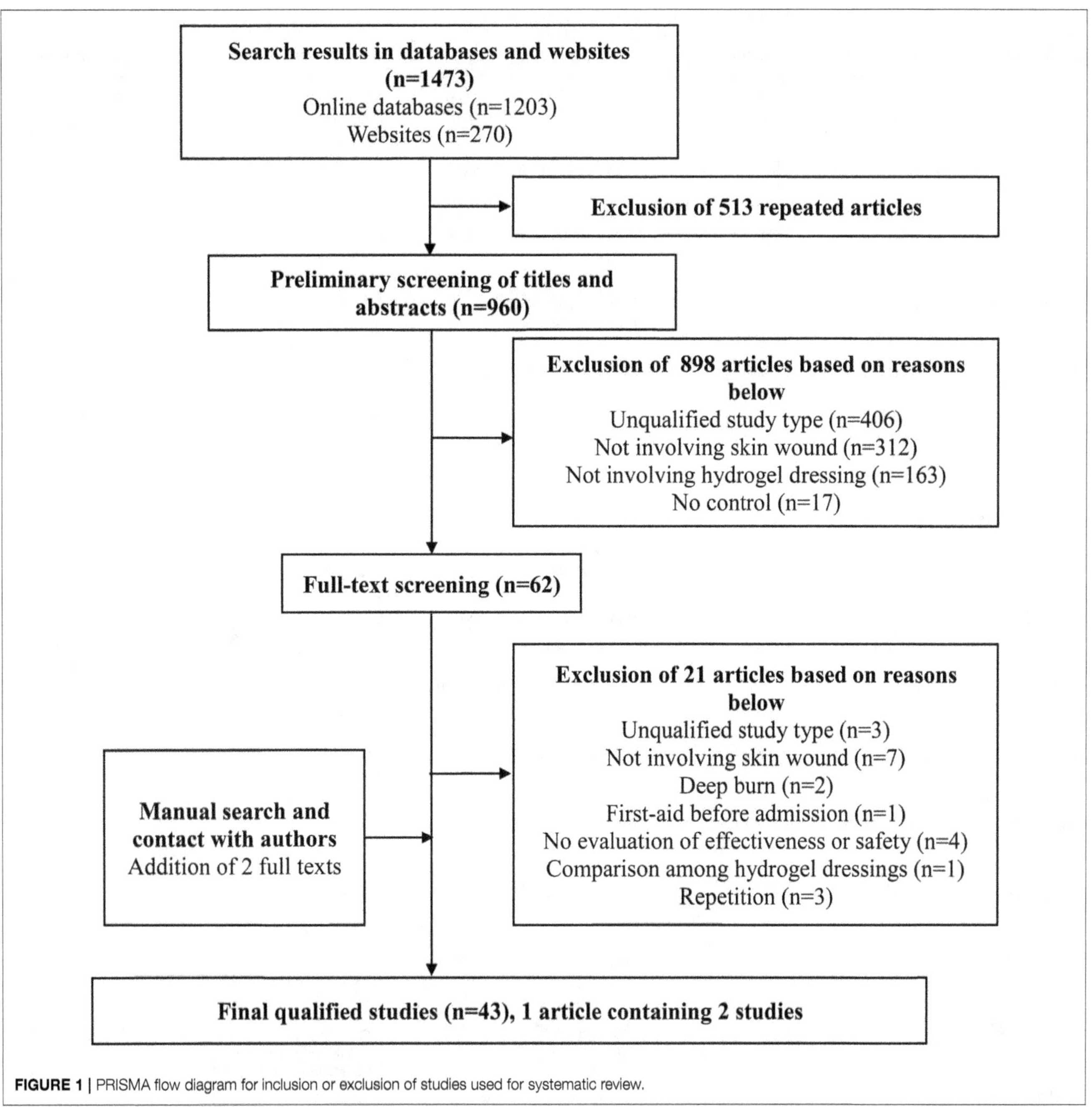

FIGURE 1 | PRISMA flow diagram for inclusion or exclusion of studies used for systematic review.

et al. (2011), Wang et al. (2013), Liu and Ye (2014), Lan and Duan (2015), Liu (2015), Shang (2015), and Jin et al. (2017), compared the healing times of degree-II deep burn wounds treated with hydrogel dressings or other therapeutics. There existed a statistical heterogeneity among the study results ($P < 0.00001$, $I^2 = 83\%$). Hence, the random effect model was applied for meta-synthesis (**Figure 2B**). The results revealed that on average the wound healing time of the hydrogel dressings group was shortened by 5.04 days as compared with the control group and that statistically this difference was highly significant (MD = −5.04, 95% CI: −5.81 to −4.26, $P < 0.00001$).

WHO Pain Ratings of Burn Wounds

Five studies, reported by Jiang et al. (2008), Jin et al. (2009), Wang et al. (2011), Jin et al. (2017), and Li and Wu (2018), compared the pain ratings difference of burn wounds after treatment with hydrogel dressings or other therapeutic means. There occurred no statistical heterogeneity among the study results ($P = 0.57$). Consequently, the fixed effect model was applied for meta-synthesis (**Figure 3**). The results brought to light that patients suffering either grade 0 or grade I pain accounted for a higher proportion among those treated with hydrogel dressings and that statistically the

TABLE 2 | Characteristics of the studies employing hydrogel dressings vs. non-hydrogel dressings.

References	Study design	Country	Participants	Sample size	Quality level
Cai et al., 2010	CCT	China	Degree-II deep burn wounds	60 patients Chitosan hydrogel = 30 SSD = 30	B
Jiang et al., 2008	RCT	China	degree-II superficial and deep burn wounds	90 patients Hydrogel = 45 SSD = 45	B
Wang et al., 2011	RCT	China	Degree-II superficial and deep burn wounds	560 patients Hydrogel with silver = 280 SSD = 280	B
Jin et al., 2009	CCT	China	Degree-II superficial and deep burn wounds	72 patients Hydrogel = 42 Iodine solution = 30	B
Wang et al., 2013	RCT	China	Degree-II burn wounds	76 patients Hydrogel = 38 Entoiodine and petrolatum gauze = 38	B
Liu, 2015	CCT	China	Degree-II superficial and deep burn wounds	120 patients Hydrogel and Lithosin solution = 60 Lithosin solution = 60	B
Jin et al., 2017	CCT	China	Degree-II superficial and deep burn wounds	92 patients Hydrogel = 48 SSD = 44	B
Diao et al., 2012	RCT	China	Degree-II superficial burn wounds	60 patients Hydrogel with silver = 30 SSD = 30	A
Lin et al., 2018	RCT	China	Degree-II superficial burn wounds	66 patients Hydrogel with silver = 33 SSD = 33	B
Liu and Ye, 2014	RCT	China	Degree-II superficial and deep burn wounds	80 patients Hydrogel = 40 Lithosin oil = 40	A
Shang, 2015	RCT	China	Degree-II deep burn wounds	68 patients Hydrogel = 34 Petrolatum gauze = 34	B
Li and Wu, 2018	CCT	China	Degree-II superficial and deep burn wounds	120 patients Hydrogel = 60 SD-Zn = 60	B
Lan and Duan, 2015	RCT	China	Degree-II deep burn wounds	60 patients Hydrogel with silver = 30 MEBO = 30	B
Gong et al., 2009	RCT	China	Degree-II superficial and deep burn wounds	104 patients Hydrogel with silver = 52 SSD and petrolatum gauze = 52	B
Cui et al., 2007	RCT	China	Degree-II superficial and deep burn wounds	44 patients Hydrogel = 22 SSD and Petrolatum gauze = 22	B
Xiang et al., 2012	CCT	China	Non-gangrenous diabetic foot ulcers	86 patients Alginate hydrogel with silver = 43 Polyvidone iodine = 43	B
Liu et al., 2017	RCT	China	Diabetic foot ulcers	30 patients Hydrogel = 15 Gentamicin dressing = 15	B
Teng, 2010	RCT	China	Diabetic foot ulcers	43 patients Hydrogel with silver = 23 Petrolatum gauze = 20	B

(Continued)

TABLE 2 | Continued

References	Study design	Country	Participants	Sample size	Quality level
Shao et al., 2015	CCT	China	Diabetic foot ulcers	78 patients Hydrogel = 39 Glauber and Lidocaine hydrochloride = 39	B
Li et al., 2015	CCT	China	Diabetic foot ulcers	40 patients Hydrogel = 20 Iodophor oil and gauze = 20	B
Nie et al., 2015	RCT	China	Diabetic foot ulcers	65 patients Hydrogel with silver = 34 Petrolatum gauze = 31	B
Wang et al., 2008	RCT	China	Diabetic foot ulcers	43 patients Hydrogel with silver = 23 Petrolatum gauze = 20	A
Mao, 2010	RCT	China	Diabetic foot ulcers	44 patients Hydrogel with silver = 22 Silver dressing = 22	B
Zhang et al., 2012	RCT	China	Diabetic foot ulcers	126 patients Hydrogel with silver = 63 Silver dressing = 63	B
Chen et al., 2015	CCT	China	Diabetic foot ulcers	66 patients Hydrogel with silver = 33 Saline and petrolatum gauze = 33	B
D'Hemecourt et al., 1998	RCT	USA	Diabetic foot ulcers	138 patients Hydrogel = 70 Non-hydrogel = 68	A
Jensen et al., 1998	RCT	USA	Diabetic foot ulcers	31 patients Hydrogel = 14 Non-hydrogel = 17	B
Vandeputte and Gryson, 1997	RCT	Belgium	Diabetic foot ulcers	31 patients Hydrogel = 14 Non-hydrogel = 17	B
Huang et al., 2017	CCT	China	Pressure ulcers	45 patients Hydrogel = 23 Iodine and gauze = 22	B
Wen, 2015	RCT	China	Pressure ulcers	40 patients Hydrogel = 20 Betadine ointment = 20	B
Jiang et al., 2018	RCT	China	Radioactive skin injuries	108 patients Hydrogel = 54 Gauze = 54	B
Hu et al., 2015	RCT	China	Radioactive skin injuries	76 patients Hydrogel = 32 Gauze = 44	B
Shi et al., 2016	CCT	China	Phlebitis patients	73 patients Hydrogel = 38 Magnesium sulfate solution = 35	B
He et al., 2008	RCT	China	Phlebitis patients	60 patients Hydrogel = 30 Saline gauze = 30	B
Huang et al., 2016	RCT	China	Traumatic skin injuries	42 patients Hydrogel = 21 Multi-source therapy device = 21	B
Chen et al., 2015	CCT	China	Traumatic skin injuries	66 patients Hydrogel with silver = 35 Multi-source therapy device = 31	B
Zeng and Li, 2016	RCT	China	Traumatic skin injuries	44 patients Hydrogel = 22 Myogenic silicone = 22	A

(Continued)

TABLE 2 | Continued

References	Study design	Country	Participants	Sample size	Quality level
Zeng and Li, 2016	RCT	China	Traumatic skin injuries	44 patients Hydrogel = 22 Myogenic cream and gauze = 22	A
Lu et al., 2017	CCT	China	Surgical wounds	62 patients Hydrogel with silver = 31 Gauze = 31	B
Fan et al., 2013	RCT	China	Surgical wounds	100 patients Hydrogel with silver = 42 Gauze = 58	A
Wang et al., 2008	RCT	China	Canine bites	40 patients Hydrogel with silver = 20 Saline and gauze = 20	A
Fang et al., 2011	CCT	China	Body surface ulcers	72 patients Hydrogel with silver = 36 Iodine, hydrogen peroxide, and petrolatum gauze = 36	B
Fan et al., 2014	RCT	China	Laser treatments	200 patients Hydrogel = 100 Non-hydrogel = 100	B

difference was highly significant (OR = 4.93, 95% CI: 4.06–5.98, $P < 0.00001$).

VAS Pain Scores of Degree-II Superficial and Deep Burn Wounds

Four studies, reported by Diao et al. (2012), Liu and Ye (2014), Liu (2015), and Lin et al. (2018), compared visual analog scale (VAS) pain scores of the burn wounds treated with hydrogel dressings or other therapeutics. There occurred a statistical heterogeneity among the study results ($P < 0.00001$, $I^2 = 87\%$). Accordingly, the random effect model was applied for meta-synthesis (**Figure 4A**). The results showed that on average the VAS score of the hydrogel dressings group was 3.31 points lower than the control group, and that the difference had a high statistical significance (MD = −3.31, 95% CI: −4.16 to −2.46, $P < 0.00001$).

Four studies, reported by Liu and Ye (2014), Lan and Duan (2015), Liu (2015), and Shang (2015), compared VAS pain scores of burn wounds treated with hydrogel dressings or other medicaments. A statistical heterogeneity turned up among the study results ($P < 0.00001$, $I^2 = 98\%$). For that reason, the random effect model was applied for meta-synthesis (**Figure 4B**). The results made clear that on average the VAS score of the hydrogel dressings group was 2.74 points lower than that of the control group and that the difference was statistically significant (MD = −2.74, 95% CI: −4.74 ∼ −0.74, $P = 0.007$).

Wound Healing Times of Diabetic Foot Ulcers

Seven studies, reported by Wang et al. (2008), Mao (2010), Teng (2010), Xiang et al. (2012), Zhang et al. (2012), Chen (2015), and Nie et al. (2015), compared the healing times of diabetic foot ulcer wounds treated with hydrogel dressing or other ministrations. There occurred a statistical heterogeneity among the study results ($P < 0.00001$, $I^2 = 99\%$). Therefore, the random effect model was applied for meta-synthesis (**Figure 5**). The results made plain that on average the healing time of the hydrogel dressings group was 7.28 days shorter than that of the control group and that the difference had a high statistical significance (MD = −7.28, 95% CI: −11.01 to −3.55, $P < 0.0001$).

Wound Cure Rates of Diabetic Foot Ulcers

Nine studies, reported by Vandeputte and Gryson (1997), D'Hemecourt et al. (1998), Jensen et al. (1998), Xiang et al. (2012), Zhang et al. (2012), Chen (2015), Li et al. (2015), Shao et al. (2015), and Liu et al. (2017), compared the wound cure rates of diabetic foot ulcers treated with hydrogel dressing or other therapeutics. There existed a statistical heterogeneity among the study results ($P = 0.002$, $I^2 = 67\%$). Hence, the random effect model was applied for meta-synthesis (**Figure 6**). The results proved that the cure rate of diabetic foot ulcers was higher in the hydrogel dressings group than in the control group and that the difference was statistically significant (RR = 1.57, 95% CI: 1.13–2.17, $P = 0.007$).

Healing Times of Traumatic Skin Injuries

Four studies, reported by Chen et al. (2015), Huang et al. (2016), and Zeng and Li (2016), compared the healing times of traumatic skin injuries treated with hydrogel dressings or other therapeutics. There occurred a statistical heterogeneity among the study results ($P < 0.00001$, $I^2 = 97\%$). Consequently, the random effect model was applied for meta-synthesis (**Figure 7**). The results revealed that on average the healing time of traumatic skin injuries was 5.28 days shorter in the hydrogel dressing group than in the control group and that the difference reached statistical significance (MD = −5.28, 95% CI: −10.49 to −0.07, $P = 0.05$).

WHO Pain Ratings of Traumatic Skin Injuries

Two studies, reported by Chen et al. (2015) and Huang et al. (2016), compared the WHO pain ratings difference

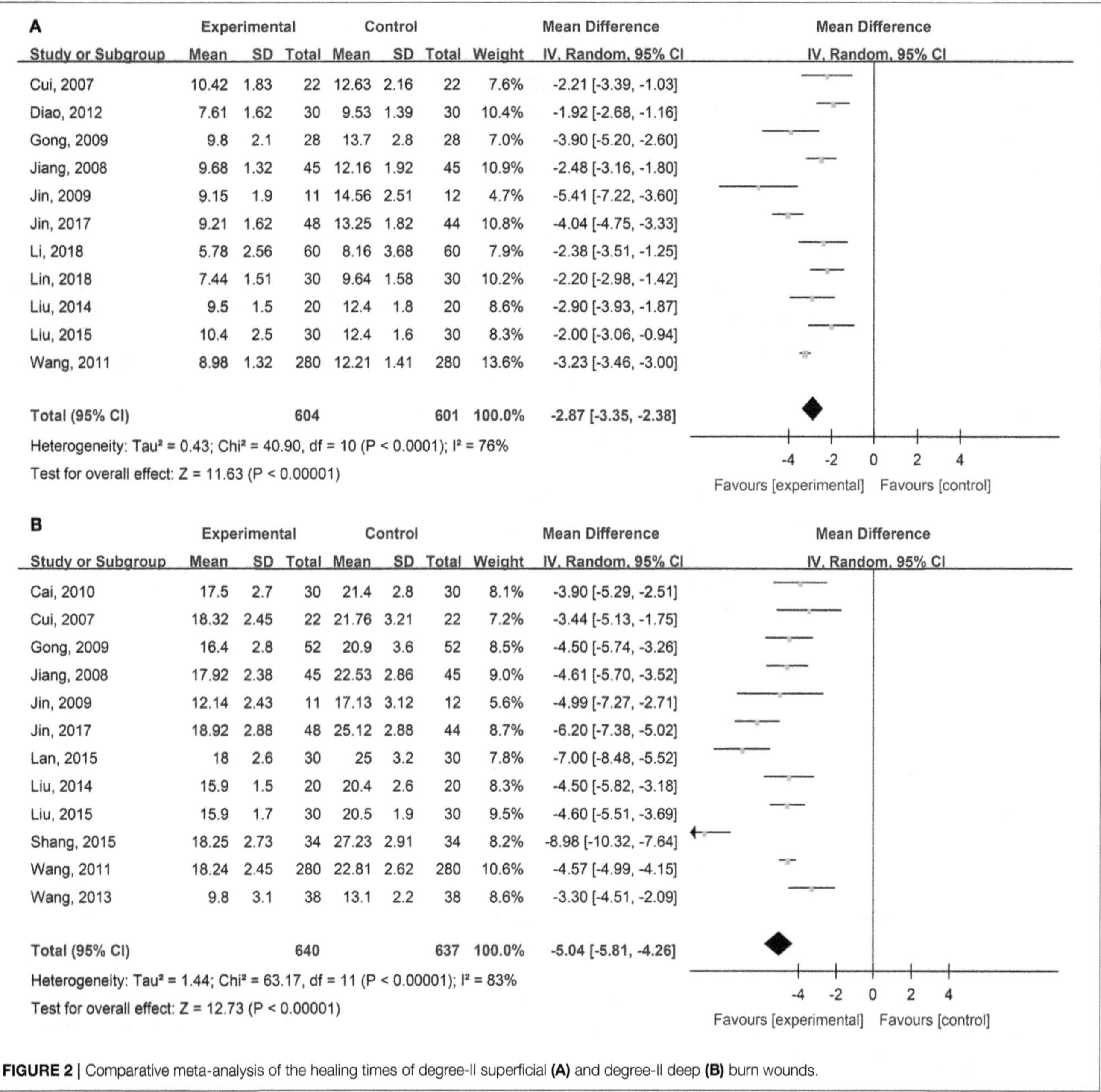

FIGURE 2 | Comparative meta-analysis of the healing times of degree-II superficial **(A)** and degree-II deep **(B)** burn wounds.

after treatment with hydrogel dressings or other therapeutic interventions. There existed no statistical heterogeneity among the study results ($P = 0.63$). In consequence, the fixed effect model was applied for meta-synthesis (**Figure 8**). The results disclosed that patients suffering grade-0 and grade-I pain accounted for a higher proportion than the control group did and that the difference was statistically significant (RR = 25.70, 95% CI: 3.33–198.43, $P = 0.002$).

Healing Times and Cure Rates of Surgical Wounds

Two studies, reported by Fan et al. (2013) and Lu et al. (2017), compared the healing times of surgical wounds treated with hydrogel dressing or other ministrations. There existed a statistical heterogeneity among the study results ($P < 0.00001$, $I^2 = 98\%$). Therefore, the random effect model was applied for meta-synthesis (**Figure 9A**). The results showed that as the healing time of surgical wounds was concerned no statistically significant difference ($P = 0.28$) intervened between the hydrogel dressings group and the control group.

Two studies, reported by Fan et al. (2013) and Lu et al. (2017), compared the cure rates of surgical wounds medicated with hydrogel dressing or other treatments. There existed no statistical heterogeneity among the study results ($P = 0.08$). Consequently, the fixed effect model was applied for meta-synthesis (**Figure 9B**). The results demonstrated that the cure rate of surgical wounds in the hydrogel dressings group was 20.85% higher than in the

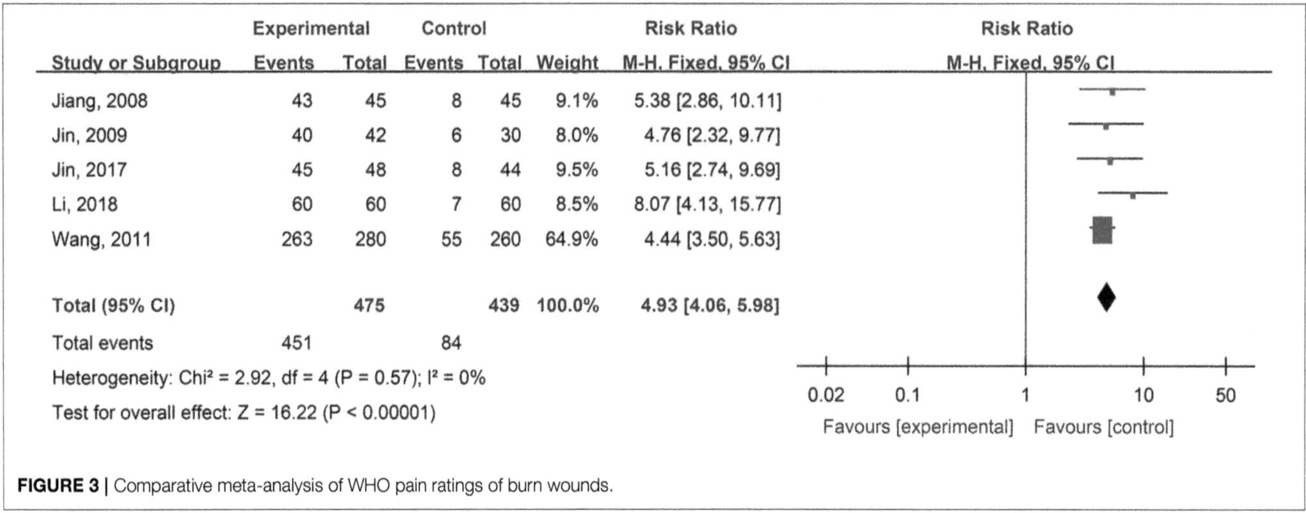

FIGURE 3 | Comparative meta-analysis of WHO pain ratings of burn wounds.

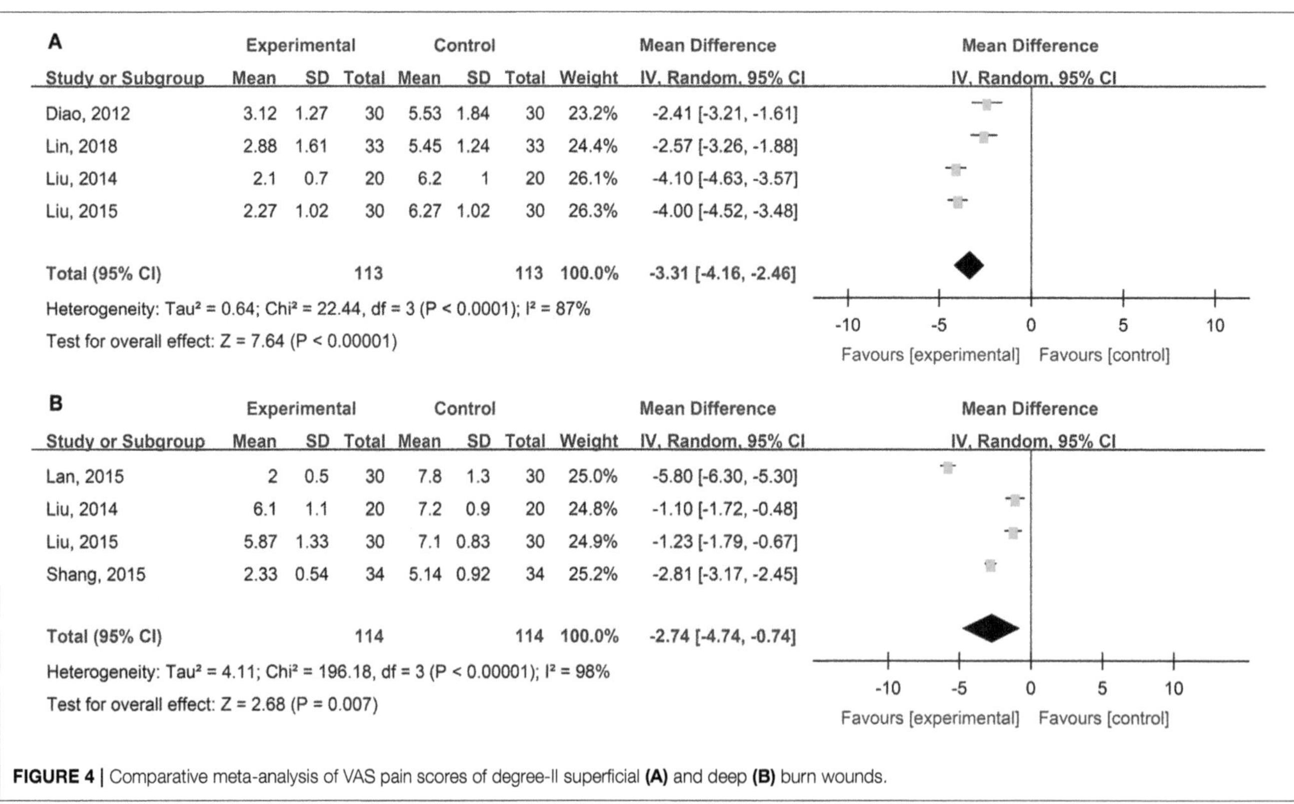

FIGURE 4 | Comparative meta-analysis of VAS pain scores of degree-II superficial **(A)** and deep **(B)** burn wounds.

control group and that statistically the difference was highly significant (MD = 20.85%, 95% CI: 20.04–21.65%, $P < 0.00001$).

The Cure Rates of Inpatients' Pressure Ulcers

Two studies, reported by Wen (2015) and Huang et al. (2017), compared the cure rates of inpatients' pressure ulcers treated with hydrogel dressings or other therapeutic means. There existed a statistical heterogeneity among the study results ($P = 0.002$, $I^2 = 81\%$). Hence, the random effect model was applied for meta-synthesis (**Figure 10**). The results revealed that there occurred no statistically significant difference between the hydrogel dressing group and the control group ($P = 0.08$) in the cure rate of inpatients' pressure ulcers.

Healing Times of Radioactive Skin Injuries

Two studies, reported by Hu et al. (2015) and Jiang et al. (2018), compared the healing times of radioactive skin injuries treated with hydrogel dressings or other medicaments. There occurred no statistical heterogeneity among the study results ($P = 0.95$). In consequence, the fixed effect model was applied for meta-synthesis (**Figure 11**). The results demonstrated that on average the healing time of the hydrogel dressings group

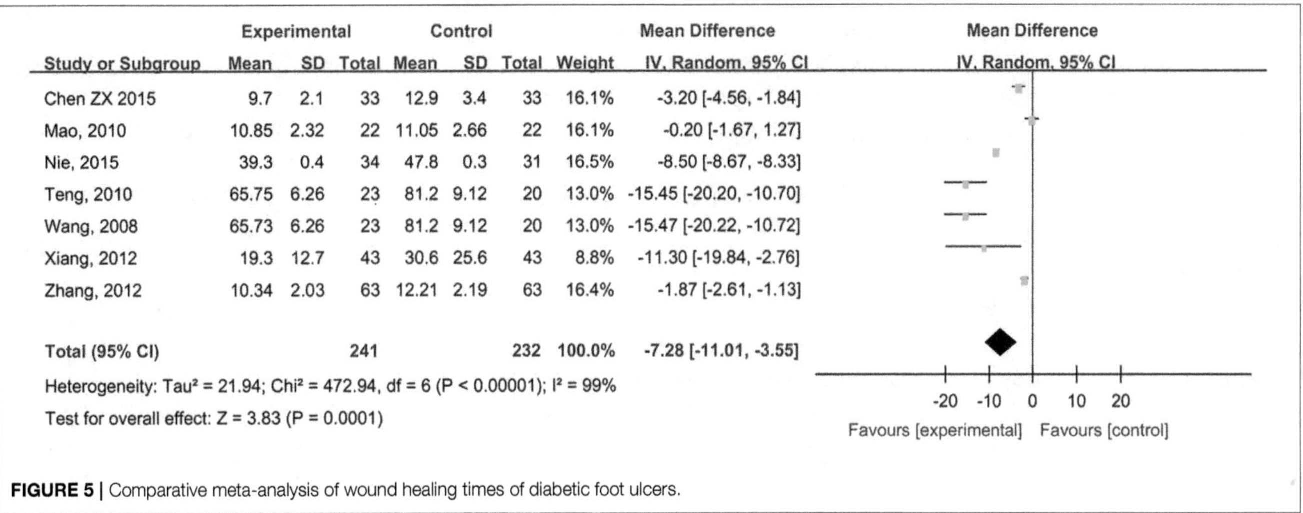

Study or Subgroup	Experimental Mean	Experimental SD	Experimental Total	Control Mean	Control SD	Control Total	Weight	Mean Difference IV, Random, 95% CI
Chen ZX 2015	9.7	2.1	33	12.9	3.4	33	16.1%	-3.20 [-4.56, -1.84]
Mao, 2010	10.85	2.32	22	11.05	2.66	22	16.1%	-0.20 [-1.67, 1.27]
Nie, 2015	39.3	0.4	34	47.8	0.3	31	16.5%	-8.50 [-8.67, -8.33]
Teng, 2010	65.75	6.26	23	81.2	9.12	20	13.0%	-15.45 [-20.20, -10.70]
Wang, 2008	65.73	6.26	23	81.2	9.12	20	13.0%	-15.47 [-20.22, -10.72]
Xiang, 2012	19.3	12.7	43	30.6	25.6	43	8.8%	-11.30 [-19.84, -2.76]
Zhang, 2012	10.34	2.03	63	12.21	2.19	63	16.4%	-1.87 [-2.61, -1.13]
Total (95% CI)			**241**			**232**	**100.0%**	**-7.28 [-11.01, -3.55]**

Heterogeneity: Tau² = 21.94; Chi² = 472.94, df = 6 (P < 0.00001); I² = 99%

Test for overall effect: Z = 3.83 (P = 0.0001)

FIGURE 5 | Comparative meta-analysis of wound healing times of diabetic foot ulcers.

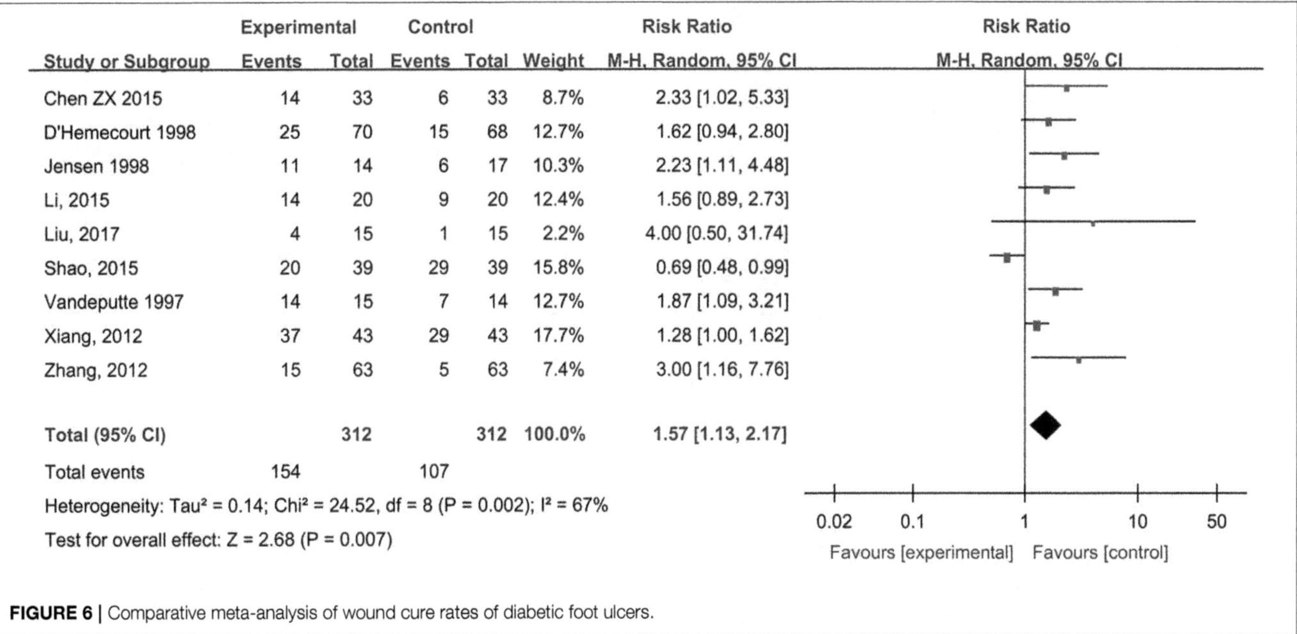

Study or Subgroup	Experimental Events	Experimental Total	Control Events	Control Total	Weight	Risk Ratio M-H, Random, 95% CI
Chen ZX 2015	14	33	6	33	8.7%	2.33 [1.02, 5.33]
D'Hemecourt 1998	25	70	15	68	12.7%	1.62 [0.94, 2.80]
Jensen 1998	11	14	6	17	10.3%	2.23 [1.11, 4.48]
Li, 2015	14	20	9	20	12.4%	1.56 [0.89, 2.73]
Liu, 2017	4	15	1	15	2.2%	4.00 [0.50, 31.74]
Shao, 2015	20	39	29	39	15.8%	0.69 [0.48, 0.99]
Vandeputte 1997	14	15	7	14	12.7%	1.87 [1.09, 3.21]
Xiang, 2012	37	43	29	43	17.7%	1.28 [1.00, 1.62]
Zhang, 2012	15	63	5	63	7.4%	3.00 [1.16, 7.76]
Total (95% CI)		**312**		**312**	**100.0%**	**1.57 [1.13, 2.17]**
Total events	154		107			

Heterogeneity: Tau² = 0.14; Chi² = 24.52, df = 8 (P = 0.002); I² = 67%

Test for overall effect: Z = 2.68 (P = 0.007)

FIGURE 6 | Comparative meta-analysis of wound cure rates of diabetic foot ulcers.

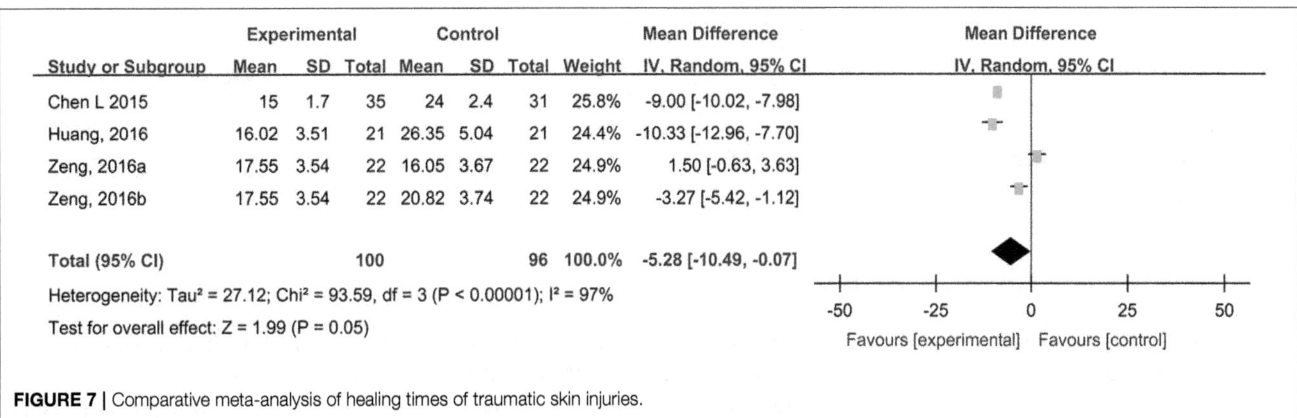

Study or Subgroup	Experimental Mean	Experimental SD	Experimental Total	Control Mean	Control SD	Control Total	Weight	Mean Difference IV, Random, 95% CI
Chen L 2015	15	1.7	35	24	2.4	31	25.8%	-9.00 [-10.02, -7.98]
Huang, 2016	16.02	3.51	21	26.35	5.04	21	24.4%	-10.33 [-12.96, -7.70]
Zeng, 2016a	17.55	3.54	22	16.05	3.67	22	24.9%	1.50 [-0.63, 3.63]
Zeng, 2016b	17.55	3.54	22	20.82	3.74	22	24.9%	-3.27 [-5.42, -1.12]
Total (95% CI)			**100**			**96**	**100.0%**	**-5.28 [-10.49, -0.07]**

Heterogeneity: Tau² = 27.12; Chi² = 93.59, df = 3 (P < 0.00001); I² = 97%

Test for overall effect: Z = 1.99 (P = 0.05)

FIGURE 7 | Comparative meta-analysis of healing times of traumatic skin injuries.

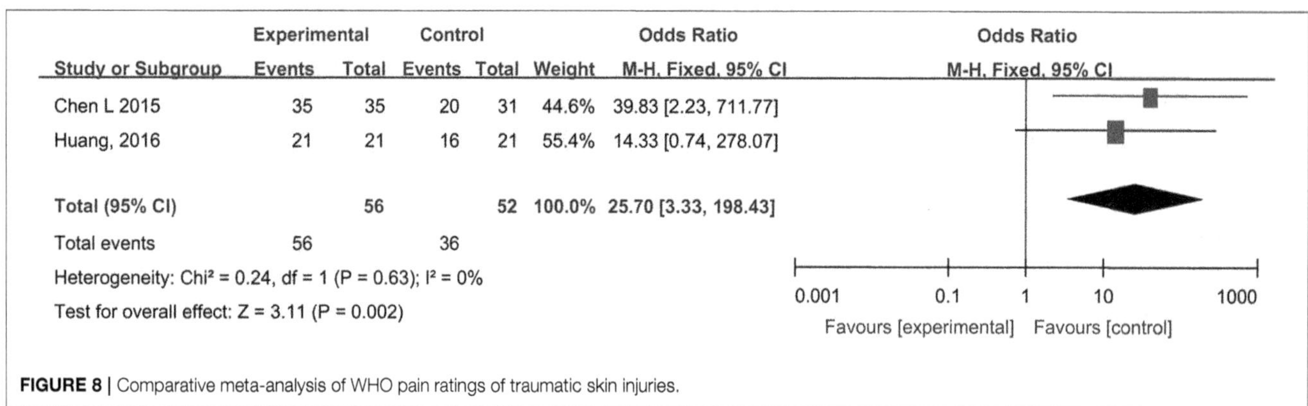

FIGURE 8 | Comparative meta-analysis of WHO pain ratings of traumatic skin injuries.

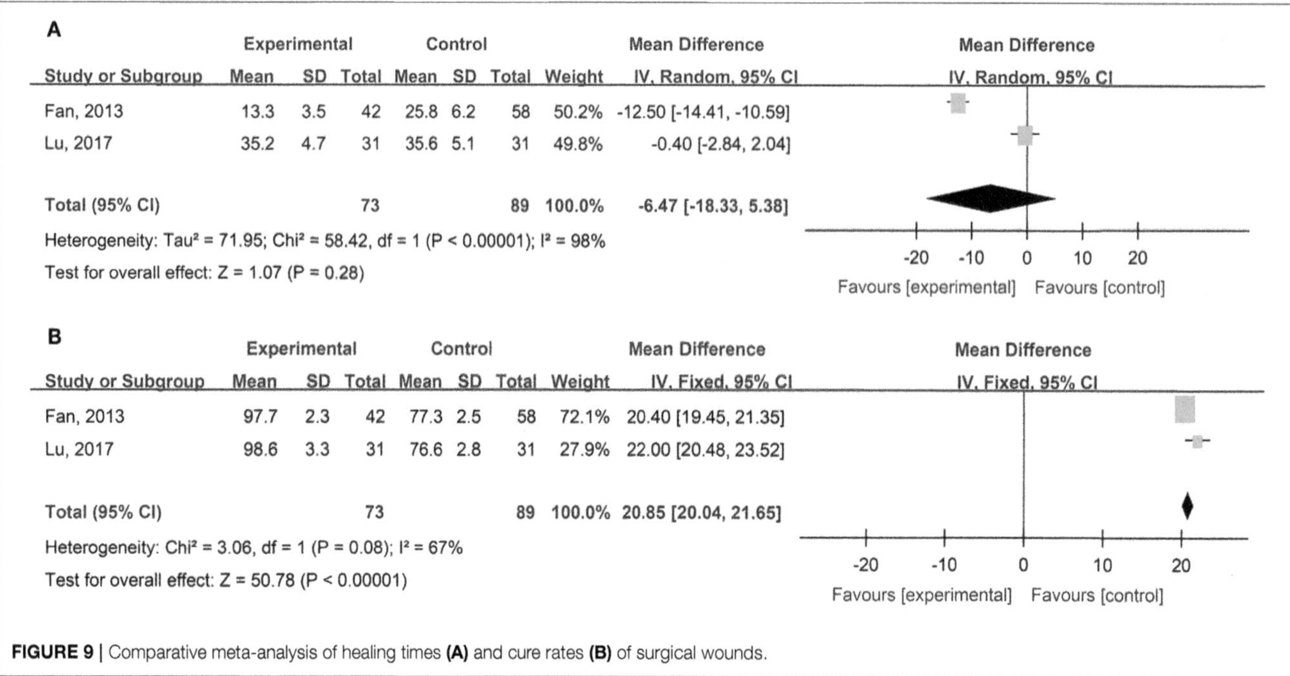

FIGURE 9 | Comparative meta-analysis of healing times **(A)** and cure rates **(B)** of surgical wounds.

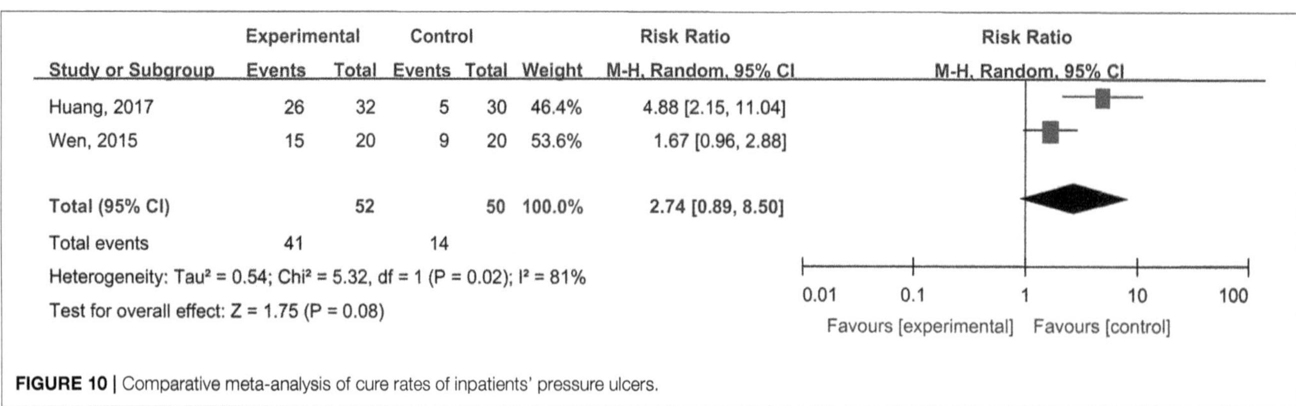

FIGURE 10 | Comparative meta-analysis of cure rates of inpatients' pressure ulcers.

was shortened by 9.46 days as compared with that of the control group and that the difference had a high statistical significance (MD = −9.46, 95% CI: −10.90 to −8.01, $P < 0.00001$).

The Cure Rates of Phlebitis Ulcers (Cure and Effectiveness)

Two studies, reported by He et al. (2008) and Shi et al. (2016), compared the cure rates of phlebitis ulcers treated with hydrogel

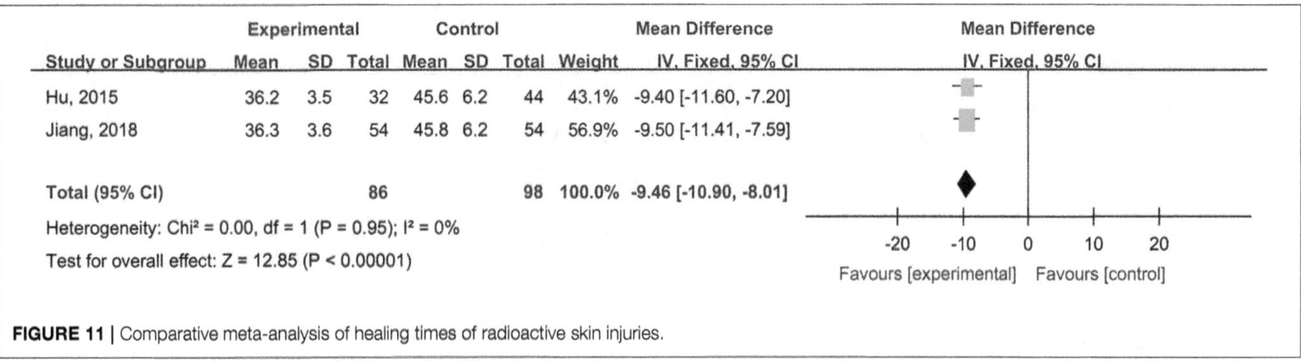

FIGURE 11 | Comparative meta-analysis of healing times of radioactive skin injuries.

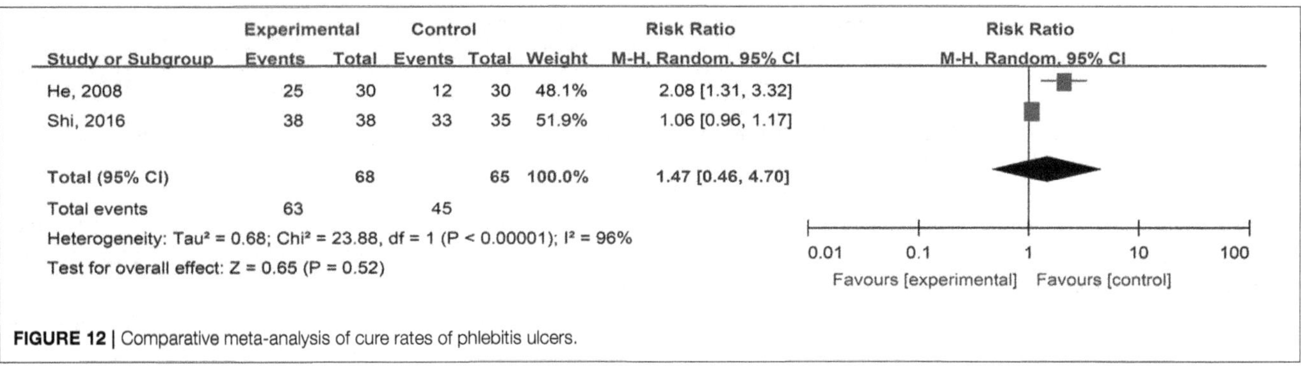

FIGURE 12 | Comparative meta-analysis of cure rates of phlebitis ulcers.

dressings and other ministrations. There existed a statistical heterogeneity among the study results ($P < 0.00001$, $I^2 = 96\%$). Consequently, the random effect model was applied for meta-synthesis (**Figure 12**). The results indicated that the difference in cure rates between the hydrogel dressings group and the control group of patients with phlebitis ulcers was not statistically significant ($P = 0.52$).

Dog Bite Wounds, Body Surface Ulcers, and Laser Treatment-Induced Wounds

Only one study, reported by Wang and Teng (2008), compared the cure rates of dog bite wounds treated with hydrogel dressings or saline gauze. The results made known that the healing time of the hydrogel dressings group was 4.0 days shorter than that of controls ($t = -16.54$, $P < 0.001$); in addition, the average cure rate of the wounds was 24.8% higher ($t = 27.8$, $P < 0.001$) than the controls.

Then again, a single study, reported by Fang et al. (2011), compared the cure rates of body surface ulcers treated with hydrogel dressings or conventional therapy with Iodophor or hydrogen peroxide plus Vaseline gauze. The results revealed that the healing time of the hydrogel dressings group was 18.4 days shorter than that of the controls ($t = -5.29$, $P < 0.001$); moreover, the total wound cure rate was also significantly higher than that of the control group ($\chi^2 = 13.78$, $P < 0.001$).

Finally, a lone study, reported by Xin et al. (2014), compared the wound care of patients categorized as hydrogel dressings group and blank control group bearing laser treatment-induced wounds. Concerning VAS scores, as contrasted with the blank control group, the pain score of the hydrogel dressings group was 1.63 lower ($t = -6.47$, $P < 0.001$), the burning sensation score was 1.10 lower ($t = -8.65$, $P < 0.001$) and the stimulating sensation score was 1.46 lower ($t = -10.78$, $P < 0.001$) than the controls.

Data Set of Complaints and Adverse Events

Data Source

Besides the mentioned above Chinese and English databases, a supplementary search was carried out in the State Monitoring System of Drug Adverse Reactions (SMSDAR; http://www.adrs.org.cn/).

Data Synthesis and Analysis

To perform Meta-analyses about the incidence rate of adverse reactions RevMan5.0 software was used and the relative risk was taken as a combined effect size. The heterogeneity of the study results was tested by χ^2-test. When the study showed a statistical homogeneity ($P > 0.1$, $I^2 < 50\%$), a fixed effect model was applied, otherwise a random effect model was adopted.

Analysis Result

Three studies, reported by Jin et al. (2009), Diao et al. (2012), and Jin et al. (2017), compared the adverse reaction rates in cases of burn wounds treated with hydrogel dressings or other therapeutics. No statistical heterogeneity was detected among the study results ($P = 0.79$). Therefore, the random effect model was applied for meta-synthesis (**Figure 13**). The results disclosed that the incidence rate of adverse reactions—including skin dryness, swelling, pruritus, and fever—was lower in the hydrogel

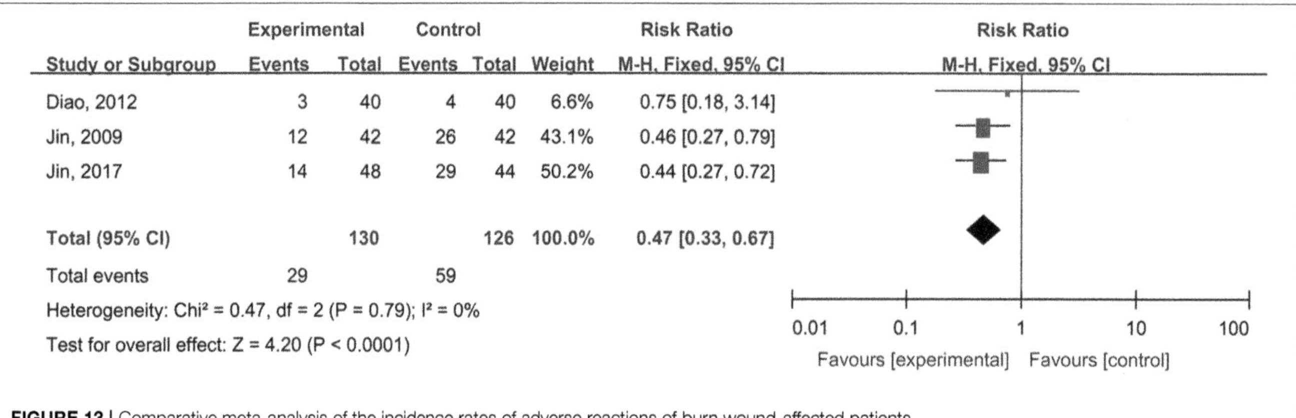

FIGURE 13 | Comparative meta-analysis of the incidence rates of adverse reactions of burn wound-affected patients.

dressings group than in the control group, and that statistically the difference was highly significant (RR = 0.47, 95% CI: 0.33–0.67, $P < 0.0001$). Other included studies reported no details about patients' adverse reactions.

No reports on adverse reactions of using medicinal hydrogels were found in the State Monitoring System of Drug Adverse Reactions (SMSDAR).

DISCUSSION

This study attempted to adopt the Cochrane systematic evaluation and Meta-analysis to assess the effectiveness and safety of hydrogel dressings employed in the management of skin wounds. The results brought to light that the application of medicinal hydrogel dressings can significantly shorten the healing time of skin wounds such as superficial degree-II burns (**Figure 2A**), deep degree-II burns (**Figure 2B**), diabetic foot ulcers (**Figure 5**), traumatic skin injuries (**Figure 7**), radioactive skin injuries (**Figure 11**), dog bites ($t = -5.29$, $P < 0.001$), and body surface ulcers ($t = -5.29$, $P < 0.001$). Hydrogel dressings can also effectively improve the cure rate of diabetic foot ulcers (**Figure 6**), surgical wounds (**Figure 9B**), dog bites ($t = 27.8$, $P < 0.001$), and body surface ulcers ($\chi^2 = 13.78$, $P < 0.001$). These advantageous effects are likely due to the nearly ideal moist environment that hydrogel dressings provide once applied to skin wounds. This promotes cell viability and physiological functioning and subsequently wound healing. In addition, hydrogel dressings reduce the loss of body fluids while absorbing wound's exudate and advancing autolytic debridement in necrotic wounds and granulating wounds. The hydrogels' swelling property has been proved to decrease the excessive fluid accumulation between the wound surface and the dressing. On the other hand, the hydrogel owns a soft texture and tends to adhere to the wound surface tightly and evenly, which prevents bacterial invasion and reduces soreness as well.

In recent years, with the appearance of new antibiotics and drugs applied to wounds, bactericidal and bacteriostatic substances such as silver ions have been combined with dressings to control local infections and accelerate wound healing. Nanocrystalline silver modulates the inflammatory response through its antimicrobial activity, thereby reducing the infections incidence and leading to an improved wound healing outcome. Furthermore, a faster re-epithelialization occurred in the wounds treated with nanocrystalline silver-coupled dressing rather than with a standard antibiotic solution (Demling and DeSanti, 2002; Nherera et al., 2017).

Study results also indicate that medicinal hydrogels can effectively alleviate the pain and burning and irritating sensations typical of skin wounds. The WHO pain rating of burn wounds (**Figure 3**) and traumatic skin injuries was significantly lower in the hydrogel dressing treatment studies. In addition, when hydrogel dressings were compared with non-hydrogel treatments, the VAS pain score was obviously lower in superficial degree-II burns (**Figure 4A**), deep degree-II burns (**Figure 4B**), and laser treatment-induced wounds. Concurrently, adverse reactions such as wound dryness, swelling, pruritus, and fever were significantly reduced (**Figure 13**). The benefits brought by hydrogel dressings to wounds might be related to the hydrogel-induced microenvironment that minimizes secondary injuries and alleviates pain by generating a cool feeling and by protecting any exposed peripheral nerve terminals. Our data also indicated that the guar gum-based hydrogel (CQ-01) is safe and can effectively alleviate the intractable pruritus otherwise affecting the patients [the score of Jun Wu scale (JW scale) pruritus rating scale for CQ-01 group was significantly lower than that of the traditional dressing group]. This further supports the clinical antipruritic effect of hydrogel dressings (Wu et al., 2016).

Meta-analysis is an observational study, thus, biases are somehow inevitable (Easterbrook et al., 1991). Among 43 original studies only 8 of them were graded A according to EPOC quality grading, which may potentially prejudice the results. Moreover, some hydrogel dressings were used in combination with other dressings, for example, silver dressings or with Lithosin solution. None of these trials assessed the effects of these combinations. It should be noted that hydrogel dressings are supposed to be applied singly rather than in combination with other therapeutics and that when used in combination their effectiveness and safety cannot be evaluated from individual dressing data. On the other hand, in the result of healing times comparison of burn wounds and others, there existed a statistical heterogeneity among the study results. The main reason for statistical heterogeneity of selected studies is that the sample size of each selected study varies greatly. In addition, clinical heterogeneity may also cause heterogeneity in statistical analysis, such as differences in baseline characteristics and medical conditions of burn patients in various studies, which may affect treatment outcomes.

The limitation of this meta-analysis is that, various dressings were applied in control groups included in this review, such as SSD, Iodine solution, Entoiodine and petrolatum gauze, Lithosin solution and oil, SD-Zn, Petrolatum gauze, Polyvidone iodine, Gentamicin dressing, etc. which may affect the outcomes and potentially add the biases to the study as well.

The main limitation of this review is the potential publication bias in terms of safety assessment of hydrogel dressings. Although we endeavored to collect quite a number of clinical trials by searching both publication databases and SMSDAR, in this systematic review only three studies compared the adverse reactions between hydrogel dressings and other medicinal products. The poor reporting of adverse reactions could be generalizable to the study purpose of clinical trials, which are commonly designed to explore the effectiveness of a dressing in promoting wound healing while they do not focus on the wound site responses to the dressing tested. On the other hand, it is sometimes hard to distinguish an adverse reaction from events related to wound healing.

CONCLUSIONS

This evidence-based systematic review and meta-analysis from RCTs and CCTs studies suggests that the use of hydrogel dressings results in a significant decrease in wound healing time, an obvious increase in cure rate, and a satisfying relief of pain as compared to non-hydrogel dressings. All the above-reported results strongly indicate that hydrogel products are effective and safe in wound management. Furthermore, there is a need for high-quality and international multi-center RCTs reporting adverse reactions to help clinicians make informed decisions on the best options for patients suffering from skin wounds.

AUTHOR CONTRIBUTIONS

Study design and conception of this manuscript were due to JW and BS. Literature retrieving and studies selection were performed by XL and JL. MY and XW carried out the quality evaluation of the study. Mathematical modeling and meta-analysis were conducted by FZha and FZho. Results analysis and interpretation were done by LZ, HY, and SQ. The manuscript was drafted by LZ and HY. All authors read and approved the final manuscript.

FUNDING

This work was supported by 100 Talents Program of Sun Yat-Sen University (Y61216), the Three-Three Project of the First Affiliated Hospital, Sun Yat-sen University (Y70214), National Natural Science Foundation of China (NSFC 81601624), China Postdoctoral Science Foundation Grant (2018M631028), and Doctoral Innovation Project of Shenzhen Health and Family Planning System Research Project (201605007).

ACKNOWLEDGMENTS

We would like to thank Prof. Ji Wang and Prof. Xuyang Feng for their useful comments.

REFERENCES

Cai, L., Lv, G., and Chen, J. (2010). Clinical study of photocrosslinked chitosan hydrogel film in the treatment of deep second degree burn wounds. *Chin. J. Inj. Repair* 5, 61–65.

Chattopadhyay, S., and Raines, R. T. (2014). Review collagen-based biomaterials for wound healing. *Biopolymers* 101, 821–833. doi: 10.1002/bip.22486

Chen, L., Ning, N., and Chen, H. (2015). Clinical observation of skin wound wet healing treatment. *Huaxi Med.* 30, 1811–1813.

Chen, Z. X. (2015). Observation on the effect of silver ion dressing combined with hydrogel in the treatment of diabetic foot. *Mod. Med.* 15, 82–83.

Cui, Z., Liu, L., and Li, J. (2007). Treatment of 42 cases of wounds in burn and plastic donor area with cold Lengningkang dressing. *Chin. J. Injury Repair Wound Healing, Electronic Edn.* 2, 36–37.

Das, S., and Baker, A. B. (2016). Biomaterials and nanotherapeutics for enhancing skin wound healing. *Front. Bioeng. Biotechnol.* 4:82. doi: 10.3389/fbioe.2016.00082

Demling, R. H., and DeSanti, M. D. L. (2002). The rate of re-epithelialization across meshed skin grafts is increased with exposure to silver. *Burns* 28, 264–266. doi: 10.1016/S0305-4179(01)00119-X

D'Hemecourt, P. A., Smiell, J. M., and Karim, M. R. (1998). Sodium carboxymethyl cellulose aqueous-based gel vs becaplermin gel in patients with nonhealing lower extremity diabetic ulcers. *Wound* 10, 69–75.

Diao, Y., Wang, S., and Chen, M. (2012). Application of hydrogel dressing Ai Kangye silver in the treatment of shallow second degree burn wounds. *J. Southeast Univ.* 31, 729–731.

Dong, R., Zhao, X., Guo, B., and Ma, P. X. (2016). Self-healing conductive injectable hydrogels with antibacterial activity as cell delivery carrier for cardiac cell therapy. *ACS Appl. Mater. Interfaces* 8, 17138–17150. doi: 10.1021/acsami.6b04911

Easterbrook, P. J., Berlin, J. A., Gopalan, R., and Matthews, D. R. (1991). Publication bias in clinical research. *Lancet*337, 867–872. doi: 10.1016/0140-6736(91)90201-Y

Fan, X., Xiao, M., and Wu, Y. (2013). A prospective study of the effect of silver ion combined with hydrogel dressing on postoperative infection wounds. *Chin. J. Basic Clin. Med.* 20, 102–104.

Fan, Z., Liu, B., Wang, J. Q., Zhang, S., Lin, Q., Gong, P., et al. (2014). A novel wound dressing based on ag/graphene polymer hydrogel: effectively kill bacteria and accelerate wound healing. *Adv. Funct. Mater.* 24, 3933–3943. doi: 10.1002/adfm.201304202

Fang, Q., Zhang, C., and Cai, X. (2011). Effect of wet therapy on the treatment of surface ulcers. *J. Nurs. Train.* 26, 2076–2077.

Garg, T., Rath, G., and Goyal, A. K. (2015). Biomaterials-based nanofiber scaffold: targeted and controlled carrier for cell and drug delivery. *J. Drug Target.* 23, 202–221. doi: 10.3109/1061186X.2014.992899

Gil, E. S., Panilaitis, B., Bellas, E., and Kaplan, D. L. (2013). Functionalized silk biomaterials for wound healing. *Adv. Healthc. Mater.* 2, 206–217. doi: 10.1002/adhm.201200192

Gong, Z., Yao, J., and Ji, J. (2009). Effects of silver ion dressing combined with hydrogel on wound healing of second-degree burns. *J. Clin. Rehabil. Tissue Eng. Res.* 13, 8373–8376.

Grice, E. A., Kong, H. H., Conlan, S., Deming, C. B., Davis, J., Young, A. C., et al. (2009). Topographical and temporal diversity of the human skin microbiome. *Science* 324 1190–1192. doi: 10.1126/science.1171700

He, Q., Wu, G., and Yu, B. (2008). Early results of wound healing hydrogel in the treatment of chronic lower extremity varicose ulcers. *Chin. J. Reconstr. Surg.* 22, 311–313.

Hu, Y., Xiao, H., and Fu, L. (2015). Study on the effect of new hydrogel dressings on the treatment of wet peeling after radiotherapy. *Chin. Nurs. Res.* 29, 1635–1637.

Huang, G., Liu, L., and Rongfen, W. (2016). Treatment and nursing observation of 42 cases of acute skin abrasion and contusion. *J. Yangtze Univ.* 13, 67–68.

Huang, Y., Han, W., and Weng, L. (2017). Application of wet healing therapy in stage III and IV severe pressure ulcers. *Modern Clin. Care* 16, 46–48.

Huang, Y., Wang, Y., Sun, L., Agrawal, R., and Zhang, M. (2015). Sundew adhesive: a naturally occurring hydrogel. *J. R. Soc. Interface* 12:12. doi: 10.1098/rsif.2015.0226

Jensen, J. L., Seeley, J., and Gilin, B. (1998). A controlled, randomized comparison of two moist wound healing protocols: carrasyn hydrogel wound dressing and wet-to-moist saline gauze. *Adv. Wound Care* 11, 323–327.

Jiang, J., Yu, S., and Shen, X. (2008). Treatment of burn wound pain by Lengningkang dressing. *Chin. J. Inj. Repair Wound Heal. (Electronic Edition)* 3, 200–202.

Jiang, X., Sun, R., and Li, J. (2018). Observation on the effect of hydrogel dressing on radiation-induced skin injury. *J. Pract. Clin. Nurs.* 3, 91–100.

Jin, A., Cai, L., and Chen, Y. (2017). Comparison of curative effect between hydrogel wound dressing and silver sulfadiazine on bromine burn wounds. *Zhejiang Med. J.* 39, 1474–1475+1482.

Jin, A., Shi, S., and Lu, J. (2009). "Application of Lengningkang in facial burn wounds," in *Zhejiang Medical Association Burns Surgery Academic Annual Conference Papers* (Zhejiang Medical Association).

Lan, Y., and Duan, N. (2015). Observation on the effect of new dressing for debridement and treatment of deep II burn wounds. *Contemp. Nurse* 5, 116–117.

Li, L., and Wu, B. (2018). Clinical study of early external HD series medical hydrogel wound dressing for small area burn wounds. *Chin. J. Damage Restor.* 13, 376–377.

Li, P., Chen, Y., and Wo, H. (2015). Clinical efficacy of Sanhuang wet compress hydrogel in the treatment of diabetic foot ulcer wounds. *Inner Mongolia Tradition. Chin. Med.* 12, 18–19.

Lin, Z., Yang, R., Shubin, R., Yan, L., Zhang, F., Xiong, X., et al. (2018). Analysis of the role of hydrogel dressing in the treatment of superficial second degree burn wounds. *J. Gannan Med. College* 38, 358–360.

Liu, B. (2015). *Comparative Study on the Clinical Efficacy of Wet Protective Dressing for the Treatment of Second Degree Burn Wounds.* Ningxia Medical University.

Liu, B., and Ye, L. (2014). Application of hydrogel dressing combined with compound comfrey oil in second degree burn wounds. *Chin. J. Aesthetic Med.* 23, 1330–1333.

Liu, L., Wang, S., and Cheng, C. (2017). Clinical observation of collagen-loaded nerve growth factor in the treatment of diabetic foot ulcer. *J. Armed Police Log. Univ.* 26, 421–423.

Lu, L., Xie, C., and Lu, J. (2017). Efficacy evaluation of cefuroxime sodium combined with silver ion and hydrogel dressing for wound healing in patients with postoperative infection. *Anti-infected Pharm.* 14, 1310–1312.

Mao, C., Xiang, Y., Liu, X., Cui, Z., Yang, X., Yeung, K. W. K., et al. (2017). Photo-inspired antibacterial activity and wound healing acceleration by hydrogel embedded with Ag/Ag@AgCl/ZnO nanostructures. *ACS Nano* 11, 9010–9021. doi: 10.1021/acsnano.7b03513

Mao, L. (2010). Therapeutic effect of silver ion dressing combined with hydrogel and moist treatment wound dressing on diabetic foot infection. *Chin. J. Misdiagn.* 10:8348.

Metcalfe, A. D., and Ferguson, M. W. (2007). Tissue engineering of replacement skin: the crossroads of biomaterials, wound healing, embryonic development, stem cells and regeneration. *J. R. Soc. Interface* 4, 413–437. doi: 10.1098/rsif.2006.0179

Mohan, Y. M., Lee, K., Premkumar, T., and Geckeler, K. E. (2007). Hydrogel networks as nanoreactors: a novel approach to silver nanoparticles for antibacterial applications. *Polymer* 48, 158–164. doi: 10.1016/j.polymer.2006.10.045

Nherera, L. M., Trueman, P., Roberts, C. D., and Berg, L. (2017). A systematic review and meta-analysis of clinical outcomes associated with nanocrystalline silver use compared to alternative silver delivery systems in the management of superficial and deep partial thickness burns. *Burns* 43, 939–948. doi: 10.1016/j.burns.2017.01.004

Nie, H., Li, K., and Zhang, Q. (2015). Application of wet dressing in dressing change of elderly diabetic foot ulcer. *Inner Mongolia Tradition. Chin. Med.* 35, 3582–3584.

Nourian Dehkordi, A., Mirahmadi Babaheydari, F., Chehelgerdi, M., and Raeisi Dehkordi, S. (2019). Skin tissue engineering: wound healing based on stem-cell-based therapeutic strategies. *Stem Cell Res. Ther.* 10:111. doi: 10.1186/s13287-019-1212-2

Purna, S. K., and Babu, M. (2000). Collagen based dressings–a review. *Burns* 26, 54–62. doi: 10.1016/S0305-4179(99)00103-5

Qiu, Y., and Park, K. (2001). Environment-sensitive hydrogels for drug delivery. *Adv. Drug Deliv. Rev.* 53, 321–339. doi: 10.1016/S0169-409X(01)00203-4

Qu, J., Zhao, X., Liang, Y., Zhang, T., Ma, P. X., and Guo, B. (2018). Antibacterial adhesive injectable hydrogels with rapid self-healing, extensibility and compressibility as wound dressing for joints skin wound healing. *Biomaterials* 183, 185–199. doi: 10.1016/j.biomaterials.2018.08.044

Roy, N., Saha, N., Kitano, T., and Saha, P. (2010). Novel hydrogels of PVP-CMC and their swelling effect on viscoelastic properties. *J. Appl. Polym. Sci.* 117, 1703–1710. doi: 10.1002/app.32056

Schwartz, V. B., Thetiot, F., Ritz, S., Puetz, S., Choritz, L., Lappas, A., et al. (2012). Antibacterial surface coatings from zinc oxide nanoparticles embedded in poly(N-isopropylacrylamide) hydrogel surface layers. *Adv. Funct. Mater.* 22, 2376–2386. doi: 10.1002/adfm.201102980

Shamseer, L., Moher, D., Clarke, M., Ghersi, D., Liberati, A., Petticrew, M., et al. (2015). Preferred reporting items for systematic review and meta-analysis protocols (PRISMA-P) 2015: elaboration and explanation. *BMJ* 350:g7647. doi: 10.1136/bmj.g7647

Shang, N. (2015). *Application of Hydrogel Dressing in Wound Healing After Grinding.* Shandong University.

Shao, M., Chen, H., and Chen, Q. (2015). Effects of pain during incision dressing on wound healing in diabetic foot. *Chin. J. Modern Nurs.* 21, 1522–1524.

Shi, S., LuTing, W., and Wang, Y. (2016). Therapeutic effect of Lengningkang HD-M hydrogel dressing on PICC-associated phlebitis. *Hainan Med. J.* 27, 2221–2222.

Sood, A., Granick, M. S., and Tomaselli, N. L. (2014). Wound dressings and comparative effectiveness *Data.* 3, 511–529. doi: 10.1089/wound.2012.0401

Teng, Y. (2010). *Evidence-Based Research on Clinical Treatment of Chronic Wounds.* Lanzhou: Lanzhou University.

Tsao, C. T., Chang, C. H., Lin, Y. Y., Wu, M. F., Wang, J. L., Han, J. L., et al. (2010). Antibacterial activity and biocompatibility of a chitosan-gamma-poly (glutamic acid) polyelectrolyte complex hydrogel. *Carbohydr. Res.* 345, 1774–1780. doi: 10.1016/j.carres.2010.06.002

Vandeputte, J., and Gryson, L. (1997). "Diabetic foot infection controlled by immuno-modulating hydrogel containing 65% glycerine. Presentation of a clinical trial," in *6th European Conference on Advances in Wound Management, Vol. 1997* (Amsterdam), 50–53.

Wang, J., and Teng, Y. (2008). Local treatment of canine bite wound III with silver ion dressing combined with hydrogel: randomized controlled group. *Chin. J. Tissue Eng. Res. Clin. Rehab.* 12, 2659–2662.

Wang, J., Yan, X., and Teng, Y. (2008). Local treatment of diabetic foot wound with silver ion dressing combined with hydrogel. *J. Chongqing Med. Univ.* 33, 747–749.

Wang, J., Yan, X., and Teng, Y. (2013). A prospective study of the effect of silver ion combined with hydrogel dressing on postoperative infection wounds. *J. Chongqing Med. Univ.* 20, 102–104.

Wang, L., Lin, X., and Xiang, X. (2011). Clinical application and safety of Lengningkang dressing in the treatment of burn wounds. *China Pharmaceutic.* 20, 64–65.

Wen, S. (2015). Nursing experience of hydrogel combined with insulin for the treatment of patients with acne. *World's Latest Med. Inform. Abst.* 15, 221–226.

Wichterle, O., and Lím, D. (1960). Hydrophilic gels for biological use. *Nature* 185, 117–118. doi: 10.1038/185117a0

Winter, G. D. (1962). Formation of the scab and the rate of epithelization of superficial wounds in the skin of the young domestic pig. *Nature* 193, 293–294. doi: 10.1038/193293a0

Wu, J., Xu, R., Zhan, R., Luo, G., Niu, X., Liu, Y., et al. (2016). Effective symptomatic treatment for severe and intractable pruritus associated with severe burn-induced hypertrophic scars: a prospective, multicenter, controlled trial. *Burns* 42, 1059–1066. doi: 10.1016/j.burns.2015.09.021

Xiang, Y., Zhang, H., and Zou, J. (2012). Clinical study on innovative dressing for the treatment of diabetic foot ulcer. *Chin. Pharm.* 23, 2063–2064.

Xin, F., Liu, L., and An, Y. (2014). Application of medical hydrogel in laser therapy and multi-center clinical efficacy observation. *J. Pract. Dermatol.* 7, 193–195.

Xu, R., Luo, G., Xia, H., He, W., Zhao, J., Liu, B., et al. (2015). Novel bilayer wound dressing composed of silicone rubber with particular micropores enhanced wound re-epithelialization and contraction. *Biomaterials* 40, 1–11. doi: 10.1016/j.biomaterials.2014.10.077

Zeng, Y., and Li, Y. (2016). Application of Shengji ointment combined with silicone dressing in wound care. *Contemp. Nurses*, 5, 78–80.

Zhang, L., Ma, J., and Zhang, H. (2012). Comparison of silver ion dressing combined with hydrogel and wet treatment wound dressing for the treatment of diabetic foot infection. *Chin. J. Nosocomiol.* 22, 4002–4003.

8

Effect of Exercise Volume on Plantar Microcirculation and Tissue Hardness in People with Type 2 Diabetes

Weiyan Ren[1†], Yijie Duan[2†], Yih-Kuen Jan[2,3], Wenqiang Ye[2], Jianchao Li[2], Wei Liu[2], Hongmei Liu[1,2], Junchao Guo[1], Fang Pu[2] and Yubo Fan[2,4*]*

[1]Key Laboratory of Rehabilitation Technical Aids for Old-Age Disability, Key Laboratory of Human Motion Analysis and Rehabilitation Technology of the Ministry of Civil Affairs, National Research Center for Rehabilitation Technical Aids, Beijing, China, [2]Key Laboratory for Biomechanics and Mechanobiology of Chinese Education Ministry, Beijing Advanced Innovation Center for Biomedical Engineering, School of Biological Science and Medical Engineering, Beihang University, Beijing, China, [3]Rehabilitation Engineering Laboratory, Department of Kinesiology and Community Health, University of Illinois at Urbana-Champaign, Champaign, IL, United States, [4]School of Engineering Medicine, Beihang University, Beijing, China

Correspondence:
Fang Pu
pufangbme@buaa.edu.cn
Yubo Fan
yubofan@buaa.edu.cn

†These authors have contributed equally to this work and share first authorship

Objective: Exercise has been reported to be beneficial for people with type 2 diabetes (T2DM), but exercise, especially weight-bearing exercise, may increase the risk of diabetic foot ulcers (DFUs). This study aimed to explore the associations between different volumes of weight-bearing physical activities and plantar microcirculation and tissue hardness in people with T2DM.

Methods: 130 elderly people with T2DM were enrolled for this cross-sectional study. They were classified into the high exercise volume group and the low exercise volume group based on their weekly energy expenditure (metabolic equivalents per week) in the past year. Weekly energy expenditure was calculated using the International Physical Activity Questionnaire and the Compendium of Physical Activities. The plantar oxygen saturation (SO_2) and soft tissue hardness of each participant's right foot were measured.

Results: A total of 80 participants completed the trial. The average exercise energy expenditure of the high exercise volume group and the low exercise volume group were significantly different ($p < 0.05$). The results showed that the SO_2 of the high exercise volume group (67.25 ± 6.12%) was significantly higher than the low exercise volume group (63.75 ± 8.02%, $p < 0.05$). The plantar tissue hardness of the high exercise volume group was lower than the low exercise volume group in the big toe, midfoot and hindfoot regions ($p < 0.05$).

Conclusion: This study demonstrates that higher volumes of exercise are associated with better plantar microcirculation and lower plantar tissue hardness in people with T2DM. The findings of this study indicate that weight-bearing exercise may not increase risk of developing diabetic foot ulcers.

Keywords: diabetic foot, weight-bearing exercise, plantar microcirculation, tissue hardness, exercise volume

INTRODUCTION

Diabetic foot ulcers (DFUs) are one of the most common and serious complications of diabetes mellitus (DM). A global survey on diabetes-related complications showed that one-third of people with diabetes suffered complications in the lower extremity (Zhang et al., 2020); and diabetes-related lower extremity amputations accounted for 30–65% of all amputations (Narres et al., 2017). DFUs can have a huge negative impact on the physical health and quality of life of people with diabetes.

Microvascular dysfunction (Greenman et al., 2005; Chao and Cheing, 2009), abnormal plantar stress (Jan et al., 2013b; Pu et al., 2018), increased plantar tissue hardness (Mithraratne et al., 2012; Jan et al., 2013a) and peripheral neuropathy (Bowering, 2001; Caselli et al., 2002) are major factors causing the development of DFUs. Research studies have shown that people with diabetes exhibit microvascular dysfunction, including a lower level of oxygen saturation of plantar tissue (Greenman et al., 2005; Chao and Cheing, 2009). Besides, the increased hardness of plantar tissue causes an increase in peak plantar pressure (Jan et al., 2013a; Teoh and Lee, 2020), which may gradually reduce the capacity to attenuate the ground impact in diabetic plantar tissue. Peripheral neuropathy can lead to a loss of protective sensation in people with diabetes, and also further aggravates microvascular dysfunction, as well as cause dry skin and musculoskeletal deformities (Armstrong et al., 2017). Although the relationships among oxygen saturation, plantar tissue hardness, neuropathy, and the occurrence of ulcerations are still unclear, these factors may play an important role in predicting and assessing the risk of DFUs.

Exercise is one of the most effective methods for managing the complications of diabetes, and has been shown to improve blood glucose levels, ankle brachial index, cardiopulmonary endurance, and muscle strength (Liao et al., 2019; Verboven et al., 2019). Moreover, weight-bearing exercise has been reported to improve tissue tolerance and significantly increase the achievable walking distance and step count of people with diabetic peripheral neuropathy (DPN) (Mueller and Maluf, 2002; Mueller et al., 2013; Kluding et al., 2017). Diloreto et al. also found that daily physical activity with an energy expenditure at 27 Mets·h/week (more than 10 Mets·h/week recommended by the American Diabetes Association) had a significant positive effect on the physical fitness of people with type 2 diabetes (Di Loreto et al., 2005; Association, 2020). However, the effects of exercise volumes of weight-bearing exercise on the risk of developing DFUs remain unclear (Liao et al., 2019). Exercise can improve endothelial function and blood circulation in the lower extremity (Mueller et al., 2013; Liao et al., 2019), which may be beneficial to improve microvascular function in people with type 2 diabetes (Mueller and Maluf, 2002; Kluding et al., 2017). On the other hand, the greater accumulated stress on plantar soft tissues caused by high volume of exercise, especially weight-bearing exercise, may increase the degree of compression of plantar tissue, and the occlusion duration of microvessels. The impaired plantar microcirculation under the accumulated stimulation of repeated mechanical loading may be more prone to cause tissue damage to the fragile foot tissue in people with type 2 diabetes (Chao et al., 2011). Particularly in people with diabetes and peripheral neuropathy, the dysfunction in the regulation of microvascular system, dry skin and musculoskeletal deformity caused by peripheral neuropathy can increase the vulnerability of plantar tissue to compressed damage during these physical activities (Mueller and Maluf, 2002; Jan et al., 2013b; Pu et al., 2018). Therefore, exploring the long-term effects of weight-bearing exercise with high exercise volume on the plantar microcirculation and soft tissue hardness in the diabetic foot may help to understand the risk of developing DFUs. This information may be used to develop appropriate exercise plans for people with type 2 diabetes.

The aim of this study was to compare the difference of plantar microcirculation and tissue hardness in people with type 2 diabetes who performed long-term weight-bearing exercise at high and low exercise volume. We hypothesized that participants with type 2 diabetes in the high exercise volume group would have better oxygen supply to the plantar foot and lower plantar hardness compared to the low exercise volume group.

MATERIALS AND METHODS

This is a cross-sectional observation study designed to explore the difference of plantar microcirculation and tissue hardness (the important factors in the development of DFUs) of the foot of people with diabetes who had habitual physical activity at high and low levels of exercise volume.

This study was conducted in accordance with clinical protocols approved by the institutional review board of Affiliated Hospital of National Research Center for Rehabilitation Technical Aids (20190101) and the Declaration of Helsinki (2013 revision). All participants were briefed on the study purposes and procedures and gave written informed consent prior to participation.

Participants

A total of 130 people with diabetes confirmed their willingness to participate in this study through a public recruitment drive in the local communities and hospitals. The inclusion criteria were: 1) diagnosed type 2 diabetes, 2) ≥40 ages, 3) no symptoms such as redness, callus, inflammation, or wounds on the skin of the feet or legs, and no history of amputation, 4) no diseases such as systematic inflammation, lower extremity edema, malignant tumor, and 5) performed regular physical activities over the course of 1 year with at least 150 min/week, with no more than two consecutive days without activity (Association, 2020) before being enrolled in this study. A total of 104 participants met the inclusion criteria and were enrolled in this study.

Physiological Information Recording and Assessment

Demographics and medical history were discussed and recorded at the initial assessment. In this study, 10 g Semmes-Weinstein monofilament and vibration perception threshold testing were used to evaluate whether participants had sensory neuropathy. For this test, 10 g monofilament was compressed perpendicular to the four areas of foot (1st, 3rd, and 5th metatarsal heads and distal hallux) for 1 s and then removed. It was considered normal large-fiber nerve function if the patient could feel the touch of the monofilament at all four areas. Moreover, a biothesiometer was placed over the dorsal hallux and the amplitude of vibration was increased until participants could detect it. The protective sensation was considered normal if a participant's vibration perception threshold was smaller than 25 V (Boulton et al., 2008). No abnormal test would rule out diabetic peripheral neuropathy. Otherwise, a participant was confirmed as a diabetic with peripheral neuropathy (Boulton et al., 2008; Schaper et al., 2020). Care was taken to avoid performing the test on callous tissue.

Assessment of Physical Activity

The type, frequency and duration of weekly physical activity performed over the course of 1 year was recorded for each participant. This was assessed using the International Physical Activity Questionnaire (IPAQ) that has been proven to be a validated tool for physical activity assessment (Mynarski et al., 2012). The level of metabolic equivalent (MET) rating was determined based on the compendium of physical activities (Ainsworth et al., 2011), including step counts, duration and distance travelled, and the type of exercise described by the participants (Mynarski et al., 2012; Lalli et al., 2013; Ainsworth, 2014). All recorded activities and corresponding MET values in this study were as follows: walking (2.5 mph-2.8 mph, and 3 Mets), brisk walking (3.5–4.0 mph, 4.3 Mets), square dancing (5 Mets), table tennis (4 Mets), tennis (4.5 Mets), golf (4.8 Mets), billiards (2.5 Mets), cycling (4 Mets), and Tai Chi (3 Mets) (Ainsworth et al., 2011).

The weekly sum of each participant's energy expenditure through physical activity was calculated using the **Eq. 1** (Knowler et al., 2002). Diloreto et al. recommended that 27 Mets·h/week can be a reasonable target of energy expenditure for sedentary people with diabetes due to its great benefits associated with HbA1c, BMI, heart rate, and 10-years coronary heart disease risk (Di Loreto et al., 2005). Therefore, people with diabetes in this study were classified into the high exercise volume (HEV) group and the low exercise volume (LEV) group according to whether their energy expenditure exceeded 27 Mets·h/week.

$$\text{Energy Expenditure} = \sum \text{Met}_i \times \text{T}_i \quad (1)$$

In which, i represents different activity models, Met_i represents the metabolic equivalent rating corresponding to different activities, and T_i represents the time spent in different activities.

Assessment of Plantar Microcirculation and Tissue Hardness

All tests were performed in a climate-controlled room at 24°C with participants in a supine position. Every participants started with a 30 min resting period before measurements. A Shore durometer (Model 1,600, Type OO, Rex Co., Buffalo Grove, United States) was used to measure the tissue hardness in the plantar regions (big toe, little toes, medial metatarsal, middle metatarsal, lateral metatarsal, medial arch, lateral arch, medial heel, and lateral heel) of each participant's right foot. It was designed to test the hardness of soft materials such as animal tissue, foams, sponge rubber, and gels. The similar durometer has been used in several studies to assess plantar hardness in people with diabetes (Thomas et al., 2003; Periyasamy et al., 2012).

During measurement, the durometer was pressed perpendicular to the plantar skin surface and expresses the hardness in degrees of Shore (unit: °shore). A lower Shore value indicates a softer material. Each region was measured 5 times sequentially and the mean was calculated for comparisons. Care was taken to avoid testing areas with prominent bones or callus tissue. The tissue hardness of the little toes was the average of the four little toes. The tissue hardness of the forefoot region was the average of the medial metatarsal, middle metatarsal and lateral metatarsal. The tissue hardness of the midfoot region was the average of the medial arch and lateral arch. The tissue hardness of the hindfoot region was the average of the medial heel and lateral heel (**Figure 1**).

After measuring the plantar tissue hardness, a moorVMS-OXY monitor (Probe OP17-1,000, Moor Instruments, Axminster, United Kingdom) was used to monitor the plantar microcirculation. This device uses a white light spectroscopy method and transmits the 6 mW white light (400–700 nm wave length) into tissue via fiber optics in order to assess tissue oxygen saturation and temperature. The probe was attached to the skin surface of the right plantar big toe area with adhesive tapes to limit movement artefacts during the measurement. The plantar tissue oxygen saturation (SO_2) and skin temperature (Temp) of each participant in the supine position were recorded for 2 min (Newton et al., 2005; Ladurner et al., 2009).

Sample Size

The required sample size was calculated using Power Analysis and Sample Size (PASS 15) software set for *t* test. This study assumed that the mean and standard deviation (SD) of cutaneous oxygen saturation in people with diabetes was equivalent to that of a prior study (64.1 ± 4.0%) (Kabbani et al., 2013), and the mean difference between two groups was equivalent to that of Charles et al.'s study (3.9%) (Ezema et al., 2019). A minimum of 24 participants per group was needed at a power of 90% and an alpha level of 0.05. This study assumed a drop-out rate of 20%, and considered that more than half of the participants may not regularly perform physical activities over the course of 1 year with at least 150 min/week (one of the inclusion criteria) (Wen et al., 2011). Therefore, at least 120 participants were recruited for this study.

Data and Statistical Analyses

The mean values of SO_2 and Temp from each participant's right plantar big toe region, and the mean values of tissue hardness in five plantar regions (big toe, little toes, forefoot, midfoot, and hindfoot) of each participant's right foot, were calculated.

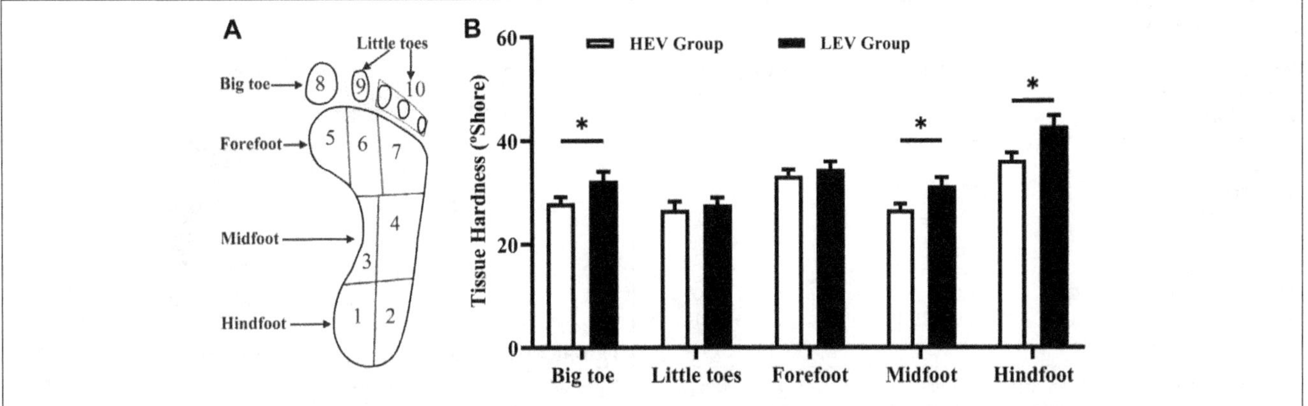

FIGURE 1 | (A) Division of the foot. **(B)** Results of tissue hardness of plantar tissue in participants (Mean with SEM). The tissue hardness of the little toes was the average of area 8 and area 9; the tissue hardness of the forefoot was the average of area 5, area 6 and area 7; the tissue hardness of the midfoot was the average of area 3 and area 4; the tissue hardness of the hindfoot was the average of area 1 and area 2. HEV: High Exercise Volume (≥27 Mets·h/week); LEV: Low Exercise Volume (<27 Mets·h/week); SEM: standard error of mean. * indicates a significant difference between the HEV group (n = 45) and LEV group (n = 35) (p < 0.05).

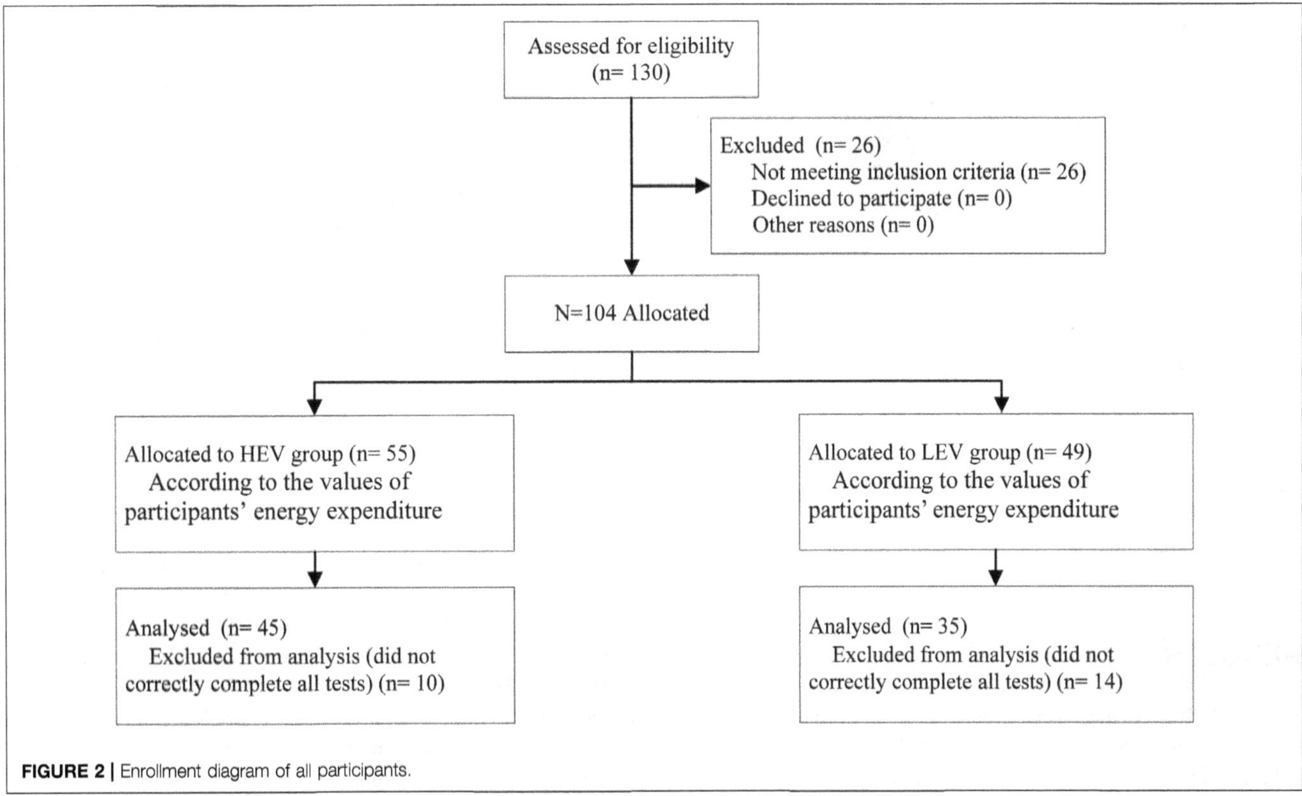

FIGURE 2 | Enrollment diagram of all participants.

Considering that peripheral neuropathy is an important factor in contributing to the development of diabetic foot ulcers (Armstrong et al., 2017), this study also preliminarily observed differences in the mean values of SO2, Temp and plantar soft tissue hardness between people with diabetic peripheral neuropathy and people without diabetic peripheral neuropathy. In addition, plantar soft tissue may be subjected to different levels of accumulated pressure stimuli under various exercise types, which may be related to the occurrence and development of diabetic foot ulcers (Burnfield et al., 2004; Lam et al., 2019). This study conducted a preliminary comparison of the mean values of SO2, Temp and plantar soft tissue hardness among people with different exercise types.

An independent t test or Mann-Whitney U test (based on the normality of the variables, as tested by a Shapiro-Wilk test) was used to evaluate differences in microcirculation and plantar hardness between the HEV group and LEV group. A Spearman or Pearson correlation analysis (based on the normality of the variables, as tested by a Shapiro-Wilk test) was used to test the relationship between tissue hardness and

TABLE 1 | Demographic and physiological information of participants in HEV and LEV groups (Mean ± SD).

Variables	HEV group	LEV group
Gender (Male/Female)	21/24	14/21
Age (years)	66.67 ± 4.55	65.85 ± 8.09
BMI (kg/m^2)	25.57 ± 3.22	26.49 ± 3.80
SBP (mmHg)	136.17 ± 14.05	132.04 ± 14.73
DBP (mmHg)	72.51 ± 8.78	72.11 ± 9.32
Heart rate (bpm)	72.94 ± 10.91	72.54 ± 9.53
Duration of diabetes (years)	13.19 ± 9.05	11.68 ± 7.61
Fasting blood glucose (mmol/L)	7.31 ± 1.51	7.63 ± 1.60
ABI	1.08 ± 0.16	1.07 ± 0.11
Diabetic peripheral neuropathy	8 (17.8%)	5 (14.3%)

HEV: high exercise volume; LEV: low exercise volume; BMI: body mass index; SBP: systolic blood pressure; DBP: diastolic blood pressure; ABI: Ankle brachial index. There was no significant difference in all parameters between the HEV, group and LEV, group.

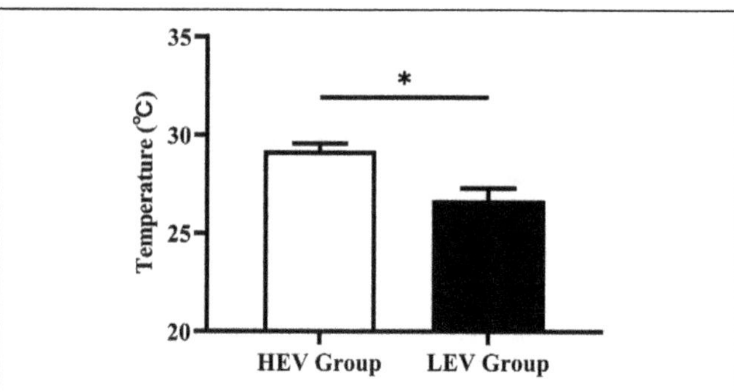

FIGURE 4 | Results of skin temperature of plantar tissue in participants (Mean with SEM). HEV: High Exercise Volume (≥27 Mets·h/week); LEV: Low Exercise Volume (<27 Mets·h/week); SEM: standard error of mean. * indicates a significant difference between the HEV group ($n < 45$) and LEV group ($n < 35$) ($p < 0.05$).

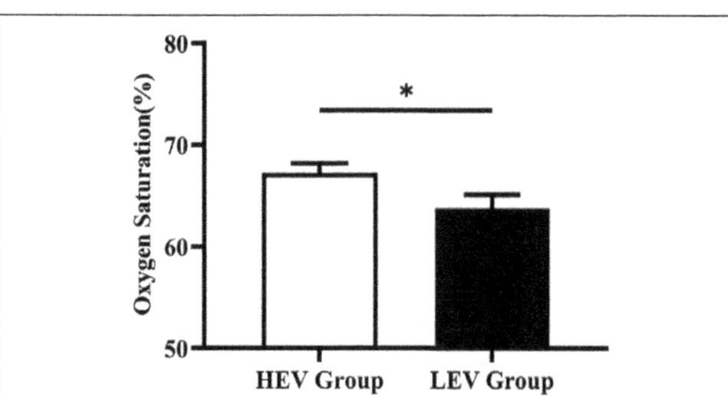

FIGURE 3 | Results of oxygen saturation of plantar tissue in participants (Mean with SEM). HEV: High Exercise Volume (≥27 Mets·h/week); LEV: Low Exercise Volume (<27 Mets·h/week); SEM: standard error of mean. * indicates a significant difference between the HEV group ($n < 45$) and LEV group ($n < 35$) ($p < 0.05$).

microcirculation. The results were expressed as mean ± SD. A statistical significance level of 0.05 was used. All statistical analyses were performed in SPSS (Version 26.0, IBM, Armonk, NY, United States).

RESULTS

A total of 80 participants completed all tests (**Figure 2**). Among them, 45 people with diabetes were classified as the HEV group, including eight people with DPN. The remaining 35 participants were classified as the LEV group, including five people with DPN. Participant characteristics are shown in **Table 1**. There was no significant difference in these parameters (age, body mass index, systolic blood pressure, diastolic blood pressure, heart rate, duration of diabetes, fasting blood glucose, and ankle brachial index) between the HEV group and LEV group. The average exercise energy expenditure of the HEV group and the LEV group were 51.69 ± 21.51 Mets·h/week and 18.34 ± 4.55 Mets·h/week ($p < 0.05$), respectively (**Table 1**).

In the HEV group, in addition to walking, 14 of the participants without DPN routinely engaged in one or more of the following weight-bearing activities; brisk walking, square dancing, ball games (table tennis, tennis, golf, and billiards), cycling, and Tai Chi. Among them, one participant did brisk walking at about 3.7 mph every day; five participants engaged in square dancing every week; four participants engaged in ball games every week; two participants went cycling daily; and two participants did Tai Chi every day. For the other 31 participants in this group, the only routine daily physical activity was walking. Similarly, in the LEV group, the only routine physical activity was walking, but with a lower energy expenditure.

Effects of Weight-Bearing Exercise on Plantar Microcirculation

The plantar oxygen saturation (SO_2) and skin temperature (Temp) of both groups were recorded and analyzed (**Figures 3, 4**). The results showed that the plantar SO_2 (67.25 ± 6.12%) and plantar Temp (29.22 ± 2.44°C) in the HEV group were both significantly higher than the LEV group (SO_2: 63.75 ± 8.02%, $p = 0.030$; Temp: 26.72 ± 3.47°C, $p = 0.001$), respectively.

Table 2 shows the SO_2 and Temp for participants without diabetic peripheral neuropathy (Non-DPN) and DPN. The mean SO_2 and Temp of participants in the HEV group was higher than the LEV group. In the HEV group, the mean SO_2 of the DPN participants was lower than the Non-DPN participants. From **Table 2**, it can be seen that the mean SO_2 and mean Temp (except for Tai Chi) for participants in the sub-group "Walking + other weight-bearing activities" was higher than participants with "Only walking".

Effect of Weight-Bearing Exercise on Plantar Tissue Hardness

Figure 1 compares the plantar tissue hardness between the HEV and LEV group. The results showed that the mean tissue hardness in the HEV group was lower than that of the LEV group, with a significant difference at the big toe region (HEV: 27.89 ± 7.72°Shore, LEV: 32.25 ± 9.94°Shore; $p = 0.030$), midfoot (HEV: 26.59 ± 7.59°Shore, LEV: 31.20 ± 9.30°Shore; $p = 0.034$),

TABLE 2 | Plantar SO_2 and Temp for Non-DPN and DPN participants in the HEV and LEV groups, and for Non-DPN participants performing different physical activities in the HEV group (Participants in LEV group did not engage in any form of exercise other than walking; Mean ± SD).

	HEV group		LEV group	
	Non-DPN (*n* = 37)	DPN (*n* = 8)	Non-DPN (*n* = 30)	DPN (*n* = 5)
SO2 (%)	67.69 ± 6.37	65.23 ± 4.52	63.78 ± 8.30	63.56 ± 6.83
Temp (°C)	29.13 ± 2.57	29.62 ± 1.76	26.77 ± 3.54	26.40 ± 3.33

	Only walking in HEV group (n = 23)	Walking + other weight-bearing activities in HEV group				
		Brisk walking (*n* = 1)	Square dancing (*n* = 5)	Ball games (n = 4)	Cycling (*n* = 2)	Tai Chi (*n* = 2)
SO2 (%)	66.07 ± 6.33	70.90	68.28 ± 8.14	70.90 ± 5.93	73.07 ± 2.77	71.38 ± 1.81
Temp (°C)	28.87 ± 2.83	31.07	29.38 ± 2.59	29.32 ± 2.11	31.57 ± 0.03	28.02 ± 1.39

DPN: diabetic peripheral neuropathy; HEV: high exercise volume; LEV: low exercise volume; SO2: plantar oxygen saturation; Temp: skin temperature.

TABLE 3 | Plantar soft tissue hardness for Non-DPN and DPN participants in the HEV and LEV groups, and for Non-DPN participants performing different physical activities in the HEV group (Participants in LEV group did not engage in any form of exercise other than walking; Mean ± SD).

		HEV group		LEV group	
		Non-DPN (*n* = 37)	DPN (*n* = 8)	Non-DPN (*n* = 30)	DPN (*n* = 5)
Soft tissue (°shore)	Big toe	26.01 ± 6.47	36.60 ± 7.34	32.19 ± 10.43	32.60 ± 7.15
	Little toes	24.62 ± 8.78	35.68 ± 13.90	27.55 ± 8.36	27.76 ± 7.56
	Forefoot	31.41 ± 7.65	40.83 ± 6.48	34.45 ± 8.85	34.37 ± 7.93
	Midfoot	24.84 ± 6.39	34.69 ± 7.80	31.53 ± 9.71	29.20 ± 6.73
	Hindfoot	33.90 ± 9.19	46.15 ± 8.66	42.81 ± 12.84	42.04 ± 8.77

		Only walking in HEV group (*n* = 23)	Walking + other weight-bearing activities in HEV group				
			Brisk walking (*n* = 1)	Square dancing (*n* = 5)	Ball games (*n* = 4)	Cycling (*n* = 2)	Tai Chi (*n* = 2)
Soft tissue (°shore)	Big toe	25.29 ± 6.94	29.40	28.64 ± 6.54	28.40 ± 5.93	20.10 ± 4.38	27.10 ± 1.27
	Little toes	23.94 ± 8.83	35.60	29.16 ± 8.54	27.15 ± 9.64	15.50 ± 0.99	19.60 ± 3.11
	Forefoot	30.81 ± 8.09	34.47	31.84 ± 6.19	36.03 ± 8.01	25.33 ± 4.81	32.57 ± 10.98
	Midfoot	24.76 ± 6.92	27.30	21.80 ± 4.08	28.48 ± 6.54	21.80 ± 5.23	27.85 ± 7.14
	Hindfoot	34.39 ± 10.24	28.60	30.64 ± 6.30	38.75 ± 7.24	28.90 ± 10.32	34.30 ± 8.91

DPN: diabetic peripheral neuropathy; HEV: high exercise volume; LEV: low exercise volume.

and hindfoot (HEV: 36.08 ± 10.17°Shore, LEV: 42.70 ± 12.23°Shore; $p = 0.010$).

It was also found that SO_2 and Temp were negatively correlated with the tissue hardness of the big toe region (SO_2: $R = -0.299$, $p = 0.007$; Temp: $R = -0.311$, $p = 0.005$).

Within the HEV group, the mean plantar tissue hardness of all regions of the foot for the DPN participants was higher than that of the Non-DPN participants. For DPN participants, the mean plantar tissue hardness in the HEV group was higher than the LEV group. Also, the plantar tissue hardness in the Non-DPN participants in the HEV group varied depending on the type of routine physical activities typically performed. Four participants who played ball games and one participant who did brisk walking had a higher tissue hardness in the forefoot region than other participants, while two participants who routinely cycled had the lowest tissue hardness (**Table 3**).

DISCUSSION

This study analyzed the association between exercise volume and plantar microcirculation and soft tissue hardness in people with type 2 diabetes. The results showed that participants with higher volume of habitual exercise had better oxygen supply and basal skin temperature and lower soft tissue hardness of the foot, compared to participants with lower volume of habitual exercise. These findings suggest that weight-bearing exercise with high exercise volume might be associated with better microcirculation function and softer plantar tissue, which may not increase the risk of developing foot ulcers.

Previous studies reported that exercise can increase insulin sensitivity in people with diabetes and promote the production of endothelium-dependent vasodilator nitric oxide, thus improving endothelial and microvascular function and promoting metabolism in the lower extremities (Kluding et al., 2017). Studies have also shown that a high stress stimulus can increase vessel diameter and arterial compliance, and was beneficial for the cardiopulmonary and vascular function (Huonker et al., 1996; Mueller and Maluf, 2002). Charles et al. also found that people with diabetes who engaged in an eight-week aerobics programme (bicycle) had a 3.9% increase in peripheral oxygen saturation compared to the control group (Ezema et al., 2019). Demachi et al. reported that skin temperature gradually increases with the duration of exercise (Demachi et al., 2013). Similarly, this current study found that the high exercise volume group (≥27 Mets·h/week) had higher plantar SO2 and basal Temp in comparison with the low exercise volume group (<27 Mets·h/week) (**Figures 3, 4**). Moreover, participants in the sub-group "Walking + other weight-bearing activities" had a higher mean SO_2 and Temp than participants with "Only walking". This may be due to the higher energy requirements when performing more than one routine exercise (Walking + other weight-bearing activities: 67.66 ± 29.55 Mets·h/week; Only walking: 41.54 ± 8.06 Mets·h/week). Sivanandam et al. demonstrated that the foot temperature of people with diabetes was significantly lower than that of healthy people (Sivanandam et al., 2012). Decreased skin temperature may be related to poor microvascular perfusion of the lower extremity in people with diabetes, which further aggravates microvascular dysfunction and leads to the occurrence of DFUs. The results of this study suggest that weight-bearing exercise with high exercise volume has a more positive effect on circulation and the nutrient supply to the plantar microvasculature, implying that the active weight-bearing exercise may be associated with lower risk of DFUs.

Some studies reported that the abnormal increase of plantar skin temperature may indicate the occurrence of some pathologic factors (e.g., peripheral neuropathy (Yavuz et al., 2019) and inflammation responses (van Netten et al., 2014)). However, the study of Kokate et al. demonstrated that the damage of deep tissue would occur under the pressure stimulus at temperature above 35°C in a reliable porcine model, and no damage was observed in the superficial or deep tissues with a temperature of 25°C under the pressure stimulus (Kokate et al., 1995). In this study, we compared the basal foot temperature of people with diabetes with different exercise volumes, none of the participants had a diabetic foot ulcer history and their plantar temperature did not exceed 35°C. Therefore, the mean temperature of the high exercise volume group was higher than that of the low exercise volume group, which may be due to the improvement of lower extremity microvascular perfusion in people with diabetes caused by higher volume of habitual exercise.

In this study, a OO Shore durometer was used to assess the plantar soft tissue hardness in people with diabetes. The results showed that compared to the low exercise volume group, people with diabetes in the high exercise volume group who actively engaged in weight-bearing exercise had a significantly lower plantar tissue hardness (**Figure 1**). According to the Physical Stress Theory proposed by Muller et al. (Mueller and Maluf, 2002; Kluding et al., 2017), tissues have different adaptive responses to external physical stress stimulation, including decreased tolerance (e.g., atrophy), maintenance, increased tolerance (e.g., hypertrophy), injury, and death. Maintenance seems to be a tissue homeostasis, physical stress stimulus below the maintenance range may result in tissue atrophy, and physical stress stimulus above the maintenance range may result in increased tolerance (Mueller and Maluf, 2002; Kluding et al., 2017). Therefore, people with diabetes in the high exercise volume group who showed a lower plantar tissue hardness may be due to the enhanced tissue adaptability under suitable repeated stress stimulus among the maintenance range. Decreased tolerance (e.g., atrophy) in the low exercise volume group may be more prone to tissue damage and cuticle thickening under mild external stress stimulus, which further leads to callus formation and an increased risk of DFUs. Some studies also reported that higher and long-term repetitive physical stress can increase collagen content and the diameter of collagen fibers, thicken skin and increase skin strength, which is beneficial to distribute plantar pressure and decrease the risk of skin breakdown (Sanders et al., 1995; Mueller and Maluf, 2002). Therefore, the mechanical stress stimulation during weight-bearing exercise in the high exercise volume group examined in this study could be expected to increase the stress tolerance threshold of plantar tissue and improve skin health.

The lower plantar tissue hardness of people with diabetes in the high exercise volume group could also be due to the improved blood circulation in the foot and enhanced protective response of tissue microvessels under stress. Mithraratne et al. demonstrated a negative correlation between the hardness of plantar tissue and the level of blood supply in the arteries of the foot (Mithraratne et al., 2012). Exercise can improve blood flow and oxygen saturation levels, which has been shown to reduce local hypoxia and waste accumulation in the foot tissue of people with diabetes (Kluding et al., 2017; Reis et al., 2019), and improve the plantar tissue viability and tolerance under an external stimulus (Jan et al., 2013b). From this study, it is evident that tissue hardness of the foot is negatively correlated with SO2 and Temp, which further confirms the above interpretation. It indicates that weight-bearing exercise with habitual high exercise volume can improve the biomechanical properties and microcirculation in the feet of people with diabetes, which can interact to play a positive role in protecting overall foot health.

In this study, eight participants were confirmed as diabetic peripheral neuropathy in the high exercise volume group (17.8%), and five participants were confirmed as diabetic peripheral neuropathy in the low exercise volume group (14.3%). This study found that the plantar SO_2 of DPN participants was slightly lower than the Non-DPN participants in the high exercise volume group (65.23 ± 4.52 vs 67.69 ± 6.37; unit: %), and the DPN participants had the highest plantar tissue hardness value (Big toe: 36.60 ± 7.34; Little toes: 35.68 ± 13.90; Forefoot: 40.83 ± 6.48; Midfoot: 34.69 ± 7.80; Hindfoot: 46.15 ± 8.66; unit: °shore). This may be due to the reduced tissue deformability and perception to external mechanical stress caused by diabetic neuropathy. For people with diabetes and neuropathy, the loss of protective sensations in the foot, dysfunction in sweat glands, bone deformities and abnormal stress distribution would further accelerate plantar tissue stiffening (Bowering, 2001; Sun et al., 2011). The impaired microvascular regulation caused by neuropathy can hinder the oxygenation capacity and waste removal capability of foot tissue under mechanical stress. This may be the reason for the decreased SO_2 and increased tissue hardness in DPN participants in the high exercise volume group (Edmonds et al., 1982; Stevens et al., 1991). Although it has been reported that moderate walking speed does not increase the incidence and recurrence of foot ulcers in people with DPN (LeMaster et al., 2008), a higher tissue hardness and lower SO_2 are thought to increase the risk of developing foot ulcers (Murray et al., 1996; Jan et al., 2013a). Therefore, neuropathy may be an important consideration when people with diabetes engage in exercise, and it is necessary for people with DPN to carefully choose the type and intensity of weight-bearing exercise. In the future, it is still necessary to expand the sample size and conduct a similar study on people with diabetic peripheral neuropathy to clarify the impact of weight-bearing exercise on the risk of diabetic foot ulcers in people with diabetic peripheral neuropathy.

In addition, the results of this study showed that participants who regularly went for brisk walk and participated in ball games had higher plantar tissue hardness in the forefoot region. Participants with brisk walking had the highest plantar tissue hardness in the hindfoot region (**Table 3**). Burnfield et al. found that faster walking increased the plantar pressure around the toes, medial metatarsal heads and heel when healthy elderly people walked at different speeds (57, 80, 97 m/min) (Burnfield et al., 2004). Similarly, Lam et al. reported that playing table tennis produced higher peak pressure in the total foot during side-step and cross-step footwork in comparison with one-step footwork (Lam et al., 2019). This suggests that the high hardness in participants of this study who routinely participated in brisk walking and ball games (table tennis, tennis, golf, and billiards) may be related to the repetitive high plantar pressure acting on the plantar soft tissues during exercise. Such a high-magnitude pressure stimulus for a brief duration may cause excessive physical stress to plantar tissue, and further cause callus formation and tissue damage (Murray et al., 1996; Mueller and Maluf, 2002). However, the effect of different types of exercise on the risk of developing DFUs needs further exploration.

There are some limitations to this study that should be noted. Firstly, the durometer works on the principle of indentation to characterize the plantar tissue hardness, ignoring the non-linear viscoelastic behaviour and tissue thickness. Subsequent studies can use ultrasound imaging to explore the biomechanical properties of plantar tissue in more detail. Secondly, this study only considered a limited number of physical activities with moderate intensity, and the predominant exercise performed across all participants was walking. The influence of accumulated stress and different activity patterns on the risk of developing DFUs needs further study. Thirdly, the impact of exercise on other DFUs risk factors such as transcutaneous oxygen tension ($TcPO_2$), the microvascular response to mechanical stress, musculoskeletal deformities and callus formation of the foot may be considered in future studies. Fourthly, participants in this study had not yet developed foot ulcers. Because the relationships between foot ulcers and tissue hardness, and oxygen saturation are still unclear, follow-up studies should determine whether lower oxygen saturation and higher plantar tissue hardness in the low exercise volume group with diabetic peripheral neuropathy is associated with higher incidence of diabetic foot ulcers.

CONCLUSION

In conclusion, this study found that higher volumes of habitual weight-bearing exercise in people with type 2 diabetes are associated with better plantar tissue oxygenation and lower plantar tissue hardness. These changes may decrease the risk of developing diabetic foot ulcers.

AUTHOR CONTRIBUTIONS

Methodology, YF, FP, and Y-KJ; formal analysis, WR and YD; investigation, WY, WL, HL, and JG; data curation, WR, YD, and WY; writing—original draft preparation, WR and YD; writing—review and editing, FP and Y-KJ; funding acquisition, WR, YF and FP. All authors have read and agreed to the published version of the manuscript.

ACKNOWLEDGMENTS

The authors thank all subjects who participated in this study.

REFERENCES

Ainsworth, B. E., Haskell, W. L., Herrmann, S. D., Meckes, N., Bassett, D. R., Jr., Tudor-Locke, C., et al. (2011). 2011 Compendium of Physical Activities. *Med. Sci. Sports Exer* 43 (8), 1575–1581. doi:10.1249/MSS.0b013e31821ece12

Ainsworth, B. E. (2014). "How to Assess the Energy Costs of Exercise and Sport," in *Sports Nutrition*. Editor R. J. Maughan. 1st ed (UK: John Wiley & Sons), 67.

Armstrong, D. G., Boulton, A. J. M., and Bus, S. A. (2017). Diabetic Foot Ulcers and Their Recurrence. *N. Engl. J. Med.* 376 (24), 2367–2375. doi:10.1056/NEJMra1615439

Association, A. D. (2020). 5. Facilitating Behavior Change and Well-Being to Improve Health Outcomes: Standards of Medical Care in Diabetes-2020. *Dia Care* 43 (1), S48–S65. doi:10.2337/dc20-S005

Boulton, A. J. M., Armstrong, D. G., Albert, S. F., Frykberg, R. G., Hellman, R., Kirkman, M. S., et al. (2008). Comprehensive Foot Examination and Risk Assessment: A Report of the Task Force of the Foot Care Interest Group of the American Diabetes Association, with Endorsement by the American Association of Clinical Endocrinologists. *Diabetes Care* 31 (8), 1679–1685. doi:10.2337/dc08-9021

Bowering, C. K. (2001). Diabetic Foot Ulcers. Pathophysiology, Assessment, and Therapy. *Can. Fam. Physician* 47 (5), 1007–1016.

Burnfield, J. M., Few, C. D., Mohamed, O. S., and Perry, J. (2004). The Influence of Walking Speed and Footwear on Plantar Pressures in Older Adults. *Clin. Biomech.* 19 (1), 78–84. doi:10.1016/j.clinbiomech.2003.09.007

Caselli, A., Pham, H., Giurini, J. M., Armstrong, D. G., and Veves, A. (2002). The Forefoot-To-Rearfoot Plantar Pressure Ratio Is Increased in Severe Diabetic Neuropathy and Can Predict Foot Ulceration. *Diabetes Care* 25 (6), 1066–1071. doi:10.2337/diacare.25.6.1066

Chao, C. Y. L., and Cheing, G. L. Y. (2009). Microvascular Dysfunction in Diabetic Foot Disease and Ulceration. *Diabetes Metab. Res. Rev.* 25 (7), 604–614. doi:10.1002/dmrr.1004

Chao, C. Y. L., Zheng, Y.-P., and Cheing, G. L. Y. (2011). *Epidermal Thickness and Biomechanical Properties of Plantar Tissues in Diabetic Foot. Ultrasound Med. Biol.* 37 (7), 1029–1038. doi:10.1016/j.ultrasmedbio.2011.04.004

Demachi, K., Yoshida, T., Kume, M., Tsuji, M., and Tsuneoka, H. (2013). The Influence of Internal and Skin Temperatures on Active Cutaneous Vasodilation under Different Levels of Exercise and Ambient Temperatures in Humans. *Int. J. Biometeorol.* 57 (4), 589–596. doi:10.1007/s00484-012-0586-y

Di Loreto, C., Fanelli, C., Lucidi, P., Murdolo, G., De Cicco, A., Parlanti, N., et al. (2005). Make Your Diabetic Patients Walk: Long-Term Impact of Different Amounts of Physical Activity on Type 2 Diabetes. *Diabetes Care* 28 (6), 1295–1302. doi:10.2337/diacare.28.6.1295

Edmonds, M. E., Roberts, V. C., and Watkins, P. J. (1982). Blood Flow in the Diabetic Neuropathic Foot. *Diabetologia* 22 (1), 9–15. doi:10.1007/bf00253862

Ezema, C. I., Omeh, E., Omeh, E., Onyeso, O. K. K., Anyachukwu, C. C., Nwankwo, M. J., et al. (2019). The Effect of an Aerobic Exercise Programme on Blood Glucose Level, Cardiovascular Parameters, Peripheral Oxygen Saturation, and Body Mass Index Among Southern Nigerians with Type 2 Diabetes Mellitus, Undergoing Concurrent Sulfonylurea and Metformin Treatment. *Malaysian J. Med. Sci.* 26 (5), 88–97. doi:10.21315/mjms2019.26.5.8

Greenman, R. L., Panasyuk, S., Wang, X., Lyons, T. E., Dinh, T., Longoria, L., et al. (2005). Early Changes in the Skin Microcirculation and Muscle Metabolism of the Diabetic Foot. *The Lancet* 366 (9498), 1711–1717. doi:10.1016/s0140-6736(05)67696-9

Huonker, M., Halle, M., and Keul, J. (1996). Structural and Functional Adaptations of the Cardiovascular System by Training. *Int. J. Sports Med.* 17 (3), S164–S172. doi:10.1055/s-2007-972919

Jan, Y.-K., Lung, C.-W., Cuaderes, E., Rong, D., and Boyce, K. (2013a). Effect of Viscoelastic Properties of Plantar Soft Tissues on Plantar Pressures at the First Metatarsal Head in Diabetics with Peripheral Neuropathy. *Physiol. Meas.* 34 (1), 53–66. doi:10.1088/0967-3334/34/1/53

Jan, Y.-K., Shen, S., Foreman, R. D., and Ennis, W. J. (2013b). Skin Blood Flow Response to Locally Applied Mechanical and thermal Stresses in the Diabetic Foot. *Microvasc. Res.* 89, 40–46. doi:10.1016/j.mvr.2013.05.004

Kabbani, M., Rotter, R., Busche, M., Wuerfel, W., Jokuszies, A., Knobloch, K., et al. (2013). Impact of Diabetes and Peripheral Arterial Occlusive Disease on the Functional Microcirculation at the Plantar Foot. *Plast. Reconstr. Surg. Glob. open* 1 (7), e48. doi:10.1097/GOX.0b013e3182a4b9cb

Kluding, P. M., Bareiss, S. K., Hastings, M., Marcus, R. L., Sinacore, D. R., and Mueller, M. J. (2017). Physical Training and Activity in People with Diabetic Peripheral Neuropathy: Paradigm Shift. *Phys. Ther.* 97 (1), 31–43. doi:10.2522/ptj.20160124

Knowler, W. C., Barrett-Connor, E., Fowler, S. E., Hamman, R. F., Lachin, J. M., Walker, E. A., et al. (2002). Reduction in the Incidence of Type 2 Diabetes with Lifestyle Intervention or Metformin. *N. Engl. J. Med.* 346 (6), 393–403. doi:10.1056/nejmoa012512

Kokate, J. Y., Leland, K. J., Held, A. M., Hansen, G. L., Kveen, G. L., Johnson, B. A., et al. (1995). Temperature-modulated Pressure Ulcers: a Porcine Model. *Arch. Phys. Med. Rehabil.* 76 (7), 666–673. doi:10.1016/s0003-9993(95)80637-7

Ladurner, R., Feilitzsch, M., Steurer, W., Coerper, S., Königsrainer, A., and Beckert, S. (2009). The Impact of a Micro-lightguide Spectrophotometer on the Intraoperative Assessment of Hepatic Microcirculation: A Pilot Study. *Microvasc. Res.* 77 (3), 387–388. doi:10.1016/j.mvr.2009.01.008

Lalli, P., Chan, A., Garven, A., Midha, N., Chan, C., Brady, S., et al. (2013). Increased Gait Variability in Diabetes Mellitus Patients with Neuropathic Pain. *J. Diabetes its Complications* 27 (3), 248–254. doi:10.1016/j.jdiacomp.2012.10.013

Lam, W.-K., Fan, J.-X., Zheng, Y., and Lee, W. C.-C. (2019). Joint and Plantar Loading in Table Tennis Topspin Forehand with Different Footwork. *Eur. J. Sport Sci.* 19 (4), 471–479. doi:10.1080/17461391.2018.1534993

LeMaster, J. W., Mueller, M. J., Reiber, G. E., Mehr, D. R., Madsen, R. W., and Conn, V. S. (2008). Effect of Weight-Bearing Activity on Foot Ulcer Incidence in People with Diabetic Peripheral Neuropathy: Feet First Randomized Controlled Trial. *Phys. Ther.* 88 (11), 1385–1398. doi:10.2522/ptj.20080019

Liao, F., An, R., Pu, F., Burns, S., Shen, S., and Jan, Y.-K. (2019). Effect of Exercise on Risk Factors of Diabetic Foot Ulcers. *Am. J. Phys. Med. Rehabil.* 98 (2), 103–116. doi:10.1097/phm.0000000000001002

Mithraratne, K., Ho, H., Hunter, P. J., and Fernandez, J. W. (2012). Mechanics of the Foot Part 2: A Coupled Solid-Fluid Model to Investigate Blood Transport in the Pathologic Foot. *Int. J. Numer. Meth. Biomed. Engng.* 28 (10), 1071–1081. doi:10.1002/cnm.2493

Mueller, M. J., and Maluf, K. S. (2002). Tissue Adaptation to Physical Stress: A Proposed "physical Stress Theory" to Guide Physical Therapist Practice, Education, and Research. *Phys. Ther.* 82 (4), 383–403. doi:10.1093/ptj/82.4.383

Mueller, M. J., Tuttle, L. J., LeMaster, J. W., Strube, M. J., McGill, J. B., Hastings, M. K., et al. (2013). Weight-Bearing versus Nonweight-Bearing Exercise for Persons with Diabetes and Peripheral Neuropathy: A Randomized Controlled Trial. *Arch. Phys. Med. Rehabil.* 94 (5), 829–838. doi:10.1016/j.apmr.2012.12.015

Murray, H. J., Young, M. J., Hollis, S., and Boulton, A. J. M. (1996). The Association between Callus Formation, High Pressures and Neuropathy in Diabetic Foot Ulceration. *Diabet. Med.* 13 (11), 979 982. doi:10.1002/(sici)1096-9136(199611)13:11<979:aid-dia267>3.0.co;2-a

Mynarski, W., Psurek, A., Borek, Z., Rozpara, M., Grabara, M., and Strojek, K. (2012). Declared and Real Physical Activity in Patients with Type 2 Diabetes Mellitus as Assessed by the International Physical Activity Questionnaire and Caltrac Accelerometer Monitor: A Potential Tool for Physical Activity Assessment in Patients with Type 2 Diabetes Mellitus. *Diabetes Res. Clin. Pract.* 98 (1), 46–50. doi:10.1016/j.diabres.2012.05.024

Narres, M., Kvitkina, T., Claessen, H., Droste, S., Schuster, B., Morbach, S., et al. (2017). Incidence of Lower Extremity Amputations in the Diabetic Compared with the Non-diabetic Population: A Systematic Review. *Plos One* 12 (8), e0182081. doi:10.1371/journal.pone.0182081

Newton, D. J., Bennett, S. P., Fraser, J., Khan, F., Belch, J. J. F., Griffiths, G., et al. (2005). Pilot Study of the Effects of Local Pressure on Microvascular Function in the Diabetic Foot. *Diabet Med.* 22 (11), 1487–1491. doi:10.1111/j.1464-5491.2005.01659.x

Periyasamy, R., Gandhi, T. K., Das, S. R., Ammini, A. C., and Anand, S. (2012). A Screening Computational Tool for Detection of Diabetic Neuropathy and Non-neuropathy in Type-2 Diabetes Subjects. *J. Med. Imaging Hlth Inform.* 2 (3), 222–229. doi:10.1166/jmihi.2012.1093

Pu, F., Ren, W., Fu, H., Zheng, X., Yang, M., Jan, Y.-K., et al. (2018). Plantar Blood Flow Response to Accumulated Pressure Stimulus in Diabetic People with Different Peak Plantar Pressure: a Non-randomized Clinical Trial. *Med. Biol. Eng. Comput.* 56 (7), 1127–1134. doi:10.1007/s11517-018-1836-x

Reis, J. F., Fatela, P., Mendonca, G. V., Vaz, J. R., Valamatos, M. J., Infante, J., et al. (2019). Tissue Oxygenation in Response to Different Relative Levels of Blood-Flow Restricted Exercise. *Front. Physiol.* 10, 407. doi:10.3389/fphys.2019.00407

Sanders, J. E., Goldstein, B. S., and Leotta, D. F. (1995). Skin Response to Mechanical Stress: Adaptation rather Than Breakdown-A Review of the Literature. *J. Rehabil. Res. Dev.* 32 (3), 214–226.

Schaper, N. C., Netten, J. J., Apelqvist, J., Bus, S. A., Hinchliffe, R. J., Lipsky, B. A., et al. (2020). Practical Guidelines on the Prevention and Management of Diabetic Foot Disease (IWGDF 2019 Update). *Diabetes Metab. Res. Rev.* 36, e3266. doi:10.1002/dmrr.3266

Sivanandam, S., Anburajan, M., Venkatraman, B., Menaka, M., and Sharath, D. (2012). Medical Thermography: a Diagnostic Approach for Type 2 Diabetes Based on Non-contact Infrared thermal Imaging. *Endocrine* 42 (2), 343–351. doi:10.1007/s12020-012-9645-8

Stevens, M. J., Edmonds, M. E., Douglas, S. L. E., and Watkins, P. J. (1991). Influence of Neuropathy on the Microvascular Response to Local Heating in the Human Diabetic Foot. *Clin. Sci.* 80 (3), 249–256. doi:10.1042/cs0800249

Sun, J.-H., Cheng, B. K., Zheng, Y.-P., Huang, Y.-P., Leung, J. Y., and Cheing, G. L. (2011). Changes in the Thickness and Stiffness of Plantar Soft Tissues in People with Diabetic Peripheral Neuropathy. *Arch. Phys. Med. Rehabil.* 92 (9), 1484–1489. doi:10.1016/j.apmr.2011.03.015

Teoh, J. C., and Lee, T. (2020). Identification of Potential Plantar Ulceration Among Diabetes Patients Using Plantar Soft Tissue Stiffness. *J. Mech. Behav. Biomed. Mater.* 103, 103567. doi:10.1016/j.jmbbm.2019.103567

Thomas, V. J., Patil, K. M., Radhakrishnan, S., Narayanamurthy, V. B., and Parivalavan, R. (2003). The Role of Skin Hardness, Thickness, and Sensory Loss on Standing Foot Power in the Development of Plantar Ulcers in Patients with Diabetes Mellitus-A Preliminary Study. *The Int. J. Lower Extremity Wounds* 2 (3), 132–139. doi:10.1177/1534734603258601

van Netten, J. J., Prijs, M., van Baal, J. G., Liu, C., van der Heijden, F., and Bus, S. A. (2014). Diagnostic Values for Skin Temperature Assessment to Detect Diabetes-Related Foot Complications. *Diabetes Technol. Ther.* 16 (11), 714–721. doi:10.1089/dia.2014.0052

Verboven, M., Van Ryckeghem, L., Belkhouribchia, J., Dendale, P., Eijnde, B. O., Hansen, D., et al. (2019). Effect of Exercise Intervention on Cardiac Function in Type 2 Diabetes Mellitus: A Systematic Review. *Sports Med.* 49 (2), 255–268. doi:10.1007/s40279-018-1003-4

Wen, C. P., Wai, J. P. M., Tsai, M. K., Yang, Y. C., Cheng, T. Y. D., Lee, M.-C., et al. (2011). Minimum Amount of Physical Activity for Reduced Mortality and Extended Life Expectancy: a Prospective Cohort Study. *The Lancet* 378 (9798), 1244–1253. doi:10.1016/s0140-6736(11)60749-6

9

Preparation of Antimicrobial Hyaluronic Acid/Quaternized Chitosan Hydrogels for the Promotion of Seawater-Immersion Wound Healing

Xinlu Wang[1,2†], *Pengcheng Xu*[2†], *Zexin Yao*[2,3], *Qi Fang*[1], *Longbao Feng*[4], *Rui Guo*[5*] and *Biao Cheng*[2*]

[1] The First Clinical Hospital of Guangzhou Medical University, Guangzhou, China, [2] Department of Plastic Surgery, General Hospital of Southern Theater Command, PLA, Guangzhou, China, [3] Department of Public Health, Guangdong Pharmaceutical University, Guangzhou, China, [4] Beogene Biotech (Guangzhou) Co., Ltd., Guangzhou, China, [5] Key Laboratory of Biomaterials of Guangdong Higher Education Institutes, Department of Biomedical Engineering, Guangdong Provincial Engineering and Technological Research Center for Drug Carrier Development, Jinan University, Guangzhou, China

***Correspondence:**
Rui Guo
guorui@jnu.edu.cn
Biao Cheng
chengbiaocheng@163.com

† These authors have contributed equally to this work

Wound immersion in seawater with high salt, high sodium, and a high abundance of pathogenic bacteria, especially gram-negative bacteria, can cause serious infections and difficulties in wound repair. The present study aimed to prepare a composite hydrogel composed of hyaluronic acid (HA) and quaternized chitosan (QCS) that may promote wound healing of seawater-immersed wounds and prevent bacterial infection. Based on dynamic Schiff base linkage, hydrogel was prepared by mixing oxidized hyaluronic acid (OHA) and hyaluronic acid-hydrazide (HA-ADH) under physiological conditions. With the addition of quaternized chitosan, oxidized hyaluronic acid/hyaluronic acid-hydrazide/quaternized chitosan (OHA/HA-ADH/O-HACC and OHA/HA-ADH/N-HACC) composite hydrogels with good swelling properties and mechanical properties, appropriate water vapor transmission rates (WVTR), and excellent stability were prepared. The biocompatibility of the hydrogels was demonstrated by *in vitro* fibroblast L929 cell culture study. The results of *in vitro* and *in vivo* studies revealed that the prepared antibacterial hydrogels could largely inhibit bacterial growth. The *in vivo* study further demonstrated that the antibacterial hydrogels exhibited high repair efficiencies in a seawater-immersed wound defect model. In addition, the antibacterial hydrogels decreased pro-inflammatory factors (TNF-α, IL-1β, and IL-6) but enhanced anti-inflammatory factors (TGF-β1) in wound. This work indicates that the prepared antibacterial composite hydrogels have great potential in chronic wound healing applications, such as severe wound cure and treatment of open trauma infections.

Keywords: quaternized chitosan, hydrogel, hyaluronic acid, seawater immersion, wound healing

INTRODUCTION

With the extensive use of high-tech weapons, especially precision-guided missiles on the battlefield, the trauma and burns caused by high-energy explosion in naval battle have become the most important and challenging healthcare issues (Zhu et al., 2017; Chen et al., 2019). In modern high-tech naval warfare, the unavoidable exposure of open traumas to seawater with high salt, high sodium, and a high abundance of pathogenic bacteria, especially gram-negative bacteria, can cause serious infections and wound-repair difficulties (Zhang et al., 2017). Current traditional antimicrobials such as antibiotics, iodine, silver, and zinc oxide are effective in preventing bacterial infection of skin wounds, but they cause resistance to last-line antibiotics and cause significant damage to vital organs (Chung et al., 2017; Lin et al., 2019). Considering these imperfect treatments, the development of new and more effective antimicrobials is still highly desired in clinical application.

Chitosan is a kind of natural polymer that has the characteristics of biodegradability, biocompatibility, and antimicrobial activity (Thattaruparambil et al., 2016; Liang et al., 2019a). It meets the requirements of environmental protection and has become one of the research hotspots in the development of natural antimicrobial agents (Sarhan et al., 2016). The antimicrobial mechanism of chitosan is based on the positive charge of the amino group at the C-2 position after protonation at a pH below 6, which can interact with the surface of bacteria and cause bacterial death (Pires et al., 2013; Yildirim-Aksoy and Beck, 2017). However, chitosan is insoluble in neutral and alkaline aqueous solutions with pH values of >6.5, which greatly limits its application (Mohamed et al., 2017). Recently, quaternized chitosan (QCS) has received more attention from researchers, as it can replace traditional antimicrobials and reduce organ damage (Thanou et al., 2002; You et al., 2016). The addition of quaternary amino groups in chitosan greatly enhances the water solubility of chitosan, and quaternized chitosan with antimicrobial activity combines with polyatomic amino groups to form double antimicrobial active groups, which greatly improves its antimicrobial field of application.

In wound treatment, wound dressing materials with superior properties are typically used to facilitate wound healing, of which hydrogels that have high water content, flexible mechanical properties, and good biocompatibility are considered promising candidates for practical application (Li et al., 2018, 2019; Yi et al., 2018). Firstly, by providing a porous structure and having a suitable swelling ratio, a hydrogel matrix can allow the presence of oxygen, remove wound exudates, and maintain a moist wound bed to promote wound healing (Kaoru et al., 2010; Rakhshaei and Namazi, 2017). Secondly, the antibacterial property of traditional dressing is endowed by antibiotics capsulated in the hydrogel matrix (Li et al., 2016). However, hydrogels with inherent antimicrobial properties have received widespread interest among biomaterial researchers (Gonzálezhenríquez et al., 2017; Zhao et al., 2017; Kumar et al., 2018). Thirdly, unlike traditional wound dressings (gauze and cotton wool), biodegraded hydrogel dressings are easy to peel off and degrade spontaneously, which avoids pain and secondary trauma during dressing changes (Yang et al., 2018).

Inspired by the concept of moist wound healing, numerous novel hydrogels have been designed, and these play an important role in the treatment of various wounds (Blacklow et al., 2019; Wang et al., 2019). The majority of hydrogels are prepared from natural polymer materials (e.g., alginate, carboxymethylcellulose, dextran, gelatin, collagen, and hyaluronic acid) and synthetic polymer materials [e.g., methoxy polyethylene glycol, poly(vinyl alcohol), peptide, and polyamidoamine] because of their excellent biocompatibility and biodegradability (Travan et al., 2016). Hyaluronic acid (HA), the main component of the extracellular membrane (ECM), can increase cell–matrix interaction and initiate the signal transduction essential for cell survival and function and has been widely used in the biomedical materials field because of its property of easily peeling, excellent biocompatibility, and high water retention (Purcell et al., 2012; Julia et al., 2013; Zhu et al., 2018a; Liang et al., 2019b).

In this work, biocompatible hydrogel wound dressings with inherent antibacterial properties were prepared by dynamic Schiff base linkage (**Scheme 1**). We furthermore demonstrated that these hydrogel dressings greatly promoted the healing process in a seawater-immersed full-thickness skin defect model. The hydrogels were prepared by mixing quaternized chitosan/hyaluronic acid-hydrazide (HA-ADH) solutions and oxidized hyaluronic acid (OHA) solution under physiological conditions. Hyaluronic acid (HA) was chosen as a hydrogel substrate due to its advantageous properties of high water retention performance and good biocompatibility (Li et al., 2017; Park et al., 2019). In this work, the addition of quaternized chitosan enhanced the mechanical properties of OHA/HA-ADH hydrogel. The hydrogels exhibited excellent antibacterial performance compared to the previous reported antibacterial hydrogels *in vitro* and *in vivo*. Furthermore, the results for the wound contraction area, bacteria in wound, histopathological examinations, collagen analysis, and pro-inflammatory factors (TNF-α, IL-1β, and IL-6) and anti-inflammatory factors (TGF-β1) in wound were employed to evaluate the *in vivo* therapeutic effect. The results indicated that these antibacterial hydrogels have good biocompatibility and show great potential as wound dressings, especially for the healing of severe wounds and open trauma infections.

MATERIALS AND METHODS

Reagents and Materials

Chitosan (CS, Mw = 3 kDa, degree of deacetylation = 95%) was obtained from Nantong Lushen Bioengineering Co., Ltd. (Jiangsu, China). Benzaldehyde, Glycidyltrimethylammonium chloride (GTMAC), (3-chloro-2-hydroxypropyl) trimethyl-ammonium chloride S, and ethylene glycol was purchased from Sinopharm Chemical Reagent Co., Ltd. (Shanghai, China). Hyaluronic acid (HA, Mw = 200 kDa) was purchased from Bloomage Freda Biopharm Co., Ltd. (Shangdong, China). Adipic dihydrazide (ADH), hydroxy-benzotriazole (HOBt), and dimethyl sulfoxide (DMSO) were purchased from Aladdin

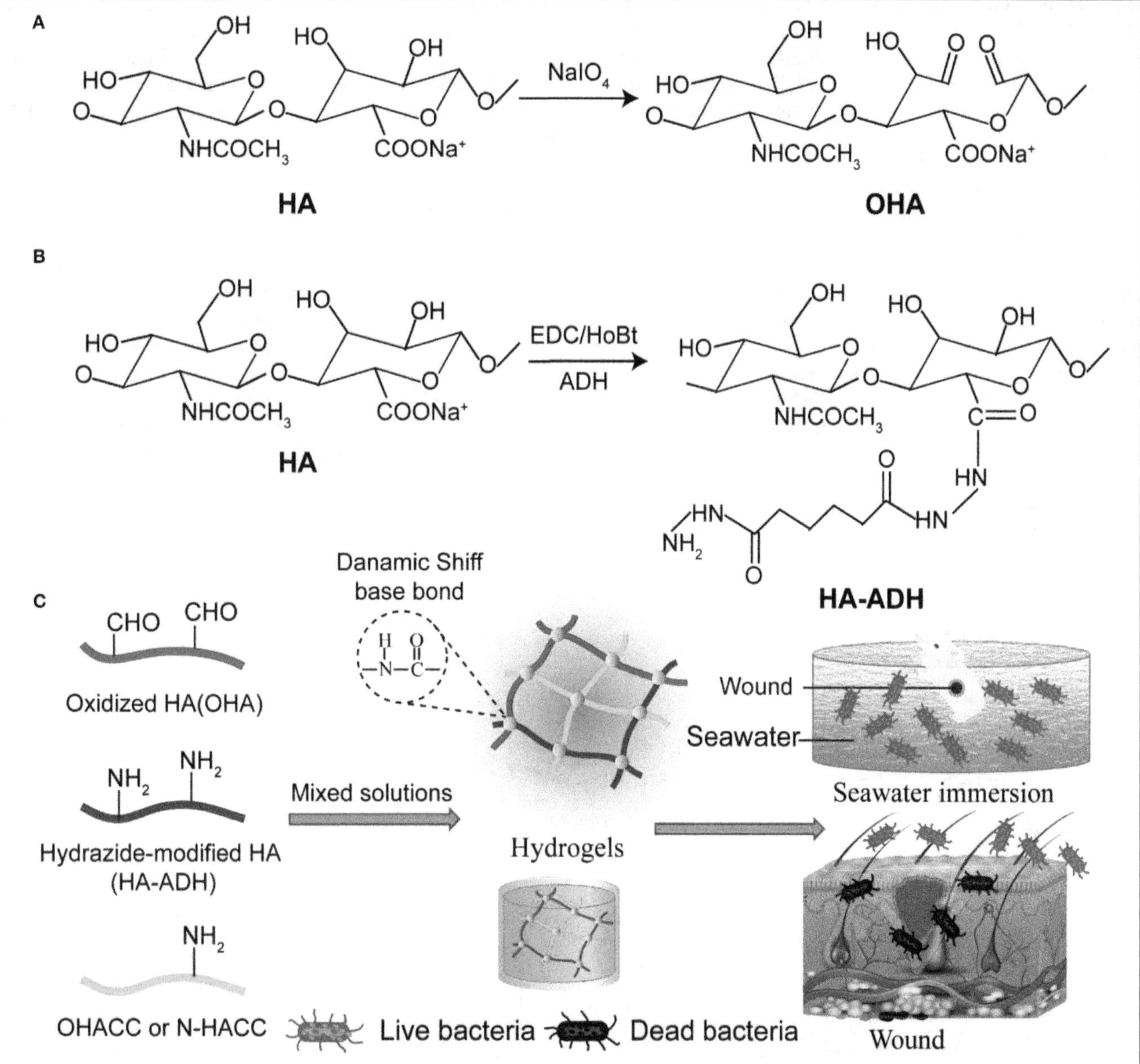

SCHEME 1 | The Davies-ENDOR pulse sequence. Schematic representation of hydrogel synthesis **(A)**. Steps of OHA synthesis. **(B)** Steps of HA-ADH synthesis. **(C)** Schematic representation of the preparation of the OHA/HA-ADH/O-HACC and OHA/HA-ADH/N-HACC hydrogels.

Chemical Company (Shanghai, China). Sodium periodate, 1-ethyl-3-(3-dimethylaminopropyl)-carbodiiminde (EDC), and hyaluronidase were obtained from Shanghai Yuanye Bio-Technology Co., Ltd. (Shanghai, China). The organic silicon film (BD film KYQ-500) was purchased from Hangzhou Baoerde New Materials Technology Co., Ltd (Hangzhou, China).

The L929 fibroblast cell line was obtained from Beogene Biotechnology Co., Ltd. (Guangzhou, China). Cell Counting Kit-8 (CCK8) was obtained from Beyotime Biotechnology Co., Ltd. (Shanghai, China). Live/dead cell staining kits were purchased from BestBio Bio-Technology Co., Ltd. (Shanghai, China). The bacteria strains of *Escherichia coli* (*E. coli*, CMCCB 44102) and *Staphylococcus aureus* (*S. aureus*, CMCCB 26003) were purchased from Guangdong Institute of Microbiology (Guangzhou, Guangdong). VRBA-MUG selection medium, Mannitol salt agar, and Pseudomonas agar base/CN-AGAR were obtained from HuanKai Microbial Biotechnology Co., Ltd (Guangzhou, China). The other reagents were listed as follows: Dulbecco's modified Eagle's medium (DMEM, Gibco, USA), fetal bovine serum (FBS, HyClone, USA), trypsin (Amresco, USA), and dimethyl sulfoxide (DMSO, Sigma-Aldrich, USA). All other reagents were analytical grade unless otherwise noted.

Synthesis of Quaternized Chitosan (QCS)

O-HACC and N-HACC were synthesized according to the previous literature with slight modifications (Hu et al., 2010; Xin et al., 2015; Mohamed et al., 2017). The synthesis route of O-HACC and N-HACC polymer is presented in **Scheme 2.**

Synthesis of O-HACC

Briefly, 0.3 g of chitosan powder was dissolved in 120 mL of 10% acetic acid for 4 h, 40 mL ethanol was added, and then 15.8 g benzaldehyde was added to the mixed solutions with continuous stirring. After the mixed solutions had been heated and reacted at 60°C for 20 h, the pH was adjusted to pH 7.0 using NaOH solution. The mixture was precipitated, filtered, and washed fully with methanol. The yellow powder chitosan imine Schiff base (Schiff-C S) was obtained by vacuum drying. A quantity of 2.5 g chitosan imine Schiff base and 7.5 g 2,3-epoxypropyl trimethylammonium chloride (ETA) were placed in a straight glass cylinder. Then, 0.02 g NaOH was dissolved in 10 mL water. The mixture was dissolved with the 10 mL 0.2 wt% NaOH solution with continuous stirring to obtain a viscous crude product. The product was precipitated by ethanol, filtered, and washed with 80% ethanol aqueous solution. The crude product was extracted by Soxhlet extractor with absolute ethyl alcohol as the solvent for 24 h and dried in a vacuum. The solid powder product was obtained and named O-HACC. The degree of quaternization (DQ) of the obtained O-HACC was 65.2%.

Synthesis of N-HACC

Briefly, 3.0 g of chitosan powder was suspended in 27 mL of isopropanol for a 4-h period at 8°C, and then 35 wt.% GTMAC was added dropwise to the suspension with continuous stirring. The pH of the mixed solutions was then adjusted to pH 7.0 using NaOH solution. After reaction at 80°C for 7 h, the mixture was poured into cold acetone, and stirring was continued for 12 h at 4°C. The mixture was washed three times with cold acetone and dialyzed in a dialysis sack (8–12 KDa molecular weight (MW) cut-off) for 3 days. The purified product was obtained by overnight lyophilization of the dialysate, and the fine powder collected was named N-HACC. The degree of quaternization (DQ) of the N-HACC obtained was 98.4%.

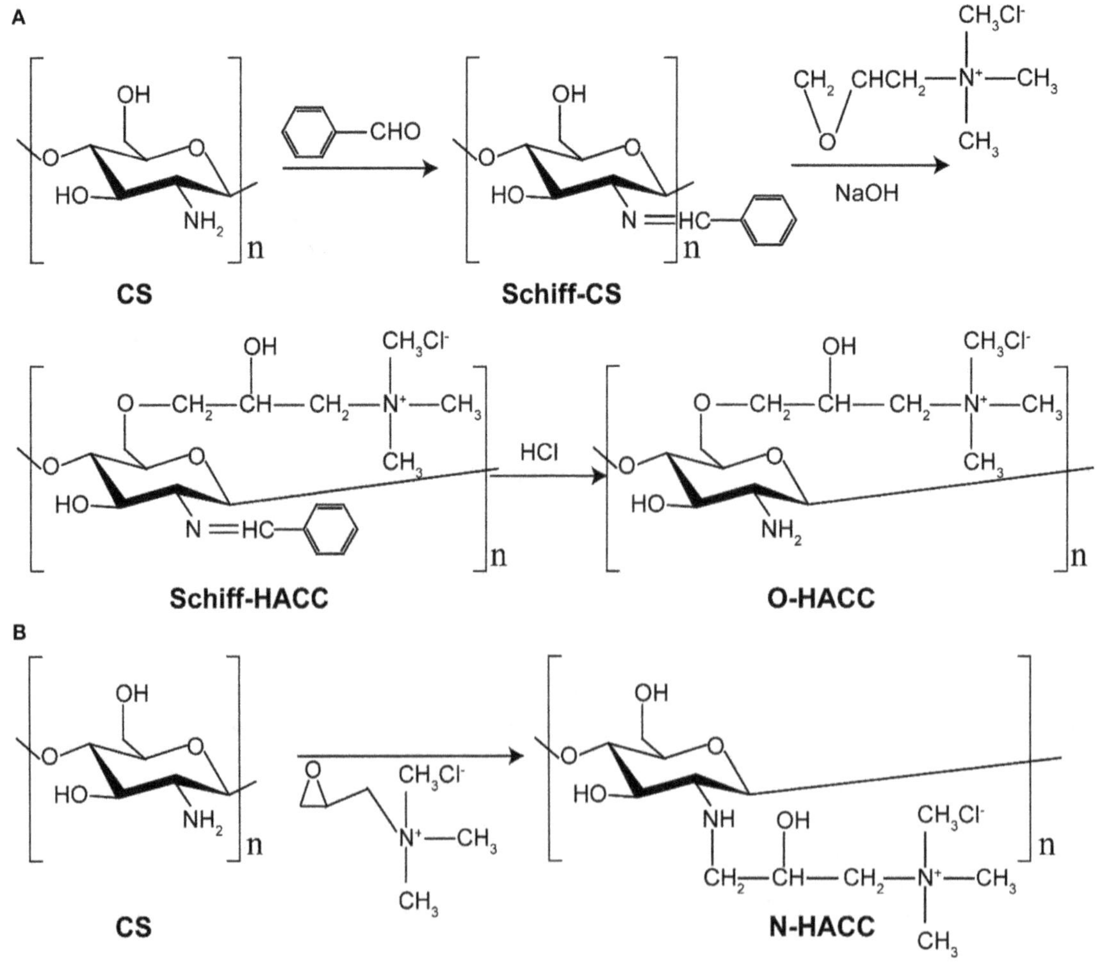

SCHEME 2 | (A) Steps of O-HACC polymer synthesis. **(B)** Steps of N-AACC polymer synthesis.

Characterization of O-HACC and N-HACC

Water Solubility

Chitosan (20 mg) was dissolved in 2 mL distilled water and 2 mL 1% (w/v) acetic acid solution at 25°C for 2 h with constant stirring, respectively. O-HACC (20 mg) and N-HACC (20 mg) was dissolved in 2 mL distilled water at 25°C for 2 h with constant stirring, respectively. The clarity of the solution was examined and photographed.

pH Dependence of the Water Solubility

The solubility was assessed for the pH range 3.0–12.0 via the turbidimetric titration method. O-HACC (40 mg) and N-HACC (40 mg) were dissolved in 20 mL of 1% acetic acid, and the solution was gradually titrated (20 μL) with NaOH (1 mol/L) to the final pH, with constant stirring. Absorbance measurements of the solutions were recorded using a UV spectrophotometer (UV-2550, Shimadzu, Tokyo, Japan) at $\lambda = 600$ nm.

Characterization of ^{1}H NMR and FT-IR

The chemical structure of the synthetic O-HACC and N-HACC was performed by ^{1}H NMR (AVANCE III 600M, Bruker, Germany). FT-IR spectral data were recorded with a Fourier transform-infrared spectrometer (FT-IR; Spectrum One, Perkin Elmer, Norwalk, USA). The samples were pressed with KBr.

Minimum Inhibitory Concentration (MIC) Measurements

The MIC of O-HACC and N-HACC were determined using a broth microdilution method, as described previously (Chin et al., 2018). Briefly, 50 μL deionized water solution of O-HACC and N-HACC with different concentrations was placed into each well of a 96-well microplate. Then, 50 μL of bacterial TSB solution (3×10^5 CFU/mL) was added into each well containing the polymer solution. A bacterial TSB solution without O-HACC and N-HACC was used as the control. The 96-well plate was kept in an incubator at 37°C under constant shaking at 100 rpm for 18 h. The MIC was taken as the concentration of the polymer at which no microbial growth was observed with unaided eyes and with the microplate reader at the end of 18-h incubation. All measurements were repeated three times in the same assay plate.

Preparation of the Antimicrobial Composite Hydrogels

Oxidized HA Synthesis (OHA)

OHA was synthesized according to a previously reported method, with a slight modification (Taichi et al., 2007). HA (1 g, 2.48 mmol) was dissolved in 150 mL distilled water, and then 5 mL $NaIO_4$ solution (0.5 mol/L) was added. The mixed solution was stirred at room temperature for 2 h, protected from light. The reaction was terminated by adding 1 mL ethylene glycol and stirring for an additional 1 h. The solution was dialyzed in a dialysis sack (MWCO 8,000–15,000) for 3 days against distilled water, changing the water three times per day, and then OHA was obtained by freeze-drying.

Hydrazide-Modified HA Synthesis (HA-ADH)

Hydrazide-modified HA (HA-ADH) was synthesized according to a previously established carbodiimide chemical process (Jia et al., 2004). In brief, HA (500 mg, 1.24 mmol) was dissolved in 125 mL distilled water, and then 8 g ADH was added. Subsequently, 10 mL DMSO/H_2O solution (V:V = 1:1) with 750 mg EDC and 660 mg HoBt was added into the previous HA solution, and the HA was reacted with ADH at a pH 4.75 for 4 h. The reaction was terminated by increasing the solution pH to 7.5 by adding NaOH solution. The HA–ADH solution was precipitated in ethanol, and the precipitate was re-dissolved in distilled water and dialyzed in a dialysis sack (MWCO 80,00–15,000) for 3 days against distilled water, changing the water three times per day, and then HA-ADH was obtained by freeze-drying.

Preparation of Composite Hydrogels

The hydrogels were fabricated by dynamic chemical bonding (Schiff base) of OHA and HA-ADH in a distilled solution. For the preparation of antimicrobial composite hydrogels, 4% (w/v) OHA and 4% (w/v) HA-ADH were fully dissolved in deionized water. Subsequently, 20 mg O-HACC (or 10 mg N-HACC) was added into 0.4 mL HA-ADH solution. After thorough gentle mixing, the mixture was transferred into a 48-well plate as a cylindrical mold. The resultant hydrogels were termed OHA/HA-ADH/O-HACC (or OHA/HA-ADH/N-HACC). The whole preparation processes of OHA/HA-ADH hydrogel was the same as for OHA/HA-ADH/O-HACC except for the addition of O-HACC.

Physical and Mechanical Properties

Swelling Ratio of the Hydrogels

The swelling behavior of the hydrogels was determined using the equilibrium swelling ratio (ESR). Briefly, hydrogels were weighed before the test and then immersed in phosphate-buffered saline (PBS) (pH 7.4, 37°C). At each measurement time point, the hydrogels were removed, gently blotted with filter paper to remove the excess surface water, and immediately weighed. The degree of swelling (DS) was calculated using the formula

$$DS = \frac{W_t - W_0}{W_0} \times 100\%$$

where W_t and W_0 are the weight of the hydrogel at time t and the weight of the hydrogel at t = 0, respectively.

Rheological Studies

Rheological measurements of the hydrogels were performed using a TA rheometer instrument (Kinexus, Ma Erwen instruments, Britain). For oscillatory time sweep experiments, the storage modulus (G′) and loss modulus (G″) were measured at a 10% strain, 1 Hz frequency, and 0.5 mm gap (CD mode) for 300 s. For the characterization of the linear viscoelastic range, a dynamic strain sweep test was run at frequencies ranging from 0.1 to 100 Hz.

Compression Test

Compression tests of the hydrogels were performed using a universal testing machine (model 5543; Instron, Norwood,

MA). The hydrogel samples (8 mm in diameter and 4 mm in thickness) were prepared in advance and equilibrated in PBS. The compressive strain rate was set at 1 mm min^{-1} with a 5 N load cell under 40% constraint. The measurements were performed three times ($n = 3$).

Water Vapor Transmission Rate (WVTR)

The moisture permeability of the hydrogels was determined by measuring their WVTR according to the American Society for Testing and Materials (ASTM) standard. Briefly, the hydrogel samples mounted on the mouth of a cylindrical vial (diameter 9.67 mm) containing 5 mL of deionized water, and then placed into a 37°C incubator at 79% relative humidity. The WVTR of the hydrogels was calculated using the formula

$$\text{WVTR}\left(\text{g/m}^2\text{day}^{-1}\right) = \frac{\Delta \text{m}}{\text{A} \times \text{time}}$$

where Δm is the weight of moisture loss for 24 h (g) and A is the effective transfer area (m^2).

In vitro Degradation of the Hydrogels

The hydrogels were placed in PBS (pH 7.4) containing either 0 or 100 U/mL of hyaluronidase solution in a horizontal shaker at 37°C for 28 days. The samples were carefully removed at predetermined time intervals of 3, 7, 14, 21, and 28 days. The remaining gels were taken out, washed with distilled water, and lyophilized. The percentage of degradation of hydrogels was calculated using the formula

$$\text{Degradation} = \frac{W_t}{W_0} \times 100\%$$

where W_0 is the initial weight of the freeze-dried hydrogels and W_t is the weight of the freeze-dried hydrogel at time t. All tests were performed on five samples ($n = 5$).

In vitro Biocompatibility Test

Hydrogels pre-treated with radiation for sterilization were immersed in DMEM with 10% fetal calf serum and 1% (v/v) penicillin/streptomycin at 37°C for 24 h to obtain the leach liquor. The L929 cells were seeded on a 96-well plate at a density of 2×10^4 cells per well and maintained with 100 μL of leach liquor. DMEM medium was cultured with L929 cells as controls. The leach liquor and DMEM medium were changed every 2 days. After 1, 2, and 3 days of incubation, the relative cell viabilities of the different experimental groups were measured via live/dead staining and CCK-8 colorimetric assay.

For the live/dead staining, the cells attached in each well were rinsed twice with PBS, and then 100 μL of live/dead staining stock solution was added to each well in a dark environment at 4°C for 15 min. Afterward, fluorescent images of the cells were examined using an inverted fluorescence microscope (TE2000-S, Nikon, Japan). For the CCK-8 assay, the cell culture medium was replaced by 100 μL of DMEM medium containing 10% CCK8 solution and was added to each well at 37°C for 1–1.5 h. The absorbance at 450 nm was read immediately on a microplate reader (SH1000, Corona, Japan).

In vitro Antimicrobial Evaluation

A 100-μL bacteria suspension (density = 10^6 CFU/mL) of *S. aureus* was added onto 400 μL of aseptically prepared OHA/HA-ADH, OHA/HA-ADH/O-HACC and OHA/HA-ADH/N-HACC hydrogels in 48-well plates and incubated for 1 h. Subsequently, 500 μL of LB broth was added to the hydrogels. After incubation for different durations (0, 8, and 16 h) at 37°C, the hydrogels were washed three times with PBS. The hydrogels were fixed with 4% (w/w) paraformaldehyde for 30 min. The hydrogels were further dehydrated with graded ethanol series (25, 50, 75, 90, and 100% ethanol) for 15 min each, and the samples were dried under a glass dryer. The specimens were pre-coated with gold and imaged using SEM.

Evaluation of the Anti-seawater Immersion and Wound Healing Efficacy of the Hydrogels *in vivo*

All animal studies were approved by the Institutional Animal Care and Use Committee (IACUC) of the General Hospital of the Southern Theater Command of the PLA, and the animals were treated according to the regulations. Adult male Sprague Dawley rats (200–250 g) were used for the study *in vivo*. Fifty receptor SD rats were randomly assigned to five groups: the organic silicon film control group (group I, the negative control without seawater), organic silicon film group (group II, the negative control with seawater), OHA/HA-ADH hydrogel group (group III with seawater), OHA/HA-ADH/O-HACC hydrogel group (group IV with seawater), and OHA/HA-ADH/N-HACC hydrogel group (group V with seawater). Prior to surgery, each rat was anesthetized with 3% pentobarbital (45 mg/kg), and the dorsal surface of the rats was shaved and disinfected with iodine. Four full-thickness skin wounds (diameter = 12 mm) were then created on the right and left sides of the backbone of each rat (see **Figure S1A**). Later, the wounded rats were soaked in seawater at a constant temperature of 28°C for 1 h. After 1 h of seawater immersion of the full-thickness skin wounds, the wounds were sewed up with their corresponding hydrogels using silicon film (see **Figure S1B**).

Wound Closure Measurement

The wounds were photographed at the different time points on day 1, 3, 7, 10, 14, and 21 post-surgery. The wound margin was traced, and the wound size was quantified using IPP 6.0 analysis software. The wound area and wound healing rate were calculated using the formulas

$$\text{Wound area} = \text{S}_t/\text{S}_0 \times 100\%$$

$$\text{Wound healing rate} = (\text{S}_0 - \text{S}_t)/\text{S}_0 \times 100\%$$

where S_0 and S_t were the area of the original wound and the area of the wound at the testing time, respectively. Rats were sacrificed on postoperative days 3, 7, 10, 14, and 21, and the tissue including the wound site and surrounding healthy skin was excised and fixed for immunohistochemical and histological evaluations.

In vivo Evaluation of the Antimicrobial Efficacy of Hydrogels

The antimicrobial efficacy of the hydrogels was explored by homogenizing skin tissue excised on day 3 for 3 min in a 5 mL centrifuge tube containing 3 mL saline. Ten-fold serial dilutions of sample solutions were prepared, and then 100 μL samples of the diluted solution were spread onto VRBA-MUG selection medium, Mannitol salt agar, and *P. aeruginosa* selection medium, respectively. VRBA-MUG selection medium was used to selectively culture *E. coli* (Red colony morphology), Mannitol salt agar was used to selectively culture *S. aureus* (yellow-gold colony morphology), and *P. aeruginosa* selection medium was used to selectively culture *P. aeruginosa* (green-yellow colony morphology). The plates were incubated for 24 h at 37°C, and the number of colonies with 5–300 CFU was counted.

Histology and Collagen Staining

The excised skin tissue was fixed by immersion in 4% paraformaldehyde solution for at least 12 h. The fixed skin grafts were dehydrated with a graded series of ethanol and then dimethyl benzene and embedded in paraffin. The paraffin-embedded wounds were cut into sections with a thickness of 4 μm using a microtome (RM2016, Leica, Shanghai, China). Sections were collected and stained with haematoxylin and eosin (H&E) for histological studies and with Sirius Red for collagen detection according to routine procedures. Finally, the skin sections were photographed by a light microscope (Vectra 3, PerkinElmer, Waltham, MA). The quantifications from Sirius Red staining was performed using IPP 6.0 software. Collagen deposition in the wound sites was calculated using the formula:

$$\text{Collagen deposition} = (\text{red} - \text{stained area of collagen}) / (\text{tissue area}).$$

Immunohistochemistry

For immunofluorescence staining, paraffin sections were stained using primary antibodies to TNF-a, TGF-β1, IL-1β, and IL-6 (Abcam, Cambridge, UK; 1:200 dilution). Subsequently, the sections were incubated with the universal secondary antibody (Abcam, ab205719, 1: 500 dilution) and VECTASTAIN Elite ABC reagent, washed in PBS, and reacted with DAB solution (Agilent Dako, Santa Clara, CA, USA). Finally, the nuclei were counterstained with hematoxylin. Images of the stained samples were photographed under a light microscope (Vectra 3, PerkinElmer, Waltham, MA). The positive marker percentage was quantified using IPP 6.0 software.

Western Blot Analysis

Tissue samples were completely homogenized in 10 times tissue volume protease inhibitors. Subsequently, the homogenates were centrifuged at 12,000 rpm for 10 min and loaded on 10–12% sodium dodecyl sulfate (SDS)-polyacrylamide gels. After being transferred to PVDF Western blot membranes, the proteins were incubated with different primary antibodies, specifically mouse anti- TGF-β1 (Abcam, ab92486, 1:1,000 dilution), rabbit anti- IL-1β (Abcam, ab108499, 1:1,000 dilution), rabbit anti-TNF-α (Abcam, ab6671, 1:1,000 dilution), and mouse anti-IL-6 (Abcam, ab9324, 1:1,000 dilution), overnight at 4°C. The membrane was further incubated with goat anti-mouse IgG H&L (HRP) conjugated secondary antibody (Abcam, ab205719, 1:5,000 dilution) for 1 h at room temperature, and was visualized via enhanced chemiluminescent reagent (Beyotime, Jiangsu, China) on X-ray film.

Assessment of Endotoxin and Inflammatory Mediators

Endotoxin was measured in blood serum. Blood was also obtained from each rat. The blood obtained was centrifuged at 5,000 rpm at 4°C for 10 min, and the upper serum was collected and stored at −80°C for subsequent evaluation. The serum was diluted 1:10 in sterile pyrogen-free water. The concentration of endotoxin (EU/mL) was measured by enzyme-linked immunosorbent assay (ELISA) techniques according to the manufacturer's protocol (Shanghai Biotechnology Co., Ltd., Shanghai, China). In this test, the detection limit of the endotoxin assay was 0–80 pg/mL (1 EU/mL = 100 pg/mL). The absorbance of each well was determined to be 450 nm using a microplate reader. The standard curve of endotoxin was constructed, and the corresponding concentration for the unknown sample was calculated. All determinations were performed in triplicate.

Statistical Analysis

Data were plotted using Origin 9.1 (OriginLab Corporation, Northampton, MA, USA). Error bars represent standard deviations (SDs). The statistical trends were analyzed by one-way analysis of variance (ANOVA). $^{*}p < 0.05$, $^{**}p < 0.01$, and $^{***}p < 0.001$ were considered to be significantly different.

RESULTS AND DISCUSSION

Synthesis of O-HACC and N-HACC

Limited solubility at pH 5.5–7.4 is one of the main disadvantages of chitosan, which restricts its application in biomedicine. The CS (water and 1% HAc, 1.0 mg/mL) and O-HACC and N-HACC derivatives (water, 1.0 mg/mL) all had the appearance of solubility (**Figure 1A**). The dependence of the solubility of CS, O-HACC, and N-HACC on pH was further investigated (**Figure 1B**). CS was completely soluble in the pH range from 3 to 5, and as the pH value reached 5.0, its solubility decreased. However, O-HACC and N-HACC were almost completely soluble in the pH range from 3 to 12. The results indicated that O-HACC and N-HACC increased solubility under different pH conditions.

The FT-IR spectra of CS, O-HACC, and N-HACC are shown in **Figure 1C**. The main bands of chitosan included a peak at 3,303 cm^{-1}, corresponding to the stretching of the O–H and N–H bonds, and the band at 1,024 cm^{-1} corresponded to the C=O bending vibration. The peak at 1,478 cm^{-1}, corresponding to the C–H bending vibration of CH_3, is presented in the infrared spectra of O-HACC and N-HACC but not that of CS (Ye et al., 2014; Xin et al., 2015).

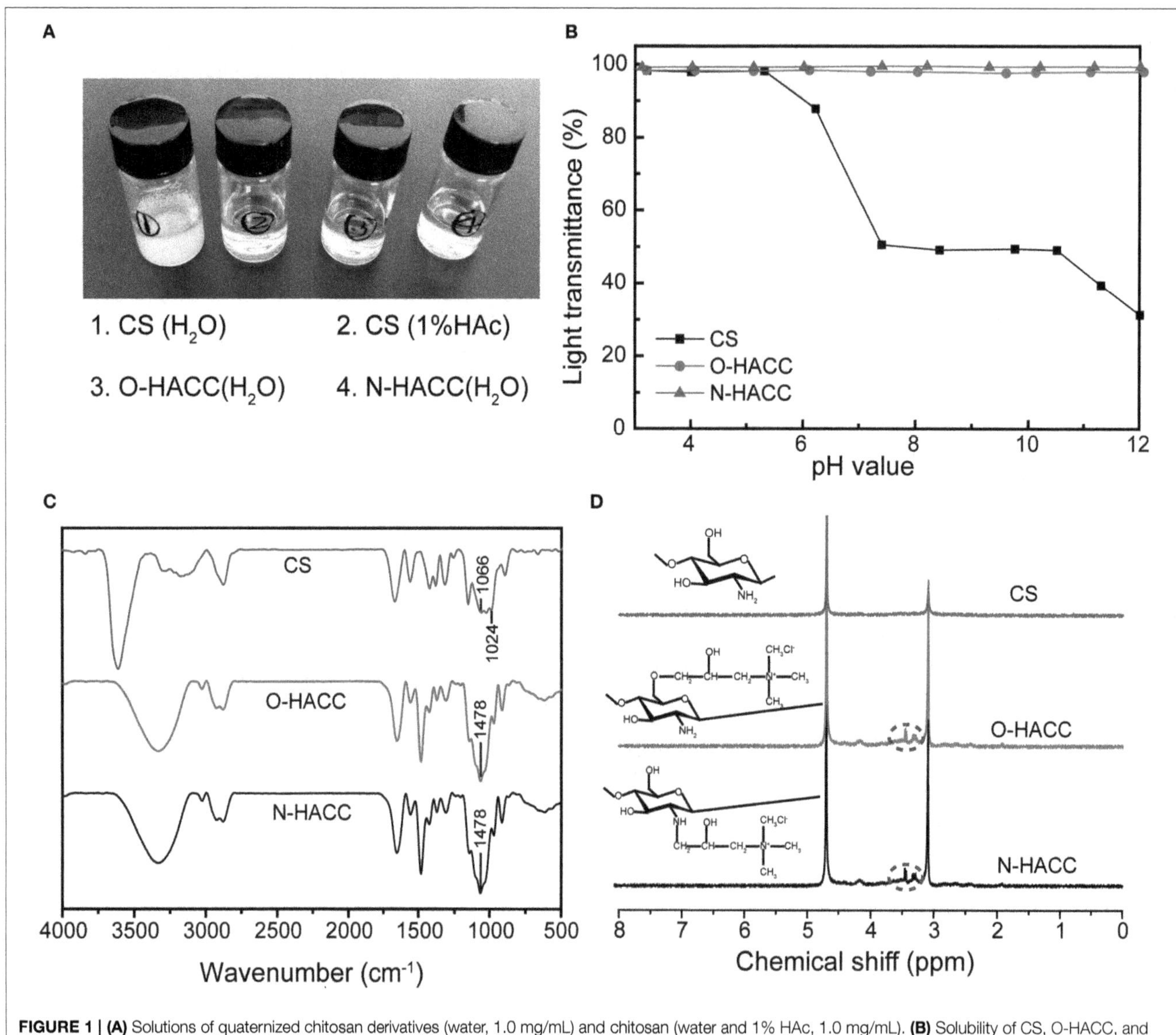

FIGURE 1 | (A) Solutions of quaternized chitosan derivatives (water, 1.0 mg/mL) and chitosan (water and 1% HAc, 1.0 mg/mL). **(B)** Solubility of CS, O-HACC, and N-HACC at pH 3–12. **(C)** FTIR spectra, and **(D)** ^{1}H NMR spectra of CS, O-HACC, and N-HACC.

This was indicative of the quaternary ammonium salt side-chain grafted onto the CS chain. In order to further determine whether the quaternary amino bond was conjugated to CS, ^{1}H NMR measurement was carried out (**Figure 1D**). Prior to the reaction with the quaternary amino group, the spectra of CS samples were determined. Compared to the spectra of the initial chitosan, a characteristic new peak in the strong-field region at $\delta = 3.2$–3.5 ppm (d, $-N^+(CH_3)_3$) indicates the presence of a trimethyl ammonium fragment in the structure of the macromolecules.

Physical and Mechanical Properties of Hydrogels

In this study, we designed a kind of hydrogel formed by dynamic Schiff's base linkage that has an appropriate swelling ratio, good compressive properties, and a comparable modulus to human soft tissue (Chen, 2017). Following the synthesis routes shown in **Schemes 1A,B**, OHA and HA-ADH macromolecules were successfully obtained.

The OHA/HA-ADH and OHA/HA-ADH/N-HACC hydrogels had a white color, while OHA/HA-ADH/O-HACC had a yellow color (**Figure 2A**). The swelling properties of the hydrogels were investigated to illustrate their water sorption capacity (Zhou et al., 2018). The results revealed that the swelling ratios of the OHA/HA-ADH, OHA/HA-ADH/O-HACC, and OHA/HA-ADH/N-HACC hydrogels in PBS reached 44.47, 6.03, and 10.96, respectively, in the first 2 h (**Figure 2B**). Compared to OHA/HA-ADH hydrogels, OHA/HA-ADH/O-HACC, and OHA/HA-ADH/N-HACC hydrogels showed a lower swelling ratio, which may be related to their higher crosslink density. The hydrogels had almost reached equilibrium swelling in 4 h, with a swelling ratio in PBS of 62.31, 14.11, and 28.84, respectively. A lower swelling ratio will not have a negative impact on the organization of the material.

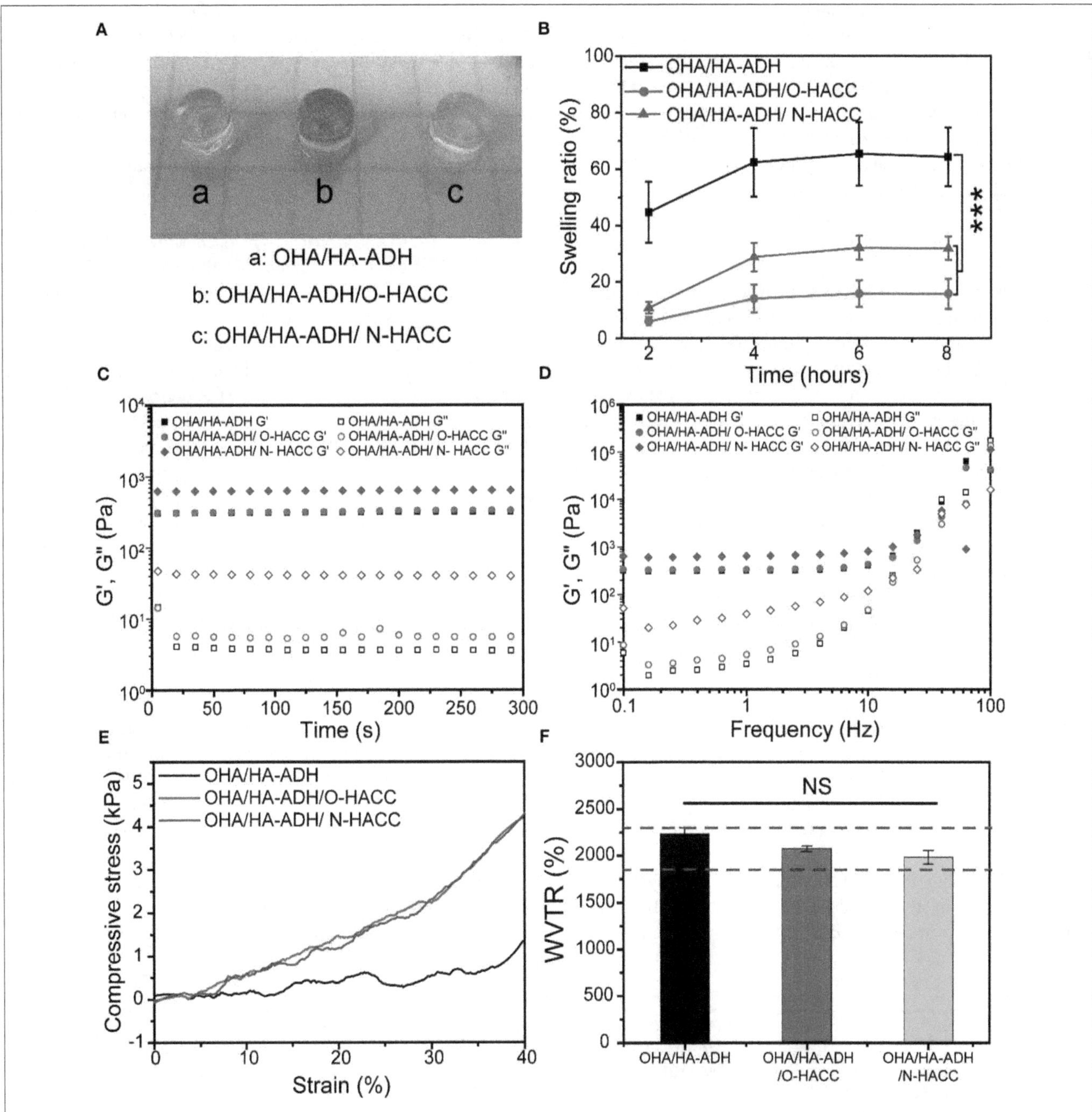

FIGURE 2 | Physical and mechanical properties of the hydrogels. **(A)** Photograph of typical hydrogels. **(B)** Swelling ratio. **(C)** Rheological properties. **(D)** Gel viscosity with frequency ranging from 0.1 to 100 Hz. **(E)** Compression modulus. **(F)** Water vapor transmission rate (WVTR); the blue dotted line represents the optimal WVTR range. $^{***}p < 0.001$.

The gelation behavior of the hydrogels was monitored by rheological analysis. As presented in **Figure 2C**, G′ surpassed G″ immediately after the addition of OHA to the HA-ADH solution due to the rapid formation of the hydrogel. This could provide hydrogel formation through diffusion of the polymer solution to the surrounding tissues when injected into the body. The final G′ of OHA/HA-ADH hydrogel can reach a plateau of 10^2-10^3 Pa, which would be able to maintain a structurally robust 3D network shape. Meanwhile, the storage modulus (G′) of OHA/HA-ADH/O-HACC and OHA/HA-ADH/N-HACC hydrogels was increased due to an increase in hydrogel concentration and dynamic Schiff's base bonding. As shown in **Figure 2D**, G′ surpassed G″ with a shear frequency from 0.1 to 100 rad/s due to the Schiff's base, which indicated that the hydrogel was stable.

An ideal hydrogel should have mechanical properties that enable it to maintain its integrity during use. The compression moduli of the hydrogels are presented in **Figure 2E**. The results showed the OHA/HA-ADH/O-HACC and OHA/HA-ADH/N-HACC hydrogels had a higher modulus (~4 kPa) than did OHA/HA-ADH hydrogel, comparable to that of human skin (Chen, 2017). This mechanical property was related to the structure of the hydrogels, i.e., the pore size of OHA/HA-ADH/O-HACC and OHA/HA-ADH/N-HACC hydrogels, which had a higher crosslinking density, was smaller than that of OHA/HA-ADH hydrogel, leading to a more compact structure. Our results showed that the compression modulus of the hydrogel could be improved by adding O-HACC or N-HACC.

Moisture control is a critical parameter in evaluating the healing process in wounds. A higher WVTR will result in dehydration of wound tissue and scarring, while a lower WVTR will cause wound maceration and harm to surrounding tissues. The WVTR values of the OHA/HA-ADH/O-HACC and OHA/HA-ADH/N-HACC hydrogels were tested to be lower than that of OHA/HA-ADH hydrogel due to their denser network structure (**Figure 2F**). This may be because the addition of quaternary ammonia chitosan leads to an increase in hydrogel concentration, resulting in a denser network structure. It is reported that the WVTR of normal skin ranges from 240 to 1,920 $g/m^2 \cdot 24\,h$, while that of an uncovered wound is in the order of 5,138 ± 202 $g/m^2 \cdot 24\,h$ (Xu et al., 2015; Yang et al., 2017). Previous studies have reported that an ideal wound dressing with a WVTR of 2,028.3 ± 237.8 $g/m^2 \cdot 24\,h$ was able to maintain a moist environment and promote exudate adsorption and that cells can also migrate more easily, promoting tissue regeneration (Xu et al., 2016). The WVTR value of the prepared hydrogels is close to that of the intact skin and ideal range, a value that avoids the risk of wound dehydration and is suitable for wound healing applications.

The weight loss curve of the prepared hydrogels when in PBS (either in the presence or absence of 100 U/mL hyaluronidase) decreased gradually as the incubation time increased (**Figures 3A,B**). All of the hydrogels degraded by 20–33% after 7 days, 50–63% after 14 days, 54–68% after 21 days, and 66–78% after 28 days (**Figure 3A**). When the hydrogels were submerged in PBS in the presence of hyaluronidase, the weight loss by degradation was significantly higher than that in PBS solution (**Figure 3B**). All of the hydrogels degraded by 82–93% after 28 days; this fast degradation rate was related to the β-elimination caused by hyaluronidase (Zhu et al., 2018b). Compared with OHA/HA-ADH, the OHA/HA-ADH/O-HACC and OHA/HA-ADH/N-HACC hydrogels shown a lower weight loss ratio. The results indicated that the addition of O-HACC and N-HACC effectively improves the enzymatic stability of the hydrogels by increasing the formation of dynamic chemical bonds (Schiff base linkage between $-NH_2$ and -CHO) (Qu et al., 2018). Therefore, the developed hydrogels could prolong the usage period and reduce replacement frequency. The MIC values of the O-HACC and N-HACC obtained were tested and are shown in **Table S1**. The results showed that the MIC values of O-HACC and N-HACC against gram-negative bacteria *E. coli* were 6.25 and 0.039 mg/mL and against gram-positive bacteria *S. aureus* were 24.2 and 0.078 mg/mL, respectively. In addition, the antibacterial effect of the O-HACC and N-HACC series against *E. coli* was stronger than that against *S. aureus*.

In vitro Biocompatibility of the Hydrogels

On the basis that the developed hydrogels had good physical properties and antibacterial activity, it was necessary to determine their biocompatibility, which is a prerequisite for well-designed biomedical materials (Wu et al., 2016; Cai et al., 2018). The cell viability ratio was evaluated by culturing murine-derived cell line L929 fibroblast cells with the leach liquor of the hydrogels. TCP and OHA/HA-ADH hydrogel without O-HACC and N-HACC were used as the control groups. It was clear that continuous increases in cell intensity from days 1 to 3 were observed for all groups, which indicated continuous proliferation of L929 fibroblast cells (**Figure 4A**). There were a large number of alive cells (green) and few dead cells (red) in all hydrogel groups,

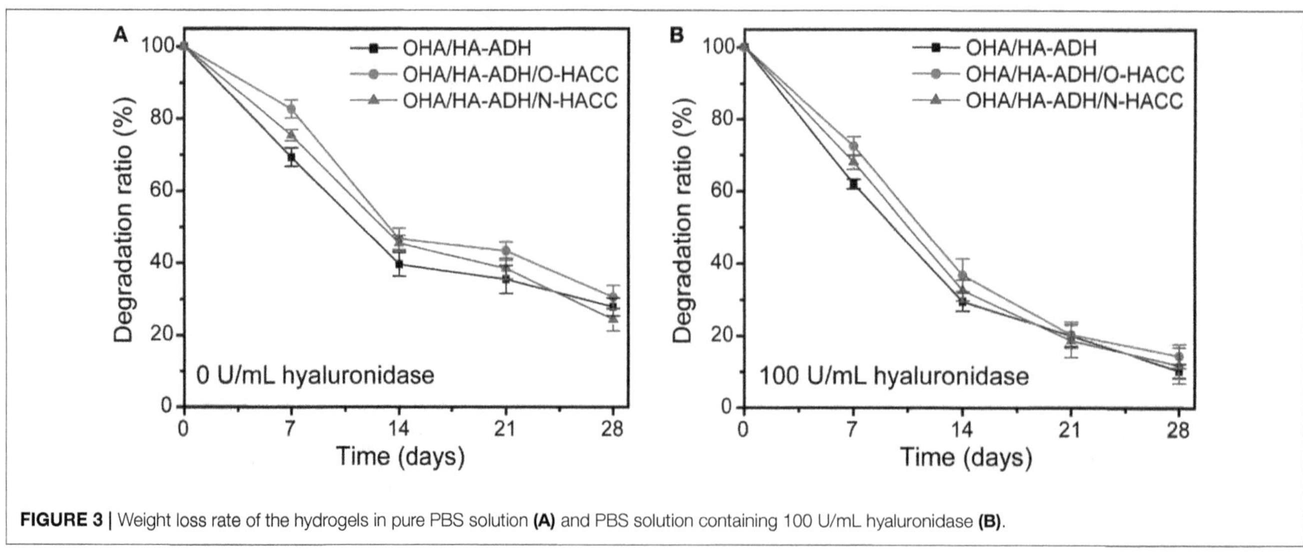

FIGURE 3 | Weight loss rate of the hydrogels in pure PBS solution **(A)** and PBS solution containing 100 U/mL hyaluronidase **(B)**.

and they showed no obvious difference from the control groups, which indicated the innate biocompatibility of the hydrogels. It is worth noting that the cell densities of the OHA/HA-ADH/O-HACC and HA/HA-ADH/N-HACC groups at predetermined time points were slightly lower than those of the OHA/HA-ADH hydrogel A and TCP groups.

The cell viability rate of L929 fibroblast cells on the hydrogel groups was further quantitatively examined in accordance with the CCK-8 assay, as shown in **Figure 4B**. For the first and second days, the cell viability of all of the hydrogel groups was comparable to the control groups. On the third day, the OHA/HA-ADH/N-HACC and OHA/HA-ADH/O-HACC groups exhibited slightly lower cell viability than the OHA/HA-ADH hydrogel and TCP groups because of the interaction between N-HACC and O-HACC, which have a positive charge, and the cells, but it still comparable with the control group (Kowapradit et al., 2011). This excellent biocompatibility can be related to the dynamic chemical bond (Schiff base linkage) of the hydrogels. All of the results confirmed that the addition of N-HACC or O-HACC to an OHA/HA-ADH hydrogel resulted

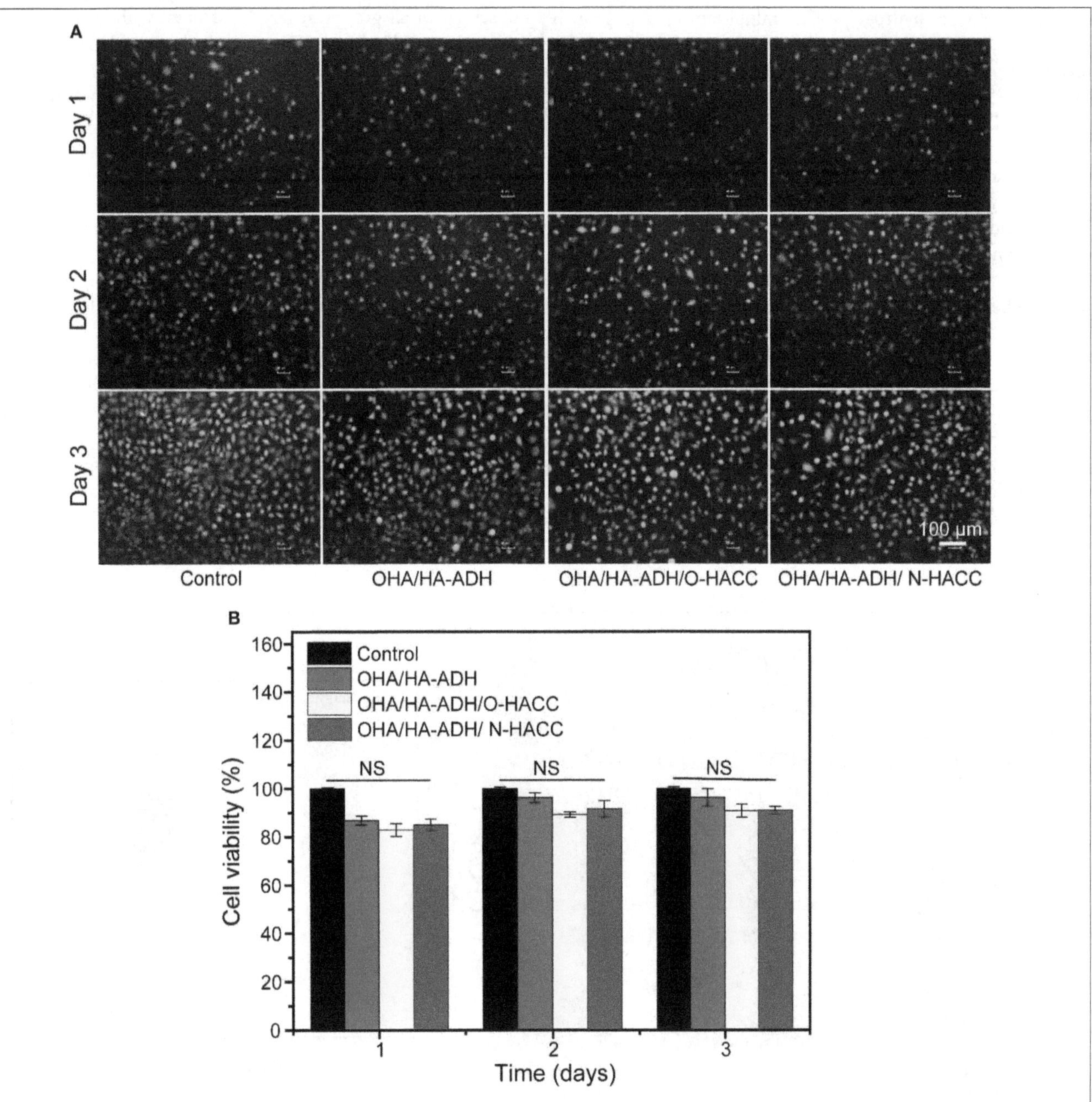

FIGURE 4 | *In vitro* biocompatibility evaluation of the hydrogels. **(A)** Fluorescence images of L929 cells after live/dead staining at day 1, day 2, and day 3. Green fluorescence indicates living cells, and red fluorescence indicates dead cells. **(B)** Cell viability of L929 cells at different culture times according to CCK-8 assay.

in satisfactory biocompatibility that was favorable for L929 cell growth and proliferation.

Bacterial Growth on the Hydrogel Surface and SEM Imaging

Besides serving as a barrier to protect wound tissues from external bacterial infections, hydrogels with inherent antimicrobial properties will be particularly attractive because they can prevent wound infections and promote the healing process (Gopinath et al., 2004). *S. aureus* was selected as a representative bacterium to evaluate the antimicrobial effect of the developed hydrogels. The inhibition of the growth of *S. aureus* by the developed hydrogels was assessed by measuring the number of *S. aureus* on the surface of the hydrogels. Bacterial growth on the hydrogels was observed using an SEM. It was clear that the OHA/HA-ADH hydrogel, which lacked antimicrobial material, had a large number of *S. aureus* attached to it, whereas *S. aureus* had significantly inhibited growth and was killed by OHA/HA-ADH/O-HACC and HA/HA-ADH/N-HACC hydrogels (**Figure 5A**). In addition, at 8 h, the number of *S. aureus* on OHA/HA-ADH was calculated to be about 179 CFU/area. However, the number of bacteria on OHA/HA-ADH/O-HACC and HA/HA-ADH/N-HACC hydrogels was 0 CFU/area for *S. aureus* (**Figure 5B**). At 24 h, the bacterial growth in the OHA/HA-ADH hydrogel increased significantly, with the bacteria number calculated to be 204 CFU/area, whereas the number of bacteria in OHA/HA-ADH/O-HACC and HA/HA-ADH/N-HACC hydrogels was only 16 and 12 CFU/area, respectively. The results indicated that *S. aureus* on the surface of the hydrogels were significantly inhibited or killed by the antimicrobial hydrogels (Peng et al., 2010).

The Hydrogels Promote Seawater-Immersion Wound Healing

The effect of the hydrogels on wound healing was further evaluated *in vivo* by using an animal wound model with seawater immersion. **Figure 6A** shows representative images of the wound surface on days 0, 3, 7, 10, 14, and 21 for each group. The wound area in all five groups became larger before 3 days, and obvious inflammation was observed in the control and OHA/HA-ADH groups with seawater immersion at day 3. Though the wound bed was infected, the wound area in the OHA/HA-ADH, OHA/HA-ADH/O-HACC, and OHA/HA-ADH/N-HACC groups became smaller with increasing time after 3 days, scab formation was observed in all groups at day 7. At day 14, the wounds of the control and OHA/HA-ADH groups had not healed well, whereas the wounds of the OHA/HA-ADH/O-HACC and OHA/HA-ADH/N-HACC groups had healed significantly. It was found that the OHA/HA-ADH/O-HACC and OHA/HA-ADH/N-HACC hydrogels significantly promoted wound healing, which could be ascribed to the combined effects of the inherent antibacterial performance of O-HACC and N-HACC and the moist wound bed provided by the OHA/HA-ADH hydrogel dressing.

The wound area percentage of the different groups at days 0, 3, 7, 10, 14, and 21 is shown in **Figure 6B**. The control group without seawater immersion showed the lowest wound area percentage of the groups. At days 3, 7, 10, and 14, the wound area percentages of the OHA/HA-ADH/O-HACC and OHA/HA-ADH/N-HACC groups were significantly lower than those of the control group and OHA/HA-ADH group with seawater immersion and were comparable with seawater immersion, which indicated that the addition of the antibacterial material (O-HACC and N-HACC) could induce bacterial death and prevent further infection. The same trend is presented through a more intuitive three-dimensional view of the wound

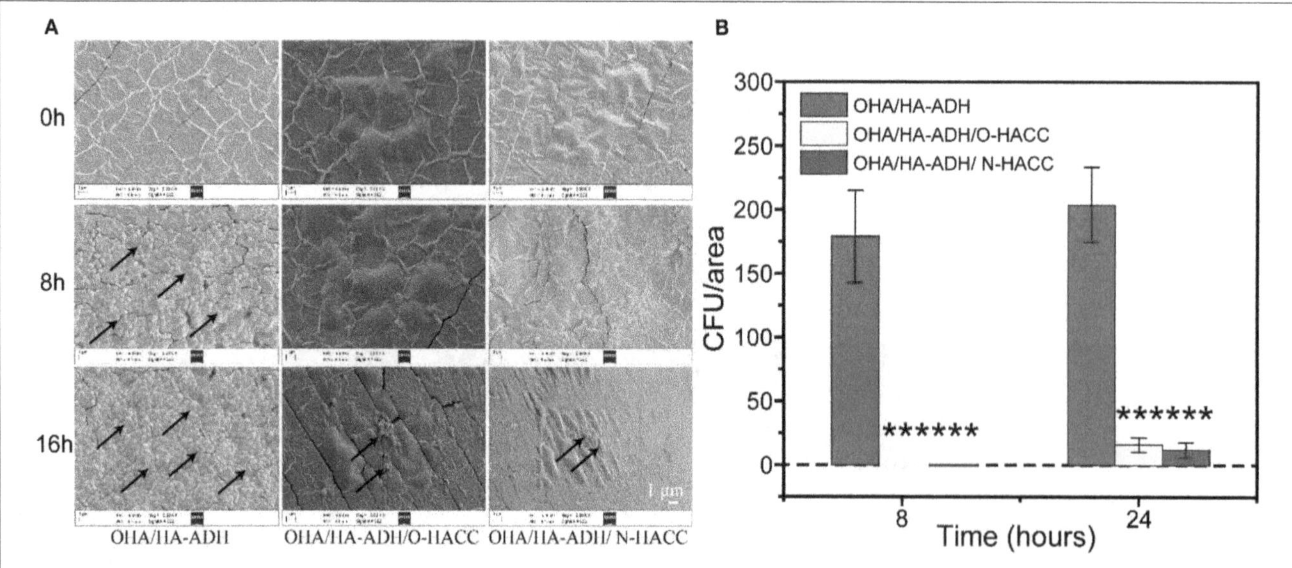

FIGURE 5 | (A) SEM images demonstrating the antibacterial activity of OHA/HA-ADH, OHA/HA-ADH/O-HACC, and OHA/HA-ADH/N-HACC hydrogels. **(B)** Quantitative analysis of the number of bacteria in each image area. $^{***}p < 0.001$.

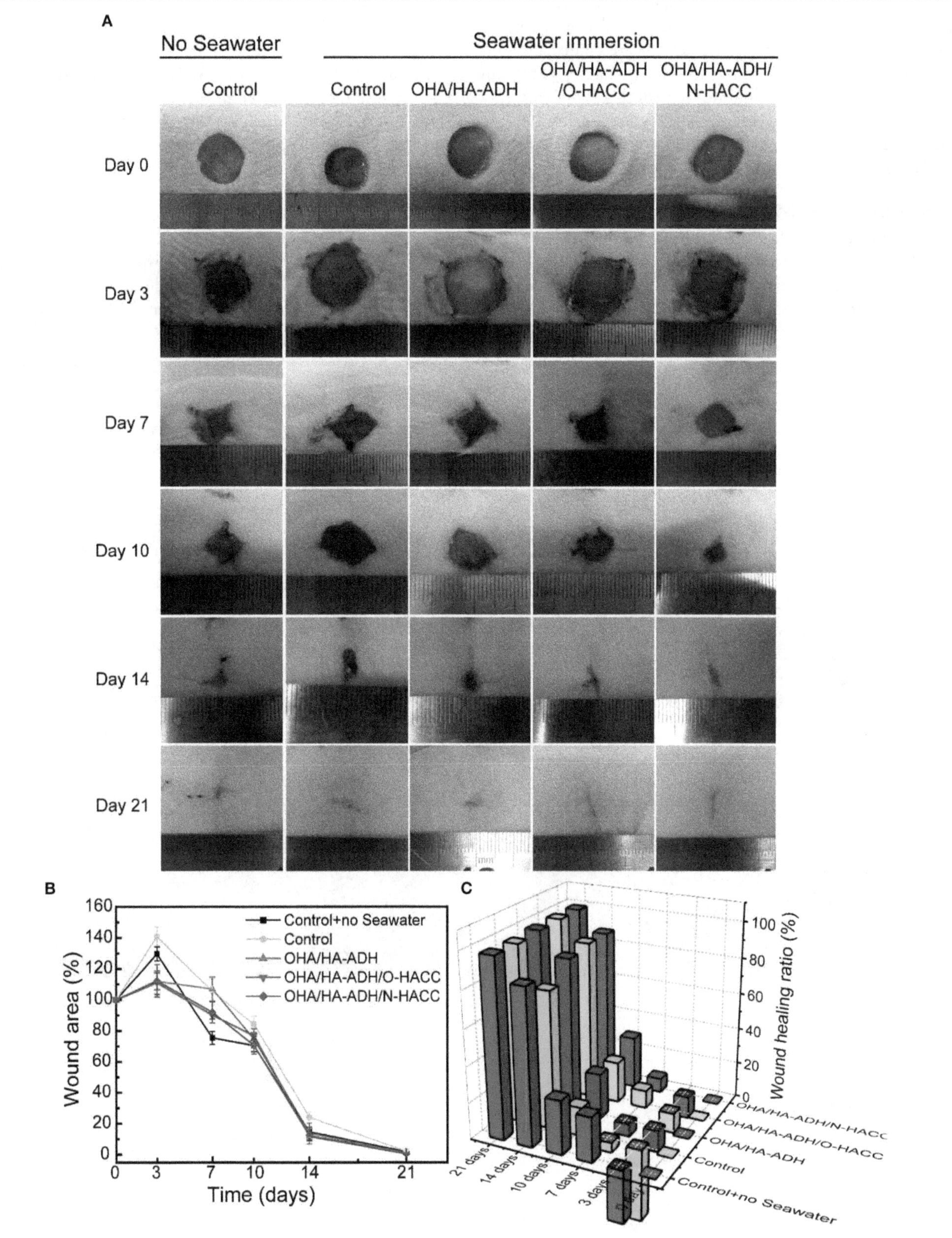

FIGURE 6 | (A) Photographs of wounds caused in the control group with or without seawater immersion and OHA/HA-ADH, OHA/HA-ADH/O-HACC, and OHA/HA-ADH/N-HACC groups with seawater immersion. **(B)** Percentage change in wound area, presented as mean ± SD. **(C)** Wound healing ratio over a 21-day period.

healing rate in **Figure 6C**. In the results, OHA/HA-ADH/O-HACC and OHA/HA-ADH/N-HACC hydrogels can be seen to accelerate and promote wound closure and re-epithelialization on the seawater-immersed wound infection of full-thickness skin wounds. Moreover, the wound-healing effect of the OHA/HA-ADH/N-HACC group was better than that of OHA/HA-ADH/O-HACC, which might be attributable to the antibacterial effect of N-HACC being stronger than that of O-HACC.

Number of Bacteria on Wound

The bacterial count on seawater-immersed wound infections of full-thickness wounds was determined at day 3. The bacteria from the wound site tissues were cultured on three selected agar media for 24 h and were then counted for further analysis (**Figure 7**). The results demonstrated that the number of bacteria on the seawater immersed wounds in the control group were approximately 6.2×10^8 CFU/wound for *E. coli*, 6.8×10^8 CFU/wound for *S. aureus*, and 2.3×10^8 CFU/wound for *P. aeruginosa*. However, the number of bacteria was significantly reduced in the OHA/HA-ADH/O-HACC group ($\sim 10^6$ CFU/wound for *E. coli*, 1.3×10^6 CFU/wound for *S. aureus*, and 2.7×10^6 CFU/wound for *P. aeruginosa*) and the OHA/HA-ADH/N-HACC group (3.0×10^6 CFU/wound for *E. coli*, 3.9×10^6 CFU/wound for *S. aureus*, and 1.6×10^6 CFU/wound for *P. aeruginosa*) at day 3. The results demonstrated that the bacteria in the wound site were inhibited or killed by the antimicrobial hydrogels. In addition, the antimicrobial hydrogels could accelerate skin wound closure and healing by

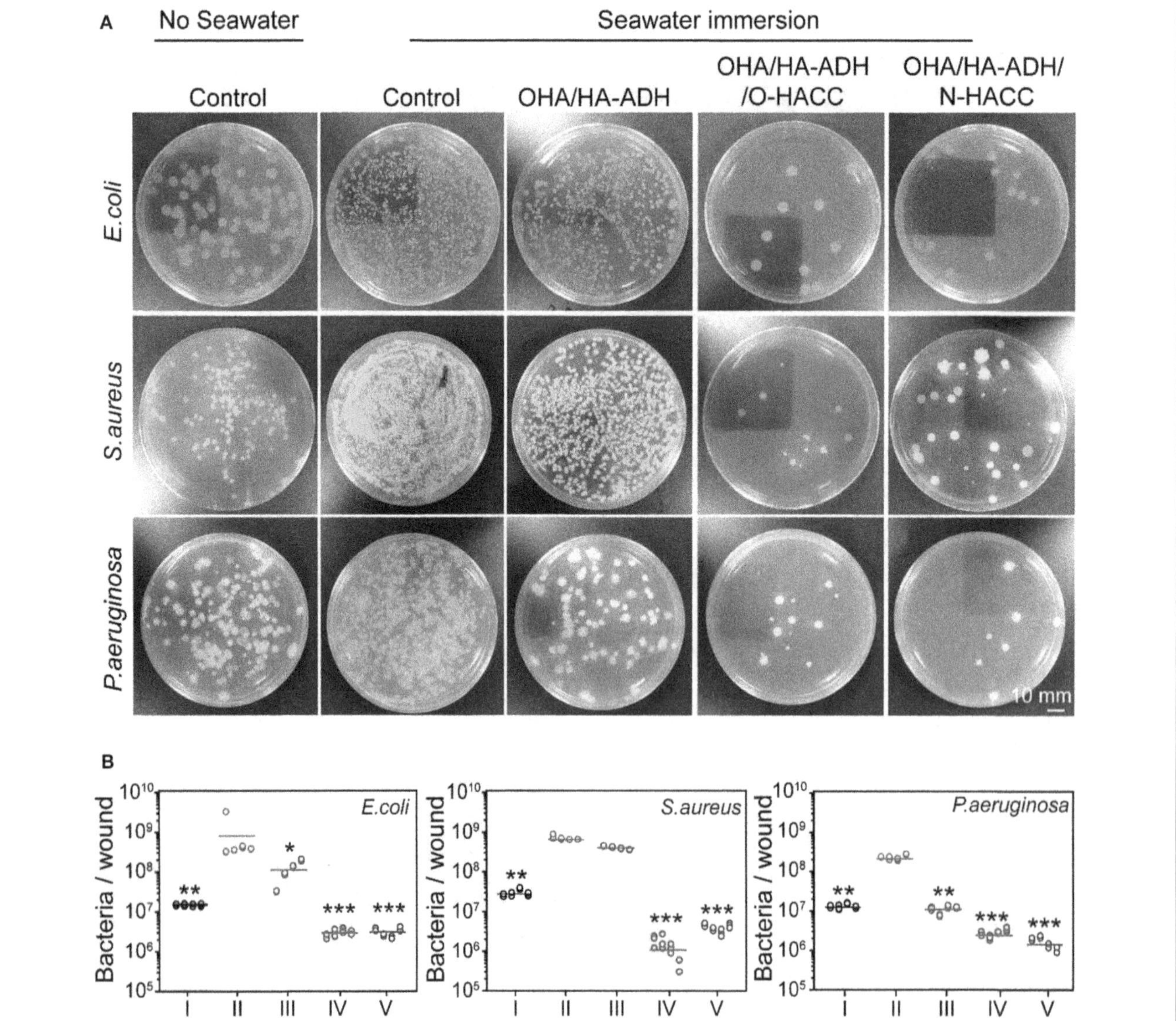

FIGURE 7 | (A) *E. coli*, *S. aureus*, and *P. aeruginosa* colonies from tissues formed on agar plates. A red ring-like morphology precipitating on VRBA-MUG selection medium means *E. coli*, a yellow-gold colony morphology on Mannitol salt agar indicates *S. aureus*, and a green-yellow colony morphology on *P. aeruginosa* selection medium represents *P. aeruginosa*. **(B)** Quantitative analysis of the number of bacteria remaining in the wound area. $^*p < 0.05$, $^{**}p < 0.01$, $^{***}p < 0.001$.

reducing the bacterial counts in seawater-immersed wounds of rats.

Histological Observations

The histologic structures of the regenerated dermis were stained with H&E to evaluate wound healing progress. The degrees of epithelial closure and granulation tissue formation in the different treatment groups were very pronounced (**Figure 8**). At day 3, a clear newly formed squamous epithelial layer was observed in OHA/HA-ADH/O-HACC and OHA/HA-ADH/N-HACC hydrogels, whereas the OHA/HA-ADH hydrogels and the control groups with seawater immersion showed an incomplete epidermal structure and a thinner dermal layer. In addition, obvious inflammatory cell infiltration was present in the wounds of the control group with seawater immersion on day 7, whereas the number of inflammatory cells on the OHA/HA-ADH/O-HACC and OHA/HA-ADH/N-HACC hydrogel groups was negligible (locally enlarged images of the tissue sections are shown in **Figure S2**). Remarkably, thick and well-formed granulation tissue was apparent in the OHA/HA-ADH/O-HACC and OHA/HA-ADH/N-HACC hydrogel-treated group on day 10, indicating that the antimicrobial hydrogels could promote rapid wound healing. At day 14, the epidermis of the new granulation tissue was integrated and thick in both the OHA/HA-ADH/O-HACC and OHA/HA-ADH/N-HACC hydrogel groups. At day 21, the OHA/HA-ADH/O-HACC and OHA/HA-ADH/N-HACC hydrogel groups developed some newly formed hair follicles in the center of the wound, which were not seen in the control group with seawater immersion. However, with respect to the microstructure of regenerated tissues, a more complete re-epithelialization and tight junction between epidermis and dermis was found in the antimicrobial hydrogel groups, which were significant for functional and scar-free tissue recovery.

Collagen Deposition

In order to gain more insight into the granulation tissue, collagen deposition and maturation were further assessed in each group by Picrosirius red staining (**Figure 9A**). Ipp 6.0 software was used to

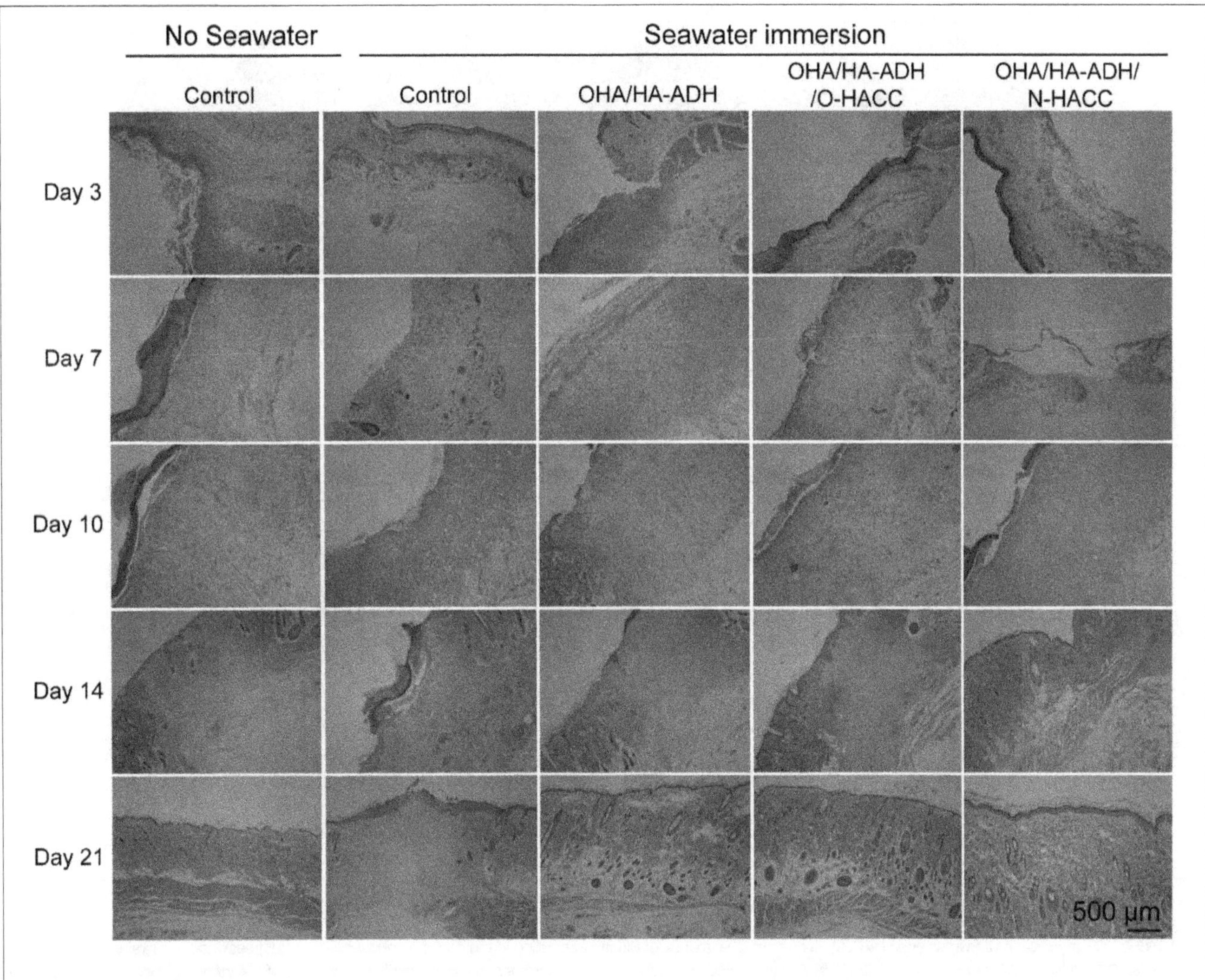

FIGURE 8 | Representative images with H&E staining of the effect of seawater immersion on wound sections at day 3, day 7, day 10, day 14, and day 21.

quantify the collagen deposition in the wound sites by calculating the intensity of the red areas in tissue area (**Figure 9B**). After 14 days of treatment, it can be seen that the OHA/HA-ADH/O-HACC and OHA/HA-ADH/N-HACC hydrogel groups not only had nearly twice as much collagen deposition as the other groups, as reflected by the Picrosirius red staining, but also had the most organized fibrous structure (local enlarged images of the wound sections are shown in **Figure S3**). In addition, at day 21, more mature fibers with regular orientation and distribution were seen in the wound sites treated with OHA/HA-ADH/O-HACC and OHA/HA-ADH/N-HACC as compared to those treated with the control with seawater immersion. With further quantitative analysis, the collagen contents in the wounds treated with OHA/HA-ADH/O-HACC and OHA/HA-ADH/N-HACC hydrogel were significantly higher than those of the OHA/HA-ADH hydrogel and control group without seawater ($p < 0.01$) and the control group with seawater ($p < 0.001$) at day 14. The enhanced collagen deposition could be attributed to the

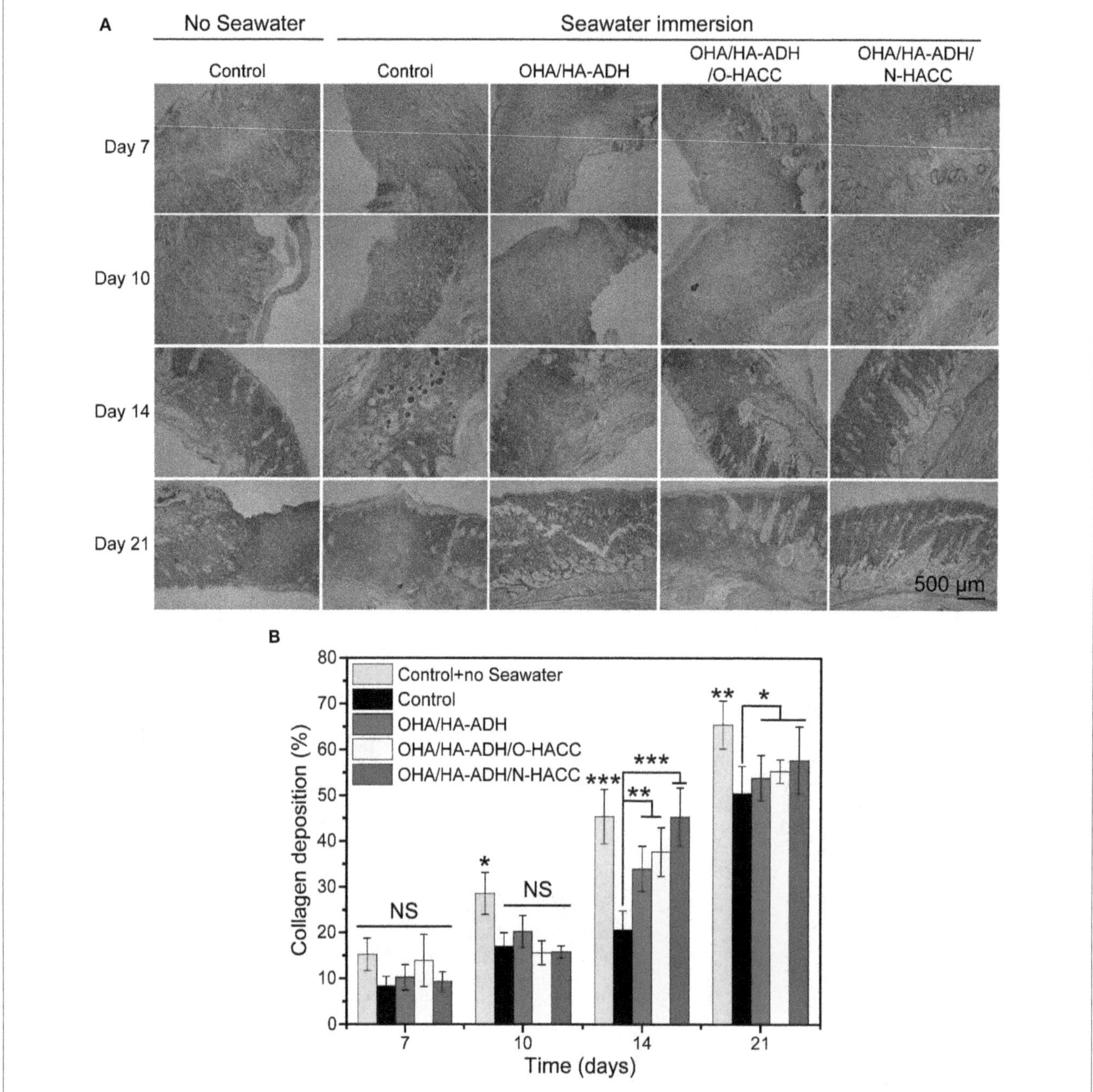

FIGURE 9 | Collagen deposition in wound sites. **(A)** Representative images of Sirius red staining in the control group with or without seawater immersion and the OHA/HA-ADH, OHA/HA-ADH/O-HACC, and OHA/HA-ADH/N-HACC groups with seawater immersion. **(B)** Quantitative analysis of collagen deposition in wound tissue. *$p < 0.05$, **$p < 0.01$, ***$p < 0.001$.

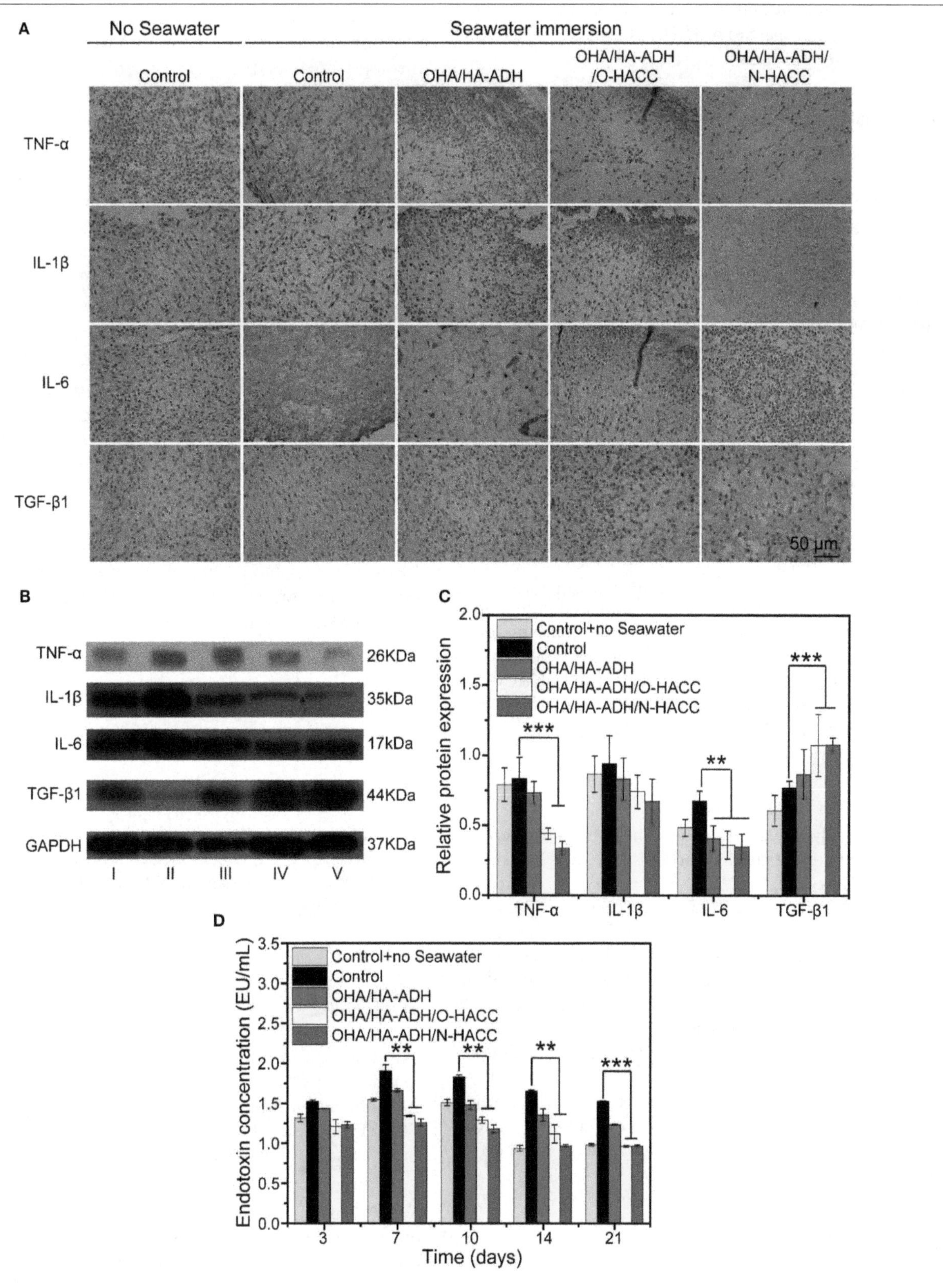

FIGURE 10 | (A) Representative images of immunohistochemistry pro-inflammatory factors (TNF-α, IL-1β, and IL-6) and anti-inflammatory factors (TGF-β1) of wound sections. **(B)** Western blot analyses were performed for TNF-α, IL-1β, IL-6, and TGF-β1. **(C)** Quantitative analysis of inflammatory factor. **(D)** Comparison of serum endotoxin concentration (EU/mL) in the different groups. $^{**}p < 0.01$, $^{***}p < 0.001$.

HA (which promotes collagen synthesis in fibroblasts) and the antibacterial properties of O-HACC or N-HACC (Kisiel et al., 2013; Hu et al., 2019).

Immunohistochemistry

The mechanism of the prepared hydrogel-promoted wound healing in the rat wound with seawater immersion model was explored by performing immunohistochemistry with pro-inflammatory factors (TNF-α, IL-1β, and IL-6) and anti-inflammatory factors (TGF-β1) in the wound (**Figure 10A**). The OHA/HA-ADH/O-HACC and OHA/HA-ADH/N-HACC hydrogel treatment decreased the expression level of pro-inflammatory factors (TNF-α, IL-1β, and IL-6) at day 7. On the other hand, the expression level of the anti-inflammatory factors (TGF-β1) was enhanced much more in the OHA/HA-ADH/O-HACC and OHA/HA-ADH/N-HACC hydrogel groups than in the OHA/HA-ADH hydrogel and control groups. The results indicated that OHA/HA-ADH/O-HACC and OHA/HA-ADH/N-HACC hydrogels reduced the expression of pro-inflammatory factors and increased that of anti-inflammatory factors in a wound with seawater immersion, which was important for the wound healing process. The Western blot analysis of TGF-β1, TNF-α, IL-1β, and IL-6 further supports these results, as less pro-inflammatory factors and more anti-inflammatory factors occurred in the antimicrobial hydrogel-treated wounds compared to the other groups (**Figures 10B,C**), which could be attributed to O-HACC and N-HACC being efficient inherently antibacterial materials capable of reducing infection (Qu et al., 2019).

Endotoxin Concentration

More specifically, the serum endotoxin levels of five groups were substantially elevated in the OHA/HA-ADH/O-HACC and OHA/HA-ADH/N-HACC groups compared to the control group with seawater (**Figure 10D**). The endotoxin concentration of the control group without seawater was about 1.0–1.5 EU/mL. However, the highest endotoxin concentration of the control group with seawater was about 1.5 EU/mL at day 3, 1.9 EU/mL at day 7, 1.8 EU/mL at day 10, 1.6 EU/mL at day 14, and 1.5 EU/mL at day 21. In addition, there was a significant decrease in endotoxin concentration in the OHA/HA-ADH/O-HACC and OHA/HA-ADH/N-HACC group compared to the control group with seawater ($P < 0.05$ at days 7, 10, and 14 and $P < 0.001$ at day 21), which was related to the bacteria numbers of their corresponding groups.

CONCLUSION

The aim of the present work was to develop biocompatible hydrogel wound dressings with inherent antibacterial properties. OHA/HA-ADH hydrogels with the addition of quaternized chitosan, OHA/HA-ADH/O-HACC and OHA/HA-ADH/N-HACC, were successfully prepared by dynamic Schiff base linkage. These hydrogels exhibited stable rheological properties, appropriate swelling properties, water vapor transmission rate, and biodegradability, inherent antibacterial properties, and good biocompatibility, meaning that they could effectively promote the wound healing process. Furthermore, the hydrogels accelerated the healing process in a seawater-immersed full-thickness skin defect model *in vivo*, as well as exhibiting excellent reepithelialization and greater granulation tissue thickness, higher-density collagen deposition, a smaller number of bacteria, a lower endotoxin level, and more balanced inflammatory infiltration than control. In particular, by reducing wound healing process-related pro-inflammatory factors (TNF-α, IL-1β, and IL-6) and upregulating anti-inflammatory factors (TGF-β1) in wound, the OHA/HA-ADH/O-HACC and OHA/HA-ADH/N-HACC antibacterial hydrogels presented the best wound healing effect among all groups. All results demonstrated that OHA/HA-ADH/O-HACC and OHA/HA-ADH/N-HACC represent promising antimicrobial hydrogel wound dressings for wound healing application, especially for open and infected traumas, due to their good bioactivity and inherent antibacterial properties.

AUTHOR CONTRIBUTIONS

RG and BC designed the experiments. XW and PX conducted most of the experiments and analyzed the data. ZY helped with cell experiments. QF and LF helped with animal experiments and *in vivo* characterization. XW, PX, RG, and BC wrote the manuscript.

FUNDING

This study was supported financially by the Natural Science Foundation of China (Nos. 81671924, 81571733, and 81272105), the National Key Research and Development Program of China (2017YFC1103301), the Science and Technology Program of Guangzhou (201508020253, 201508020115, 201604020094, 201601010270, 2017010160489, 201704030083, 201907010032, 201907010037), the Science and Technology Project of Guangdong Province (2014B020212010, 2015B020233012, 2017A010103009, 2017B020227009, 2015A010101313, 2017A050506011, 2017B090911012, 2018A050506021, 2018A050506019, 2018A050506040), the Military Medical Innovation Special Projects (18CXZ029), and the Joint Logistic Support Force Project (CWH17J023).

REFERENCES

Blacklow, S. O., Li, J., Freedman, B. R., Zeidi, M., Chen, C., and Mooney, D. J. (2019). Bioinspired mechanically active adhesive dressings to accelerate wound closure. *Sci. Adv.* 5:eaaw3963. doi: 10.1126/sciadv.aaw3963

Cai, X., Hu, S., Yu, B., Cai, Y., Yang, J., Li, F., et al. (2018). Transglutaminase-catalyzed preparation of crosslinked carboxymethyl chitosan/carboxymethyl cellulose/collagen composite membrane for postsurgical peritoneal adhesion prevention. *Carbohydr. Polym.* 201, 201–210. doi: 10.1016/j.carbpol.2018.08.065

Chen, X. (2017). Making electrodes stretchable. *Small Methods* 1:1600029. doi: 10.1002/smtd.201600029

Chen, Y., Qiu, H., Dong, M., Cheng, B., Jin, Y., Tong, Z., et al. (2019). Preparation of hydroxylated lecithin complexed iodine/carboxymethyl chitosan/sodium alginate composite membrane by microwave drying and its applications in infected burn wound treatment. *Carbohydr. Polym.* 206, 435–445. doi: 10.1016/j.carbpol.2018.10.068

Chin, W. G., Zhong, Q., Pu, C., Yang, W., Lou, P. F. D., Sessions, B., et al. (2018). A macromolecular approach to eradicate multidrug resistant bacterial infections while mitigating drug resistance onset. *Nat. Commun.* 9:917. doi: 10.1038/s41467-018-03325-6

Chung, E. M. C., Dean, S. N., Propst, C. N., Bishop, B. M., and Hoek, M. L. V. (2017). Komodo dragon-inspired synthetic peptide DRGN-1 promotes wound-healing of a mixed-biofilm infected wound. *NPJ Biofilms Microbiomes* 3:9. doi: 10.1038/s41522-017-0017-2

Gonzálezhenríquez, C. M., Sarabiavallejos, M. A., and Rodriguezhernandez, J. (2017). Advances in the fabrication of antimicrobial hydrogels for biomedical applications. *Materials* 10:232. doi: 10.3390/ma10030232

Gopinath, D. M, Rafiuddin, A., Gomathi, K., Chitra, K., Sehgal, P. K., and Jayakumar, R. (2004). Dermal wound healing processes with curcumin incorporated collagen films. *Biomaterials* 25, 1911–1917. doi: 10.1016/S0142-9612(03)00625-2

Hu, H., Yu, L., Tan, S., Tu, K., and Wang, L. Q. (2010). Novel complex hydrogels based on N -carboxyethyl chitosan and quaternized chitosan and their controlled *in vitro* protein release property. *Carbohydr. Res.* 345, 462–468. doi: 10.1016/j.carres.2009.11.029

Hu, S., Cai, X., Qu, X., Yu, B., Yan, C., Yang, J., et al. (2019). Preparation of biocompatible wound dressings with long-term antimicrobial activity through covalent bonding of antibiotic agents to natural polymers. *Int. J. Biol. Macromol.* 123, 1320–1330. doi: 10.1016/j.ijbiomac.2018.09.122

Jia, X., Colombo, G. R., Langer, R., and Kohane, D. S. (2004). Prolongation of sciatic nerve blockade by *in situ* cross-linked hyaluronic acid. *Biomaterials* 25, 4797–4804. doi: 10.1016/j.biomaterials.2003.12.012

Julia, D., Andreas, K., Lena, M. L., George, K., Markus, M. W., Astrid, D., et al. (2013). Fully defined *in situ* cross-linkable alginate and hyaluronic acid hydrogels for myocardial tissue engineering. *Biomaterials* 34, 940–951. doi: 10.1016/j.biomaterials.2012.10.008

Kaoru, M., Hiroshi, A., Shingo, N., Shin-Ichiro, N., Megumi, T., Motoaki, H., et al. (2010). Hydrogel blends of chitin/chitosan, fucoidan and alginate as healing-impaired wound dressings. *Biomaterials* 31, 83–90. doi: 10.1016/j.biomaterials.2009.09.031

Kisiel, M., Martino, M. M., Ventura, M., Hubbell, J. A., Hilborn, J., and Ossipov, D. A. (2013). Improving the osteogenic potential of BMP-2 with hyaluronic acid hydrogel modified with integrin-specific fibronectin fragment. *Biomaterials* 34, 704–712. doi: 10.1016/j.biomaterials.2012.10.015

Kowapradit, J., Opanasopit, P., Ngawhirunpat, T., Rojanarata, T., and Sajomsang, W. (2011). Structure–activity relationships of methylated -aryl chitosan derivatives for enhancing paracellular permeability across Caco-2 cells. *Carbohydr. Polym.* 83, 430–437. doi: 10.1016/j.carbpol.2010.08.005

Kumar, A., Boyer, C., Nebhani, L., and Wong, E. H. H. (2018). Highly bactericidal macroporous antimicrobial polymeric gel for point-of-use water disinfection. *Sci. Rep.* 8:7965. doi: 10.1038/s41598-018-26202-0

Li, M., Chen, J., Shi, M., Zhang, H., Ma, P. X., and Guo, B. (2019). Electroactive anti-oxidant polyurethane elastomers with shape memory property as non-adherent wound dressing to enhance wound healing. *Chem. Eng. J.* 375:121999. doi: 10.1016/j.cej.2019.121999

Li, S., Dong, S., Xu, W., Tu, S., Yan, L., Zhao, C., et al. (2018). Antibacterial hydrogels. *Adv. Sci.* 5:1700527. doi: 10.1002/advs.201700527

Li, Y., Han, M., Liu, T., Cun, D., Fang, L., and Yang, M. (2017). Inhaled hyaluronic acid microparticles extended pulmonary retention and suppressed systemic exposure of a short-acting bronchodilator. *Carbohydr. Polym.* 172:197. doi: 10.1016/j.carbpol.2017.09.038

Li, Z., He, C., Yuan, B., Dong, X., and Chen, X. (2016). Injectable polysaccharide hydrogels as biocompatible platforms for localized and sustained delivery of antibiotics for preventing local infections. *Macromol. Biosci.* 17:1600347. doi: 10.1002/mabi.201600347

Liang, Y., Zhao, X., Hu, T., Chen, B., Yin, Z., Ma, P. X., Guo, B. (2019b). Adhesive hemostatic conducting injectable composite hydrogels with sustained drug release and photothermal antibacterial activity to promote full-thickness skin regeneration during wound healing. *Small* 15:e1900046. doi: 10.1002/smll.201900046

Liang, Y., Zhao, X., Ma, P. X., Guo, B., Du, Y., Han, X. (2019a). pH-responsive injectable hydrogels with mucosal adhesiveness based on chitosan-grafted-dihydrocaffeic acid and oxidized pullulan for localized drug delivery. *J. Colloid Interface Sci.* 536:224–234. doi: 10.1016/j.jcis.2018.10.056

Lin, Z., Wu, T., Wang, W., Li, B., Wang, M., Chen, L., et al. (2019). Biofunctions of antimicrobial peptide-conjugated alginate/hyaluronic acid/collagen wound dressings promote wound healing of a mixed-bacteria-infected wound. *Int. J. Biol. Macromol.* 140, 330–342. doi: 10.1016/j.ijbiomac.2019.08.087

Mohamed, R. R., Elella, M. H., and Sabaa, M. W. (2017). Cytotoxicity and metal ions removal using antibacterial biodegradable hydrogels based on N-quaternized chitosan/poly(acrylic acid). *Int. J. Biol. Macromol.* 98:302. doi: 10.1016/j.ijbiomac.2017.01.107

Park, T. Y., Jeon, E. Y., Kim, H. J., Choi, B. H., and Cha, H. J. (2019). Prolonged cell persistence with enhanced multipotency and rapid angiogenesis of hypoxia pre-conditioned stem cells encapsulated in marine-inspired adhesive and immiscible liquid micro-droplets. *Acta Biomater.* 86, 257–268. doi: 10.1016/j.actbio.2019.01.007

Peng, Z. X., Wang, L., Du, L., Guo, S. R., Wang, X. Q., and Tang, T. T. (2010). Adjustment of the antibacterial activity and biocompatibility of hydroxypropyltrimethyl ammonium chloride chitosan by varying the degree of substitution of quaternary ammonium. *Carbohydr. Polym.* 81, 275–283. doi: 10.1016/j.carbpol.2010.02.008

Pires, N. R., Cunha, P. L. R., Maciel, J. S., Angelim, A. L., Melo, V. M. M., Paula, R. C. M. D., et al. (2013). Sulfated chitosan as tear substitute with no antimicrobial activity. *Carbohydr. Polym.* 91, 92–99. doi: 10.1016/j.carbpol.2012.08.011

Purcell, B. P., Elser, J. A., Anbin, M., Margulies, K. B., and Burdick, J. A. (2012). Synergistic effects of SDF-1α chemokine and hyaluronic acid release from degradable hydrogels on directing bone marrow derived cell homing to the myocardium. *Biomaterials* 33, 7849–7857. doi: 10.1016/j.biomaterials.2012.07.005

Qu, J., Zhao, X., Liang, Y., Xu, Y., Ma, P. X., and Guo B. (2019). Degradable conductive injectable hydrogels as novel antibacterial, anti-oxidant wound dressings for wound healing. *Chem. Eng. J.* 362:548–560. doi: 10.1016/j.cej.2019.01.028

Qu, J., Zhao, X., Liang, Y., Zhang, T., Ma, P. X., and Guo, B. (2018). Antibacterial adhesive injectable hydrogels with rapid self-healing, extensibility and compressibility as wound dressing for joints skin wound healing. *Biomaterials* 183, 185–199. doi: 10.1016/j.biomaterials.2018.08.044

Rakhshaei, R., and Namazi, H. (2017). A potential bioactive wound dressing based on carboxymethyl cellulose/ZnO impregnated MCM-41 nanocomposite hydrogel. *Mater. Sci. Eng. C Mater. Biol. Appl.* 73:456. doi: 10.1016/j.msec.2016.12.097

Sarhan, W. A., Azzazy, H. M., and El-Sherbiny, I. M. (2016). Honey/chitosan nanofiber wound dressing enriched with allium sativum and cleome droserifolia: enhanced antimicrobial and wound healing activity. *ACS Appl. Mater. Interfaces* 8, 6379–6390. doi: 10.1021/acsami.6b00739

Taichi, I., Yoon, Y., Highley, C. B., Evangelia, B., Benitez, C. A., and Kohane, D. S. (2007). The prevention of peritoneal adhesions by *in situ* cross-linking hydrogels of hyaluronic acid and cellulose derivatives. *Biomaterials* 28, 975–983. doi: 10.1016/j.biomaterials.2006.10.021

Thanou, M., Florea, B. I., Geldof, M., Junginger, H. E., and Borchard, G. (2002). Quaternized chitosan oligomers as novel gene delivery vectors in epithelial cell lines. *Biomaterials* 23, 153–159. doi: 10.1016/S0142-9612(01)00090-4

Thattaruparambil, R. N., Baranwal, G., Mavila, C. B., Biswas, R., and Jayakumar, R. (2016). Anti-staphylococcal activity of injectable nano tigecycline/chitosan-PRP composite hydrogel using drosophila melanogaster model for infectious wounds. *ACS Appl. Mater. Interfaces* 8, 22074–22083. doi: 10.1021/acsami.6b07463

Travan, A., Scognamiglio, F., Borgogna, M., Marsich, E., Donati, I., Tarusha, L., et al. (2016). Hyaluronan delivery by polymer demixing in polysaccharide-based hydrogels and membranes for biomedical applications. *Carbohydr. Polym.* 150, 408–418. doi: 10.1016/j.carbpol.2016.03.088

Wang, W., Liu, S., Chen, B., Yan, X., Li, S., Ma, X., et al. (2019). DNA-inspired adhesive hydrogels based on the biodegradable polyphosphoesters tackified by nucleobase. *Biomacromolecules* 20, 3672–3683. doi: 10.1021/acs.biomac.9b01446

Wu, Y., Ling, W., Guo, B., Shao, Y., and Ma, P. X. (2016). Electroactive biodegradable polyurethane significantly enhanced Schwann cells myelin gene expression and neurotrophin secretion for peripheral nerve tissue engineering. *Biomaterials* 87, 18–31. doi: 10.1016/j.biomaterials.2016.02.010

Xin, Z., Peng, L., Guo, B., and Ma, P. X. (2015). Antibacterial and conductive injectable hydrogels based on quaternized chitosan-graft-polyaniline/oxidized dextran for tissue engineering. *Acta Biomater.* 26, 236–248. doi: 10.1016/j.actbio.2015.08.006

Xu, R., Xia, H., He, W., Li, Z., Zhao, J., Liu, B., et al. (2016). Controlled water vapor transmission rate promotes wound-healing via wound re-epithelialization and contraction enhancement. *Sci. Rep.* 6:24596. doi: 10.1038/srep24596

Xu, Z., Shi, L., Yang, M., Zhang, H., and Zhu, L. (2015). Fabrication of a novel blended membrane with chitosan and silk microfibers for wound healing: characterization, *in vitro* and *in vivo* studies. *J. Mater. Chem. B* 3, 3634–3642. doi: 10.1039/C5TB00226E

Yang, Y., Bechtold, T., Redl, B., Caven, B., and Hong, H. (2017). A novel silver-containing absorbent wound dressing based on spacer fabric. *J. Mater. Chem. B* 5, 6786–6793. doi: 10.1039/C7TB01286A

Yang, Z., Hideyoshi, S., Jiang, H., Matsumura, Y., Dziki, J. L., Lopresti, S. T., et al. (2018). Injectable, porous, biohybrid hydrogels incorporating decellularized tissue components for soft tissue applications. *Acta Biomater.* 73:112–126. doi: 10.1016/j.actbio.2018.04.003

Ye, W., Yi, D., Wen, X., Ling, Y., Li, H., Wang, X., et al. (2014). Interface behavior of quaternized chitosan on cellulosic substrates. *Fibers Polym.* 15, 1450–1455. doi: 10.1007/s12221-014-1450-y

Yi, X., He, J., Wang, X., Zhang, Y., Tan, G., Zhou, Z., et al. (2018). Tunable mechanical, antibacterial, and cytocompatible hydrogels based on a functionalized dual network of metal coordination bonds and covalent crosslinking. *ACS Appl. Mater. Interfaces* 10, 6190–6198. doi: 10.1021/acsami.7b18821

Yildirim-Aksoy, M., and Beck, B. H. (2017). Antimicrobial activity of chitosan and a chitosan oligomer against bacterial pathogens of warmwater fish. *J. Appl. Microbiol.* 122:1570. doi: 10.1111/jam.13460

You, J., Xie, S., Cao, J., Hao, G., Min, X., Zhang, L., et al. (2016). Quaternized chitosan/poly(acrylic acid) polyelectrolyte complex hydrogels with tough, self-recovery, and tunable mechanical properties. *Macromolecules* 49, 1049–1059. doi: 10.1021/acs.macromol.5b02231

Zhang, J., Ma, Y., Liang, X., and Bing, S. (2017). Applications of vacuum sealing drainage in treating seawater-immersed sulfur mustard injury. *Toxicol. Env. Chem.* 99, 975–986. doi: 10.1080/02772248.2017.1338702

Zhao, X., Wu, H., Guo, B., Dong, R., Qiu, Y., and Ma, P. X. (2017). Antibacterial anti-oxidant electroactive injectable hydrogel as self-healing wound dressing with hemostasis and adhesiveness for cutaneous wound healing. *Biomaterials* 122, 34–47. doi: 10.1016/j.biomaterials.2017.01.011

Zhou, F., Hong, Y., Zhang, X., Yang, L., and Zhang, S. (2018). Tough hydrogel with enhanced tissue integration and *in situ* forming capability for osteochondral defect repair. *Appl. Mater. Today* 13, 32–44. doi: 10.1016/j.apmt.2018.08.005

Zhu, H., Li, X., and Zheng, X. (2017). A descriptive sudy of open fractures contaminated by seawater: infection, pathogens, and antibiotic resistance. *Biomed Res. Int.* 2017:2796054. doi: 10.1155/2017/2796054

Zhu, J., Li, F., Wang, X., Yu, J., and Wu, D. (2018a). Hyaluronic acid and polyethylene glycol hybrid hydrogel encapsulating nanogel with hemostasis and sustainable antibacterial property for wound healing. *ACS Appl. Mater. Interfaces* 10, 13304–13316. doi: 10.1021/acsami.7b18927

Zhu, Q., Ming, J., Qiang, L., Yan, S., and Rui, G. (2018b). Enhanced healing activity of burn wound infection by dextran-HA hydrogel enriched with sanguinarine. *Biomater. Sci.* 6, 2472–2486. doi: 10.1039/C8BM00478A

10

Hypertension and Stroke Cardiovascular Control Evaluation by Analyzing Blood Pressure, Cerebral Blood Flow, Blood Vessel Resistance and Baroreflex

Shoou-Jeng Yeh*[1]*, Chi-Wen Lung*[2,3]*, Yih-Kuen Jan*[3]*, Fang-Chuan Kuo*[4] *and Ben-Yi Liau*[5]*

[1]Section of Neurology and Neurophysiology, Cheng-Ching General Hospital, Taichung, Taiwan, [2]Department of Creative Product Design, Asia University, Taichung, Taiwan, [3]Rehabilitation Engineering Lab, Kinesiology and Community Health, Computational Science and Engineering, University of Illinois at Urbana-Champaign, Champaign, IL, United States, [4]Department of Physical Therapy, Hungkuang University, Taichung, Taiwan, [5]Department of Biomedical Engineering, Hungkuang University, Taichung, Taiwan

***Correspondence:**
Ben-Yi Liau
byliau@hk.edu.tw

Cardiovascular diseases have been the leading causes of mortality in Taiwan and the world at large for decades. The composition of cardiovascular and cerebrovascular systems is quite complicated. Therefore, it is difficult to detect or trace the related signs of cardiovascular and cerebrovascular diseases. The characteristics and changes in cardiopulmonary system disease can be used to track cardiovascular and cerebrovascular disease prevention and diagnosis. This can effectively reduce the occurrence of cardiovascular and cerebrovascular diseases. This study analyzes the variability in blood pressure, cerebral blood flow velocity and the interaction characteristics using linear and nonlinear approaches in stroke, hypertension and healthy groups to identify the differences in cardiovascular control in these groups. The results showed that the blood pressure and cerebral blood flow of stroke patients and hypertensive patients were significantly higher than those of healthy people (statistical differences ($p < 0.05$). The cerebrovascular resistance (CVR) shows that the CVR of hypertensive patients is higher than that of healthy people and stroke patients ($p < 0.1$), indicating that the cerebral vascular resistance of hypertensive patients is slightly higher. From the patient's blood flow and vascular characteristics, it can be observed that the cardiovascular system is different from those in healthy people. Baroreflex sensitivity (BRS) decreased in stroke patients ($p < 0.05$). Chaotic analysis revealed that the blood pressure disturbance in hypertensive patients has a higher chaotic behavior change and the difference in initial state sensitivity. Cross-correlation (CCF) analysis shows that as the course of healthy→hypertension→stroke progresses, the maximum CCF value decreases significantly ($p < 0.05$). That means that blood pressure and cerebral blood flow are gradually not well controlled by the self-regulation mechanism. In conclusion, cardiovascular control performance in hypertensive and stroke patients displays greater variation. This can be observed by the bio-signal analysis. This analysis could identify a measure for detecting and preventing the risk for hypertension and stroke in clinical practice. This is a pilot study to analyze cardiovascular control variation in healthy, hypertensive and stroke groups.

Keywords: cardiovascular control, hypertension, stroke, blood pressure, cerebral blood flow, blood vessel resistance, baroreflex

1 INTRODUCTION

Cardiovascular diseases (CVD) have become a leading health care burden in many areas of the world. It was reported that high blood pressure is the main risk factor to induce CVD. Most deaths are caused by ischemic heart disease and ischemic stroke (Roth et al., 2020). Therefore, systolic blood pressure variability could be assessed as a stroke and CVD risk predictor in the hypertensive population (Pringle et al., 2003). Because CVD is common in most areas of the world, WHO established a CVD risk prediction chart to reduce the medical burden (WHO CVD risk chart working group, 2019). Moreover, blood pressure is highly related to CVD (Fuchs and Ethlton, 2020). Hypertension is high blood pressure in the blood vessels. In the brain, high blood pressure induces hypertrophy and remodels smooth muscle cells in the cerebral arteries (Yu et al., 2011). The changes in blood vessel wall composition leads to greater cerebral artery stiffness. Aortic stiffness could be an independent predictor of hypertensive-stroke patient (Baumbach et al., 1988; Laurent et al., 2003, Laurent et al., 2005; Benjo et al., 2007). The change in blood pressure is the earliest sign of abnormal cardiopulmonary circulation. The change in blood pressure causes considerable variation in the physiological feedback mechanism. The relationship between blood pressure and cerebral blood flow in the brain is cerebral autoregulation (CA). Cerebral autoregulation maintains cerebral blood flow to protect the brain by reducing the effect of blood pressure variation. Previous studies reported that impaired CA may be associated with higher stroke risk (Shekhar et al., 2017; Castro et al., 2018). Therefore, CA assessment is also important to predict and reduce CVD risk. CA measurement and evaluation may obtain a predictive value for the development of delayed cerebral ischemia and radiographic vasospasm (Tiecks et al., 1995; Aoi wt al., 2012; Oeinck et al., 2013; Ma et al., 2016; Crippa et al., 2018). Although some non-invasive approaches (ex. Cross-correlation function, chaotic analysis etc.) and devices (ex. Near-infrared spectroscopy, transcranial Doppler etc.) have been developed to assess CA, measuring CA is difficult and standard measurement is not currently available (Tiecks et al., 1995; Liau et al., 2010; Rivera-Lara et al., 2017; Xiong et al., 2017). On the other hand, few studies revealed the differences in physiological signals and properties between hypertension and stroke. The changes in the cardiovascular disease physiological parameter development process (healthy→hypertension→stroke) are not clear. The objective of this study was to apply linear and nonlinear physiological signal analysis methods to assess multiple blood pressure signal correlation effects on cerebral blood flow signals, blood vessel properties, baroreflex and CA in healthy people, hypertension and stroke patients. To the best of our knowledge, this is the first study to investigate bio-signal performance and differences. The findings from multiple views could be used to better understand the effects of various cardiovascular diseases on bio-signal variation and tissue properties as assessed using multi-correlation approaches.

2 MATERIALS AND METHODS

2.1 Subjects and Measurement

In this study, 3 groups were enrolled: 1) 11 healthy subjects (57.4 ± 8.4 years) that have no history of related cardiovascular diseases. 2) 11 hypertensive patients (50.8 ± 10.3 years) from the Neurology Section of Cheng-Ching General Hospital, Taiwan. Hypertension was according to WHO, 2003 that clinic blood pressure ≥140/90 mmHg (WHO, 2003). 3) 10 hypertensive stroke outpatients (56 ± 10.16 years) from the Neurology Section of Cheng-Ching General Hospital were enrolled in this study. These stroke patients have to qualify blood pressure level defined as a clinic blood pressure ≥140/90 mmHg (WHO, 2003). National Institutes of Health Stroke Scale, NIHSS <15. Stroke more than 7 days. The subjects in 3 groups were age-matched and none of the subjects were receiving any medication during the study period. Informed consent was received from all subjects prior to entry into the study. This study was approved by the Research Ethics Committee of Cheng-Ching General Hospital, Taiwan. Continuous arterial blood pressure signals were acquired via using the Finapres (Model 2,300, Ohemda, Englewood, CO, United States). Cerebral blood flow velocity signals were obtained through TCD (transcranial Doppler ultrasound, EME TC 2020, Nicolet instrument, Warwick, United Kingdom) in conjunction with a 5-MHz transducer fixed over the temporal bones by an elastic headband. Subjects lied down on a tilt-table that enabled a motor-driven change from a supine to an upright position at 75° within 4 s. Data acquisition was started after a 10-min relaxation period in the supine position. After that, continuous arterial blood pressure and cerebral blood flow velocity signals were acquired during both supine and 75° head-up tilt positions and then returned to supine and rest for 5 minutes. The experimental devices included a general-purpose data acquisition board with a computer and LabVIEW program for acquiring signal processing. This equipment was developed in our previous study (Chiu et al., 2007; Liau et al., 2010).

2.2 BP and CBFV Signals

Mean value estimation is based on every waveform peak and valley location. The mean arterial blood pressure (MABP) value was calculated using each pulse as follows:

$$MABP_i = \frac{1}{P_{i+1} - P_i} \sum_{k=P}^{P_{i+1}} BP(k) \tag{1}$$

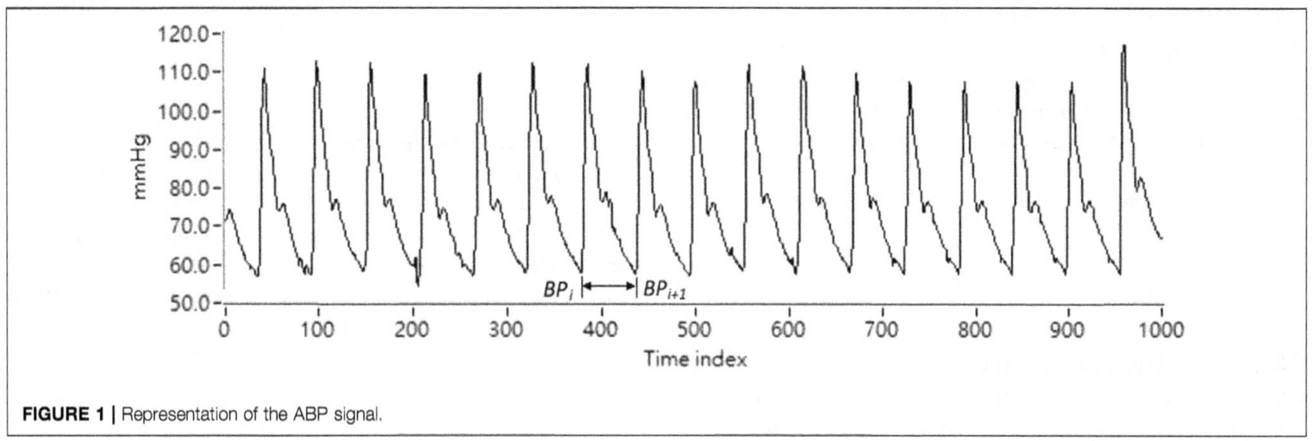

FIGURE 1 | Representation of the ABP signal.

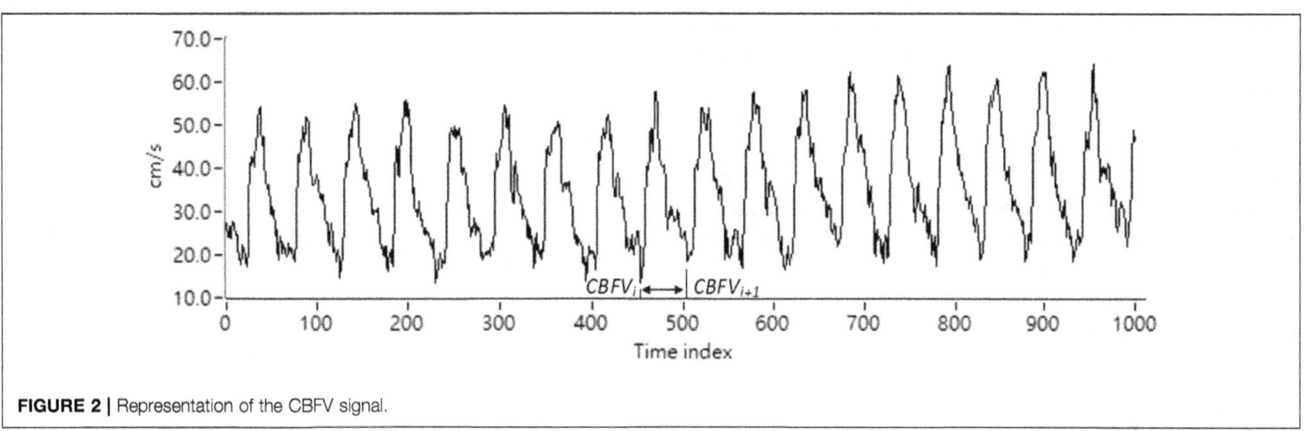

FIGURE 2 | Representation of the CBFV signal.

where *BP*(⊠)in **Eq. 1** is the arterial blood pressure pulse signal acquired by Finapres continuously. P_i is the wave-through time index in the *i*th BP pulse beat. Therefore, $MABP_i$ is the mean BP value calculated by the *i*th pulse beat. Representation of the BP signal is shown as **Figure 1**.On the other hand, mean cerebral blood flow velocity (MCBFV) could be obtained using **Eq. 2** as follows.

$$MCBFV_i = \frac{1}{V_{i+1} - V_i} \sum_{k=V}^{V_{i+1}} CBFV(k) \tag{2}$$

where *CBFV*(⊠) is the CBFV pulse signal continuously acquired by the TCD. *Vi* is the time index of the wave-through in the CBFV signal corresponding to the *i*th pulse beat. *MCBFVi* is the mean CBFV value for the *i*th pulse beat. The CBFV signal representation is shown as **Figure 2**.

2.3 Methodology

2.3.1 Resistance Index

Resistance index is a measure of peripheral blood flow resistance. Low vascular resistance has a higher diastolic blood flow velocity characteristic, and will have a lower RI. A high vascular resistance has a lower diastolic blood flow velocity characteristic, and will produce a higher RI. RI can be calculated using the following formula, SCBFV is the systolic blood flow velocity, and DCBFV is the diastolic blood flow velocity. RI can be obtained by **Eq. 3** as below (Hilz et al., 2004).

$$\mathrm{RI} = \frac{SCBFV - DCBFV}{SCBFV} \tag{3}$$

2.3.2 Pulsatility Index

The pulsation index is a measurement that describes the type of signal waveform. Low intracranial vascular resistance will reduce PI, and rising intracranial pulsations have been found to be related to rising intracranial pressure. The normal PI range is between 0.5 and 1.4, less than 0.5 may be an ischemic flow pattern under vascular dilation, and greater than 1.5 may be a decrease in vascular compliance or an increase in intracranial pressure. PI can be calculated using the following formula, SCBFV is the systolic blood flow velocity, DCBFV is the diastolic blood flow velocity, and MCBFV is the average blood flow velocity. *PI* can be obtained by **Eq. 4** (Hilz et al., 2004)

$$\mathrm{PI} = \frac{\mathrm{SCBFV} - \mathrm{DCBFV}}{\mathrm{MCBFV}} \tag{4}$$

2.3.3 Cerebrovascular Resistance

The cerebrovascular resistance can be expressed as the ratio of the average pressure to the average cerebral blood flow rate. The unit is mmHg/(cm/s). CVR can be calculated using the following formula, where MABP is the average blood pressure and MCBFV is the average cerebral blood flow. *CVR* can be obtained using **Eq. 5** (Hilz et al., 2004)

$$CVR = \frac{MABP}{MCBFV} \tag{5}$$

2.3.4 Cross-Correlation Analysis

Cross-correlation analysis mainly observes the correlation between the two signals in the time domain. Taking the average cerebral blood flow signal and the average blood pressure signal as an example, the correlation and phase relationship between the average cerebral blood flow signal and the average blood pressure signal can be determined by the brain. The phase relationship between blood flow and blood pressure is used to explore the blood flow regulation mechanism using the cardiovascular system. Let the cross-correlation function be expressed as CCF(k), W is the length of the window, k is the number of peak-to-peak displacement points, N is the total length of the signal, and the MABP time series normalized with the average value is expressed as x(n), MCBFV time series is expressed as y(n), the time series of x(n) after band-pass filtering is expressed as, and the time series of y(n) after band-pass filtering is expressed as, then cross-correlation The analyzed formula is as follows (Chiu et al., 2001; Chiu et al., 2005; Liau et al., 2010; Fan et al., 2019):

$$CCF_i(k) = \frac{R^i_{\hat{x}\hat{y}}(k)}{\left[R^i_{\hat{x}\hat{x}}(0)R^i_{\hat{y}\hat{y}}(0)\right]^{\frac{1}{2}}}, \quad k = 0, \pm 1, \pm 2, \ldots, \quad i = 1 \text{ to } N - W + 1 \tag{6}$$

where

$$R^i_{\hat{x}\hat{y}}(k) = \begin{cases} \dfrac{1}{W}\displaystyle\sum_{j=i}^{i+W} \hat{x}(j)\hat{y}(j+k), & k = 0, 1, 2, \ldots \\ \dfrac{1}{W}\displaystyle\sum_{j=i}^{i+W} \hat{x}(j-k)\hat{y}(j), & k = 0, -1, -2, \ldots \end{cases}$$

$$R^i_{\hat{x}\hat{x}}(0) = \frac{1}{W}\sum_{j=i}^{i+W}[\hat{x}(j)]^2, \text{and } R^i_{\hat{y}\hat{y}}(0) = \frac{1}{W}\sum_{j=i}^{i+W}[\hat{y}(j)]^2$$

2.3.5 Baroreflex Sensitivity

The index is used to evaluate the pressure-sensitive reflex. In order to observe the changes in heart rate and blood pressure at the same time, the baroreflex sensitivity index observes the relationship between the heart rate signal and the blood pressure signal. Assuming that the systolic blood pressure sequence SBP is S(n), and the heartbeat interval RR interval is R(n), the baroreflex sensitivity (BRS) T(n) can be expressed as: (Karemaker and Wesseling, 2008):

$$T(n) = \sum_{k=1}^{n} \frac{R(k)}{S(k)} \tag{7}$$

2.3.6 Correlation Dimension

The correlation dimension (CD) can quantify the properties of the attractors from the time series and determine the singularity of the attractors, which is estimated by the correlation function by calculating the pairs of points where the attractors fall on the radius of the "sphere". The correlation function Cd(R) is defined as (Grassberger and Procaccia, 1983; Liau et al., 2008; Gao et al., 2011; Bolea et al., 2014):

$$C_d(R) = \lim_{N\to\infty}\left[\frac{1}{N^2}\sum_{i,j=1, i\neq j} H_E\left(R - |X_i - X_j|\right)\right] \tag{8}$$

N:number of points
H_E:Heaviside step function
$H_E = 1$, if R-| X_i- X_j | ≧ 0
$H_E = 0$, otherwise
(X_i, X_j)The Euclidean distance of an attractor in 1 dm dimension is:

$$|X_i - X_j| = \left[\left(x_{i,1} - x_{j,1}\right)^2 + \left(x_{i,2} - x_{j,2}\right)^2 + \cdots\left(x_{i,dm} - x_{j,dm}\right)^2\right]^{1/2}$$

The relationship between the correlation integral and R is: Cd(R)~R^{dc}, the logarithm of both sides can be obtained:

$$\log C_d(R) = d_c \log R + \text{constant}$$

2.3.7 Lyapunov Exponent

The Lyapunov exponent (LE) is used to quantitatively analyze the chaotic behavior by measuring the sensitivity of the attractor initial state. Its physical meaning is the exponential rate of the divergence of adjacent trajectories in the attractor. It is used to measure the degree of attraction or separation between two adjacent trajectories in phase space. For example: the initial distance between two points of adjacent trajectories is d_L (0), and then the distance becomes d_L(t) due to the trajectory divergence at time t, so$d_L(t) = d_L(0)e^{\lambda t}$. A positive LE value indicates that the system dynamic behavior is chaotic, and a negative value or zero indicates regular behavior. For an N-dimensional attractor, there will be N LE values. The algorithm for calculating LE is to obtain the maximum positive LE (that is, λ_1) in the time series. This method calculates the divergence rate of the reference trajectory and adjacent trajectories in the attractor. The maximum positive LE of the time series can be expressed as (Eckhardt and Yao, 1993; Rozenbaum et al., 2017):

$$\lambda_1 = \lim_{N\to\infty}\frac{1}{t_m - t_0}\sum_{i=1}^{m}\ln\frac{d_L^{'}(t_i)}{d_L(t_{i-1})} \tag{9}$$

t_0:initial timet_m:the *m*th time.

2.3.8 Kolmogorov Entropy (K2)

Kolmogorov entropy is a quantitative method for measuring the degree of chaotic behavior. It can also be used to distinguish the characteristics of dynamic systems: chaotic or non-chaotic. "Entropy" is adopted from the concept of thermodynamics as a method for expressing information characteristics, that is, the prediction of an uncertain system. The Kolmogorov entropy concept can be expressed as:

$$S(t_2) = S(t_1) + K(t_2 - t_1) \tag{10}$$

K stands for Kolmogorov entropy. The unit is bit/s. $S(t_1,t_2)$ is the amount of change in the time development information predicted by the initial information $S(t_1)$ after one (t_2—t_1) time. Assume that the initial entropy information is $S(t_1)$, after a time interval t_2—t_1, the information change to become $S(t_2)$. The change difference information is $K(t_2—t_1)$. Thus, it can be derived: $S(t_2) = S(t_1) + K(t_2—t_1)$. When $S(t_1) > S(t_2)$, so $K(t_2—t_1) = S(t_1)—S(t_2)$. Assume $S(t_1) = \ln C_d(R)$, $S(t_2) = \ln C_{d+1}(R)$. $C_d(R)$ is the signal correlation function. The equation for $K2$ is derived as below (Grassberger 1983; Zhang 2017):

$$K2 = \ln \frac{C_d(R)}{C_{d+1}(R)} \tag{11}$$

t-test was used to determine the significance of difference between healthy group and patient groups. The significance level was set to 0.05. All statistical tests were performed using SPSS 26 (IBM, Somers, NY, United States).

3 RESULTS

3.1 Blood Pressure and Cerebral Blood Flow

Figure 3 showed the comparison of differences in blood pressure and cerebral blood flow while in supine position among groups. From the systolic arterial blood pressure (SABP) and mean arterial blood pressure (MABP), it can be observed that stroke patients (SABP:177.0 ± 21.25 mmHg; MABP: 127.95 ± 18.66 mmHg)>hypertension patients (SABP:146.07 ± 26.04 mmHg; MABP: 106.55 ± 19.72 mmHg)>healthy people (SABP:120.94 ± 7.74 mmHg; MABP: 88.11 ± 7.76 mmHg). Both of these differences were significant ($p < 0.05$). Diastolic arterial blood pressure (DABP) is statistically different in stroke patients (DABP: 101.69 ± 18.02 mmHg) as opposed to hypertensive patients (DABP: 87.01 ± 18.16 mmHg) ($p < 0.05$). It can be seen that cardiovascular diseases (hypertension, stroke) do have obvious changing factors and trends to increase blood pressure. The systolic cerebral blood flow velocity (SCBFV) and mean cerebral blood flow velocity (MCBFV) showed that the value of stroke patients (SCBFV: 118.37 ± 60.42 cm/s; MCBFV: 73.99 ± 39.20 cm/s) was significantly higher than that of hypertension patients (SCBFV: 67.19 ± 21.84 cm/s; MCBFV: 36.84 ± 16.55 cm/s) and healthy people (SCBFV: 58.73 ± 9.62 cm/s; MCBFV: 38.82 ± 7.84 cm/s), and there was a statistical difference ($p < 0.05$). Diastolic cerebral blood flow velocity (DCBFV) is statistically different between stroke patients (DCBFV: 45.12 ± 24.78 cm/s) and healthy people (DCBFV: 23.69 ± 6.90 cm/s) ($p < 0.05$), and there is no significant difference in diastolic cerebral blood flow between hypertensive patients and stroke patients. **Figure 3** indicated the significant differences in blood pressure and cerebral blood flow while in supine position among healthy people, hypertensive patients, and stroke patients.

Figure 4 revealed the blood pressure and cerebral blood flow differences comparison in healthy people, hypertensive patients, and stroke patients in head-up tilt position. After interference induced by the tilting table, it can be seen that the SABP, MABP, and DABP values of stroke patients are significantly ($p < 0.05$) higher than those in healthy people ($SABP_{stroke}$:163.97 ± 19.55 mmHg; $MABP_{stroke}$:116.90 ± 12.78 mmHg; $DABP_{stroke}$: 94.71 ± 12.38 mmHg; $SABP_{healthy}$:128.83 ± 18.18 mmHg; $MABP_{healthy}$:95.0 ± 11.79 mmHg; $DABP_{healthy}$:76.30 ± 11.49 mmHg). On the other hand, the BP values of hypertensive patients between healthy and stroke patients were without significant difference and this might indicate an increasing BP trend toward abnormal. The cerebral blood flow velocity of stroke patients is higher than that of healthy people. The systolic cerebral blood flow velocity values revealed a significant statistical difference ($SCBFV_{stroke}$:114.18 ± 60.65 cm/s; $SCBFV_{healthy}$:60.87 ± 14.05 cm/s, $p < 0.05$).

3.2 Resistance Index, Pulsation Index) and Cerebrovascular Resistance

Figures 5, 6 show the resistance index (RI), pulsation index (PI), and cerebrovascular resistance (CVR) analysis results of the three groups in both supine and tilting positions, respectively. There is no obvious difference in movement and progress in RI and PI during position change. The CVR values indicated a slight statistical difference between healthy people and hypertensive patients ($CVR_{healthy}$: 2.32 ± 0.32; $CVR_{hypertension}$: 3.9 ± 2.78), hypertensive patients vs. stroke patients ($CVR_{hypertension}$: 3.9 ± 2.78; $CVR_{hypertension}$: 2.13 ± 1.03) while in supine position ($p < 0.1$). There was no significant difference in PI in the subjects tested this time. Only the PI values of hypertensive patients and stroke patients tended to be slightly higher than normal. The cerebrovascular resistance index CVR shows that the CVR of hypertensive patients is higher than that of normal people and stroke patients ($p < 0.1$), which shows that the cerebral vascular resistance of hypertensive patients is higher, but it is speculated that once a stroke develops, the cerebral vascular lesions Instead, it reduces the vascular resistance in the brain.

3.3 Analysis of Baroreflex

The pressure-sensitive reflex degree—baroreflex sensitivity (BRS) (also known as the pressure-sensitive reflex gain) is used as a measure of the autonomous control of the cardiovascular system. Usually BRS is a measure of the response of autonomic effectors to a given change in arterial pressure. When the position of a person changes from supine to a head-up position, blood pressure drops. This decreasing blood pressure can be compensated by the baroreflex through the conduction of the vagus nerve reflex. The sensory signal caused by the pressure receptor can inhibit the activity of the parasympathetic nerve and promote the activity of the sympathetic nerve, which increases the heart rate and

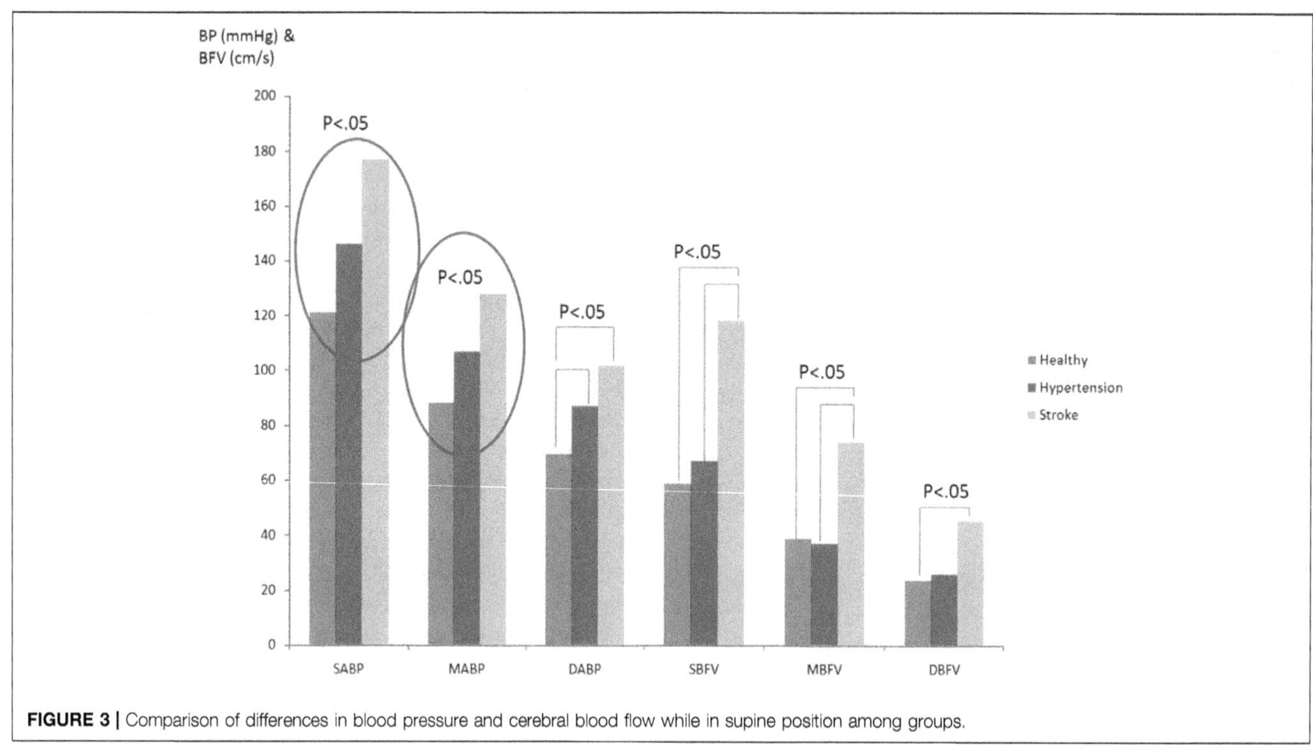

FIGURE 3 | Comparison of differences in blood pressure and cerebral blood flow while in supine position among groups.

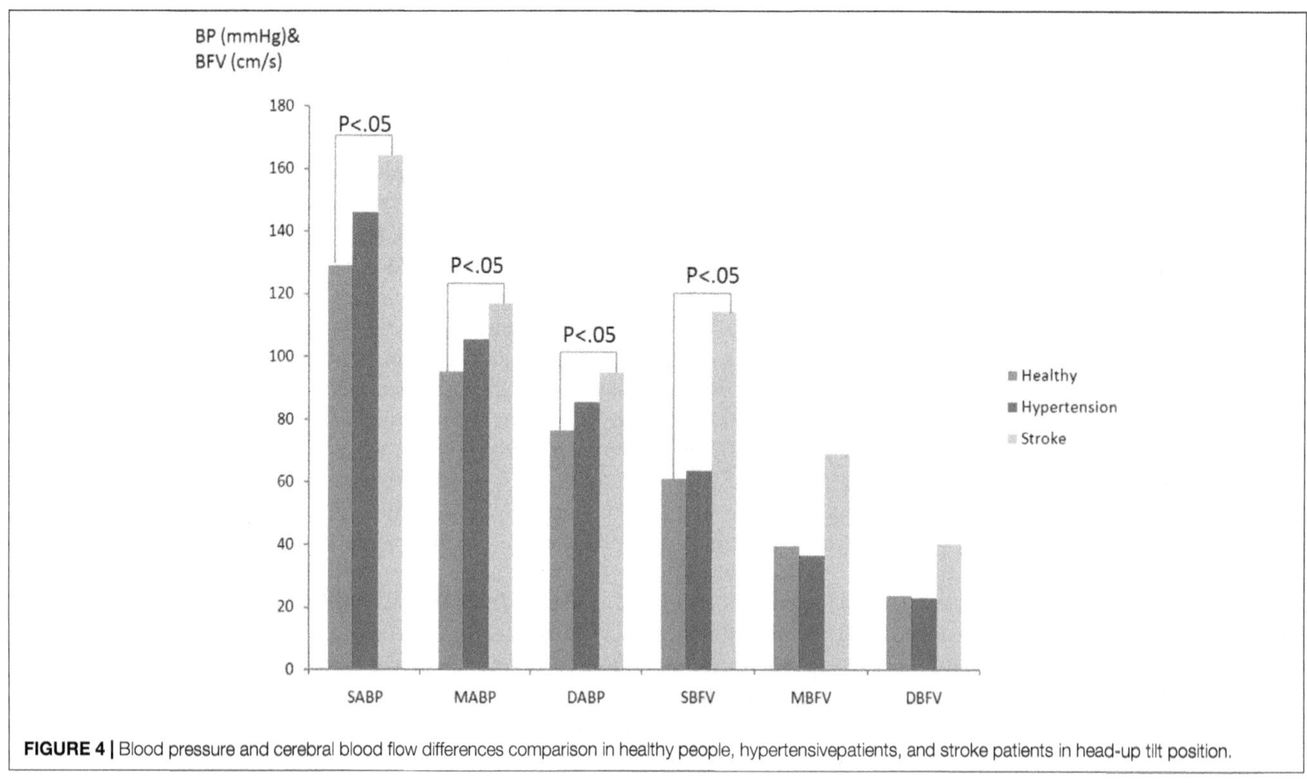

FIGURE 4 | Blood pressure and cerebral blood flow differences comparison in healthy people, hypertensivepatients, and stroke patients in head-up tilt position.

vasoconstriction, helping to maintain proper blood pressure when standing. **Figure** 7 shows the baroreflex sensitivity analysis results of healthy people, hypertensive patients, and stroke patients. It shows that as the course of healthy→hypertension→stroke progresses, $BRS_{healthy} > BRS_{hypertension} > BRS_{stroke}$, and BRS decreases accordingly. Healthy people vs. hypertension (supine: $BRS_{healthy}$: 7.29 ± 0.88, $BRS_{hypertension}$: 6.1 ± 1.49; tilting: $BRS_{healthy}$: 6.43 ± 0.98,

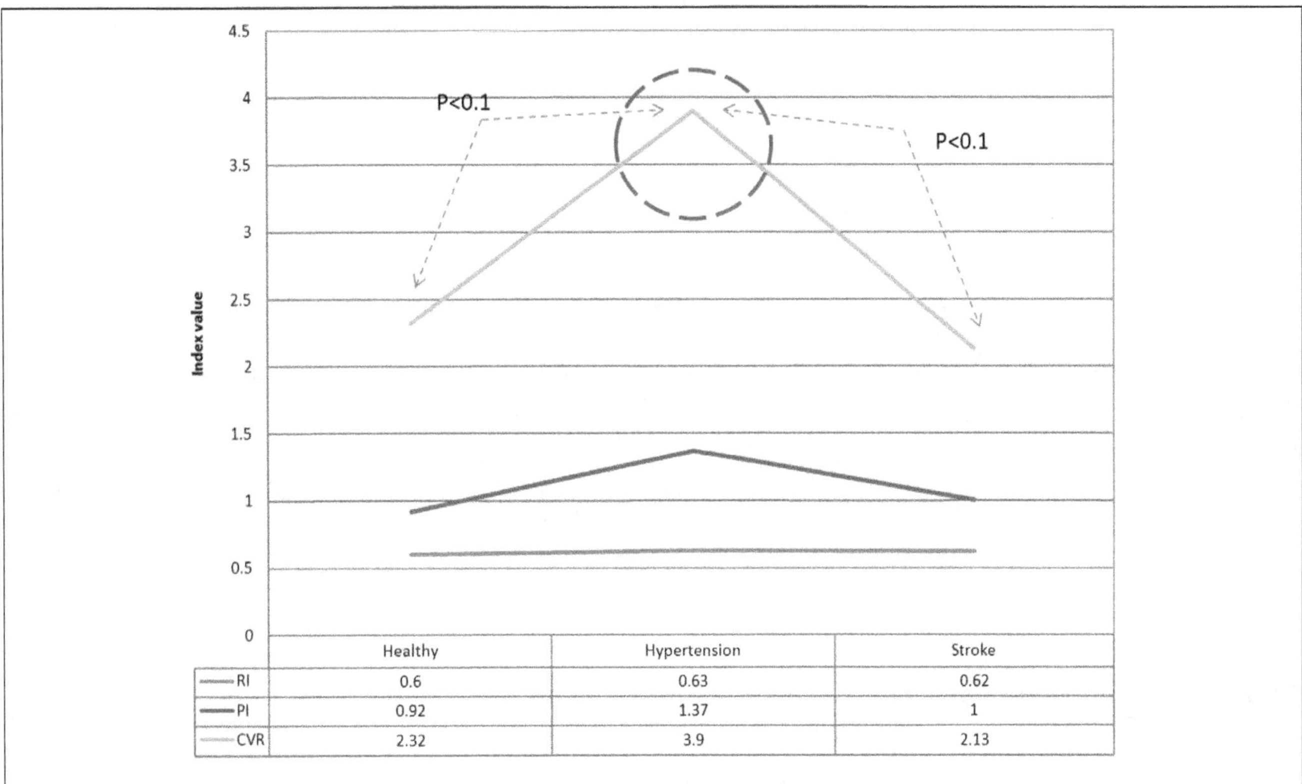

FIGURE 5 | Comparison of differences in vascular resistance indexes between healthy people, hypertension patients, and stroke patients in supine position.

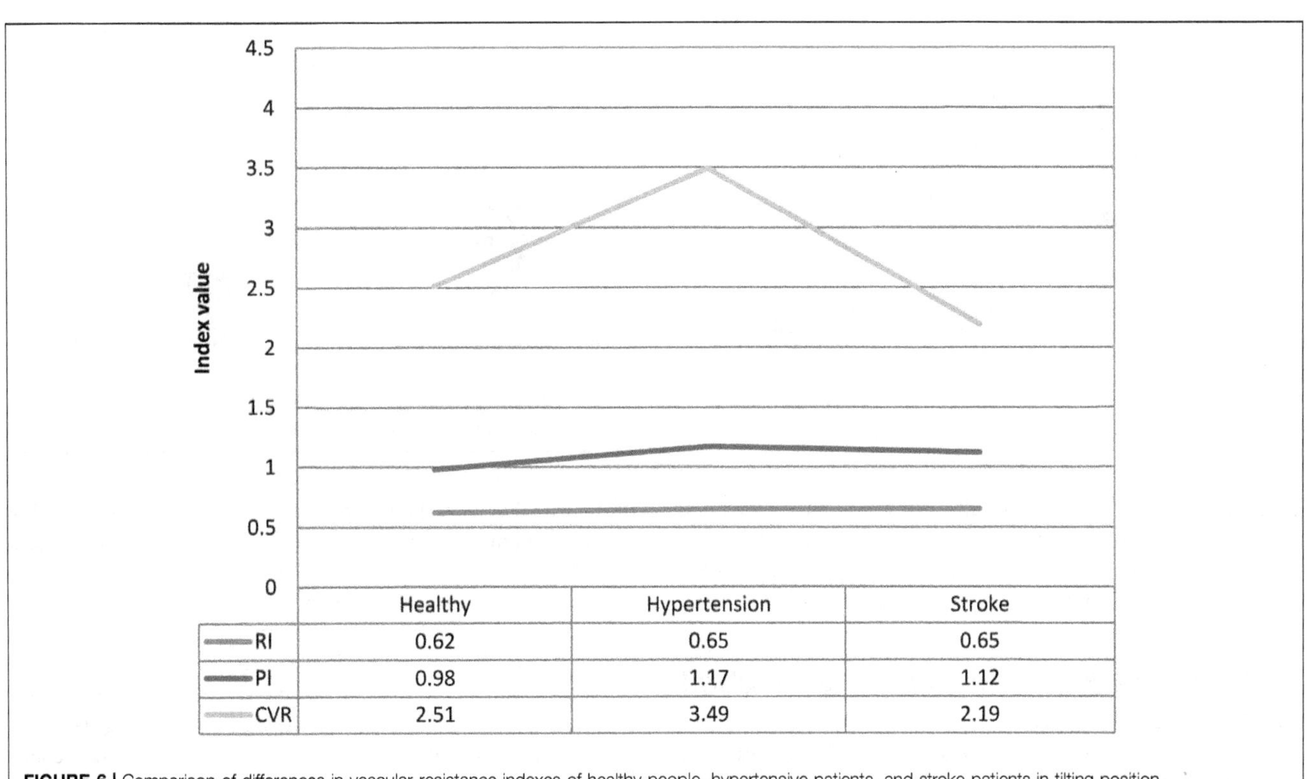

FIGURE 6 | Comparison of differences in vascular resistance indexes of healthy people, hypertensive patients, and stroke patients in tilting position.

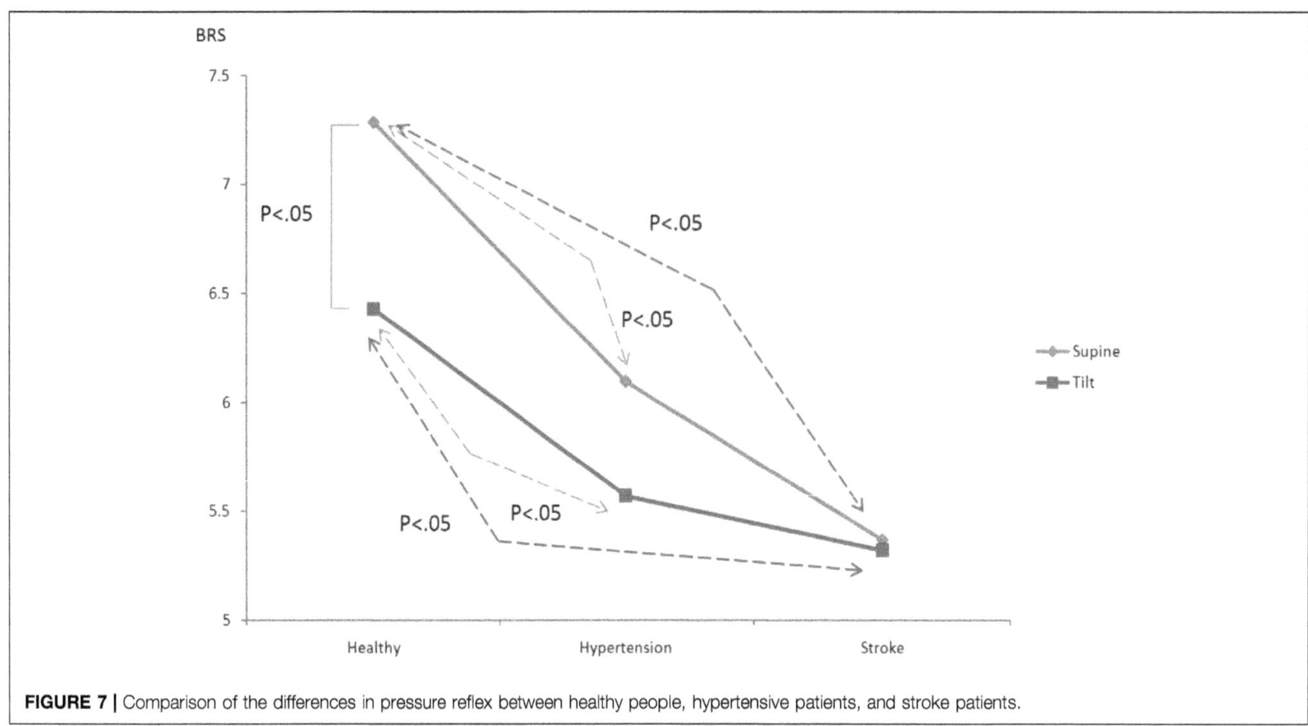

FIGURE 7 | Comparison of the differences in pressure reflex between healthy people, hypertensive patients, and stroke patients.

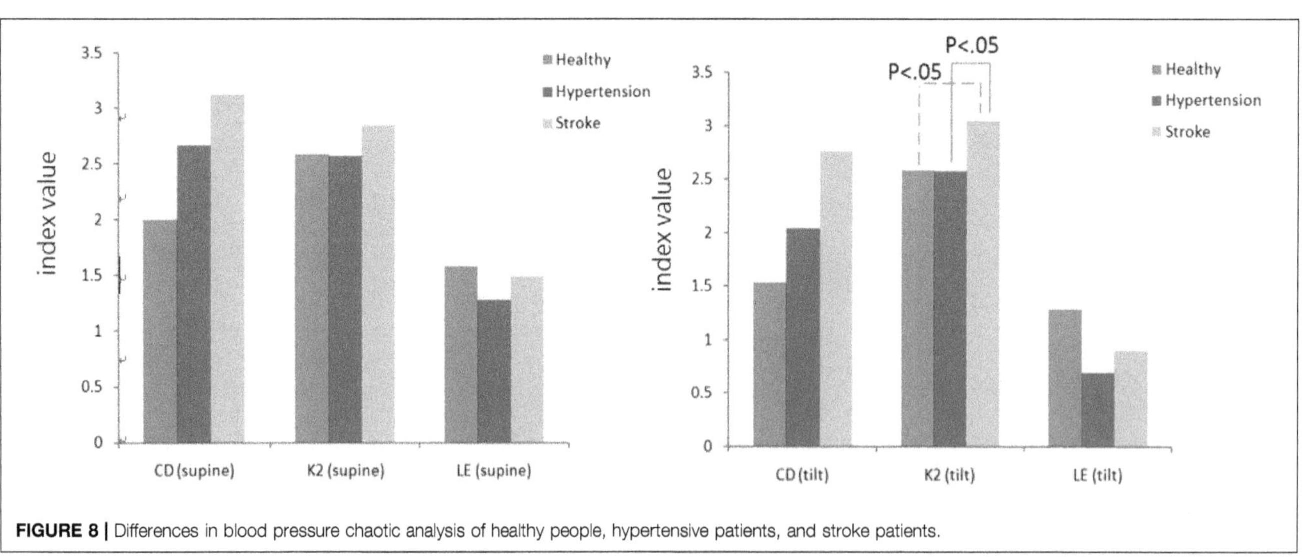

FIGURE 8 | Differences in blood pressure chaotic analysis of healthy people, hypertensive patients, and stroke patients.

$BRS_{hypertension}$: 5.57 ± 0.86), healthy people vs. stroke (supine: $BRS_{healthy}$: 7.29 ± 0.88, BRS_{stroke}: 5.37 ± 1.33; tilting: $BRS_{healthy}$: 6.43 ± 0.98, $BRS_{stroken}$: 5.32 ± 1.22), there are significant differences in both supine and tilting positions ($p < 0.05$).

3.4 Nonlinear Blood Pressure and Cerebral Blood Flow Analysis

There are three main parameters in chaotic analysis: 1. Correlation dimension (CD) represents the complexity of a system, and the higher the CD value, the higher the system complexity. 2. Lyapunov exponent (LE) represents the sensitivity of the initial system state. A positive LE value indicates that the system dynamic behavior is chaotic, and a negative value or zero indicates regular behavior. 3. Kolmogorov entropy (K2) is a quantitative method for the degree of chaotic behavior. It is used to predict the information loss rate of future behavior, that is, the degree of unpredictability. For a regular system, K2 is zero. For a completely random system, the K2 value is infinite. For a chaotic system, the K2 value is finite and positive. **Figure 8** is a comparison chart of the differences in blood pressure chaos analysis between healthy people, hypertensive .patients, and stroke patients. It can be observed that the change trend between supine and head-up positions is close. After head-up

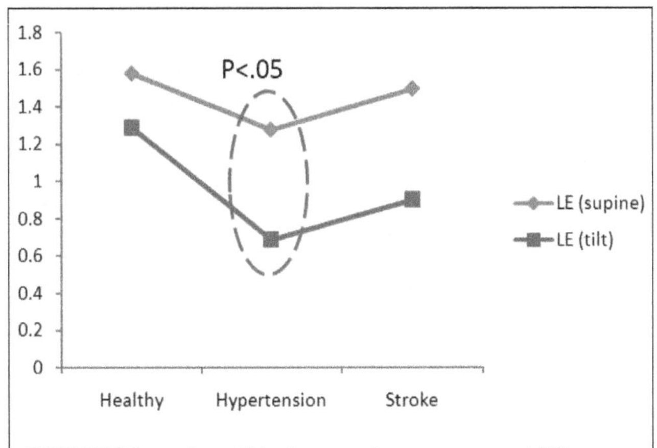

FIGURE 9 | Comparison of blood pressure Lyapunov exponent (LE) analysis of healthy people, hypertension patients, and stroke patients.

tilting, the K2 value of stroke patients is greater than that of hypertension patients and healthy people ($K2_{stroke}$:3.04 ± 0.28, $K2_{hypertension}$:2.58 ± 0.39, $K2_{healthy}$:2.59 ± 1.11), and there are statistical differences ($p < 0.05$) as shown in **Figure 8**. On the other hand, when the LE value changes posture in hypertensive patients, there is a statistically significant difference (Supine-$LE_{hypertension}$:1.28 ± 0.67,Tilt-$LE_{hypertension}$:0.69 ± 0.43$p < 0.05$), such as shown in **Figure 9**.

Figure 10 is a comparison chart of the chaotic analysis of cerebral blood flow in healthy people, hypertensive patients, and stroke patients. It can be observed that there is a significant difference ($p < 0.05$) in the K2 index between supine and tilting positions. While in supine position, the K2 value of stroke was higher than that of healthy people, with a statistical difference ($K2_{stroke}$: 3.74 ± 0.42, $K2_{healthy}$: 3.14 ± 0.59, $p < 0.05$). After head-up tilting, the K2 values of stroke patients were higher than those in hypertension patients and healthy people, and there was a statistical difference ($K2_{stroke}$:3.87 ± 1.03; $K2_{hypertension}$:3.24 ± 0.3; $K2_{healthy}$:2.80 ± 0.46, $p < 0.05$) as shown in **Figure 10**. When the LE value during changes posture in hypertensive patients, there is a statistically significant difference (supine $LE_{hypertension}$:1.11 ± 0.43; tilting $LE_{hypertension}$:0.64 ± 0.25, $p < 0.05$).

TABLE 1 | Correlation analysis results for blood pressure and cerebral blood flow in each group.

	Supine			Tilting		
	Max CCF	**Index**	**SD**	**Max CCF**	**Index**	**SD**
Healthy	0.57	−1.9	015	0.53	−1.6	0.18
Hypertension	0.43*	−2.2	0.16	0.40^	−2.5	0.19
Stroke	0.40**	−0.11	0.20	0.34^	−3.52	0.22

*Max CCF, in supine (Healthy vs. Hypertension, *p < 0.05; Healthy vs. Stroke, **p < 0.05); max CCF, in tilting (Healthy vs. Hypertension, ^p < 0.05; Healthy vs. Stroke, ^p < 0.05).*

3.5 Cross-Correlation Function Analysis

3.5.1 Blood Pressure and Cerebral Blood Flow

Table 1 shows the correlation analysis results for blood pressure and cerebral blood flow in healthy people, hypertensive patients, and stroke patients. **Figure 11** shows the comparison of the maximum CCF differences between blood pressure and cerebral blood flow in healthy people, hypertensive patients, and stroke patients. The results show that as the course of healthy→ hypertension → stroke progresses with the maximum CCF value decreases indicated significantly differences (Healthy vs. Hypertension; Healthy vs. Stroke, $p < 0.05$). That means the relationship between blood pressure and cerebral blood flow decreased, reaching a statistical difference ($p < 0.05$). **Figures 12–14** show the correlation analysis between blood pressure and cerebral blood flow in typical healthy people, hypertensive patients, and stroke patients.

4 DISCUSSION

The time domain analysis results indicate that high blood pressure is one of the most important factors influencing the

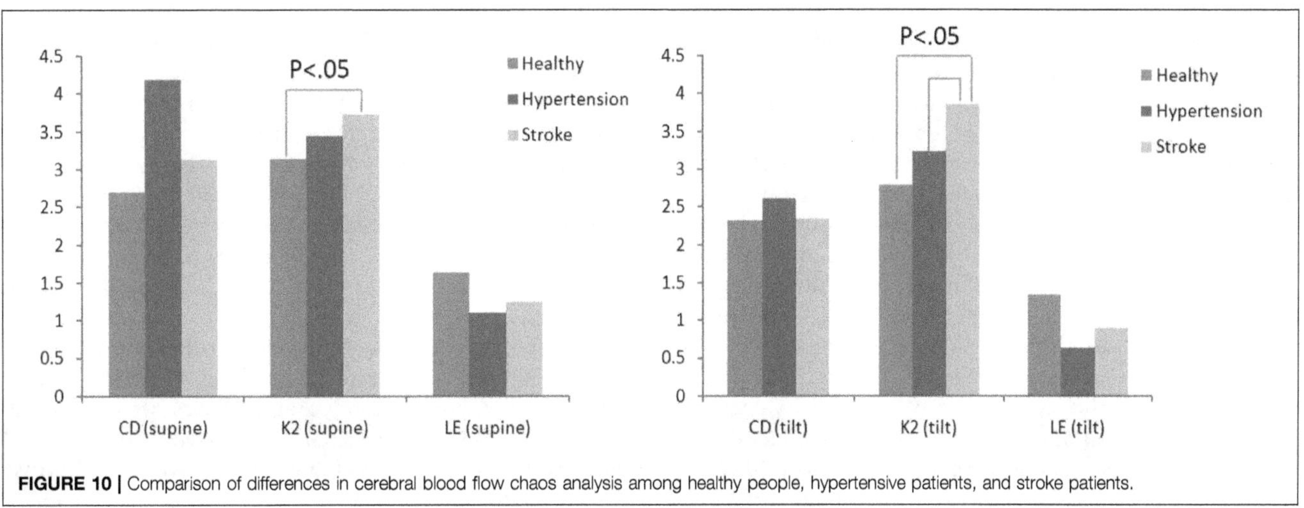

FIGURE 10 | Comparison of differences in cerebral blood flow chaos analysis among healthy people, hypertensive patients, and stroke patients.

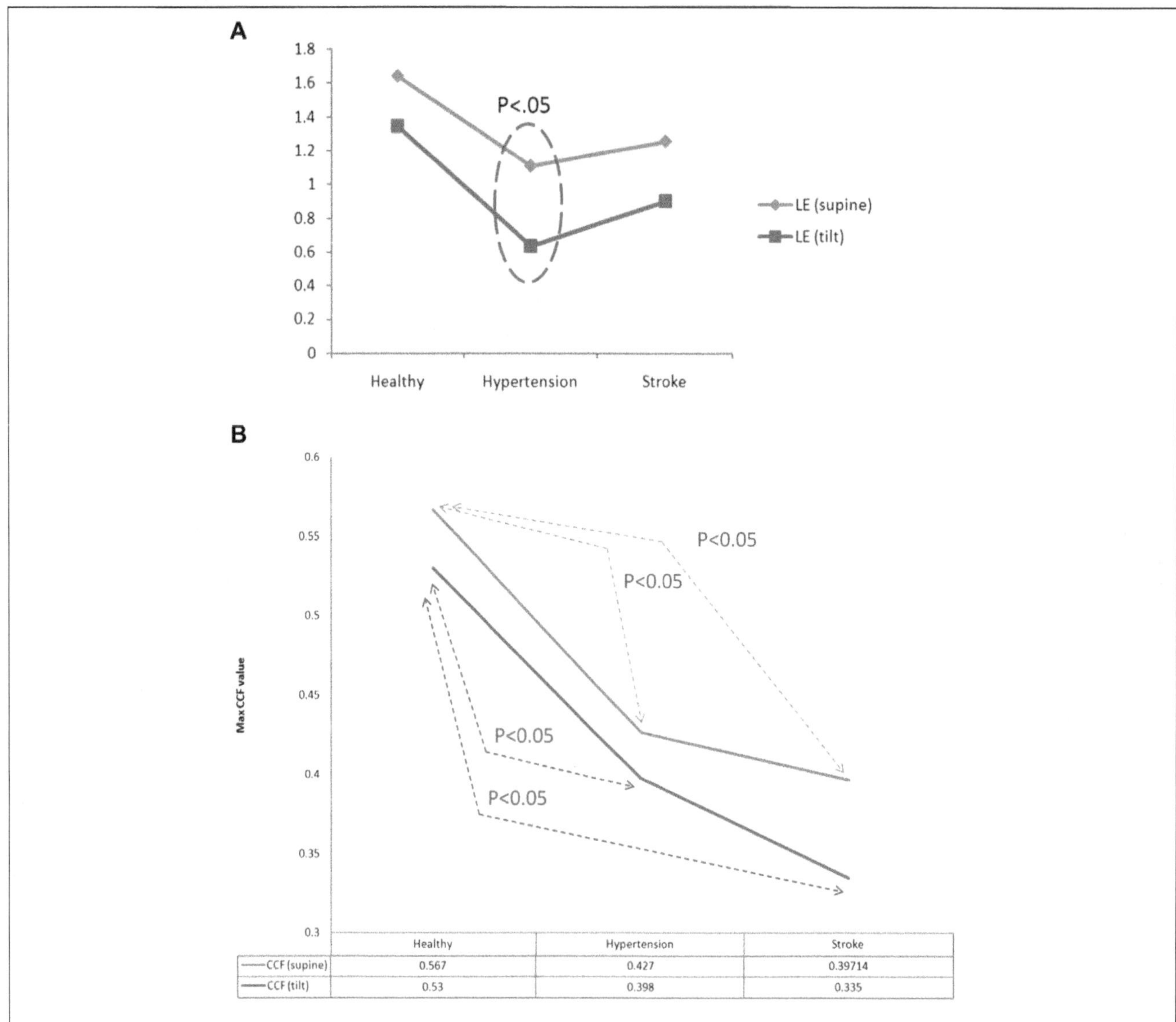

	Healthy	Hypertension	Stroke
CCF (supine)	0.567	0.427	0.39714
CCF (tilt)	0.53	0.398	0.335

FIGURE 11 | (A) Comparison of Lyapunov exponent (LE) analysis of cerebral blood flow in healthy people, hypertensive patients, and stroke patients. **(B)** Comparison of maximum CCF differences between blood pressure and cerebral blood flow in healthy people, hypertensive patients, and stroke patients.

stroke process. Higher blood pressure and blood flow increase the risk for stroke (Fuchs and Ethlton, 2020). Although there is no statistical difference between the average cerebral blood flow and the diastolic cerebral blood flow, it can be clearly observed that the CBFV value of stroke patients is higher than those in healthy and hypertensive patients. Therefore, it can also be inferred that the increase in blood pressure and blood flow is accompanied by a high risk for hypertension and stroke due to hypertrophy and smooth muscle cells remodeling (Yu et al., 2011). On the other hand, the blood vessel resistance index (RI) is a measure of peripheral blood flow resistance. Low vascular resistance has a higher diastolic blood flow velocity characteristic, and will have a lower RI value, and a high vascular resistance has a lower diastolic blood flow velocity characteristic and will induce a higher RI value (Hilz et al., 2004). The results showed that there was no significant difference in RI among the groups in this study. The pulsation index (PI) is a measurement that describes the type of signal waveform. Low intracranial vascular resistance will reduce PI, and rising intracranial pulsations have been found to be related to rising intracranial pressure. The general PI range is between 0.5 and 1.4, less than 0.5 may be an ischemic flow pattern under vascular dilation. PI range greater than 1.5 may indicate a decrease in vascular compliance or an increase in intracranial pressure (Hilz et al., 2004). Because the CVR value in the hypertension group is higher than those in other groups, it would indicate that blood vessel resistance increased and blood vessel characteristics were changed. Moreover, average PI value in hypertension group is 1.37 close to 1.4, it may reveal high blood pressure decrease

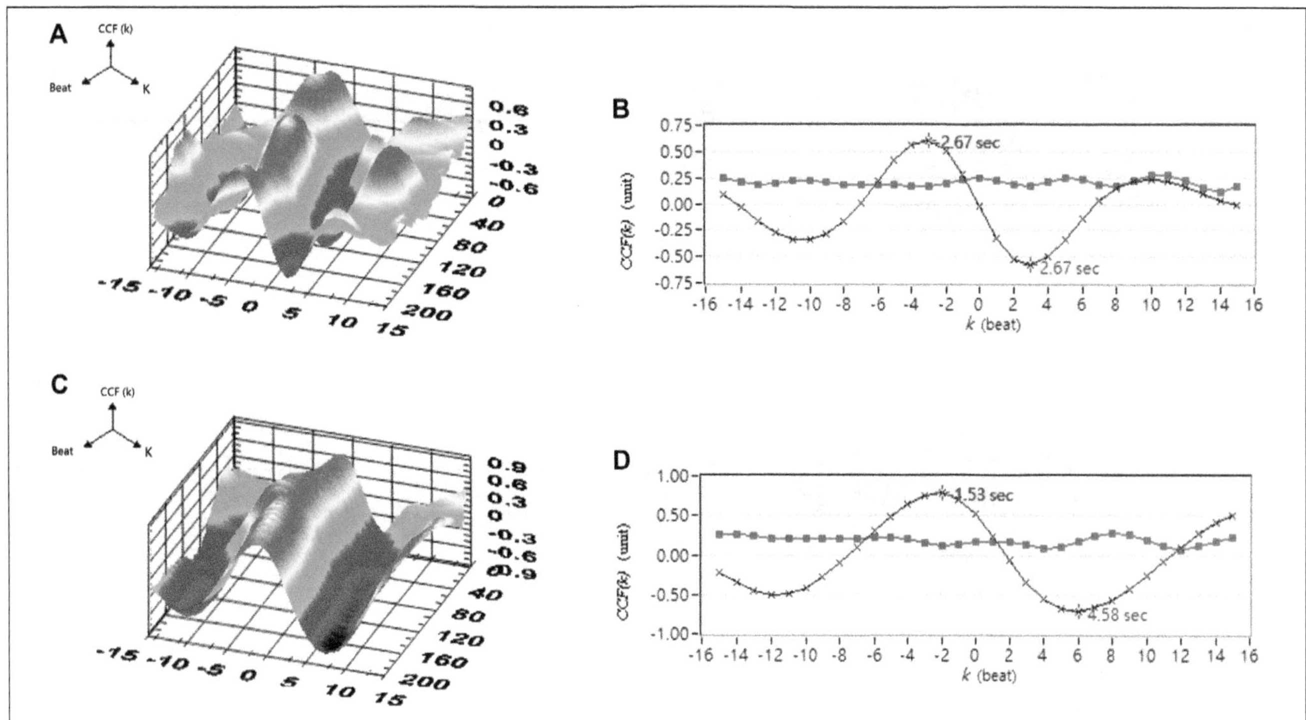

FIGURE 12 | A typical healthy person's blood pressure and cerebral blood flow correlation analysis. **(A)** 3D representative CCF figures in supine position. **(B)** 2D representative figures of CCF in supine position. **(C)** 3D representative figures of CCF in head-up tilt position. **(D)** 2D representative figures of CCF in head-up tilt position. CCF(k) is the CCF value in the time indices. The mean (–x–) and standard deviation (–■–) of CCF value in each time index k.

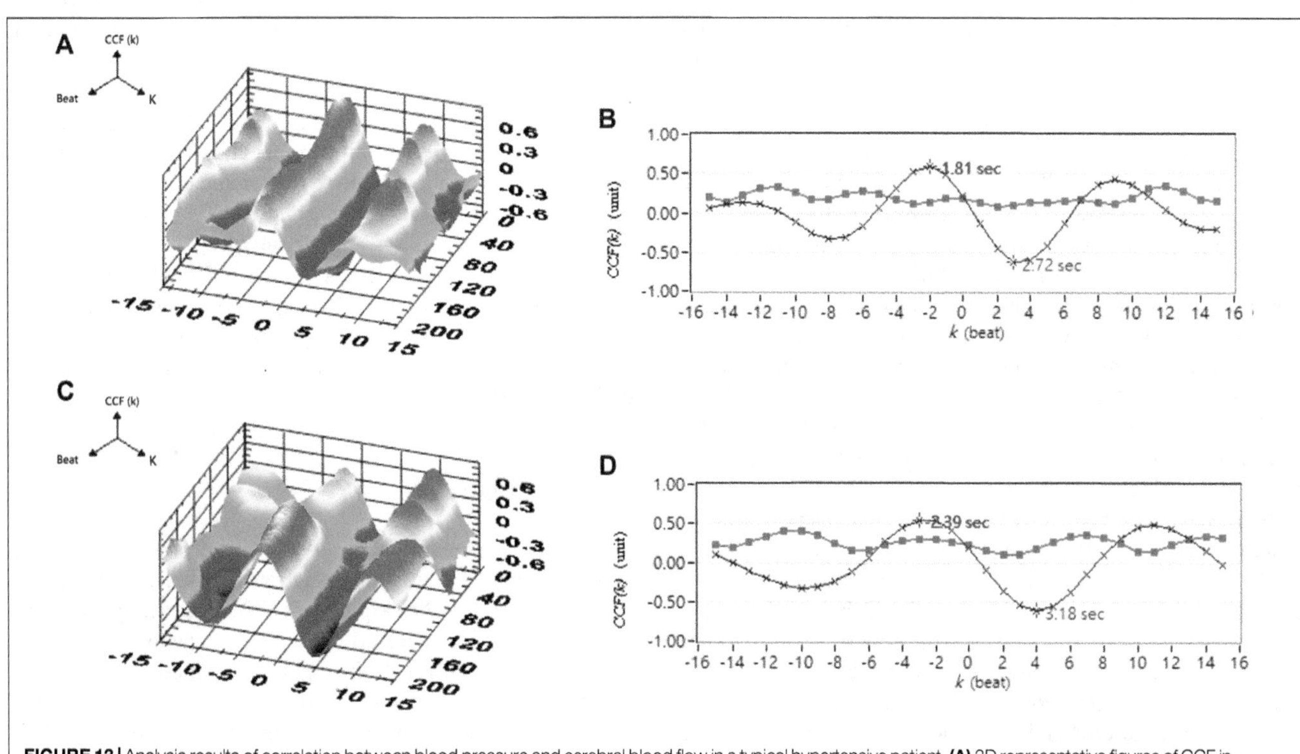

FIGURE 13 | Analysis results of correlation between blood pressure and cerebral blood flow in a typical hypertensive patient. **(A)** 3D representative figures of CCF in supine position. **(B)** 2D representative figures of CCF in supine position. **(C)** 3D representative CCF figures in head-up tilt position. **(D)** 2D representative CCF figures in head-up tilt position. CCF(k) is the CCF value in the time indices. The mean (–x–) and standard deviation (–■–) of CCF value in each time index k.

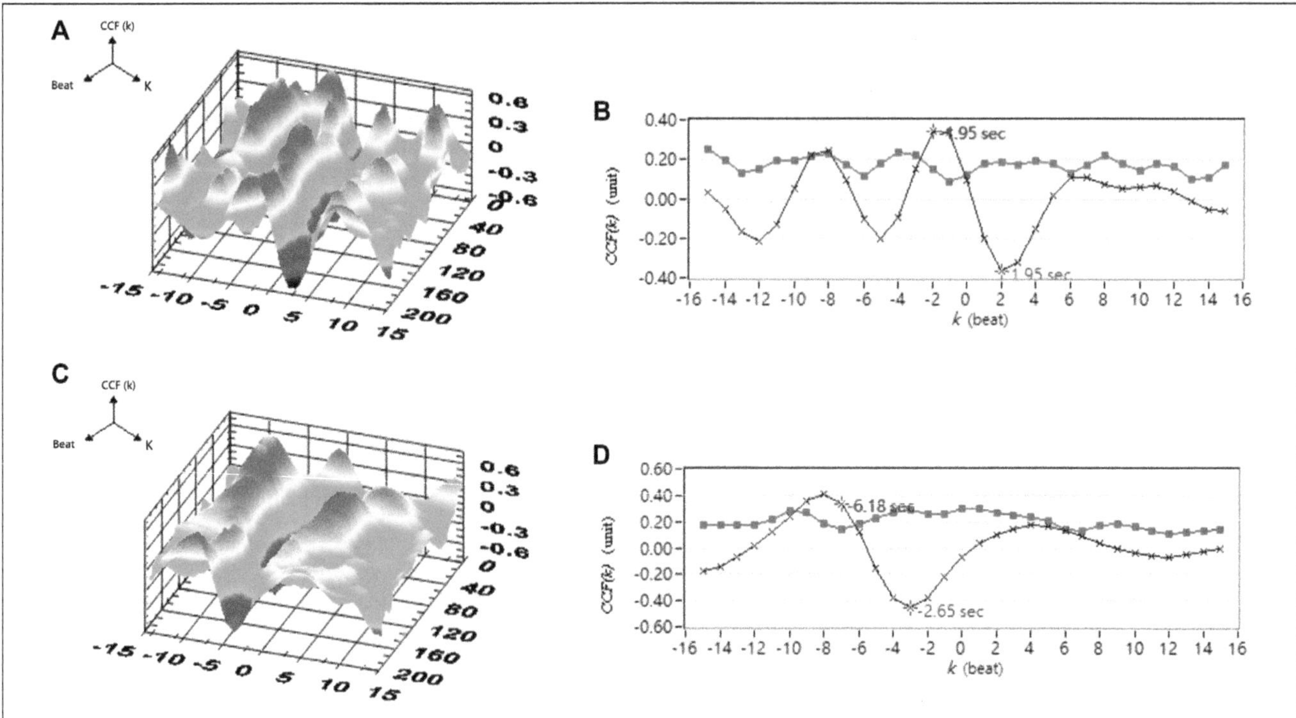

FIGURE 14 | Analysis results for the correlation between blood pressure and cerebral blood flow in a typical stroke patient. **(A)** 3D representative figures of CCF in supine position. **(B)** 2D representative figures of CCF in supine position. **(C)** 3D representative CCF figures in head-up tilt position. **(D)** 2D representative CCF figures in head-up tilt position. CCF(k) is the CCF value in the time indices. The mean (–x–) and standard deviation (–■–) of CCF value in each time index k.

vascular compliance or increase intracranial pressure (Hilz et al., 2004). From the baroreflex results, it can be inferred that the BRS receptor sensitivity in patients with hypertension and stroke is reduced, and it is unable to effectively sense the changes in blood pressure and regulate the cardiovascular system. If high blood pressure occurs, hypertension exceeds the normal pressure reflex receptor operating range (The average blood pressure is 60–120 mmHg), the individual cannot adjust their heartbeat, blood vessel radius and other factors through the autonomic nervous system to maintain normal cardiovascular system regulation. Therefore, dysfunctional baroreflex and hypertension would lead to stroke risk according to the results and previous studies (Kuusela et al., 2002; Yu et al., 2011; Fuchs et al., 2020).

Chaotic analysis can extract hidden behavior in a system. The K2 value is finite and positive for a chaotic system. Using the BP K2 results in chaotic analysis, it can be speculated that the changes in blood pressure in stroke patients are more unpredictable than in healthy people and hypertensive patients (Grassberger 1983; Zhang 2017). According to previous studies (Eckhardt and Yao, 1993; Rozenbaum et al., 2017), the difference in LE indicated that the blood pressure disturbance in hypertensive patients has a higher change in chaotic behavior and a difference in initial state sensitivity. On the other hand, nonlinear analysis of cerebral blood flow infers that the changes in cerebral blood flow in stroke patients is more unpredictable than in healthy people and hypertensive patients. This revealed that cerebral blood flow disturbance in hypertensive patients has a higher change in chaotic behavior and a difference in initial state sensitivity. Summarizing the chaotic analysis and baroreflex results, due to lower BRS value mean dysfunction baroreflex and it would induced circulation system to be more complicated (Kuusela et al., 2002), it can be inferred that changes in blood pressure and cerebral blood flow in patients with hypertension and stroke lead to higher chaotic behavior and changes in initial state sensitivity. CCF analysis indicated the interaction of circulation subsystems and it showed maximum CCF value decreasing significant in hypertension and stroke group respect to healthy group. This means that blood pressure and cerebral blood flow are gradually not affected by the autoregulation mechanism, and that the buffer between blood pressure and cerebral blood flow is dysfunctional. It can also be speculated that the incidence of stroke is increased.

5 CONCLUSION

This study demonstrated the results from assessing the link change in linear and nonlinear analysis in healthy, hypertensive and stroke groups. The significant differences might indicate high blood pressure would be a critical factor that affects cardiovascular control with regulation function and blood vessel properties in hypertension and stroke subjects. The results from this study revealed the time domain analysis included BP and BFV levels, BRS, CVR and CCF. The nonlinear measures included LE, and K2, which are suitable parameters to explore the hidden components of circulation characteristics and performance in hypertensive and stroke patients. We speculate that an irregular cardiovascular system would tend toward dysfunction in various sub-systems and less predictable behavior. This could be as a measure for detecting and preventing the risk for hypertension and stroke in clinical practice (Faure and Korn, 1998; Rivera-Lara et al., 2017).

AUTHOR CONTRIBUTIONS

Conceptualization and methodology, B-YL and S-JY; formal analysis, B-YL and Y-KJ; writing, B-YL, C-WL, F-CK, and Y-KJ; project administration, B-YL and S-JY All authors have read and agreed to the published version of the manuscript.

ACKNOWLEDGMENTS

The authors would like to thank the National Science Council, Taiwan, ROC, for supporting this research under Contract Nos. MOST 108-2221-E-241-008 and MOST 110-2637-E-241-002.

REFERENCES

Aoi, M. C., Hu, K., Lo, M.-T., Selim, M., Olufsen, M. S., and Novak, V. (2012). Impaired Cerebral Autoregulation Is Associated with Brain Atrophy and Worse Functional Status in Chronic Ischemic Stroke. *PLoS ONE* 7 (10), e46794. doi:10.1371/journal.pone.0046794

Baumbach, G. L., and Heistad, D. D. (1988). Cerebral Circulation in Chronic Arterial Hypertension. *Hypertension* 12 (2), 89–95. doi:10.1161/01.hyp.12.2.89

Benjo, A., Thompson, R. E., Fine, D., Hogue, C. W., Alejo, D., Kaw, A., et al. (2007). Pulse Pressure Is an Age-independent Predictor of Stroke Development after Cardiac Surgery. *Hypertension* 50, 630–635. doi:10.1161/HYPERTENSIONAHA.107.095513

Bolea, J., Laguna, P., Remartínez, J. M., Rovira, E., Navarro, A., and Bailón, R. (2014). Methodological Framework for Estimating the Correlation Dimension in HRV Signals. *Comput. Math. Methods Med.* 2014, 129248. doi:10.1155/2014/129248

Castro, P., Azevedo, E., and Sorond, F. (2018). Cerebral Autoregulation in Stroke. *Curr. Atheroscler. Rep.* 20, 37. doi:10.1007/s11883-018-0739-5

Chiu, C.-C., and Yeh, S.-J. (2001). Assessment of Cerebral Autoregulation Using Time-Domain Cross-Correlation Analysis. *Comput. Biol. Med.* 31 (6), 471–480. doi:10.1016/s0010-4825(01)00015-4

Chiu, C. C., Yeh, S. J., and Chen, C. H. (2007). Self-organizing Arterial Pressure Pulse Classication Using Neural Networks: Theoretical Considerations and Clinical Applicability. *Comput. Biol. Med.* 30, 71–88.

Chiu, C. C., Yeh, S. J., and Liau, B. Y. (2005). Assessment of Cerebral Autoregulation Dynamics in Diabetics Using Time-Domain Cross-Correlation Analysis. *J. Med. Biol. Eng.* 25 (2), 53–59.

Crippa, I. A., Subirà, C., Vincent, J.-L., Fernandez, R. F., Hernandez, S. C., Cavicchi, F. Z., et al. (2018). Impaired Cerebral Autoregulation Is Associated with Brain Dysfunction in Patients with Sepsis. *Crit. Care* 22, 327. doi:10.1186/s13054-018-2258-8

Eckhardt, B., and Yao, D. (1993). Local Lyapunov Exponents in Chaotic Systems. *Physica D: Nonlinear Phenomena* 65, 100–108. doi:10.1016/0167-2789(93)90007-n

Fan, X., Li, X., and Yin, J. (2019). Dynamic Relationship between Carbon price and Coal price: Perspective Based on Detrended Cross-Correlation Analysis. *Energ. Proced.* 158, 3470–3475. doi:10.1016/j.egypro.2019.01.925

Faure, P., and Korn, H. (1998). A New Method to Estimate the Kolmogorov Entropy from Recurrence Plots: its Application to Neuronal Signals. *Physica D: Nonlinear Phenomena* 122, 265–279. doi:10.1016/s0167-2789(98)00177-8

Fuchs, F. D., and Whelton, P. K. (2020). High Blood Pressure and Cardiovascular Disease. *Hypertension* 75 (2), 285–292. doi:10.1161/hypertensionaha.119.14240

Gao, J., Hu, J., and Tung, W.-w. (2011). Facilitating Joint Chaos and Fractal Analysis of Biosignals through Nonlinear Adaptive Filtering. *PLoS ONE* 6 (9), e24331. doi:10.1371/journal.pone.0024331

Grassberger, P., and Procaccia, I. (1983). Estimation of the Kolmogorov Entropy from a Chaotic Signal. *Phys. Rev. A.* 28 (4), 2591–2593. doi:10.1103/physreva.28.2591

Grassberger, P., and Procaccia, I. (1983). Measuring the Strangeness of Strange Attractors. *Physica D: Nonlinear Phenomena* 9, 189–208. doi:10.1016/0167-2789(83)90298-1

Hilz, M. J., Kolodny, E. H., Brys, M., Stemper, B., Haendl, T., and Marthol, H. (2004). Reduced Cerebral Blood Flow Velocity and Impaired Cerebral Autoregulation in Patients with Fabry Disease. *J. Neurol.* 251 (5), 564–570. doi:10.1007/s00415-004-0364-9

Karemaker, J. M., and Wesseling, K. H. (2008). Variability in Cardiovascular Control: The Baroreflex Reconsidered. *Cardiovasc. Eng.* 8, 23–29. doi:10.1007/s10558-007-9046-4

Kuusela, T. A., Jartti, T. T., Tahvanainen, K. U. O., and Kaila, T. J. (2002). Terbutaline-Induced Heart Rate and Blood Pressure Changes. *Am. J. Physiol. Heart Circ. Physiol.* 282, H773–H781.

Laurent, S., Katsahian, S., Fassot, C., Tropeano, A.-I., Gautier, I., Laloux, B., et al. (2003). Aortic Stiffness Is an Independent Predictor of Fatal Stroke in Essential Hypertension. *Stroke* 34, 1203–1206. doi:10.1161/01.STR.0000065428.03209.64

Laurent, S. p., and Boutouyrie, P. (2005). Arterial Stiffness and Stroke in Hypertension. *CNS Drugs* 19 (1), 1–11. doi:10.2165/00023210-200519010-00001

Liau, B.-Y., Yeh, S.-J., Chiu, C.-C., and Tsai, Y.-C. (2008). Dynamic Cerebral Autoregulation Assessment Using Chaotic Analysis in Diabetic Autonomic Neuropathy. *Med. Bio Eng. Comput.* 46, 1–9. doi:10.1007/s11517-007-0243-5

Liau, B. Y., Chiu, C. C., and Yeh, S. J. (2010). Assessment of Dynamic Cerebral Autoregulation Using Spectral and Cross-Correlation Analyses of Different Antihypertensive Drug Treatments. *J. Med. Biol. Eng.* 30 (3), 169–176.

Ma, H., Guo, Z.-N., Liu, J., Xing, Y., Zhao, R., Yang, Y., et al. (2016). Temporal Course of Dynamic Cerebral Autoregulation in Patients with Intracerebral Hemorrhage. *Stroke* 47, 674–681. doi:10.1161/STROKEAHA.115.011453

Oeinck, M., Neunhoeffer, F., Buttler, K.-J., Meckel, S., Schmidt, B., Czosnyka, M., et al. (2013). Dynamic Cerebral Autoregulation in Acute Intracerebral Hemorrhage. *Stroke* 44, 2722–2728. doi:10.1161/STROKEAHA.113.001913

Pringle, E., Phillips, C., Thijs, L., Davidson, C., Staessen, J. A., de Leeuw, P. W., et al. (2003). Systolic Blood Pressure Variability as a Risk Factor for Stroke and Cardiovascular Mortality in the Elderly Hypertensive Population. *J. Hypertens.* 21, 2251–2257. doi:10.1097/00004872-200312000-00012

Rivera-Lara, L., Zorrilla-Vaca, A., Geocadin, R. G., Healy, R. J., Ziai, W., and Mirski, M. A. (2017). Cerebral Autoregulation-Oriented Therapy at the Bedside. *Anesthesiology* 126 (6), 1187–1199. doi:10.1097/aln.0000000000001625

Rivera-Lara, L., Zorrilla-Vaca, A., Geocadin, R., Ziai, W., Healy, R., Thompson, R., et al. (2017). Predictors of Outcome with Cerebral Autoregulation Monitoring. *Crit. Care Med.* 45 (4), 695–704. doi:10.1097/CCM.0000000000002251

Roth, G. A., Mensah, G. A., Johnson, C. O., Addolorato, G., Ammirati, E., Baddour, L. M., et al. (2020). Global Burden of Cardiovascular Diseases and Risk Factors, 1990-2019: Update from the GBD 2019 Study. *J. Am. Coll. Cardiol.* 76 (5), 2982–3021. doi:10.1016/j.jacc.2020.11.010

Rozenbaum, E. B., Ganeshan, S., and Galitski, V. (2017). Lyapunov Exponent and Out-Of-Time-Ordered Correlator's Growth Rate in a Chaotic System. *Phys. Rev. Lett.* 118, 086801. doi:10.1103/PhysRevLett.118.086801

Shekhar, S., Liu, R., Travis, O. K., Roman, R. J., and Fan, F. (2017). Cerebral Autoregulation in Hypertension and Ischemic Stroke: a Mini Review. *J. Pharm. Sci. Exp. Pharmacol.* 2017 (1), 21–27.

Tiecks, F. P., Lam, A. M., Aaslid, R., and Newell, D. W. (1995). Comparison of Static and Dynamic Cerebral Autoregulation Measurements. *Stroke* 26 (6), 1014–1019. doi:10.1161/01.str.26.6.1014

WHO CVD risk chart working group (2019). World Health Organization Cardiovascular Disease Risk Charts: Revised Models to Estimate Risk in 21 Global Regions. *Lancet Glob. Health* 7 (10), e1332–e1345. doi:10.1016/S2214-109X(19)30318-3

WHO (2003), International Society of Hypertension Writing Group. *J. Hypertens.* 21 (11), 1983–1992.

Xiong, L., Liu, X., Shang, T., Smielewski, P., Donnelly, J., Guo, Z.-n., et al. (2017). Impaired Cerebral Autoregulation: Measurement and Application to Stroke. *J. Neurol. Neurosurg. Psychiatry* 88, 520–531. doi:10.1136/jnnp-2016-314385

Yu, J.-G., Zhou, R.-R., and Cai, G.-J. (2011). From Hypertension to Stroke: Mechanisms and Potential Prevention Strategies. *CNS Neurosci. Ther.* 17, 577–584. doi:10.1111/j.1755-5949.2011.00264.x

Zhang, X. D. (2017). "Entropy for the Complexity of Physiological Signal Dynamics,". Editor B. Shen (Springer Nature Singapore Pte Ltd.), Adv. Exp. Med. Biol., 1028, 39–53. doi:10.1007/978-981-10-6041-0_3

11

Application of 3D Printed Models of Complex Hypertrophic Scars for Preoperative Evaluation and Surgical Planning

Peng Liu[1,2†], Zhicheng Hu[1†], Shaobin Huang[1†], Peng Wang[1], Yunxian Dong[1], Pu Cheng[1], Hailin Xu[1], Bing Tang[1] and Jiayuan Zhu[1*]*

[1] Department of Burn Surgery, The First Affiliated Hospital of Sun Yat-sen University, Guangzhou, China, [2] Department of Burn and Plastic Surgery, Guangzhou Red Cross Hospital, Medical College, Jinan University, Guangzhou, China

***Correspondence:**
Bing Tang
tangbing@mail.sysu.edu.cn
Jiayuan Zhu
zhujiay@mail.sysu.edu.cn

† These authors have contributed equally to this work

Background: Complex hypertrophic scar is a condition that causes multiple joint contractures and deformities after trauma or burn injuries. Three-dimensional (3D) printing technology provides a new evaluation method for this condition. The objective of this study was to print individualized 3D models of complex hypertrophic scars and to assess the accuracy of these models.

Methods: Twelve patients with complex hypertrophic scars were included in this study. Before surgery, each patient underwent a computed tomography (CT) scan to obtain cross-sectional information for 3D printing. Mimics software was used to process the CT data and create 3D printed models. The length, width, height, and volume measurements of the physical scars and 3D printed models were compared. Experienced surgeons used the 3D models to plan the operation and simulate the surgical procedure. The hypertrophic scar was completely removed for each patient and covered with skin autografts. The surgical time, bleeding, complications, and skin autograft take rate were recorded. All patients were followed up at 12 months. The surgeons, young doctors, medical students, and patients involved in the study completed questionnaires to assess the use of the 3D printed models.

Results: The 3D models of the hypertrophic scars were printed successfully. The length, width, height, and volume measurements were significantly smaller for the 3D printed models than for the physical hypertrophic scars. Based on preoperative simulations with the 3D printed models, the surgeries were performed successfully and each hypertrophic scar was completely removed. The surgery time was shortened and the bleeding was decreased. On postoperative day 7, there were two cases of subcutaneous hemorrhage, one case of infection and one case of necrosis. On postoperative day 12, the average take rate of the skin autografts was 97.75%. At the 12-month follow-up, all patients were satisfied with the appearance and function.

Conclusion: Accurate 3D printed models can help surgeons plan and perform successful operations, help young doctors and medical students learn surgical methods, and enhance patient comprehension and confidence in their surgeons.

Keywords: 3D printed models, hypertrophic scars, preoperative evaluation, surgical planning, wound scarring prevention

INTRODUCTION

Complex hypertrophic scar is a condition caused by trauma or burn injuries that may cause multiple joint contractures and deformities (Butzelaar et al., 2015; Anthonissen et al., 2016; Seo and Jung, 2016). The treatment of complex hypertrophic scars can dramatically improve a patient's quality of life. At present, many conservative methods are used to treat complex hypertrophic scars; however, the outcomes are poor for patients with multiple skeletal deformities and scar contractures. Therefore, surgery is often the first treatment choice for patients with complex hypertrophic scars. When there are abnormal anatomical structures around the complex hypertrophic scar caused by skeletal deformities and soft tissue contractures, it is difficult for doctors to identify and assess the size of the scar clearly. Preoperative evaluation of complex hypertrophic scars is important for effective surgical treatment.

Currently, preoperative evaluation of complex hypertrophic scars depends exclusively on traditional, two-dimensional (2D) images, namely X-rays, computed tomography (CT), and magnetic resonance imaging (MRI). These types of imaging are used to evaluate the limits of complex hypertrophic scars and bone deformities; however, it is difficult to establish precise limits with 2D images (Ploch et al., 2016; Pfeil et al., 2017). Furthermore, it is also difficult to provide spatial anatomical information and tactile feedback for surgeons using these techniques.

Recently, 3D printing has been widely applied in orthopedic surgery, stomatology, and other medical fields because it has advantages in terms of individualization, tactility, and visualization (Cutroneo et al., 2016; Fitzhugh et al., 2016; Gu et al., 2016; Rashaan et al., 2016; Schepers et al., 2016). In this study, we made 3D models of complex hypertrophic scars to measure their dimensions preoperatively. We evaluated the accuracy of the 3D printed models. In addition, we assessed whether the 3D printed models were useful to surgeons in planning the operation, if they were helpful in the training of young doctors and medical students, and if they were useful tools for explaining the disease and operation to patients. Lastly, we assessed the clinical effect after surgery.

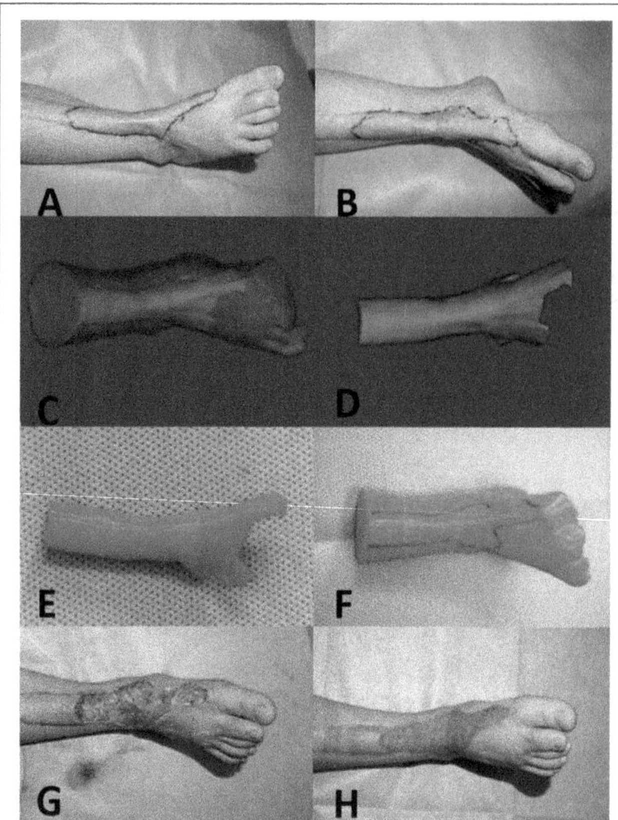

FIGURE 1 | Three-year-old girl with a complex hypertrophic scar. **(A,B)** Preoperative images of the hypertrophic scar, which resulted in a loss of flexure and extension of the right ankle. **(C,D)** A 3D model of the hypertrophic scar was designed using reconstruction software. **(E,F)** The 3D model of the hypertrophic scar on the right ankle was printed for surgery simulation and anatomical measurement. **(G)** Based on the 3D printed model, the hypertrophic scar on the right ankle was completely removed surgically, and the wound was covered with razor-thin autologous skin. **(H)** At the 12-month follow-up visit, the appearance and function of right ankle were recovered.

MATERIALS AND METHODS

Patients

Twelve patients who were hospitalized with complex hypertrophic scars from 1 December 2014 to 1 December 2015 were enrolled in this study. All patients experienced a loss of joint function and activity and exhibited severe deformity due to a complex hypertrophic scar (**Figures 1**, **2A,B**). The study protocol was approved by the Institutional Review Board of The First Affiliated Hospital of Sun Yat-sen University, and informed consent was obtained from all participants.

Image Processing and 3D Printing

A 64-slice spiral CT (Toshiba-Aquilion Corporation, Japan) was utilized to acquire serial cross-sectional data for each hypertrophic scar. Hypertrophic scar tissues were segmented from the optimal cross-sectional images with a thresholding tool using reconstruction software. Next, the 3D geometric models of the hypertrophic scar were exported as stereolithography (STL) format files for 3D printing (**Figures 1**, **2C,D**). The STL format files were imported to PST-ZB (PST Photon Technology Co., Ltd., China), a rapid prototyping 3D printer with fused deposition modeling (FDM) principles. The printing material is polylactic acid (PLA), which is obtained by extracting starch from plants such as corn and cassava through multiple processes, fermenting it into lactic acid by microorganisms, and then polymerizing it. PLA is safer, lower in carbon, and greener compared with traditional materials. The printing parameters: printing speed 150 mm/s, temperature 200°C, and layer thickness 0.1 mm. The 3D scar models produced by the 3D printer were used preoperatively by experienced surgeons to simulate the surgical procedure to remove the hypertrophic scar. The printing process is shown in **Figure 3**.

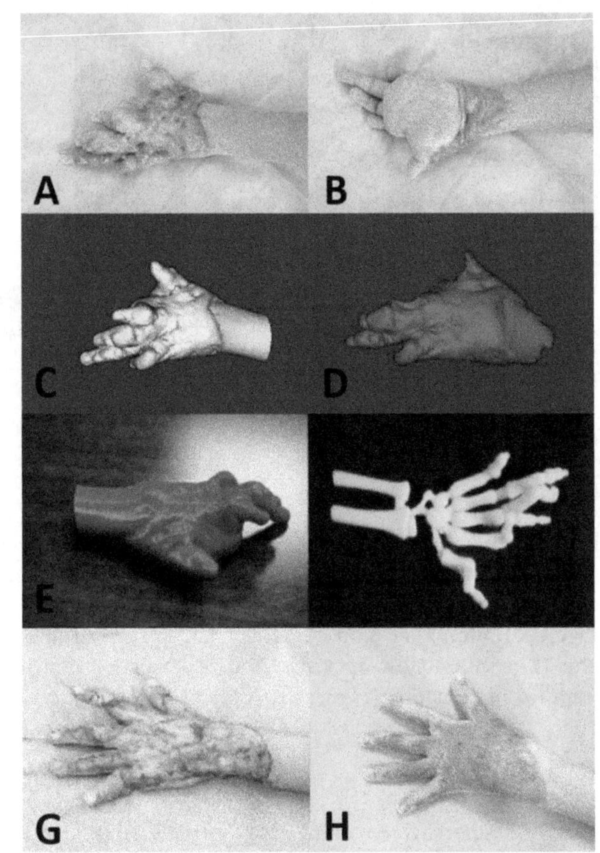

FIGURE 2 | Five-year-old boy with a complex hypertrophic scar. **(A,B)** Preoperative images of the hypertrophic scar, which resulted in a loss of flexure and extension of the left hand. **(C,D)** A 3D model of the hypertrophic scar was designed using reconstruction software. **(E,F)** The 3D model of the hypertrophic scar on the left hand was printed for surgery simulation and anatomical measurement. **(G)** Based on the 3D printed model, the hypertrophic scar on the left hand was completely removed surgically, and the deformed bones were corrected with Kirschner wires. **(H)** At the 12-month follow-up visit, the appearance and function of the left hand were recovered.

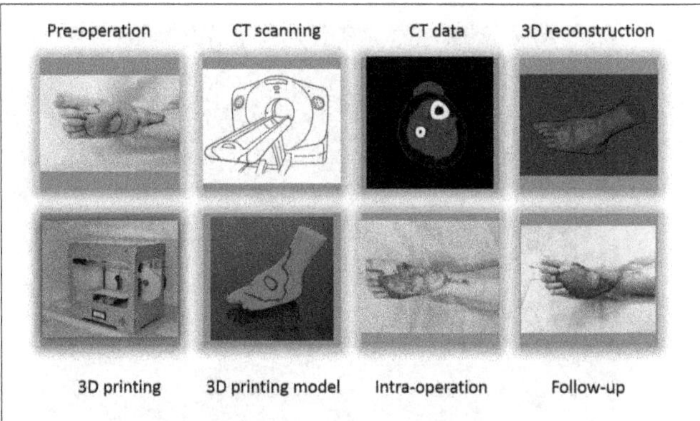

FIGURE 3 | The workflow showing preoperation image acquisition, printing the 3D model, and follow-up.

Validating Accuracy of the 3D Printed Models

The length, width, and height of each hypertrophic scar were measured manually using rulers for the physical scar and with reconstructive software for the 3D printed model. Then the measurements of the physical scar and 3D printed model were compared as shown in **Figure 4** (Olszewski et al., 2014; Yong et al., 2014; Lee et al., 2015; Wu et al., 2015; Yin et al., 2015). The volume of each 3D printed model was calculated automatically by Gemagic Quality software, and the volume of each 3D printed model was measured using the drainage method. These parameters were statistically analyzed by SPSS 13.0.

Surgical Procedure and Postoperative Visits

Hypertrophic scar resection was performed for all 12 patients by the same group of experienced surgeons. Each hypertrophic scar was completely removed according to the measurement data and preoperative surgical simulation on the 3D printed models. A nurse recorded the surgery time and bleeding for each patient. Razor-thin skin autografts were harvested from the inner thigh to cover the scar area. The autografts were placed over human acellular dermal matrix scaffold (Jie-Ya Life Tissue Engineering, Beijing, China) intraoperatively and sutured to the graft area. Pressure was applied on the graft area. The 12 patients were followed up for 12 months after they were discharged from the hospital. At the 12-month follow-up visit, the skin autografts were assessed for skin color, appearance, elasticity, and texture at the suture.

Evaluation of the 3D Models

The surgeons, young doctors, medical students, and patients evaluated the 3D printed models with specially designed feedback questionnaires. The responses to the questions were made on a 5-point Likert scale where 1 represents strongly disagree, 2 represents disagree, 3 represents neither agree nor disagree, 4 represents agree, and 5 represents strongly agree. The surgeons assessed the use of the models as surgical aids in terms of their visual appearance, quality, size, and surgical anatomy. The young doctors and medical students evaluated the use of the models for surgery simulation and training as well as the quality and size of the models. The patients assessed whether the use of the 3D printed models helped illustrate and explain the disease and helped them understand the surgical process and risks.

Statistical Analysis

Statistical significance between groups was determined by paired t-test. All data were analyzed using SPSS version 16.0 software (IBM, Armonk, NY, United States).

RESULTS

Before surgery, individualized 3D models of the hypertrophic scars and deformed bones were successfully printed (**Figures 1, 2E,F**). The size and depth of the hypertrophic scar could be measured accurately on the 3D printed models.

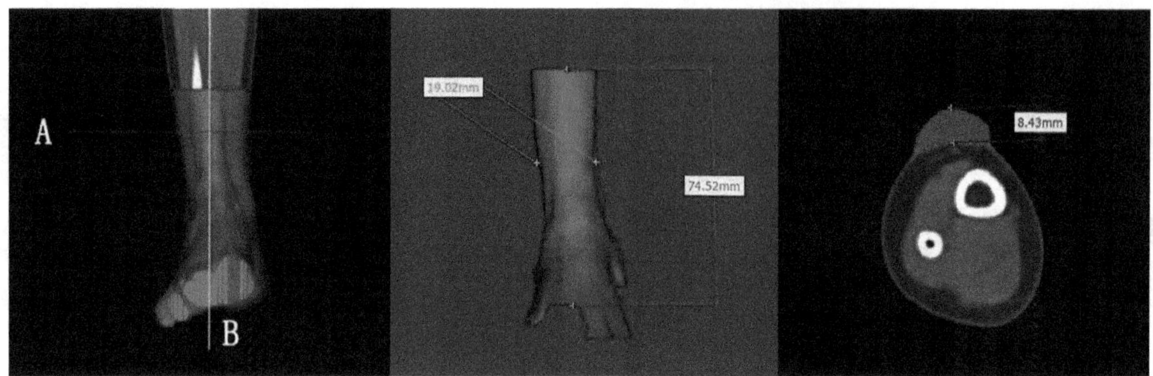

FIGURE 4 | The length, width, and height of each hypertrophic scar were measured manually with rulers. These dimensions were measured with reconstruction software on the 3D printed models.

The average length, width, height, and volume of the physical hypertrophic scars and 3D printed models are presented in **Table 1**. The average length, width, and height of the 3D printed models were significantly smaller than the measurements of the physical scars. The average volume of the 3D scar models was significantly smaller than the average volume of the physical scars.

For each patient, surgery was completed according to the planned simulation by the same group of experienced surgeons, and the results were satisfactory. The medical students indicated that they had an improved comprehension of many surgical skills for resecting hypertrophic scars because of the simulated operations using the 3D printed models. The patients indicated that the explanations using the 3D printed models improved their understanding of the surgery and increased their trust of the surgeons. The average score of the evaluation about 3D printed models in each group on was greater than 3 points, which indicated that all of the groups were satisfied with the surgical simulations using the 3D printed models (**Figure 5**).

All patients successfully underwent hypertrophic scar resection according to the surgical simulations using the 3D printed models. The hypertrophic scar tissue was completely removed, and deformed bones were corrected according to the preoperative surgical plan (**Figures 1, 2G**). The surgical time was shortened and the bleeding was decreased. On postoperative day 7, there were two cases of subcutaneous hemorrhage, one case of infection and one case of necrosis, which may have been caused by excessive postoperative activity. On postoperative day 12, the average take rate of the skin autografts was 97.75% (**Table 2**). At the 12-month follow-up visit, all patients had satisfactory appearance and function (**Figures 1, 2H**).

TABLE 1 | Measurements of the patient scars and 3D printed models.

Parameter	Physical hypertrophic scar	3D printed model	*p*-value
Length (cm)	7.16 ± 2.17	7.10 ± 2.16	0.001*
Width (cm)	4.68 ± 1.40	4.57 ± 1.32	0.002*
Height (cm)	1.14 ± 0.37	1.10 ± 0.36	0.000*
Volume (ml)	38.22 ± 19.94	38.08 ± 19.94	0.001*

*The maximum length, width, and height of the hypertrophic scar were measured with rulers and reconstruction software. The volume of the hypertrophic scar was measured using the water displacement method with a 5 L container. n = 12. *p < 0.05; paired t-test.*

DISCUSSION

Surgery is generally recommended for the treatment of hypertrophic scars. For surgery to be successful, it is important to identify the precise size of the hypertrophic scar (So et al., 2011; Amici, 2014; Lim et al., 2014; Orgill and Ogawa, 2014). The present study applied 3D printing to produce personalized models and observe the spatial position of the hypertrophic scar and bone deformity (Srougi et al., 2016). Using the models, anatomical measurements were made of the hypertrophic scar, including its length, width, and height (Silberstein et al., 2014). Our results suggest that 3D printed models of hypertrophic scars may guide surgeons to identify the surgical cutting plane that marks the limit between scar tissue and normal tissue. Knowledge of the surgical cutting plane can influence surgical effectiveness and potentially reduce complications (**Figure 6**).

Although 3D printing technology has been applied in many fields, it is necessary to evaluate its accuracy to meet clinical requirements. In the present study, the 3D printed models had a significantly smaller average length, width, height, and volume compared with the physical scars. These differences were caused by shrinkage of the material during printing, which affected the accuracy of the 3D models. The results of our study were similar to those of Lee et al. (2015; Wu et al., 2015). Although these differences were statistically significant, they were regarded as clinically insignificant. The 3D models served as valuable references for measuring anatomical parameters of the hypertrophic scar preoperatively, for planning the surgery, and for guiding the intraoperative manipulations.

The preoperative method for surgical resection of hypertrophic scar was direct measurement mainly to measure the size of hypertrophic scar, and the flap covered the wound

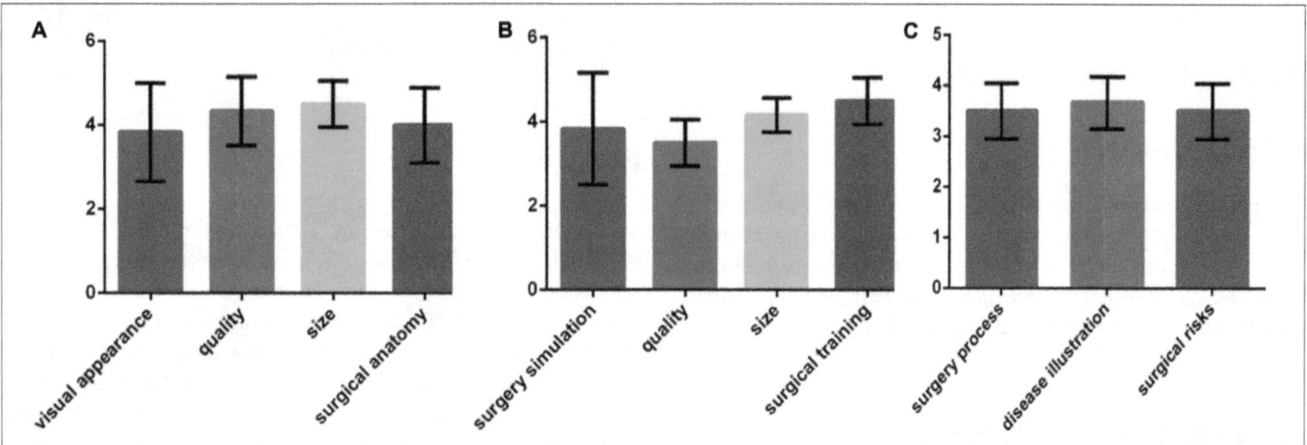

FIGURE 5 | Assessments of the 3D printed models. **(A)** Evaluations by surgeons. **(B)** Evaluations by young doctors and medical students. **(C)** Evaluations by patients.

TABLE 2 | Patient characteristics and the take rate after surgery.

Patient	Sex	Age (years)	Cause of injury	Location	Injury time (years)	Take rate (%)*	Complication
1	Male	5	Hot water	Left hand	4	98	None
2	Female	19	Hot water	Left foot	10	97	Hematoma
3	Female	3	Flame	Right foot	2	99	None
4	Male	2	Hot water	Right hand	1	98	Hematoma
5	Male	16	Hot water	Left elbow joint	11	97	None
6	Female	4	Hot water	Right foot	2	98	Infection
7	Male	18	Hot water	Left hand	15	97	None
8	Female	3	Hot water	Right foot	2	97	Necrosis
9	Male	22	Flame	Left foot	14	98	None
10	Female	5	Hot water	Left hand	3	99	None
11	Female	26	Hot water	Left foot	18	97	None
12	Male	18	Flame	Right foot	9	99	None

**The take rates of skin autografts were recorded on postoperative day 12.*

after scar removal (Alali et al., 2015; Hwang et al., 2015; Martelli et al., 2016). However, this method lacked important parameters such as scar depth and volume, and cannot assess the anatomical relationship between scars and important anatomical structures such as nerves, blood vessels, and tendons, which in turn affects preoperative planning. Furthermore, we also successfully printed 3D models of deformed bones before surgery in the present study, measured the angle of the skeletal deformity, and corrected the angle of the deformity, which would be more helpful for surgeons to preoperative surgical evaluation and surgical planning (**Figure 2F**).

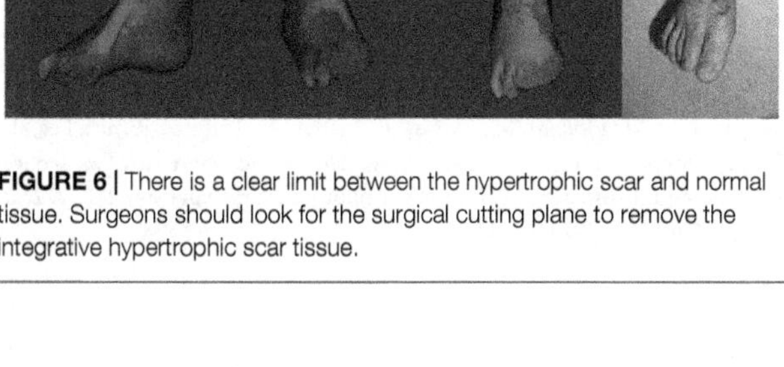

FIGURE 6 | There is a clear limit between the hypertrophic scar and normal tissue. Surgeons should look for the surgical cutting plane to remove the integrative hypertrophic scar tissue.

Many studies reported that 3D printed models were used in clinical practice and achieved good clinical results (Matsumoto et al., 2015; Rose et al., 2015; Powers et al., 2016; Youssef et al., 2016). Valverde et al. (2015) also used a Likert scale to assess the effect of 3D printed models by two experts for treatment of aortic hypoplasia and that it could reduce complications and operative time. Liu et al. (2014) demonstrated that the use of 3D printed models led to a 20% reduction in operating time. In this study, preparation of such 3D models for each hypertrophic scar patient can be feasible for surgeons. Preparation of 3D models has the following advantages. First, 3D printing can provide physiologically, anatomically, and tactilely realistic models before surgery. Second, individualized 3D models can be used for preoperative evaluation to reduce the operation time and bleeding, which can shorten hospital stay and reduce hospitalization costs. Third, individualized 3D models provide an effective way to improve communication and build trust between patients and doctors. Fourth, individualized 3D models may be used to simulate surgery and to teach new doctors (Alali et al., 2015; Hwang et al., 2015; Matsumoto et al., 2015; Rose et al., 2015; Martelli et al., 2016; Powers et al., 2016).

CONCLUSION

Preoperative 3D printing technology can provide accurate 3D models to help surgeons plan operations to resect hypertrophic scars, help young doctors and medical students learn surgical methods, enhance communication and trust between patients and surgeons, and achieve good clinical effects.

AUTHOR CONTRIBUTIONS

JZ and BT designed the research, and reviewed and edited the manuscript. PL, ZH, SH, BT, JZ, PW, YD, PC, and HX performed the experiment. PL, ZH, and SH wrote the manuscript. BT, JZ, ZH, and PL researched the data.

FUNDING

This work was supported by research grant 81471875 (JZ), 81571908 (BT), 81871565 (BT), and 81501675 (ZH) from the National Natural Science Foundation of China, research grant 2016B090916001 (JZ) from the Science and Technology Planning Project of Guangdong Province, research grant 2019A1515012208 (ZH) from the Guangdong Provincial Natural Science Foundation of China, research grant 19ykpy66 (ZH) from the Fundamental Research Funds for the Central Universities of Sun Yat-sen University, and research grant 2013001 (JZ) and 2018003 (BT) from the Sun Yat-sen University Clinical Research 5010 Program.

REFERENCES

Alali, A. B., Griffin, M. F., and Butler, P. E. (2015). Three-dimensional printing surgical applications. *Eplasty* 15:e37.

Amici, J. M. (2014). Early hypertrophic scar after surgery on the nasal region: value of long-acting corticosteroid injections. *Ann. Dermatol. Venereol.* 141, 7–13. doi: 10.1016/j.annder.2013.09.167

Anthonissen, M., Daly, D., Janssens, T., and Kerckhove, E. (2016). The effects of conservative treatments on burn scars: a systematic review. *Burns* 42, 508–518. doi: 10.1016/j.burns.2015.12.006

Butzelaar, L., Ulrich, M. M., Mink, V. D. M. A., Niessen, F. B., and Beelen, R. H. J. (2015). Currently known risk factors for hypertrophic skin scarring: a review. *J. Plast. Reconstr. Aesthet. Surg.* 69, 163–169. doi: 10.1016/j.bjps.2015.11.015

Cutroneo, G., Bruschetta, D., Trimarchi, F., Alberto, C., Maria, C., Antonio, D., et al. (2016). In Vivo CT direct volume rendering: a three-dimensional anatomical description of the heart. *Pol. J. Radiol.* 81, 21–28. doi: 10.12659/PJR.895476

Fitzhugh, A., Naveed, H., Davagnanam, I., and Ashraf, M. (2016). Proposed three-dimensional model of the orbit and relevance to orbital fracture repair. *Surg. Radiol. Anat.* 38, 557–561. doi: 10.1007/s00276-015-1561-1

Gu, X., Yeoh, G. H., and Timchenko, V. (2016). Three-dimensional modeling of flow and deformation in idealized mild and moderate arterial vessels. *Comput. Methods Biomech. Biomed. Eng.* 19, 1395–1408. doi: 10.1080/10255842.2016.1145211

Hwang, T. J., Kiang, C., and Paul, M. (2015). Surgical applications of 3-dimensional printing and precision medicine. *JAMA Otolaryngol. Head Neck Surg.* 141, 305–306.

Lee, K. Y., Cho, J. W., Chang, N. Y., Chae, J. M., Kang, K. H., Kim, S. C., et al. (2015). Accuracy of three-dimensional printing for manufacturing replica teeth. *Korean J. Orthod.* 45, 217–225. doi: 10.4041/kjod.2015.45.5.217

Lim, A. F., Weintraub, J., Kaplan, E. N., Januszyk, M., Cowley, C., McLaughlin, P., et al. (2014). The embrace device significantly decreases scarring following scar revision surgery in a randomized controlled trial. *Plast. Reconstr. Surg.* 133, 398–405. doi: 10.1097/01.prs.0000436526.64046.d0

Liu, Y. F., Xu, L. W., Zhu, H. Y., and Liu, S. S. (2014). Technical procedures for template-guided surgery for mandibular reconstruction based on digital design and manufacturing. *Biomed. Eng. Online* 23:63. doi: 10.1186/1475-925X-13-63

Martelli, N., Serrano, C., van den Brink, H., Pineau, J., Prognon, P., Borget, I., et al. (2016). Advantages and disadvantages of 3-dimensional printing in surgery: a systematic review. *Surgery* 159, 1485–1500. doi: 10.1016/j.surg.2015.12.017

Matsumoto, J. S., Morris, J. M., Foley, T. A., Williamson, E. E., Leng, S., McGee, K. P., et al. (2015). Three-dimensional physical modeling: applications and experience at mayo clinic. *Radiographics* 35, 1989–2006. doi: 10.1148/rg.2015140260

Olszewski, R., Szymor, P., and Kozakiewicz, M. (2014). Accuracy of three-dimensional, paper-based models generated using a low-cost, three-dimensional printer. *J. Craniomaxillofac. Surg.* 42, 1847–1852. doi: 10.1016/j.jcms.2014.07.002

Orgill, D. P., and Ogawa, R. (2014). Discussion: the embrace device significantly decreases scarring following scar revision surgery in a randomized controlled trial. *Plast. Reconstr. Surg.* 133, 406–407. doi: 10.1097/01.prs.0000436812.73412.a4

Pfeil, A., Haugeberg, G., Renz, D. M., Li, R., Christian, J., Marcus, F., et al. (2017). Digital X-ray radiogrammetry and its sensitivity and specificity for the identification of rheumatoid arthritis-related cortical hand bone loss. *J. Bone Miner. Metab.* 35, 192–198. doi: 10.1007/s00774-016-0741-3

Ploch, C. C., Mansi, C. S., Jayamohan, J., and Ellen, K. (2016). Using 3D printing to create personalized brain models for neurosurgical training and preoperative planning. *World Neurosurg.* 90, 668–674. doi: 10.1016/j.wneu.2016.02.081

Powers, M. K., Lee, B. R., and Silberstein, J. (2016). Three-dimensional printing of surgical anatomy. *Curr. Opin. Urol.* 26, 283–288. doi: 10.1097/MOU.0000000000000274

Rashaan, Z. M., Stekelenburg, C., van der Wal, M. B., Euser, A. M., Hagendoorn, B. J. M., Zuijlen, P., et al. (2016). Three-dimensional imaging: a novel, valid, and reliable technique for measuring wound surface area. *Skin Res. Technol.* 22, 443–450. doi: 10.1111/srt.12285

Rose, A. S., Webster, C. E., Harrysson, O. L., Formeister, E. J., Rawal, R. B., and Iseli, C. E. (2015). Pre-operative simulation of pediatric mastoid surgery with 3D-printed temporal bone models. *Int. J. Pediatr. Otorhinolaryngol.* 79, 740–744. doi: 10.1016/j.ijporl.2015.03.004

Schepers, R. H., Kraeima, J., Vissink, A., Lahoda, L. U., Roodenburg, J. L. N., Reintsema, H., et al. (2016). Accuracy of secondary maxillofacial reconstruction with prefabricated fibula grafts using 3D planning and guided reconstruction. *J. Craniomaxillofac. Surg.* 44, 392–399. doi: 10.1016/j.jcms.2015.12.008

Seo, B. F., and Jung, S. N. (2016). The immunomodulatory effects of mesenchymal stem cells in prevention or treatment of excessive scars. *Stem Cells Int.* 2016:6937976. doi: 10.1155/2016/6937976

Silberstein, J. L., Maddox, M. M., Dorsey, P., Feibus, A., Thomas, R., and Lee, B. R. (2014). Physical models of renal malignancies using standard cross-sectional imaging and 3-dimensional printers: a pilot study. *Urology* 84, 268–272. doi: 10.1016/j.urology.2014.03.042

So, K., Mcgrouther, D. A., Bush, J. A., Durani, P., Taylor, L., Skotny, G., et al. (2011). Avotermin for scar improvement following scar revision surgery: a randomized, double-blind, within-patient, placebo-controlled, phase II clinical trial. *Plast. Reconstr. Surg.* 128, 163–172. doi: 10.1097/PRS.0b013e318217429b

Srougi, V., Rocha, B. A., Tanno, F. Y., Almeida, M., Baroni, B., Mendonça, B., et al. (2016). The use of three-dimensional printers for partial adrenalectomy: estimating the resection limits. *Urology* 90, 217–221. doi: 10.1016/j.urology.2015.11.043

Valverde, I., Gomez, G., Coserria, J. F., Suarez-Mejias, C., Uribe, S., Sotelo, J., et al. (2015). 3D printed models for planning endovascular stenting intransverse aorticarch hypoplasia. *Catheter. Cardiovasc. Interv.* 85, 1006–1012. doi: 10.1002/ccd.25810

Wu, A. M., Shao, Z. X., Wang, J. S., Yang, X. D., Weng, W. Q., Wang, X. Y., et al. (2015). The accuracy of a method for printing three-dimensional spinal models. *PLoS One* 10:124291. doi: 10.1371/journal.pone.0124291

Yin, H., Dong, X., and Yang, B. (2015). A new three-dimensional measurement in evaluating the cranial asymmetry caused by craniosynostosis. *Surg. Radiol. Anat.* 37, 989–995. doi: 10.1007/s00276-015-1430-y

Yong, W. J., Tan, J., Adikrishna, A., Lee, H. Y., Jung, J. W., Cho, D. W., et al. (2014). Morphometric analysis of the proximal ulna using three-dimensional computed tomography and computer-aided design: varus, dorsal, and torsion angulation. *Surg. Radiol. Anat.* 36, 763–768. doi: 10.1007/s00276-014-1260-3

Youssef, R. F., Spradling, K., Yoon, R., Dolan, B., Chamberlin, J., Okhunov, Z., et al. (2016). Applications of three-dimensional printing technology in urological practice. *BJU Int.* 116, 697–702. doi: 10.1111/bju.13183

12

The Role of Cutaneous Microcirculatory Responses in Tissue Injury, Inflammation and Repair at the Foot in Diabetes

Gayathri Victoria Balasubramanian, Nachiappan Chockalingam and Roozbeh Naemi *

Centre for Biomechanics and Rehabilitation Technologies, Staffordshire University, Stoke-on-Trent, United Kingdom

***Correspondence:**
Roozbeh Naemi
r.naemi@staffs.ac.uk

Diabetic foot syndrome is one of the most costly complications of diabetes. Damage to the soft tissue structure is one of the primary causes of diabetic foot ulcers and most of the current literature focuses on factors such as neuropathy and excessive load. Although the role of blood supply has been reported in the context of macro-circulation, soft tissue damage and its healing in the context of skin microcirculation have not been adequately investigated. Previous research suggested that certain microcirculatory responses protect the skin and their impairment may contribute to increased risk for occlusive and ischemic injuries to the foot. The purpose of this narrative review was to explore and establish the possible link between impairment in skin perfusion and the chain of events that leads to ulceration, considering the interaction with other more established ulceration factors. This review highlights some of the key skin microcirculatory functions in response to various stimuli. The microcirculatory responses observed in the form of altered skin blood flow are divided into three categories based on the type of stimuli including occlusion, pressure and temperature. Studies on the three categories were reviewed including: the microcirculatory response to occlusive ischemia or Post-Occlusive Reactive Hyperaemia (PORH); the microcirculatory response to locally applied pressure such as Pressure-Induced Vasodilation (PIV); and the interplay between microcirculation and skin temperature and the microcirculatory responses to thermal stimuli such as reduced/increased blood flow due to cooling/heating. This review highlights how microcirculatory responses protect the skin and the plantar soft tissues and their plausible dysfunction in people with diabetes. Whilst discussing the link between impairment in skin perfusion as a result of altered microcirculatory response, the review describes the chain of events that leads to ulceration. A thorough understanding of the microcirculatory function and its impaired reactive mechanisms is provided, which allows an understanding of the interaction between functional disturbances of microcirculation and other more established factors for foot ulceration.

Keywords: diabetic foot, foot ulcer, microvessels, post-occlusive reactive hyperaemia, pressure-induced vasodilation, LDI flare, plantar soft tissues

---

Abbreviations: PORH, Post-Occlusive reactive hyperaemia; PIV, Pressure-Induced Vasodilation; LDI, Laser Doppler Imager; GDP, Gross Domestic Product.

DIABETES IS A GLOBAL HEALTH ISSUE

Diabetes is a common condition which has a considerable impact on the health and economy of nations around the world. There is an annual upsurge in the number of patients being diagnosed with diabetes. The International Diabetes Federation estimates that total global health-care spending on diabetes more than tripled over the period 2003 to 2013 (World Health Organization, 2016). The estimated direct annual cost of diabetes to the world is more than US$ 827 billion and the projected losses in gross domestic product (GDP) for the period 2011 to 2030 is a total of US$ 1.7 trillion worldwide incurred by both the direct and indirect costs (World Health Organization, 2016). This indicates that diabetes imposes a large economic burden on the global health-care system and the wider global economy. As diabetes is a chronic condition, many complications arise as the disease progresses.

DIABETES COMPLICATIONS AND THE ROLE OF MICROCIRCULATION

Microcirculation is vital for the efficient exchange of gases and nutrients and the removal of the waste products of metabolism. In addition, the cutaneous microcirculation plays an important role in thermoregulation (Flynn and Tooke, 1992). Some of the common complications of diabetes are retinopathy, neuropathy, nephropathy, peripheral vascular diseases, and diabetic foot syndrome. One of the important aspects that resonate with all these complications is microcirculation. Endothelial damage and dysfunction of the microvasculature have been observed in various parts of the body such as the eyes, kidneys and the foot in people with diabetes (Goldenberg et al., 1959; Flynn and Tooke, 1992; Hile and Veves, 2003; Williams et al., 2004; Boulton et al., 2006; Schramm et al., 2006; Körei et al., 2016). Both structural and functional microvascular disturbances (known as microangiopathy or disease to small blood vessels) are commonly observed in people with diabetes as a result of glycation related changes that occur due to the prolonged hyperglycaemic state (Boulton et al., 2006; Singh et al., 2014; Stirban et al., 2014). Besides, glycation related direct changes in the microvessels, both sensory and autonomic neuropathies contribute to the functional changes of the microvasculature (Schramm et al., 2006). As early as in 1983 Parving et al. introduced the "haemodynamic theory" to explain microangiopathy in diabetes (Flynn and Tooke, 1992; Veves et al., 2006; Chao and Cheing, 2009). The theory proposes that the increased microvascular blood flow triggers endothelial injury response, followed by microvascular sclerosis (Flynn and Tooke, 1992; Veves et al., 2006). This, in turn, may lead to functional abnormalities such as impaired maximum hyperaemic response, reduced tissue response to injury or trauma, autoregulation of blood flow and changes to vascular tone (Flynn and Tooke, 1992; Boulton et al., 2006; Veves et al., 2006).

DIABETIC FOOT DISEASE AS A SIGNIFICANT COMPLICATION AND THE ROLE OF MICROCIRCULATION

In the foot, the adverse complications of diabetes are ulceration and amputation. The annual population-based incidence of diabetic foot ulcers is estimated to be 1.9–2.2% (Levin et al., 2008). Once the skin on the foot is ulcerated, it is susceptible to infections leading to an urgent medical problem (Bakker et al., 2016). It is estimated that only two-thirds of diabetic foot ulcers will eventually heal, but approximately 28% may result in some form of lower extremity amputation (Bakker et al., 2016). Hence, understanding the risks associated with foot ulcer development and its course is crucial. While the role of peripheral vascular disease and neuropathy resulting in diabetic foot ulcers is well-established, more research is needed to understand the contribution of microcirculation (Schaper et al., 2016).

The role of microcirculation in diabetic foot ulcers is a continuing area of research, where there are many theories put forth by several studies on microcirculation and the concept of "small vessel disease" was proposed (Goldenberg et al., 1959). Although this theory of an exclusive microvascular disease is widely debated, historical evidence for structural and functional microcirculation and related disturbances exist (Boulton et al., 2006). Also, studies have shown that capillary pressure is increased in the foot of people with diabetes due to arteriovenous shunting caused by sympathetic denervation (Deanfield et al., 1980; Flynn and Tooke, 1992; Boulton, 2000; Korzon-Burakowska & Edmonds, 2006). Collectively, these studies outline a critical role for microcirculation in ulceration.

With respect to diabetic foot ulcers, it is proposed that the impaired microcirculatory response may induce microcirculatory failure, resulting in tissue necrosis and ulceration (Flynn and Tooke, 1992; Korzon-Burakowska & Edmonds, 2006). Although microvascular disease may not be the single cause of pathogenesis of diabetic foot ulcers, the co-existence of abnormal microcirculatory function with both peripheral arterial disease and neuropathy may be associated with tissue damage (Flynn and Tooke, 1990; Boulton et al., 2006). This is supported by the evidence from studies that demonstrate the role of microcirculation in the development of ulceration, gangrene, necrosis and wound healing (Flynn and Tooke, 1992; Boulton et al., 2006; Levin et al., 2008; Lanting et al., 2017). Therefore, understanding functional abnormalities is of importance when studying diabetic foot ulcers.

INJURY, INFLAMMATION AND SOFT-TISSUES

To gain a better understanding of microcirculatory function and recognise appropriate methods to evaluate it, it is important to look at the bigger picture of the body's defence, injury, inflammation and repair mechanisms. In the host defence mechanism, both lymphatic and blood vessels play an important role in an inflammatory response (Granger and Rodrigues, 2016; Parnham, 2016). Changes in the inflammatory mediators are known to correlate with the risk of developing a diabetic foot ulcer and inflammation is one of the earliest signs of ulcer (Lanys et al., 2021). Inflammation is a microcirculation-dependent tissue response to extrinsic and intrinsic stimuli (Granger and Rodrigues, 2016). During such an inflammatory response, the cardinal signs of inflammation that can be observed are heat (calor), pain (dolor), redness (rubor), and swelling (tumor), which may eventually lead to the loss of tissue function. In general, microcirculation is highly reactive to inflammatory response and plays a pivotal role in it as all components of the microvasculature such as the arterioles, capillaries, and venules respond and work towards the delivery of inflammatory cells to the injured or infected tissue/site (Granger and Senchenkova, 2010). The microvasculature isolates the infected or injured region from the healthy tissue and the systemic circulation, to facilitate tissue repair and regeneration (Johnson, 1973; Granger and Senchenkova, 2010; Bentov and Reed, 2014). The inflammatory responses of microcirculation include impaired vasomotor function, reduced capillary perfusion, leukocytes and platelets adhesion, activation of the coagulation cascade, enhanced thrombosis, increased vascular permeability, and an increased proliferation rate of blood and lymphatic vessels (Granger and Senchenkova, 2010). Other common microcirculatory changes result in shunting and hypoxia (reduced oxygen capacity of the tissues) caused by endothelial cell injury induced by a severe form of infection like sepsis, stasis of red blood cells due to vascular resistance, increased distances in oxygen diffusion in case of oedema owing to capillary leak syndrome (Guven et al., 2020).

In the foot, defence mechanisms (stimulation–response) plays a vital role. The role of microcirculation in wound repair and healing is well-realised (Shapiro and Nouvong, 2011; Ambróży et al., 2013). Evidence suggests that despite the reasons behind an ulcer incident, the microcirculatory role in the process of healing remains the same and that the subpapillary perfusion plays a major role in the formation of granulation tissue, which was studied through the use of Laser Doppler Flowmetry system in patients with venous ulcers (Ambróży et al., 2013). Microvasculature aids with tissue perfusion, fluid homeostasis, cutaneous oxygen delivery and recruiting collateral vessels to facilitate healing process (Bentov and Reed, 2014). Transcutaneous Oxygen Pressure (TcPo2) technique allows the measurement of cutaneous oxygen supply, which is found to be reduced in type 2 diabetic patients with the foot at risk of ulceration (Zimny et al., 2001). This was related to an impaired neurogenic blood flow regulation, which may contribute to capillary hypertension, endothelial dysfunction leading to oedema and skin damage (Zimny et al., 2001). Other non-invasive methods such as the measurement of skin perfusion pressure allow to assess healing (wound is likely to heal if pressure is above 30 mmHg) and to determine amputation levels (Sarin et al., 1991; Shapiro and Nouvong, 2011). Newer technology such as Laser Speckle Perfusion Imaging allows visualising the blood in the microvaculatore in and around the ulcer area, which may indicate the ability to heal (Shapiro and Nouvong, 2011). However, this device images cutaneous circulation to a depth no greater than 1 mm (Shapiro and Nouvong, 2011). While recent research focuses on assessing microcirculation to predict ulcer outcomes, further studies are needed to gain a deeper understanding of the microcirculatory changes in the ulcers with respect to the stages of healing for better prediction of wound healing.

Although the responses of the inflammatory system are regarded as defence mechanisms (stimulation–response) it may also be considered as a homeostatic system that operates continually to maintain organ and organism function (Tracy, 2006). Based on the dual nature of inflammation, stimulation–response and homeostatic, research suggest the use of biomarkers such as C-reactive protein or interleukin-6 to assess the activity level of the inflammatory process (Tracy, 2006). These biomarkers may represent normal homeostatic function, a response to a pathological condition or to both, which can take place to varying degrees depending on the differences in the person, time and condition (Tracy, 2006). Whilst in younger, healthier people, the biomarkers may likely represent the ongoing homeostatic activity, with increasing age and in the presence of underlying pathology such as chronic inflammatory changes due to diabetes or triggered atherosclerotic changes in cardiovascular conditions, these biomarkers may indicate a stimulation–response type inflammation (Payne, 2006; Tracy, 2006; Pahwa et al., 2020). Overall, there is consensus that inflammation biomarkers are independent predictors of the future occurrence of chronic disease outcomes and events (Tracy, 2006). Similarly, physiological markers such as skin temperature, galvanic skin response and perfusion measurements that indicate homeostatic and stimulation-response in relation to microcirculation may be pertinent to predict the future occurrences of chronic disease outcomes or events such as ulcers.

ASSESSMENT OF MICROCIRCULATION

Diabetic foot ulcers are multifactorial and there are new and emerging technologies that enable the assessment of these factors to aid prevention and management. Some of the methods are various nerve function tests (quantitative sensory testing, vibration perception, galvanic skin response and sudomotor activity testing), temperature measurement (infrared thermography), biomechanical properties measurements (plantar pressure and ultrasound indentation tests/ elastography), macrovascular assessments (ankle-brachial index and toe brachial index) and microvascular assessments (TCPO2, laser doppler flowmetry, hyperspectral imaging and laser speckle contrast imager) and such (Pham et al., 2000; Naemi et al., 2017; Balasubramanian et al., 2020; Lung et al., 2020). However, in this review the main focus would be to discuss the assessment of microcirculation in tissue injury and inflammation to better understand its role in ulceration.

In the past, the key signs of inflammation were predominantly detected through mere observation. However, nowadays contactless and pain-free non-invasive techniques have facilitated objective assessment of inflammatory signs, tissue injury responses, repairs and healing. Laser Doppler flowmetry (LDF) technique is one such non-invasive technique, which allows assessment of microvascular blood flow when reflection and scattering of the laser light occurs due to the movement of the red blood cells (Nakamoto et al., 2012; Balasubramanian et al., 2020). Although the depth the laser penetrates is relatively low (~1 mm), it is a useful device for the evaluation of cutaneous microcirculation. This device is gaining popularity in the field of research in diabetes, cerebrovascular conditions, Raynaud's phenomenon and others. The use of LDF is being explored in dentistry as well, especially for perioperative procedures to gain a better understanding of soft tissue diagnosis. Apart from LDF, other non-invasive methods used to evaluate microcirculation are Laser Speckle Contrast Imager (LSCI) and photo-plethysmography. At times, since small fibre nerve functions and thermal changes influence microcirculation, methods such as quantitative sensory testing, skin electrodermal activity assessment and thermography are also used in conjunction with microvascular testing.

SCOPE OF THIS REVIEW

This narrative review of literature focuses on key microcirculatory responses in relation to diabetic foot in order to understand some of the functional aspects of microcirculation. Firstly, search terms such as "Post-Occlusive Reactive Hyperaemia", "PORH" "pressure-induced vasodilation", "PIV" and "skin blood flow" "local application of pressure", "LDI flare" and "axon-mediated flare" were listed and used to identify articles (the search was not limited to these terms only). PubMed and Medline databases were searched to identify relevant publications in journals. Secondly, the reference lists of the selected articles were scrutinised to find additional studies. However, the data sources were not limited to articles published in journals, but also included grey literature. The sources for grey literature included: 1) Reports from International Diabetes Federation and Diabete UK 2) Websites of equipment manufacturers (Perimed AB, Moor Instruments, FLIR and Impeto Medical Solutions) 3) OpenGrey, and 4) Google. The articles of interest from MEDLINE, PubMed, and PubMed Central (PMC) included in the review were identified through the initial phase of title and abstract sifting. Subsequently, after the title and abstract sifting, relevant articles that adequately described cutaneous microcirculatory responses were retrieved for further study. Later, the data were extracted from relevant articles. Specific insights generated from the literature are presented and discussed below.

VARIOUS MICROCIRCULATORY RESPONSES AND THEIR ASSOCIATION IN DIABETES FOOT-RELATED COMPLICATIONS

The foot is continuously under mechanical stress due to weight-bearing activities of daily living such as walking, exercise, and standing. It is exposed to various trauma, physical injury due to sudden or violent action, exposure to dangerous toxins or repetitive mechanical stress. Some of the extrinsic factors for trauma are thermal (Example: hot surfaces), mechanical (Example: repetitive damage from ill-fitted shoes), and chemical (Example: corn treatments) (Boulton, 2000; Armstrong and Lavery, 2005; Boulton et al., 2006; Vanderah, 2007; Hawke and Burns, 2009). On the other hand, some of the intrinsic factors that contribute to the risk of trauma are foot deformity and glycation related changes in case of diabetes.

Both neuro and vascular aspects are essential for healthy foot function. The nerves of the feet can respond to the thermal, mechanical and chemical stimuli, provoking a reflex withdrawal from the respective harmful stimulus (Hawke and Burns, 2009). For instance, jerking the foot away from a sharp object. This protective mechanism may be absent due to neuropathy in people with diabetes (Boulton et al., 2006; Hawke and Burns, 2009). On the other hand, microcirculation is important for tissue injury response to stimuli such as local heat or pressure (Abraham et al., 2001; Korzon-Burakowska & Edmonds, 2006). Such neurovascular mechanisms of the foot appear to play a vital role to prevent tissue injuries.

Previous research shows that there are certain protective microcirculatory responses to stimuli, which are controlled by neural mechanisms, metabolic aspects, hormones and chemicals (Guyton, 1991). A microcirculatory hyperaemic response is induced on the application of a stimulus. This transient hyperaemic response to various stimuli, witnessed by an increase in blood perfusion is one of the measures to assess microcirculatory function known as reactive hyperaemia. Reactive hyperaemia is an indicator of the intrinsic ability of an organ or tissue to locally autoregulate its blood supply, which is found to be impaired in people with diabetes (Flynn and Tooke, 1992; Korzon-Burakowska & Edmonds, 2006; Merrill, 2008; Klabunde, 2012). For the purpose of this review, based on the select stimuli, the microcirculatory responses observed are stratified into:

1) Vasodilation in response to occlusive ischemia or Post-Occlusive Reactive Hyperaemia (PORH)
2) Microcirculatory response to locally applied pressure;
   (a) Pressure-induced vasodilation (PIV);
   (b) Reduced skin blood flow;
3) Interplay between microcirculation and temperature -vasodilation in response to local heating

The reviewed studies demonstrate the inability of cutaneous microcirculation to respond normally to non-painful stimulation, such as the application of pneumatic pressure, local pressure and local heating in people with diabetes (Fromy et al., 2002). This may be significant in understanding tissue response to injuries. During incidents of prolonged pressure, injury or infection, more demands are made upon the capillary circulation (Flynn and Tooke, 1992; Abraham et al., 2001). Owing to the microcirculatory dysfunction, the hyperaemic response may be impaired and tissue demands are not met (Flynn and Tooke, 1992). Vascular insufficiency to the tissues that leads to breakdown may contribute to adverse complications and increase the risk of ulceration (Flynn and Tooke, 1992).

Nevertheless, there are very limited studies that evaluate the vasodilatory responses to stimuli in subjects with diabetes. Furthermore, only a handful number of research articles address these vasodilatory responses in diabetic foot syndrome, including ulcerated and non-ulcerated cohorts. Key articles on this subject were appraised and discussed in this review.

Vasodilation in Response to Occlusion or Post Occlusive Reactive Hyperaemia (PORH)

Reactive hyperaemia to occlusion is the transient increase in blood flow in the organ or tissue that occurs following a brief period of arterial occlusion. During the process of occlusion, the blood flow goes to a biological zero that is defined as the "no flow" Laser Doppler signal during a PORH test. Following the release of the occlusion, blood flow rapidly increases, which is reactive hyperaemia (Klabunde, 2012). This process is known as post-occlusive reactive hyperaemia (PORH). During the hyperaemia, the tissue becomes re-oxygenated and reperfusion occurs. Simultaneously, the vasodilator metabolites are removed from the tissue, which restores the vascular tone of the resistant vessels causing the blood flow to return to normal (Klabunde, 2012). The longer the period of occlusion, the greater the metabolic stimulus for vasodilation leading to an increase in peak reactive hyperaemia and duration of hyperaemia (Guyton, 1991; Larkin and Williams, 1993; Klabunde, 2012). Based on the time taken to occlude the blood supply to the tissue from few seconds to several hours, the blood flow post-occlusion increases four to seven times in the tissue than normal and lasts from few seconds to hours in relation to the initial occlusion time (Guyton, 1991). Additionally, depending upon the organ or tissue, maximal vasodilation as indicated by peak flow varies (Klabunde, 2012).

PORH is predominantly an endothelial-dependent process, however, it also aids combined assessment of both endothelial-dependent and independent function (Maniewski et al., 2014; Lanting et al., 2017). Hyperaemia occurs because of the shear stress, the tangential frictional force-acting at the endothelial cell surface caused by arterial occlusion (Maniewski et al., 2014). A mechanical stimulation occurs when the shear stress vector is directed perpendicular to the long axis of the arterial vessel (Maniewski et al., 2014). The endothelium responds to this mechanical stimuli, thereby, releasing vasodilatory substances (Maniewski et al., 2014). The factors that are known to contribute to vasodilation are myogenic, neurogenic, and other local factors, such as potassium ions, hydrogen ions, carbon dioxide, catecholamines, prostaglandins, and adenosine (Maniewski et al., 2014; Lanting et al., 2017). Few studies mention that endothelial nitric oxide and other endothelium-derived agents, such as prostaglandins and endothelium-derived hyperpolarizing factors are known to be involved in the mechanism of PORH (Maniewski et al., 2014; Carasca et al., 2017; Marche et al., 2017). However, some researchers contend that nitric oxide and prostaglandins may not be contributing to the mechanism (Cracowski et al., 2011; Maniewski et al., 2014). It is argued that whilst nitric oxide is known to play a major role in the vasodilation of macrovessels, endothelium-derived hyperpolarizing factors are found to play a substantial role in the dilation of microvessels (Quyyumi and Ozkor, 2006; Cracowski et al., 2011). Apart from these substances, the sensory nerves make a vital contribution to the PORH mechanism (Larkin and Williams, 1993; Lorenzo and Minson, 2007; Cracowski et al., 2011; Lanting et al., 2017; Marche et al., 2017). To summarise, various studies have shown that PORH response is elicited with temporary tissue hypoxia upon occlusion through the accumulation of vasodilators (substances that cause the blood vessels to dilate or expand) and other complex factors that are myogenic, endothelial, neurogenic and metabolic (Guyton, 1991; Klabunde, 2012; Lanting et al., 2017).

The PORH test has a wide range of applications. Previously, PORH has been used to assess microcirculatory function in people with arterial diseases, certain ophthalmologic conditions and cardiovascular disorders (Morales et al., 2005; Maniewski et al., 2014; Carasca et al., 2017). It is impaired in people with peripheral arterial disease and has been associated with increased cardiovascular risk (Morales et al., 2005). The test was observed to be useful as an early marker of cardiovascular damage (Busila et al., 2015). PORH test is also used to assess the altered microvascular reactivity in patients with advanced renal dysfunction (Busila et al., 2015). Besides, the use of the PORH test has also been explored in the area of diabetes.

A limited amount of research has been conducted in people with diabetes using PORH measures, both in type 1 and 2. PORH vasodilation is significantly decreased in patients with type 1 diabetes (Marche et al., 2017). In 1986, Rayman et al. demonstrated the impaired hyperaemic response to injury in people with diabetes for the first time (Rayman et al., 1986). Prolongation of the hyperaemic reaction and decrease in response was observed in patients with insulin-dependent diabetes and peripheral occlusive arterial disease (Maniewski et al., 2014). PORH is known to be impaired not only in adults but also in children with type 1 diabetes (Schlager et al., 2012). The results from children in terms of diabetic foot complications is as important as the studies conducted in adults because of two main reasons. Firstly, although this segment of the population is less likely to be vulnerable to foot complications at a younger age, but they are likely to develop complications as they advance in age. Therefore, understanding the microvascular reactivity from an earlier period may prove to be useful. Secondly, this particular study explored other less commonly assessed variables such as biological zero and reperfusion time, which can shed more light on understanding PORH. It was identified that peak perfusion was higher and biological zero was lower in children with type 1 diabetes in comparison to the controls. A key implication from this study was that higher peak perfusion might reflect a decline in the vasoconstrictive ability of arteriolar smooth muscle cells upstream of capillary beds in children with type 1 diabetes (Schlager et al., 2012).

Few studies have explored PORH more specifically in diabetic foot complications (Cheng et al., 2004; Barwick et al., 2016; Lanting et al., 2017). The presence of peripheral sensory neuropathy in people with type 2 diabetes is found to be associated with altered PORH in the foot (Barwick et al.,

2016). A study on the relationship between active or previous foot complication and PORH measured by LDF in people with type 2 diabetes revealed that the increase in time to Peak, which is a variable that shows the time taken for a maximum flux post occlusion, increased the likelihood of a participant having a history of foot complication by 2% (Lanting et al., 2017). This association was not reflected in people with an active foot ulcer (Lanting et al., 2017). These findings in a cohort with type 2 diabetes with a previous history or existing foot-related complications support the need for further investigation into the relationship between measures of microvascular function and development of diabetic foot complications, prospectively (Lanting et al., 2017). Considering this evidence, it seems that PORH is an interesting microcirculatory mechanism that may be useful to assess a foot at risk. In future, their application may be a useful indicator for determining the future risk of diabetic foot complications, especially with ulcer prediction and prevention of amputation.

Microcirculation in Response to Local Application of Pressure

In the foot, the areas prone to high pressure such as the heel, the great toe and areas under the metatarsal heads are at risk of ulceration (Veves et al., 1992; Ledoux et al., 2013). Based on this, many weight-bearing activities were considered to be a contraindication to people with neuropathy (Kluding et al., 2017). However, this has recently changed as there is emerging evidence of positive adaptations of the musculoskeletal and integumentry system to overload stress (Kluding et al., 2017). Literature suggests that peripheral neuropathy may no longer be a hindrance to promoting weight-bearing activity as it did not lead to significant increases in foot ulcers (LeMaster et al., 2008). However, in people with diabetes various other factors may interplay with pressure such as increased stiffness of tissues, aging related changes, presence of other comorbidities, mobility and vascular issues. Studies show that the accumulated mechanical stimulus affected blood perfusion in the foot and should be considered when assessing the risk of developing ulcers (Ledoux et al., 2013; Pu et al., 2018). However, more understanding on the relationship between pressure stimulus and microvascular responses could shed more light on the effect of different levels of accumulated mechanical stimulus on microvascular response and their significance in an ulcer incident.

Responses to local mechanical stresses are mediated through a considerable number and variety of cutaneous receptors and some of these receptors are connected to the small fibres (Abraham et al., 2001). The vasodilation to pressure strains not only occur for noxious stimuli but also non-noxious stimuli applied over a period (Abraham et al., 2001). Local pressure strain to the skin is recognised to play a vital role in cutaneous microcirculatory impairment (Fromy et al., 2000; Abraham et al., 2001). It is presumed that this may be linked to the development of cutaneous lesions such as pressure sores and diabetic foot ulcers (Abraham et al., 2001; Fromy et al., 2002). Two important microcirculatory responses to locally applied pressure identified through the literature review are discussed below.

Pressure-induced Vasodilation

The transient increase in cutaneous blood flow initially before it decreases in response to a progressive locally applied pressure strain is known as pressure-induced vasodilation (PIV). This microcirculatory response appears to be a protective cutaneous response that relies on the excitation of unmyelinated afferent nerve fibres (Fromy et al., 2002; Koïtka et al., 2004; Körei et al., 2016). PIV is considered to be more than a transient phenomenon and an important physiological response allowing the skin to respond adequately to mechanical stimuli (Abraham et al., 2001). Cutaneous receptors in the skin respond to local mechanical stresses such as local pressure strain and these receptors are found to be of mechanothermal nature (Fromy et al., 2002). This response is noted to be compromised in the aging population (Fromy et al., 2010; Fouchard et al., 2019). Furthermore, the impairment of PIV is postulated to contribute to the development of lesions such as pressure ulcers and diabetic foot ulcers (Abraham et al., 2001; Saumet, 2005; Vouillarmet et al., 2019).

The interplay between biomechanical factors and physiological responses is well-realised in the development of pressure ulcers, including in people with diabetes. Current studies highlight PIV in relation to the development of pressure ulcers or decubitus ulcers in the sacral region. As discussed above, one of the key implications from the studies on PIV is that it is a protective mechanism without which certain pressure-associated lesions may develop and plausibly this could explain the high risk of decubitus and plantar ulcers in people with diabetes (Abraham et al., 2001; Fromy et al., 2002; Bergstrand, 2014). Although pressure ulcers and plantar ulcers may differ in many ways, one of the key causal pathways to foot ulceration is somatic motor neuropathy that leads to small muscle wasting, foot deformities, loss of sensation, increased plantar pressure and repetitive trauma resulting in neuropathic foot ulcer (Armstrong and Lavery, 2005). This suggests that local pressure strain increases the vulnerability of the foot to ulcerate. Similar to pressure ulcer development, reduced physiological responses may induce local ischaemia and reperfusion injury in the foot (Flynn and Tooke, 1992; Coleman et al., 2014). A similar role of reduced microcirculatory responses in foot ulcer development is widely discussed in the literature (Flynn and Tooke, 1992; Boulton et al., 2006; Korzon-Burakowska & Edmonds, 2006). This knowledge can potentially be translated to diabetic foot ulcer prediction to see if the microcirculatory response to local pressure and plantar pressure have any association. This also accords with other observations, which showed that people with impaired or absent PIV are known to be at a higher risk to develop pressure ulcers (Fromy et al., 2002; Braden and Blanchard, 2007; Bergstrand, 2014). Evidence shows that decreased hyperaemic response and absence of PIV is known to increase the risk of pressure ulcers (Bergstrand et al., 2014). However, very limited research is available on PIV in human hand and feet in relation to diabetes (Abraham et al., 2001; Koïtka et al., 2004).

A particular study by Koitka et al. (2004) observed PIV at the foot level in people type 1 diabetes (Koïtka et al., 2004). Since low skin temperature in people with diabetes is known to interfere with microcirculation, this research was performed in warm conditions of 29.5± 0.2°C (Koïtka et al., 2004). The cutaneous blood flow was studied at warm conditions using laser Doppler flowmetry on the first metatarsal head in response to applied pressure at 5.0 mmHg/min and PIV was found to be absent at foot level in people with type 1 diabetes whereas it existed in healthy subjects at 29.5±0.2°C (Koïtka et al., 2004). These findings were attributed to an interaction between functional changes in C-fibres and the endothelium in people with diabetes (Koïtka et al., 2004). A similar study found PIV to be absent at low skin temperature even in healthy subjects (28.7±0.4°C) (Fromy et al., 2002). It was explained that a skin temperature close to 34°C was optimal for the evaluation of skin vasomotor reflexes in the lower limb and the nervous receptors involved in the PIV development are mechanothermal, and not only mechanical (Fromy et al., 2002). The results from Koitka et al. (2004) revealed that in the same subjects the non-endothelial-mediated response to sodium nitroprusside was preserved, whereas the endothelial-mediated response to acetylcholine was impaired (Koïtka et al., 2004). Therefore, suggesting the relevance of endothelial dysfunction to PIV. Also, a previous study on PIV found that the absence of vasodilatory axon reflex response to local pressure strain when the capsaicin-sensitive nerve terminals were pre-treated with local anaesthetic or chronically applied capsaicin (Fromy et al., 1998). The capsaicin-sensitive nerve fibres are the small nerve fibres and their role in neuropathic pain and related complications, especially in people with diabetes is well-established (Boulton et al., 2006). Thus, the researchers speculated that the PIV, which is associated with the stimulation of small fibre nerves, could be a missing link between neuropathy and foot ulcers in diabetes (Koïtka et al., 2004). In support of this, several studies have demonstrated that damage to C-fibres have a great impact on skin, with disrupted blood flow predisposing to foot ulcers (Vinik et al., 2001; Caselli et al., 2003; Boulton et al., 2006; Themistocleous et al., 2014). As previously discussed, impaired microcirculatory response to local pressure strain may potentially make people with diabetes more vulnerable to pressure strains and explain the high prevalence of foot ulcer that occurs in diabetic patients (Koïtka et al., 2004).

The insights from the above-discussed studies suggest that PIV is absent at the foot level in people with diabetes. Identifying the point or stage of the disappearance of PIV in the foot, during the disease progression through prospective studies, may help in understanding the progression of neurovascular dysfunction in the foot. On the other hand, since PIV may be absent from an earlier stage, its capability to indicate risk for ulceration is disputable and needs further research. Also, the current study has observed PIV only at two sites, which was the head of the first metatarsus and the area over the internal ankle bone in a small sample size. More research is required to explore various regions of the plantar aspect of the foot, especially in areas subject to increased plantar pressure. The findings from such research can aid to comprehend the association between PIV and plantar ulcers and help identify foot at risk. Furthermore, it may aid to bridge the research gap to understand the role of microcirculation in the development of diabetic foot ulcers.

Reduced Skin Blood Flow to Locally Applied Pressure

As discussed earlier, PIV allows the skin blood flow to increase in response to locally applied pressure. In the absence of the transient PIV response, the cutaneous blood flow is observed to progressively decrease with the application of increasing local pressure (Fromy et al., 2002). The observed cutaneous blood flow in response to locally applied pressure is found to be impaired in people with diabetes owing to the combined effects of low cutaneous temperature and alterations in microcirculatory function (Fromy et al., 2002). Additionally, the presence of neuropathy may aggravate the condition (Fromy et al., 2002). This study used a laser Doppler flowmetry system and applied local pressure using a specially designed apparatus at the internal anklebone allowing for a 5.0 mmHg/min rate of pressure increase (Fromy et al., 2000; Fromy et al., 2002). The skin blood flow decreased significantly from baseline at much lower applied pressure of 7.5 mmHg in people with diabetes in groups without neuropathy and with subclinical or clinical neuropathy at 6.3 mmHg in comparison to the healthy controls at 48.8 mmHg (Fromy et al., 2002). The large difference between these pressures reported within this study indicate a plausible association between decreased skin blood flow to local pressure and the development of decubitus and plantar ulcers (Fromy et al., 2002). This hypothesis is consistent with the one proposed by Koitka et al. (2004) who suggested an association between microcirculatory dysfunction and the high prevalence of foot ulcer (Koïtka et al., 2004). They also postulate that the arterial wall and surrounding tissues are very compressible in people with diabetes making them vulnerable to the development of pressure ulcers (Fromy et al., 2002; Coleman et al., 2014). The application of this knowledge to understand the role of microcirculation in foot ulceration may potentially be useful.

Although the collated findings reveal the possibility of decreased skin blood flow and PIV to be associated with pressure ulcer development, more research is needed to understand the mechanism in relation to diabetic foot complications. The aetiology for decubitus ulcer and plantar ulcers may vary, nevertheless, pressure remains as a common contributing factor in both the incidents. Studies suggest pressure-induced local ischaemia and reperfusion injuries in relation to both pressure ulcers and diabetic foot ulcers (Flynn and Tooke, 1992; Korzon-Burakowska & Edmonds, 2006; Coleman et al., 2014; Shahwan, 2015). Understanding PIV, reduced skin flow and other microcirculatory responses in various regions prone to diabetic foot ulcers and in relation to plantar pressure during standing or walking are important. The need for such a study is further supported by the evidence from a study that identified subjects who lacked PIV and reactive hyperaemia in response to locally applied pressure, to be particularly vulnerable to pressure exposure (Bergstrand, 2014; Bergstrand et al., 2014). These subjects were stratified to be at a higher risk for pressure ulcer development (Bergstrand, 2014; Bergstrand et al., 2014). Thereby, translating the knowledge generated from the studies on microcirculatory responses in the development of pressure ulcers to diabetic foot ulcers can prove to be useful.

Interplay Between Microcirculation and Temperature - Vasodilation in Response to Local Heating

While specific literature on the microcirculatory responses and temperature changes in response to plantar skin tissue injuries and healing are limited, previous studies reviewed microcirculatory assessments in various organs in people with diabetes. The knowledge of microcirculatory responses to temperature changes in other organs, can reveal that external stimuli causes an increased microvascular demand. This showcases the role of cutaneous microcirculatory response in tissue injuries and healing.

When injuries and repair occur, monitoring the conditions between the skin, soft tissues or even after skin grafts can aid better prognosis. A study explored the proposed theory that conducive interface conditions between soft tissue and prostheses are necessary for a better outcome with prosthodontic treatment. This study by Nakamoto et al. (2012) focused on the gingiva and mucosa surrounding anterior implants and both LDF and thermographs were concurrently used to elucidate the relationship between temperature and blood flow as peri-implant soft tissues are often portrayed to have decreased blood flow because of the lack of blood supply from the periodontal ligament. The study also analysed the morphological changes of the cutaneous microvasculature and temperature changes between participants with and without bone grafting associated with implant placement. The findings suggested that soft tissue around implants showed decreased blood flow compared with periodontal tissue in adjacent natural teeth, despite the absence of clinical signs such as chronic inflammation. The study also highlighted the significance of bone quality to maintain blood flow in the soft as the area around implants with bone grafting showed significantly reduced blood flow. Many research studies suggest that microcirculatory blood flow is influenced by thermal changes and reportedly increases in proportion to temperature to an extent, which is not limited to dentistry but also in studies on other cutaneous microcirculation (Molnár et al., 2015). However, the observed results by Nakamoto et al. (2012) were contrary to this popular idea. The suggested explanation for this was the involvement of deeper structures that modified the thermal properties and the usually observed increase in temperature was often associated with inflammation due to infection such as periodontitis but not in case of tissue surrounding implants (Baab et al., 1990).

Although the skin and the oral mucosa have certain similarities and differences anatomically, they have some comparable physiological properties. For instance, they play a crucial role in the prevention of infections and act as a barrier against exogenous or endogenous substances, pathogens, and mechanical stresses (Liu et al., 2010). The dysfunction of these barriers can compromise the integrity of the underlying tissue as well. The combination of findings from the study provides some support for the conceptual premise that the simultaneous measurements of blood flow and temperature are useful to evaluate the microcirculation of soft tissue behaviour in injury and healing, and its significane even in the absence of noticeable signs chronic inflammation. A similar study compared the peripheral blood flow in the lower limbs during the local heating tests with different temperature protocols in people with diabetes mellitus and healthy participants (Filina et al., 2017). The LDF was used to evaluate the adaptive changes of the microvascular bed during thermal tests and the detection of the preclinical stage of trophic disorders owing to disruption in nutritional or nerve supply (Filina et al., 2017). Research suggest that in the feet of patients with diabetic neuropathy, total skin blood flow is increased due to an increased shunt flow due to denervation (Harpuder et al., 1940; Schaper et al., 2008). Further study in the area has shown that the increased anastomotic shunt flow lead to either under- or over perfused nutritive capillaries (Netten et al., 1996). Skin temperature measurements and LDF were performed to record mainly shunt flow and capillaroscopy to study nailfold capillary blood flow (Netten et al., 1996). The study showed that in insulin-dependent diabetic patients with neuropathy, the baseline skin temperature and capillary blood-cell velocity was higher in comparison to those without neuropathy and healthy control subjects (Netten et al., 1996). The findings from the study highlighted the presence of hyperperfused nutritive capillary circulation in the feet of patients with diabetic neuropathy favouring the previously discussed hyperdynamic hypothesis and in contradiction to the capillary steal phenomenon to explain the decreased healing potential in diabetic neuropathic foot ulceration.

As suggested by previous research, microcirculatory and temperature measurements might become useful techniques to evaluate healthy, infected, injured, inflamed and treated skin and soft tissues of the foot (Netten et al., 1996; Gatt et al., 2018; Gatt et al., 2020). But, there is abundant room for further progress in determining if these two measurements may be useful for the diagnosis or prognosis of foot ulcers. Such research may aid to draw a margin between the compromised tissue and the surrounding healthy tissue when determining the course of treatment, surgery or even amputation. Furthermore, comparative studies conducted on healthy vs inflamed/injured tissue in the foot can help to identify early signs of dysfunction, inflammation and injury in a foot in order to effectively manage the condition. For instance, Ren et al. (2021) explored the stimulation of microcirculation using simple thermal stimuli such as infrared and warm bath in healthy adults to explore the options in hope to design interventions to promote better circulation in the lower extremities of the body in the geriatric population and those suffering from diabetes who are likely to have impaired microcirculation (Ren et al., 2021).

The vasodilation in response to local heating and the neurogenic flare response to nociceptive stimuli is mediated by an axon reflex involving C-fibres. This is studied using the laser Doppler imager (LDI) and the induced flare response is known as the LDI flare. The LDI flare area which is the area with the hyperaemic response is known to be reflective of the small fibre function. Therefore, the size of the LDI flare is known to be dependent on the C-fibre function and the underlying skin small fibre neural network and its extent (Green et al., 2010; Vas et al., 2012). Whereas, the LDI max (perfusion) in the skin immediately beneath the heating probe is shown to be mediated by non-neurogenic means and to reflect the endothelial function (Green et al., 2010; Vas et al., 2012). Therefore, the intensity of the hyperaemic response depends on the microvascular ability to vasodilate. The site commonly studied is the dorsum of the feet because the underlying skin is less influenced by the thermoregulatory blood flow due to the absence of arteriovenous anastomoses (Braverman, 2000). The method used to assess this reflex involves local skin heating to 44°C for 20 min or 6 min in a stepwise fashion: 44°C for 2 min, 46°C for 1 min and finally 47°C for 3 min in a temperature-controlled room to evoke the flare followed by scanning the site using an LDI to measure the area (Krishnan and Rayman, 2004; Green et al., 2010; Vas et al., 2012). Another technique is also known to be used to observe the hyperaemic response to local heating. This involves the use of a skin-heating probe filled with deionized water and heating to 44 °C to assess heat-induced vasodilation. In summary, the LDI flare test in subjects shows reduced microcirculatory response as well as a neurogenic flare in people with either type 1 or two diabetes (Krishnan and Rayman, 2004; Vas et al., 2012). It facilitates early diagnosis of C-fibre dysfunction even before its detection by other available methods such as the quantitative sensory testing, which focuses on the testing of sensory abnormalities in the areas of temperature change sensation, vibration, and pain threshold testing (Example: Using equipment named Computer Aided Sensory Evaluator–IV - case IV) (Krishnan and Rayman, 2004). Therefore, the heat provocation or LDI flare test is commonly used with a focus on LDI flare for the assessment of C-fibre function than with a concentration on the LDI max for evaluating the microcirculatory function. However, the test can be used to assess not only C-fibre function but also microcirculation, and additionally investigate their association in neuropathy (Vas et al., 2012; Marche et al., 2017). This can further clarify the link between microcirculation impairment and tissue damage in light of impaired sensation.

CONCLUSION

Microcirculation plays a vital role in homeostatic and defence states during tissue injury and inflammation. Firstly, the most obvious finding to emerge from this review is the protective role of microcirculation. Secondly, the impairment of microcirculation and the possibility of it being the missing link in the chain of events that leads to foot ulceration in people with diabetes is clearly supported by the current findings. Thirdly, assessment of microcirculatory structural damages might be complex, however, the insights emerged from this review has shown that there are responses such as post-occlusive reactive hyperaemia, pressure-induced vasodilation and vasodilation to local heating (LDI flare) that are simple to assess. In conclusion, a thorough understanding of the microcirculatory function and its impaired reactive mechanisms is imperative and will contribute extensively to understanding the soft tissue biomechanics and aid to devise strategies for comprehensive assessment of the diabetic foot. This, in turn, will aid in prevention and early diagnosis of ulcers, thereby, reducing amputations.

AUTHOR CONTRIBUTIONS

GB: Conducted the literature review and wrote the first draft of the manuscript. NC: Reviewed the manuscript draft and provided comments. RN: Developed the concept and contributed to revising the draft and shaping the manuscript.

REFERENCES

Abraham, P., Fromy, B., Merzeau, S., Jardel, A., and Saumet, J.-L. (2001). Dynamics of Local Pressure-Induced Cutaneous Vasodilation in the Human Hand. *Microvasc. Res.* 61 (1), 122–129. doi:10.1006/MVRE.2000.2290

Ambrózy, E., Waczulíková, I., Willfort, A., Böhler, K., Cauza, K., Ehringer, H., et al. (2013). Healing Process of Venous Ulcers: The Role of Microcirculation. *Int. Wound J.* 10 (1), 57–64. doi:10.1111/j.1742-481X.2012.00943.x

Armstrong, D. G., and Lavery, L. A. (2005). *Clinical Care of the Diabetic Foot.* American Diabetes Association.

Baab, D. A., Öberg, Å., and Lundström, Å. (1990). Gingival Blood Flow and Temperature Changes in Young Humans with a History of Periodontitis. *Arch. Oral Biol.* 35 (2), 95–101. doi:10.1016/0003-9969(90)90169-B

Bakker, K., Apelqvist, J., Lipsky, B. A., Van Netten, J. J., and Schaper, N. C. (2016). The 2015 IWGDF Guidance Documents on Prevention and Management of Foot Problems in Diabetes: Development of an Evidence-Based Global Consensus. *Diabetes Metab. Res. Rev.* 32, 2–6. doi:10.1002/dmrr.2694

Balasubramanian, G., Vas, P., Chockalingam, N., and Naemi, R. (2020). A Synoptic Overview of Neurovascular Interactions in the Foot. *Front. Endocrinol.* 11, 308. doi:10.3389/fendo.2020.00308

Barwick, A. L., Tessier, J. W., Janse de Jonge, X., Ivers, J. R., and Chuter, V. H. (2016). Peripheral Sensory Neuropathy Is Associated with Altered Postocclusive Reactive Hyperemia in the Diabetic Foot. *BMJ Open Diab Res. Care* 4, e000235. doi:10.1136/bmjdrc-2016-000235

Bentov, I., and Reed, M. J. (2014). Anesthesia, Microcirculation, and Wound Repair in Aging. *Anesthesiology* 120 (3), 760–772. doi:10.1097/ALN.0000000000000036

Bergstrand, S., Källman, U., Ek, A.-C., Lindberg, L.-G., Engström, M., Sjöberg, F., et al. (2014). Pressure-induced Vasodilation and Reactive Hyperemia at Different Depths in Sacral Tissue under Clinically Relevant Conditions. *Microcirculation* 21 (8), 761–771. doi:10.1111/micc.12160

Bergstrand, S. (2014). *Preventing Pressure Ulcers by Assessment of the Microcirculation in Tissue Exposed to Pressure.* Doctoral dissertation, (Linköping, Sweden): Linköping University Electronic Press. doi:10.3384/diss.diva-109960

Boulton, A. J. (2000). *The Diabetic Foot.* South Dartmouth: MDText.com, Inc. Available at: http://www.ncbi.nlm.nih.gov/pubmed/28121117 (Accessed February 18, 2018).

Boulton, A. J. M., Cavanagh, P. R., and Rayman, G. (2006). *The Foot in Diabetes.* Wiley.

Braden, B., and Blanchard, S. (2007). "Risk Assessment in Pressure Ulcer Prevention," in *Chronic Wound Care A Clin Source B Healthc Prof,* 593–608.

Braverman, I. M. (2000). The Cutaneous Microcirculation. *J. Invest. Dermatol. Symp. Proc.* 5 (1), 3–9. doi:10.1046/j.1087-0024.2000.00010.x

Busila, I., Onofriescu, M., Gramaticu, A., Hogas, S., Covic, A., and Florea, L. (2015). ENDOTHELIAL DYSFUNCTION ASSESSED BY LASER DOPPLER POST-OCCLUSIVE HYPEREMIA IN CHRONIC KIDNEY DISEASE PATIENTS. *Rev. Med. Chir Soc. Med. Nat. Iasi* 119 (4), 1001–1009.

Carasca, C., Magdas, A., Tilea, I., and Incze, A. (2017). Assessment of Post-Occlusive Reactive Hyperaemia in the Evaluation of Endothelial Function in Patients with Lower Extremity Artery Disease. *Acta Med. Marisiensis* 63 (3), 129–132. doi:10.1515/amma-2017-0024

Caselli, A., Rich, J., Hanane, T., Uccioli, L., and Veves, A. (2003). Role of C-Nociceptive Fibers in the Nerve Axon Reflex-Related Vasodilation in Diabetes. *Neurology* 60, 297–300. doi:10.1212/01.wnl.0000040250.31755.f9

Chao, C. Y. L., and Cheing, G. L. Y. (2009). Microvascular Dysfunction in Diabetic Foot Disease and Ulceration. *Diabetes Metab. Res. Rev.* 25 (7), 604–614. doi:10.1002/dmrr.1004

Cheng, X., Mao, J. M., Xu, X., Elmandjra, M., Bush, R., Christenson, L., et al. (2004). Post-occlusive Reactive Hyperemia in Patients with Peripheral Vascular Disease. *Clin. Hemorheol. Microcirc.* 31 (1), 11–21. Available at: http://www.ncbi.nlm.nih.gov/pubmed/18644817.

Coleman, S., Nixon, J., Keen, J., Wilson, L., McGinnis, E., Dealey, C., et al. (2014). A New Pressure Ulcer Conceptual Framework. *J. Adv. Nurs.* 70 (10), 2222–2234. doi:10.1111/jan.12405

Cracowski, J. L., Gaillard-Bigot, F., Cracowski, C., Roustit, M., and Millet, C. (2011). Skin Microdialysis Coupled with Laser Speckle Contrast Imaging to Assess Microvascular Reactivity. *Microvasc. Res.* 82 (3), 333–338. doi:10.1016/j.mvr.2011.09.009

Deanfield, J. E., Daggett, P. R., and Harrison, M. J. G. (1980). The Role of Autonomic Neuropathy in Diabetic Foot Ulceration. *J. Neurol. Sci.* 47 (2), 203–210. doi:10.1016/0022-510X(80)90004-0

Filina, M. A., Potapova, E. V., Makovik, I. N., Zharkih, E. V., Dremin, V. V., Zherebtsov, E. A., et al. (2017). Functional Changes in Blood Microcirculation in the Skin of the Foot during Heating Tests in Patients with Diabetes Mellitus. *Hum. Physiol.* 43 (6), 693–699. doi:10.1134/S0362119717060020

Flynn, M. D., and Tooke, J. E. (1992). Aetiology of Diabetic Foot Ulceration: a Role for the Microcirculation? *Diabet Med. A. J. Br. Diabet Assoc.* 9 (4), 320–329. doi:10.1111/j.1464-5491.1992.tb01790.x

Flynn, M. D., and Tooke, J. E. (1990). Microcirculation and the Diabetic Foot. *Vasc. Med. Rev.* 1 (2), 121–138. doi:10.1177/1358836X9000100204

Fouchard, M., Misery, L., Le Garrec, R., Sigaudo-Roussel, D., and Fromy, B. (2019). Alteration of Pressure-Induced Vasodilation in Aging and Diabetes, a Neuro-Vascular Damage. *Front. Physiol.* 10, 862. doi:10.3389/fphys.2019.00862

Fromy, B., Abraham, P., and Saumet, J. L. (1998). Non-nociceptive Capsaicin-Sensitive Nerve Terminal Stimulation Allows for an Original Vasodilatory Reflex in the Human Skin. *Brain Res.* 811 166 doi:10.1016/S0006-8993(98)00973-1

Fromy, B., Abraham, P., Bouvet, C., Bouhanick, B., Fressinaud, P., and Saumet, J. L. (2002). Early Decrease of Skin Blood Flow in Response to Locally Applied Pressure in Diabetic Subjects. *Diabetes* 51 (4), 1214–1217. doi:10.2337/DIABETES.51.4.1214

Fromy, B., Abraham, P., and Saumet, J.-L. (2000). Progressive Calibrated Pressure Device to Measure Cutaneous Blood Flow Changes to External Pressure Strain. *Brain Res. Protoc.* 5 (2), 198–203. doi:10.1016/S1385-299X(00)00013-1

Fromy, B., Sigaudo-Roussel, D., Gaubert-Dahan, M.-L., Rousseau, P., Abraham, P., Benzoni, D., et al. (2010). Aging-associated Sensory Neuropathy Alters Pressure-Induced Vasodilation in Humans. *J. Invest. Dermatol.* 130 (3), 849–855. doi:10.1038/jid.2009.279

Gatt, A., Falzon, O., Cassar, K., Ellul, C., Camilleri, K. P., Gauci, J., et al. (2018). Establishing Differences in Thermographic Patterns between the Various Complications in Diabetic Foot Disease. *Int. J. Endocrinol.* 2018, 1–7. doi:10.1155/2018/9808295

Gatt, A., Mercieca, C., Borg, A., Grech, A., Camilleri, L., Gatt, C., et al. (2020). Thermal Characteristics of Rheumatoid Feet in Remission: Baseline Data. *PLoS One* 15, e0243078. doi:10.1371/journal.pone.0243078

Goldenberg, S., Alex, M., Joshi, R. A., and Blumenthal, H. T. (1959). Nonatheromatous Peripheral Vascular Disease of the Lower Extremity in Diabetes Mellitus. *Diabetes* 8 (4), 261–273. doi:10.2337/diab.8.4.261

Granger, D. N., and Senchenkova, E. (2010). "Inflammation and the Microcirculation," in *Colloquium Series On Integrated Systems Physiology: From Molecule To Function* (Morgan & Claypool Life Sciences) Vol. 2, 1–87. Available at: https://www.ncbi.nlm.nih.gov/books/NBK53373/ (Accessed June 27, 2021).

Granger, D. N., and Rodrigues, S. F. (2016). "Microvascular Responses to Inflammation," in *Compendium of Inflammatory Diseases* (Springer Basel), 942–948. doi:10.1007/978-3-7643-8550-7_178

Green, A. Q., Krishnan, S., Finucane, F. M., and Rayman, G. (2010). Altered C-Fiber Function as an Indicator of Early Peripheral Neuropathy in Individuals with Impaired Glucose Tolerance. *Diabetes Care* 33 (1), 174–176. doi:10.2337/dc09-0101

Guven, G., Hilty, M. P., and Ince, C. (2020). Microcirculation: Physiology, Pathophysiology, and Clinical Application. *Blood Purif.* 49 (1-2), 143–150. doi:10.1159/000503775

Guyton, A. C. (1991). *Textbook of Medical Physiology*. Philadelphia: Saunders.

Harpuder, K., Stein, I. D., and Byer, J. (1940). The Role of the Arteriovenous Anastomosis in Peripheral Vascular Disease. *Am. Heart J.* 20 (5), 539–545. doi:10.1016/S0002-8703(40)90932-2

Hawke, F., and Burns, J. (2009). Understanding the Nature and Mechanism of Foot Pain. *J. Foot Ankle Res.* 2, 1. doi:10.1186/1757-1146-2-1

Hile, C., and Veves, A. (2003). Diabetic Neuropathy and Microcirculation. *Curr. Diab Rep.* 3 (6), 446–451. doi:10.1007/s11892-003-0006-0

Johnson, P. C. (1973). The Microcirculation of normal and Injured Tissue. *Adv. Exp. Med. Biol.* 33 (0), 45–51. doi:10.1007/978-1-4684-3228-2_5

Klabunde, R. E. (2012). *Cardiovascular Physiology Concepts*. Lippincott Williams & Wilkins/Wolters Kluwer. Available at: https://books.google.co.uk/books/about/Cardiovascular_Physiology_Concepts.html?id=27ExgvGnOagC&redir_esc=y (Accessed July 24, 2018).

Kluding, P. M., Bareiss, S. K., Hastings, M., Marcus, R. L., Sinacore, D. R., and Mueller, M. J. (2017). Physical Training and Activity in People with Diabetic Peripheral Neuropathy: Paradigm Shift. *Phys. Ther.* 97 (1), 31. doi:10.2522/PTJ.20160124

Koïtka, A., Abraham, P., Bouhanick, B., Sigaudo-Roussel, D., Demiot, C., and Saumet, J. L. (2004). Impaired Pressure-Induced Vasodilation at the Foot in Young Adults with Type 1 Diabetes. *Diabetes* 53 (3), 721–725. doi:10.2337/DIABETES.53.3.721

Körei, A. E., Istenes, I., Papanas, N., and Kempler, P. (2016). Small-Fiber Neuropathy. *Angiology* 67 (1), 49–57. doi:10.1177/0003319715583595

Korzon-Burakowska, A., and Edmonds, M. (2006). Role of the Microcirculation in Diabetic Foot Ulceration. *The Int. J. Lower Extremity Wounds* 5 (3), 144–148. doi:10.1177/1534734606292037

Krishnan, S. T. M., and Rayman, G. (2004). The LDIflare: a Novel Test of C-Fiber Function Demonstrates Early Neuropathy in Type 2 Diabetes. *Diabetes Care* 27 (12), 2930–2935. Available at: http://www.ncbi.nlm.nih.gov/pubmed/15562209 (Accessed May 10, 2018).

Lanting, S. M., Barwick, A. L., Twigg, S. M., Johnson, N. A., Baker, M. K., Chiu, S. K., et al. (2017). Post-occlusive Reactive Hyperaemia of Skin Microvasculature and Foot Complications in Type 2 Diabetes. *J. Diabetes its Complications* 31 (8), 1305–1310. doi:10.1016/j.jdiacomp.2017.05.005

Lanys, A., Moore, Z., and Avsar, P. (2021). What Is the Role of Local Inflammation in the Development of Diabetic Foot Ulcers? A Systematic Review - DiabetesontheNet. DiabetesontheNet. Available at: https://diabetesonthenet.com/diabetic-foot-journal/what-is-the-role-of-local-inflammation-in-the-development-of-diabetic-foot-ulcers-a-systematic-review/(Accessed August 15, 2021).

Larkin, S. W., and Williams, T. J. (1993). Evidence for Sensory Nerve Involvement in Cutaneous Reactive Hyperemia in Humans. *Circ. Res.* 73 (1), 147–154. doi:10.1161/01.RES.73.1.147

Ledoux, W. R., Shofer, J. B., Cowley, M. S., Ahroni, J. H., Cohen, V., and Boyko, E. J. (2013). Diabetic Foot Ulcer Incidence in Relation to Plantar Pressure Magnitude and Measurement Location. *J. Diabetes its Complications* 27 (6), 621–626. doi:10.1016/J.JDIACOMP.2013.07.004

LeMaster, J. W., Mueller, M. J., Reiber, G. E., Mehr, D. R., Madsen, R. W., and Conn, V. S. (2008). Effect of Weight-Bearing Activity on Foot Ulcer Incidence in People with Diabetic Peripheral Neuropathy: Feet First Randomized Controlled Trial. *Phys. Ther.* 88 (11), 1385–1398. doi:10.2522/ptj.20080019

Levin, M. E., O'Neal, L. W., Bowker, J. H., and Pfeifer, M. A. (2008). *Levin and O'Neal's the Diabetic Foot*. St. Louis: Mosby/Elsevier.

Liu, J., Bian, Z., Kuijpers-Jagtman, A. M., and Von den Hoff, J. W. (2010). Skin and Oral Mucosa Equivalents: Construction and Performance, *Orthod. Craniofac. Res.*, 13, 11–20. doi:10.1111/j.1601-6343.2009.01475.x

Lorenzo, S., and Minson, C. T. (2007). Human Cutaneous Reactive Hyperaemia: Role of BKCachannels and Sensory Nerves. *J. Physiol.* 585 (Pt 1), 295–303. doi:10.1113/jphysiol.2007.143867

Lung, C.-W., Wu, F.-L., Liao, F., Pu, F., Fan, Y., and Jan, Y.-K. (2020). Emerging Technologies for the Prevention and Management of Diabetic Foot Ulcers. *J. Tissue Viability* 29 (2), 61–68. doi:10.1016/j.jtv.2020.03.003

Maniewski, R., Wojtkiewicz, S., Zbieć, A., Wierzbowski, R., Liebert, A., and Maniewski, R. (2014). Prolonged Postocclusive Hyperemia Response in Patients with normal-tension Glaucoma. *Med. Sci. Monit.* 20, 2607–2616. doi:10.12659/MSM.891069

Marche, P., Dubois, S., Abraham, P., Parot-Schinkel, E., Gascoin, L., Humeau-Heurtier, A., et al. (2017). Neurovascular Microcirculatory Vasodilation Mediated by C-Fibers and Transient Receptor Potential Vanilloid-Type-1 Channels (TRPV 1) Is Impaired in Type 1 Diabetes. *Sci. Rep.* 7 (1). 44322 doi:10.1038/srep44322

Merrill, G. F. (2008). *Our Marvelous Bodies : An Introduction to the Physiology of Human Health.* Rutgers University Press.

M. J. Parnham (2016). *Compendium of Inflammatory Diseases* Springer Basel. doi:10.1007/978-3-7643-8550-7

Molnár, E., Lohinai, Z., Demeter, A., Mikecs, B., Tóth, Z., and Vág, J. (2015). Assessment of Heat Provocation Tests on the Human Gingiva: The Effect of Periodontal Disease and Smoking. *Acta Physiol. Hungarica* 102 (2), 176–188. doi:10.1556/036.102.2015.2.8

Morales, F., Graaff, R., Smit, A. J., Bertuglia, S., Petoukhova, A. L., Steenbergen, W., et al. (2005). How to Assess post-occlusive Reactive Hyperaemia by Means of Laser Doppler Perfusion Monitoring: Application of a Standardised Protocol to Patients with Peripheral Arterial Obstructive Disease. *Microvasc. Res.* 69 (1-2), 17–23. doi:10.1016/j.mvr.2005.01.006

Naemi, R., Chatzistergos, P., Suresh, S., Sundar, L., Chockalingam, N., and Ramachandran, A. (2017). Can Plantar Soft Tissue Mechanics Enhance Prognosis of Diabetic Foot Ulcer? *Diabetes Res. Clin. Pract.* 126, 182–191. doi:10.1016/j.diabres.2017.02.002

Nakamoto, T., Kanao, M., Kondo, Y., Kajiwara, N., Masaki, C., Takahashi, T., et al. (2012). Two-dimensional Real-Time Blood Flow and Temperature of Soft Tissue Around Maxillary Anterior Implants. *Implant Dent* 21 (6), 522–527. doi:10.1097/ID.0b013e318272fe81

Netten, P. M., Wollersheim, H., Thien, T., and Lutterman, J. A. (1996). Skin Microcirculation of the Foot in Diabetic Neuropathy. *Clin. Sci. (Lond).* 91 (5), 559–565. doi:10.1042/CS0910559

Pahwa, R., Goyal, A., Bansal, P., and Jialal, I. (2020). "Chronic Inflammation," in *StatPearls* Treasure Island: StatPearls. Available at: https://www.ncbi.nlm.nih.gov/books/NBK493173/(Accessed June 27, 2021).

Payne, G. W. (2006). Effect of Inflammation on the Aging Microcirculation: Impact on Skeletal Muscle Blood Flow Control. *Microcirculation* 13 (4), 343–352. doi:10.1080/10739680600618918

Pham, H., Armstrong, D. G., Harvey, C., Harkless, L. B., Giurini, J. M., and Veves, A. (2000). Screening Techniques to Identify People at High Risk for Diabetic Foot Ulceration: a Prospective Multicenter Trial. *Diabetes Care* 23 (5), 606–611. doi:10.2337/diacare.23.5.606

Pu, F., Ren, W., Fu, H., Zheng, X., Yang, M., Jan, Y.-K., et al. (2018). Plantar Blood Flow Response to Accumulated Pressure Stimulus in Diabetic People with Different Peak Plantar Pressure: a Non-randomized Clinical Trial. *Med. Biol. Eng. Comput.* 56 (7), 1127–1134. doi:10.1007/s11517-018-1836-x

Quyyumi, A. A., and Ozkor, M. (2006). Vasodilation by Hyperpolarization. *Hypertension* 48 (6), 1023–1025. doi:10.1161/01.HYP.0000250965.03934.15

Rayman, G., Williams, S. A., Spencer, P. D., Smaje, L. H., Wise, P. H., and Tooke, J. E. (1986). Impaired Microvascular Hyperaemic Response to Minor Skin Trauma in Type I Diabetes. *Bmj* 292 (6531), 1295–1298. Available at: http://www.ncbi.nlm.nih.gov/pubmed/2939920 (Accessed August 8, 2018).

Ren, W., Xu, L., Zheng, X., Pu, F., Li, D., and Fan, Y. (2021). Effect of Different thermal Stimuli on Improving Microcirculation in the Contralateral Foot. *Biomed. Eng. Online* 20 (1), 1–10. doi:10.1186/s12938-021-00849-9

Sarin, S., Shami, S., Shields, D. A., Scurr, J. H., and Coleridge Smith, P. D. (1991). Selection of Amputation Level: a Review. *Eur. J. Vasc. Surg.* 5 (6), 611–620. doi:10.1016/s0950-821x(05)80894-1

Saumet, J. L. (2005). [Cutaneous Vasodilation Induced by Local Pressure Application: Modifications in Diabetes]. *Bull. Acad. Natl. Med.* 189 (1), 99–105. Available at: http://ezproxy.staffs.ac.uk/login?url=http://search.ebscohost.com/login.aspx? direct=true&db=cmedm&AN=16119883&site=ehost-live.

Schaper, N. C., Huijberts, M., and Pickwell, K. (2008). Neurovascular Control and Neurogenic Inflammation in Diabetes. *Diabetes Metab. Res. Rev.* 24 (Suppl. 1), S40–S44. doi:10.1002/dmrr.862

Schaper, N. C., Van Netten, J. J., Apelqvist, J., Lipsky, B. A., and Bakker, K. (2016). Prevention and Management of Foot Problems in Diabetes: A Summary Guidance for Daily Practice 2015, Based on the IWGDF Guidance Documents. *Diabetes Metab. Res. Rev.* 32, 7–15. doi:10.1002/dmrr.2695

Schlager, O., Hammer, A., Willfort-Ehringer, A., Fritsch, M., Rami-Merhar, B., Schober, E., et al. (2012). Microvascular Autoregulation in Children and Adolescents with Type 1 Diabetes Mellitus. *Diabetologia* 55 (6), 1633–1640. doi:10.1007/s00125-012-2502-8

Schramm, J. C., Dinh, T., and Veves, A. (2006). Microvascular Changes in the Diabetic Foot. *Int. J. Lower Extremity Wounds* 5 (3), 149–159. doi:10.1177/1534734606292281

Shahwan, S. (2015). Factors Related to Pressure Ulcer Development with Diabetic Neuropathy. *Clin. Res. Trial* 1 (4). 102–105. doi:10.15761/CRT.1000124

Shapiro, J., and Nouvong, A. (2011). "Assessment of Microcirculation and the Prediction of Healing in Diabetic Foot Ulcers," in *Topics in the Prevention, Treatment and Complications of Type 2 Diabetes* (Riijeka, Croatia: IntechOpen), 215–226. doi:10.5772/21967

Singh, V. P., Bali, A., Singh, N., and Jaggi, A. S. (2014). Advanced Glycation End Products and Diabetic Complications. *Korean J. Physiol. Pharmacol.* 18 (1), 1–14. doi:10.4196/kjpp.2014.18.1.1

Stirban, A., Gawlowski, T., and Roden, M. (2014). Vascular Effects of Advanced Glycation Endproducts: Clinical Effects and Molecular Mechanisms. *Mol. Metab.* 3 (2), 94–108. doi:10.1016/j.molmet.2013.11.006

Themistocleous, A. C., Ramirez, J. D., Serra, J., and Bennett, D. L. H. (2014). The Clinical Approach to Small Fibre Neuropathy and Painful Channelopathy. *Pract. Neurol.* 14 (6), 368–379. doi:10.1136/practneurol-2013-000758

Tracy, R. P. (2006). The Five Cardinal Signs of Inflammation: Calor, Dolor, Rubor, Tumor And Penuria (Apologies to Aulus Cornelius Celsus, De Medicina, C. A.D. 25). *Journals Gerontol. Ser. A: Biol. Sci. Med. Sci.* 61 (10), 1051–1052. doi:10.1093/gerona/61.10.1051

Vanderah, T. W. (2007). Pathophysiology of Pain. *Med. Clin. North America* 91 (1), 1–12. doi:10.1016/j.mcna.2006.10.006

Vas, P. R. J., Green, A. Q., and Rayman, G. (2012). Small Fibre Dysfunction, Microvascular Complications and Glycaemic Control in Type 1 Diabetes: a Case-Control Study. *Diabetologia* 55 (3), 795–800. doi:10.1007/s00125-011-2417-9

Veves, A., Giurini, J. M., and LoGerfo, F. W. (2006). *The Diabetic Foot.* Totowa: Humana Press.

Veves, A., Murray, H. J., Young, M. J., and Boulton, A. J. M. (1992). The Risk of Foot Ulceration in Diabetic Patients with High Foot Pressure: a Prospective Study. *Diabetologia* 35 (7), 660–663. doi:10.1007/bf00400259

Vinik, A. I., Erbas, T., Stansberry, K. B., and Pittenger, G. L. (2001). Small Fiber Neuropathy and Neurovascular Disturbances in Diabetes Mellitus. *Exp. Clin. Endocrinol. Diabetes* 109, S451–S473. doi:10.1055/s-2001-18602

Vouillarmet, J., Josset-Lamaugarny, A., Michon, P., Saumet, J. L., Koitka-Weber, A., Henni, S., et al. (2019). Neurovascular Response to Pressure in Patients with Diabetic Foot Ulcer. *Diabetes*, 68 832. doi:10.2337/DB18-0694

Williams, D. T., Norman, P. E., and Stacey, M. C. (2004). Comparative roles of microvascular and nerve function in poof ulceration in type 2 diabetes: Response to Krishnan et al. [9] (multiple letters). *Diabetes Care* 27 (12), 1343–1348. doi:10.2337/diacare.27.12.3026

World Health Organization (2016). *Global Report on Diabetes.* Geneva: WHO, 83.

Zimny, S., Dessel, F., Ehren, M., Pfohl, M., and Schatz, H. (2001). Early Detection of Microcirculatory Impairment in Diabetic Patients with Foot at Risk. *Diabetes Care* 24 (10), 1810–1814. doi:10.2337/diacare.24.10.1810

13

Electrospun Biomaterials in the Treatment and Prevention of Scars in Skin Wound Healing

*Eoghan J. Mulholland**

Gastrointestinal Stem Cell Biology Laboratory, Wellcome Trust Centre for Human Genetics, University of Oxford, Oxford, United Kingdom

Electrospinning is a promising method for the rapid and cost-effective production of nanofibers from a wide variety of polymers given the high surface area morphology of these nanofibers, they make excellent wound dressings, and so have significant potential in the prevention and treatment of scars. Wound healing and the resulting scar formation are exceptionally well-characterized on a molecular and cellular level. Despite this, novel effective anti-scarring treatments which exploit this knowledge are still clinically absent. As the process of electrospinning can produce fibers from a variety of polymers, the treatment avenues for scars are vast, with therapeutic potential in choice of polymers, drug incorporation, and cell-seeded scaffolds. It is essential to show the new advances in this field; thus, this review will investigate the molecular processes of wound healing and scar tissue formation, the process of electrospinning, and examine how electrospun biomaterials can be utilized and adapted to wound repair in the hope of reducing scar tissue formation and conferring an enhanced tensile strength of the skin. Future directions of the research will explore potential novel electrospun treatments, such as gene therapies, as targets for enhanced tissue repair applications. With this class of biomaterial gaining such momentum and having such promise, it is necessary to refine our understanding of its process to be able to combine this technology with cutting-edge therapies to relieve the burden scars place on world healthcare systems.

***Correspondence:**
Eoghan J. Mulholland
eoghan.mulholland@well.ox.ac.uk

Keywords: nanofibers, nanotechnology, electrospinning, polymer, drug delivery, tissue engineering, wound healing, scars

INTRODUCTION

Pathological scar formation is the physiological conclusion of wound healing, and so it is important to understand its underlying cellular and molecular processes in order to apprehend how a scar is formed, but also for the exploration of potential therapeutic targets. Currently, scarring is a huge burden on world healthcare, and the global scar treatment market is projected to represent as much as $34.9 billion by the year 2023[1]. Indeed, scarring can lead to many adverse side effects such as reduced mobility, compromised function in organs such as the liver or kidney, and the development of functional disabilities such as the psychological stress (Krafts, 2010; Sarrazy et al., 2011). A plethora of treatment options are available for scarring including topical treatments and

[1]https://www.prnewswire.com/news-releases/global-scar-treatment-market-2013-2018--2023---rise-in-online-retailing-of-scar-treatment-products-300698219.html

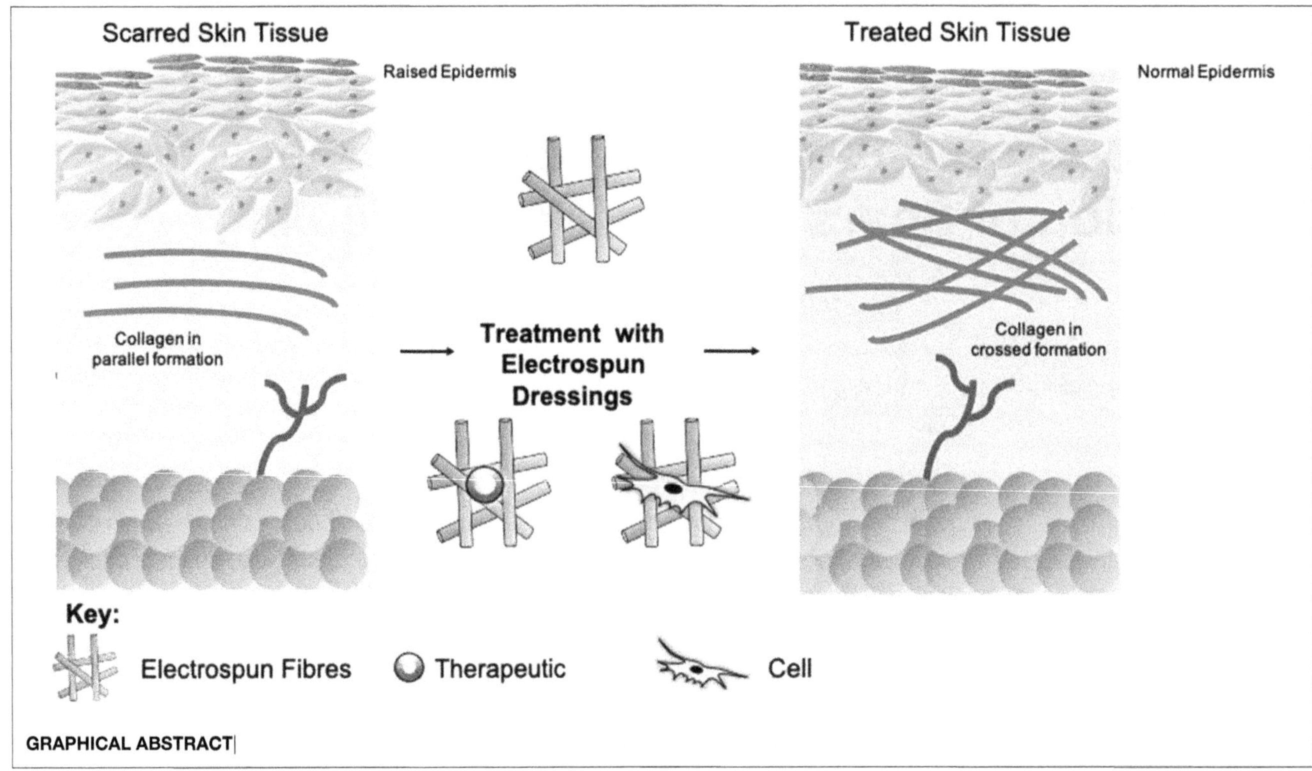

GRAPHICAL ABSTRACT|

dressings but are met with many limitations and are proving ineffective. This review will explore the use of electrospun nanofibers as novel instruments for efficient wound healing and reducing scar formation. The large surface area to volume ratio make electrospun fibers attractive options as they offer therapeutic incorporation capabilities whilst also being absorptive. A key focus of this review will be how these nanofibers can be applied alone, but also in conjunction with pharmacotherapies and cells for effective skin repair.

WOUND HEALING

Wound healing is a highly complex process which stems from three well-defined phases: inflammation, proliferation, and remodeling. Inflammation is the immediate response phase, commencing with the contact of platelets from blood with exposed collagen at the site of injury (Qin, 2016). This contact initiates the formation of a fibrin clot, comprised of the platelets, thrombin, and fibronectin. The fibrin clot acts as a reservoir of cytokines and growth factors, stimulating inflammatory mediators to migrate to the wound, while also providing an architecture for infiltrating cells (Hsieh et al., 2017). For example, transforming growth factors (TGF-α, TGF-β) is a highly significant signaling pathway initiated by platelets within the fibrin clot (Ramirez et al., 2014). TGFs draw leukocytes to the injury site and initiate the inflammatory stage (Kryczka and Boncela, 2015). These leukocytes support the secretion of additional cytokines, e.g., platelet-derived growth factor (PDGF), interleukin-1 (IL-1), and fibroblast growth factor (FGF) (Grove and Kligman, 1983). During proliferation, the secondary stage of wound healing, TGF signaling becomes increasingly crucial, especially in cell types such as keratinocytes, macrophages, and fibroblasts, essential for the transcription of collagen, fibronectin, and proteoglycan. Additionally, TGFs prevent the release of protease enzymes responsible for the degradation of the matrix and activates inhibitors of protease production (Broughton et al., 2006). As proliferation progresses, fibroblasts are the principal cell type. Fibroblasts are of mesenchymal origin and are accountable for new matrix production, resulting in the restoration of tissue homoeostasis (Darby et al., 2014). Remodeling, the final stage, can last up to 1-year after injury. Collagenase enzymes secreted from fibroblasts, macrophages, and neutrophils, cleave the molecules of collagen, thereby breaking it down (Caley et al., 2015). This results in Type I collagen gradually replacing Type III collagen, which in time increases the tensile strength of the new tissue (Longaker et al., 2008). The collagen fibers in the wound tissue are thinner than that of normal dermal collagen. These thinner fibers will gradually thicken over time and organize along the stress lines of the injury. This resulting scar tissue, however, will never be as strong as the preceding normal tissue (White et al., 1971; Schilling, 1976; Corr et al., 2009). Many studies suggest that variations in inflammation during the wound healing process are directly related to the extent of scar tissue formation (Lim et al., 2006). For example, fetal wound healing presents with a lack of typical inflammatory markers and is "*scarless*" up to a certain age (Longaker et al., 2008). In adult wound healing, polymorphonuclear leukocytes are recruited to the site of injury, followed by macrophages and lymphocytes. Contrastingly, fetal wounds are void of polymorphonuclear leukocytes, and as healing progresses, fetal macrophages enter the wound site but in lesser numbers than that of an adult (Mackool et al., 1998). This characteristic lack of an inflammatory response may be credited to a dearth in appropriate signaling in fetal wounds, and the fundamentally immature condition of fetal inflammatory cell populations. Many non-healing wounds fail to switch from the inflammatory phase into the proliferative phase, thus resulting in abnormal wound repair.

SCAR FORMATION

Scars present as a significant burden to healthcare systems, and so are a catalyst for global research for prevention and reduction (Mirastschijski et al., 2015; Barnes et al., 2018). A mature scar consists predominantly of Type I collagen (Marshall et al., 2018). Within scar tissue, this collagen is arranged in bundles parallel to the skins surface, as opposed to a non-parallel conformation in normal skin. This parallel configuration in scar tissue equates to an overall reduction in tensile strength (van Zuijlen et al., 2003). The epidermal basement membrane presents with a more flattened nature as opposed to normal skin, as it does not contain the rete pegs which typically infiltrate the dermis (Monaco and Lawrence, 2003). Furthermore, scar tissue is void of other classic dermal adjuncts such as hair follicles or sweat glands (Fu et al., 2005; Kiani et al., 2018). Upon maturation, the concentration of fibroblasts with the scar tissue depletes, which in combination with the lack of dermal adjuncts results in a dermal layer comprising of few cells. The extracellular matrix (ECM) of this tissue has less elastin than healthy tissue, which contributes to the loss in tensile strength, and means that re-injury is more probable (Kordestani, 2019).

The extent of fibrosis post-injury varies between organs and tissues. When the molecular regulation of the remodeling phase of wound healing is inefficient or disturbed, more problematic scars occur: hypertrophic scars and keloids. Hypertrophic scars typically develop post-surgery or from other trauma such as burns (Carswell and Borger, 2019). Keloids contrast from hypertrophic scars in that they grow beyond the natural margins of the initial damaged tissue (Berman et al., 2017). These keloidal scars do not naturally revert, as opposed to hypertrophic scares which typically regress to a degree within 6 months. Histologically speaking, keloid, and hypertrophic scars are distinguishable by a difference in collagen fiber architecture, presence of myofibroblasts which are alpha-smooth muscle actin-positive, and the degree of angiogenesis (Carswell and Borger, 2019). Keloids are characterized by thick fibers of collagen, while hypertrophic scars encompass thin fibers organized in nodules. The dysregulation to normal collagen maturation is a central influencer on excessive scar formation. Hypertrophic scars contain high concentrations of microvessels, attributed to excess proliferation and loss of functionality of endothelial cells. This phenomenon can be traced back to myofibroblast hyperactivity and the resulting excess collagen fabrication. Myofibroblasts are the principal cell type responsible for scar contraction (Li and Wang, 2011), and are derived from fibroblasts ~2 weeks post-wounding (Singer and Clark, 1999). PDGF and TGF-β stimulate this cellular differentiation and the resultant contractile force exerted by the myofibroblasts enables wound edges in humans to come together, at a rate of ~0.75 mm a day (**Figure 1**) (Werner and Grose, 2003; Storch and Rice, 2005). Of course, in normal scars this wound contraction is an essential process; however, myofibroblasts typically go through apoptosis post-epithelialization, thus halting contractive pathways (Desmoulière et al., 2005). In hypertrophic scars, these myofibroblasts do not apoptose beyond epithelialization and so cause persistent contraction, resulting in functional implications to the skin (Ehrlich et al., 1994). Keloid scars, however, are smooth muscle actin negative (Ehrlich et al., 1994). This can be attributed to the presence of protomyofibroblasts in keloids, which can manufacture large quantities of ECM but not the force to contract lesions. This explains why functional defects resulting from contraction are only observed in hypertrophic scarring. Typically, the granulation tissue continues to expand and secrete growth factors, while lacking molecules essential for apoptosis or ECM remodeling such as cleaved-caspase 3,–8, and-9 (Yang et al., 2016). Indeed, upregulation of p53 expression has been reported in scarring phenotypes, a protein important for the inhibition of apoptosis (Tanaka et al., 2004).

Most lab-based *in vivo* assessment of wound closure and development is performed in rodents. This is mainly due to the high-throughput and low costs of these systems. However, it is important to understand that rodent wounds close differently to that of human's, primarily due to the process of contraction. This is mainly owed to an extensive subcutaneous striated muscle layer known as the panniculus carnosus that is virtually non-existent in humans. In rodents however, the panniculus carnosus allows the skin to move independently of the deeper muscles and is accountable for the rapid contraction of skin following injury. This physiological difference therefore creates difficulties to replicate the wound closure processes of human skin. This is a universal problem, one that is noted in much recent literature (Wang et al., 2013; Hu et al., 2018). Wang et al. discussed this problem, proposing an alternative model which involved splinting rodent wounds to inhibit contraction and force re-epithelization. Nevertheless, this model also encountered limitations including inflammation induced from sutures used to anchor the splint to the mouse skin which could influence any molecular changes (Dunn et al., 2013). Formerly published reports utilizing the splinted wound model lack descriptive details of splint management and exclusion criteria for removing animals from analysis in cases where splints might have been incompletely secured due to suture rupture or damage to the splint by the animal.

Another alternative method is the direct suturing of a scaffold to the edges of the experimental wounds. Anjum et al. conducted wounding experiments of this nature with (Nu/Nu) mice and found that contraction is still observed in all wounds, however a more reepithelialization route was observed in the central wound regions (Anjum et al., 2017). However, limitations of this method again point to the provoking of an inflammatory response and coincidently with an increased risk of surgical site infections (He et al.,

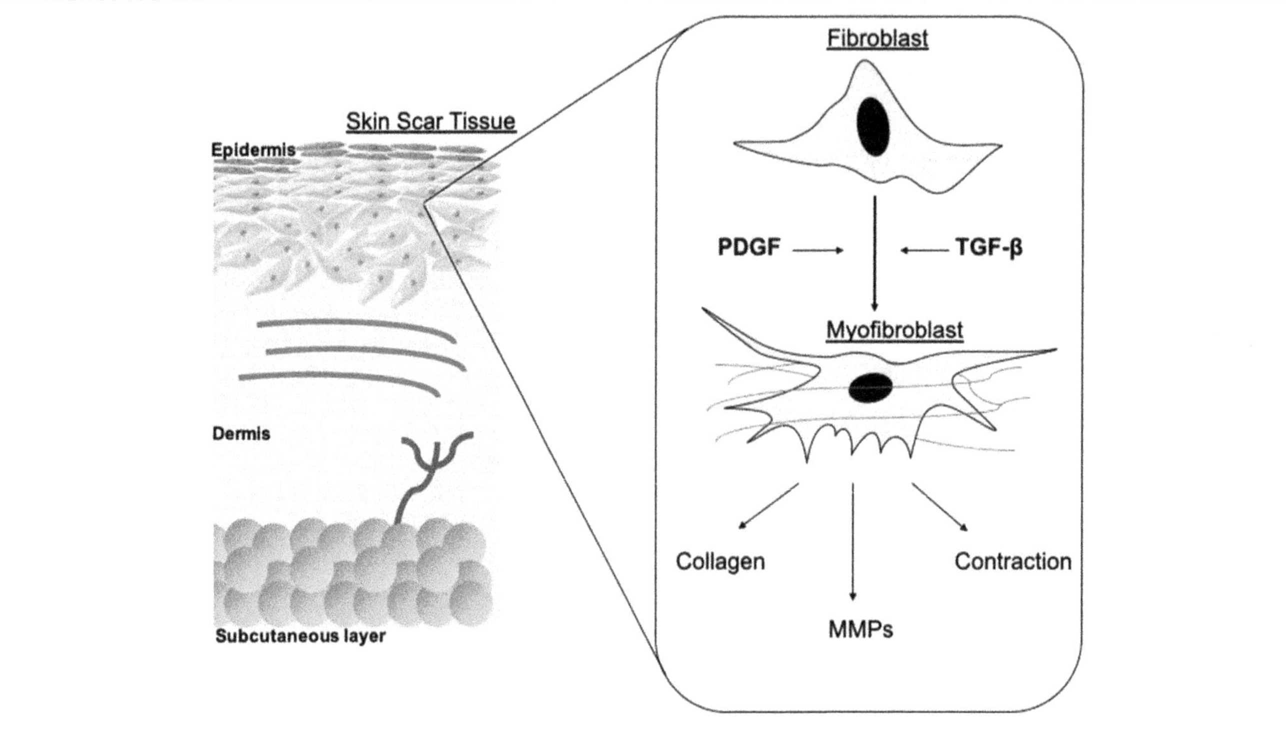

FIGURE 1 | Schematic of fibroblast differentiation into myofibroblasts within scar tissue. TGF-β and PDGF stimulate the differentiation of myofibroblasts from fibroblasts, thus contributing to wound contraction. The contractile force is delivered by the myofibroblasts until re-epithelialisation is complete then they go through apoptosis. MMPs are also released and are essential in the remodeling phase of wound healing and scar formation. However, in hypertrophic scarring this myofibroblast depletion is not well-orchestrated, resulting in functional defects.

2009). Suture knots, for example, can act as platforms for bacterial colonization and reproduction (Mashhadi and Loh, 2011).

To overcome these limitations, porcine models of wound healing are often used. Pigs are anatomically and physiologically similar to humans, and therefore can be considered excellent models of human diseases (Seaton et al., 2015; Acevedo et al., 2019). Indeed, the skin of pigs and humans are similar in that they have a relatively thick epidermis and dermal papillae (Montagna and Yun, 1964).

CURRENT SCAR TREATMENTS

There is a vast array of current treatments for scars which come in a variety of forms. Topical treatments such as Mederma® Skin Care gel (Merz Pharmaceuticals, Greensboro, NC, USA)[2] is available over the counter. The active ingredients of Mederma® gel include onion extract; however, this product displayed no benefit when tested in a trial involving patients subjected to Mohs microsurgery (Jackson and Shelton, 1999).

Surgical revision is sometimes utilized for hypertrophic or normal scars. It is common practice in the clinic to wait several months before surgically excising scars, allowing them to become fully mature (Thomas and Somenek, 2012). The most direct excision technique for scar removal is surgical removal followed by linear closure of the skin. Surgery as a treatment, however, can result in excessive tension across the wound area or infection (Marshall et al., 2018). There are also many injectable treatments which can be used for scar treatment, including corticosteroids which is common therapy for keloid and hypertrophic scars (Thomas and Somenek, 2012).

A further example is Botulinum toxin [BOTOX® Cosmetic (onabotulinumtoxinA)[3], Allergan, Irvine, CA], which is linked with improving scar appearance (Gassner et al., 2000). However, in a clinical trial in humans who presented with forehead wounds in an emergency department and were treated with botox or placebo, there was no difference in scar appearance in 3 of 4 visual scales upon suturing (Ziade et al., 2013).

Dressings are the traditional treatment mode for wound healing and scar reduction as a means of protecting the wounds, keeping a moist microenvironment, and offloading tension from the skin (Commander et al., 2016). Indeed, the use of simple paper tape alone has shown promise. When paper tape was applied to patients with cesarean section wounds for 12 weeks post-surgery, there was a reduction in scar formation, and it decreased the probability of the patient developing hypertrophic scars (Atkinson et al., 2005).

[2]https://www.mederma.com/

[3]https://hcp.botoxcosmetic.com/Contact

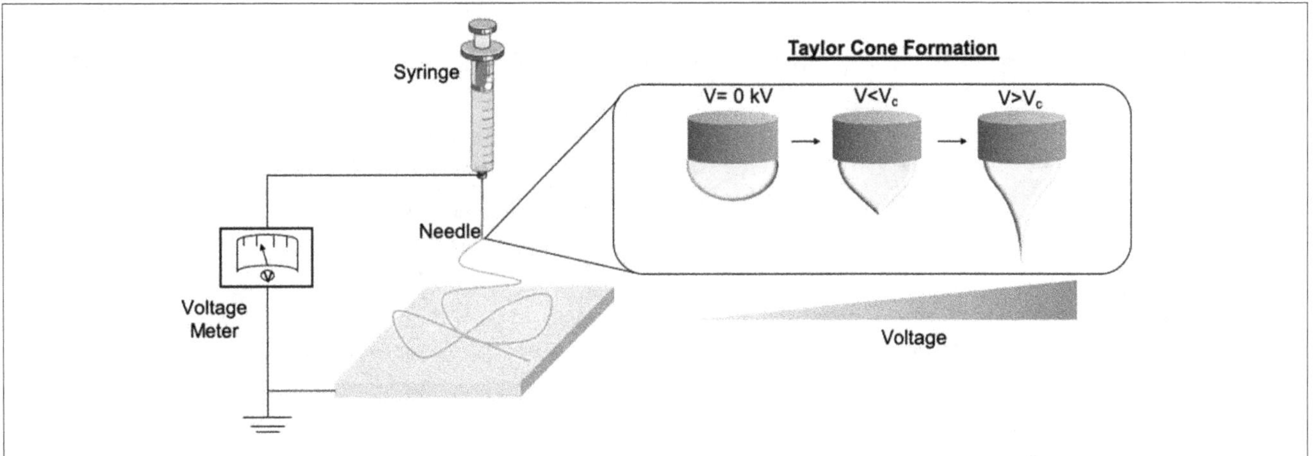

FIGURE 2 | Schematic of the formation of the Taylor Cone. As the voltage supply to the electrospinning rig increases and surpasses the critical voltage (V_C), the repulsion within the charged polymer overcomes its surface tension, fabricating solid nanofibers onto the collector. This is known as the Taylor Cone effect.

With current treatments offering varying degrees of efficacy it is imperative to develop novel modalities of treatment. The electrospinning of polymers holds potential in this regard.

ELECTROSPINNING

Electrospinning forms fibres through the application of an electrostatic field to a polymer solution (Cui et al., 2007; Bhardwaj and Kundu, 2010; Lagaron et al., 2017). The process of electrospinning can produce fibers right down to nanoscale and have applications in various fields, for example, wound dressings, drug delivery, and tissue engineering devices. The process itself is rapid and can be scaled to meet industrial demands to continuously produce fibers. This technique involves the use of a high voltage field strength from as low as 1 kV cm^1, to charge the surface of a polymer solution droplet, subsequently inducing the ejection of a liquid jet toward a grounded surface. When the voltage reaches the optimal threshold [critical voltage (V_C)] by radial charge repulsion, the single jet will divide into multiple filaments; this is recognized as the Taylor cone effect (**Figure 2**). This cone formation results in the construction of solidified fibers as the solvent evaporates. The V_C value varies between polymers due to alterations in chemical properties (Quinn et al., 2018). Solution properties such as viscosity, concentration, and dielectric constant, and operational parameters including the strength of the applied voltage, jet to collector distance, and flux, will all affect the morphology of the resulting fibers (Sencadas et al., 2012; Haider et al., 2015). Electrospun fibers possess high surface area to volume ratios, meaning they exhibit many of the desirable properties of an effective wound dressing such as protection from mechanical stimuli and providence of excellent gaseous exchange, and as such a lot of research has gone into optimizing them for this application. The following sections, therefore, explore the use of electrospun fibers in the treatment of scars and the potential future applications this technology could hold as a therapeutic (**Table 1**).

Electrospinning is a versatile process which encompasses many different modes of fabrication for the incorporation of therapeutics (**Figure 3**). Blending is the predominant method for drug incorporation into electrospun nanofibers. The process of blending consists of drug or drug precursors encapsulated by means of dissolving or dispersing it into the polymer solution, before subsequent electrospinning. As the drug itself is in direct contact with the polymer, the drug-polymer interaction must be analyzed to ensure functionality is retained and that the drug can be adequately released from the product fibers. For example, Yang et al. investigated the use of gold nanoparticles modified with an antibacterial intermediate (6-aminopenicillanic acid) for wound healing applications. The gold nanoparticles were assimilated into electrospun nanofibers composed of polycaprolactone (PCL) and gelatin by blending. The nanoparticles release profile was investigated by nanofiber dipping into saline. The results showed that after Day 1 20.4% of the gold had been released, increasing to 65.7% by Day 7. Burst release was apparent within the initial days which can be attributed to a percentage of the gold existing near the surface of the fibers (Yang et al., 2017).

Modification of nanofiber surfaces to allow incorporation of therapeutics is another method for drug and cell loading (Prabhakaran et al., 2008; Ma et al., 2011; Wakuda et al., 2018). This method is advantageous for avoiding burst discharge of therapeutics and results in a more gradual release profile (Im et al., 2010). This technique is particularly beneficial for biomolecular therapeutics such as enzymes as surface conjugation, and slow-release helps to preserve functionality (Zamani et al., 2013). Plasma treatment of polymers is a typical method of surface modification. Nanofiber treatment with plasma in the presence of oxygen, ammonia, or air has resulted in the generation of amine or carboxyl groups on the surface of the fibers (Baker et al., 2006; Yan et al., 2013). This process functionalizes fibers for a variety of applications, such as the adhesion of the collagen or gelatin, which are key proteins found in the extracellular matrix, and so can improve cell adhesion and proliferation (He et al., 2005; Koh et al., 2008). It has been shown that poly(lactic-co-glycolic acid) PLGA nanofibers can be transformed to contain carboxylic acid groups through plasma glow discharge in the presence of oxygen and gaseous

TABLE 1 | Therapeutic potential of various electrospun polymers including therapy loaded nanofibers and tissue engineering options.

Electrospun devices	Electrospun polymers	Incorporated therapeutics	Therapeutic outcomes	References
Polymers	Recombinant Human Collagen, Chitosan and PEO	–	This dressing resulted in elevated levels of collagen III *in vivo* 14 days post-surgery in normal male SD rats compared to control groups, which is indicative of less scar tissue formation.	Deng et al., 2018
	Collagen Type I and PCL	-	Significantly reduced the area of scar tissue formation in back skin wounds of Sprague-Dawley rat compared to controls as determined via H&E staining.	Bonvallet et al., 2014
	Silk fibroin/gelatin	-	This dressing inhibited scar tissue formation *in vivo* via stimulating wound closure ($p < 0.05$), enhancing angiogenesis, and successfully refining collagen organization.	Shan et al., 2015
	Silk fibroin/PEO	-	This dressing stimulated rapid collagen production with a similar architecture to normal skin.	Ju et al., 2016
Polymers + therapeutic agents	Collagen (Col, mimicking protein), PCL	Bioactive glass nanoparticles	This dressing delivered bioglass nanoparticles resulting in enhanced endothelial cell attachment and proliferation *in vitro*. This translated to well organized collagen deposition and skin appendages *in vivo* compared to controls without nanoparticles in specific pathogen-free male Sprague-Dawley rats.	Gao et al., 2017
	PELA and PEG	pbFGF and PEI	This dressing after 4 weeks resulted in fully differentiated epidemic cells, closely arranged basal cells and elevated occurrences of hair and sebum, consistent with the epithelial structure of normal skin.	Yang et al., 2012
	Poly(ε-caprolactone) (PCL)/gelatin	TGF-β1 inhibitor (SB-525334)	This dressing released PGT to effectively inhibit fibroblast proliferation *in vitro* and this translated to the successful prevention of hypertrophic scar formation *in vivo* in a full-thickness wound model on the ear of female New Zealand white rabbits.	Wang et al., 2017
Polymers + cells	Recombinant Human Tropoelastin	Adipose derived stem cells (ADSC)	This dressing significantly improved wound closure and enhanced epithelial thickness *in vivo* in a murine excisional wound model compared to controls. It is hypothesized that the device could persist within the skin after healing and improve the overall tensile strength of the resulting scar tissue.	Machula et al., 2014
	Collagen and PCL	Keratinocytes and Fibroblasts	This layered dressing becoming unrecognizable after Day 21 post-implantation, indicative of high grafting efficiency.	Mahjour et al., 2015
	PLGA and Collagen	Bone marrow-derived MSCs (BM-MSCs)	This dressing resulted in faster wound closure times *in vivo* in full-thickness wound models in rats, with wounds closing 8 days earlier than controls.	Ma et al., 2011

acrylic acid (Park et al., 2007). These fibers exhibited enhanced fibroblast cell adhesion and proliferation, desirable properties for wound healing.

The fabrication of core/shell nanofibers is another attractive method of bioactive incorporation into electrospun nanofibers. The production of electrospun core-shell nanofibers is accomplished through either co-axial or emulsion electrospinning. Co-axial electrospinning is a two-stream process that results in the fabrication of multipolymer fibers with the inner stream being the "core," and the outer polymer passed stream forms the shell (Jiang et al., 2014). This method is auspicious for the incorporation of fragile cargos (e.g., DNA or growth factors) as the therapeutic interaction with the shell polymer blend which may be produced with harsh solvents is minimized, therefore preserving the cargo (Ghosh et al., 2008; Xie et al., 2016; Cheng et al., 2019). Wei et al. utilized this technique for the development of a wound dressing, comprising a PCL core and collagen shell nanofibers. The shell was blended with silver nanoparticles to take advantage of the anti-bacterial activity, and the core permeated with vitamin A, which has been shown to help with wound healing by increasing intra- and extracellular hydration (Campos et al., 1999; Wei et al., 2016). Emulsion electrospinning produces nanofibers of core/shell morphology by first introducing an emulsion into an initial

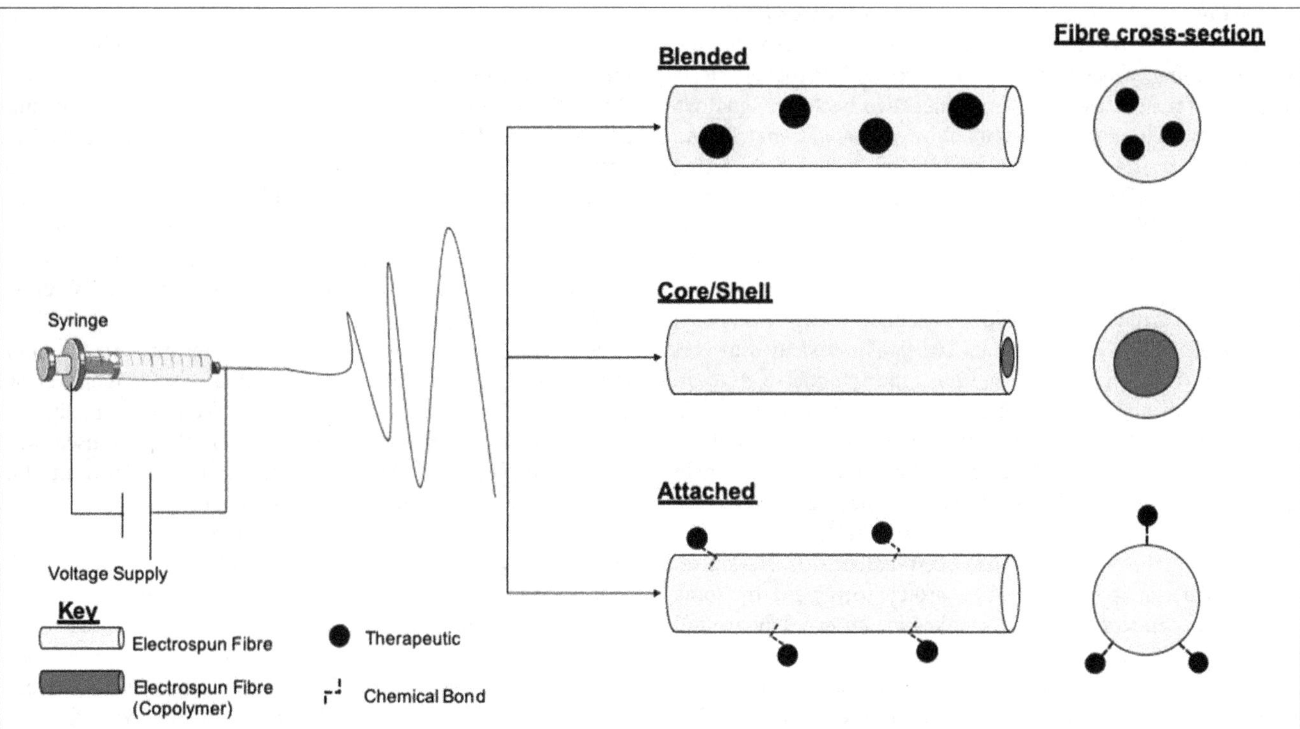

FIGURE 3 | Schematic of electrospinning equipment and the resultant fibers and therapy loaded variants. The electrospinning set-up comprises a high voltage (V) supply which is connected to a syringe loaded with a polymer solution. Within the blending technique therapeutics or therapeutic precursors are mixed with polymer solutions before electrospinning. Either co-axial or emulsion electrospinning produces core/shell morphology fibers. This method allows for the encapsulation of therapeutics in either layer. Therapeutic attachment to fibers post-electrospinning allows for the loading of fragile molecules which cannot endure the electrospinning process.

polymer solution before the addition of a surfactant to isolate the different phases from each other (Liao et al., 2009). Castro et al. manufactured nanofibers composed of PCL and PCL/gelatin, which retained and delivered ketoprofen by solution and emulsion electrospinning, respectively. It was reported that using emulsion electrospinning of PCL/gelatin could diminish the burst release of ketoprofen compared with single PCL nanofibers, and sustained drug release for >100 h. Furthermore, the combination of gelatin into the nanofibers resulted in an increase in the cell proliferation of L929 fibroblast cells (murine) (Basar et al., 2017). It should be noted however that emulsion electrospinning can cause damage to molecules such as DNA via interface tension between the organic and aqueous phases within the emulsion (He et al., 2012).

ELECTROSPINNING POLYMERS FOR SCAR TREATMENT

With the process of electrospinning being so versatile, a plethora of both synthetic and natural polymers can be processed to form fibrous structures with the potential to promote scar-free wound healing. Expectedly, not every polymer can be easily electrospun. Many factors influence this ability, including polymer viscosity, concentration, and entanglement. For polymers with inadequate characteristics for electrospinning, a copolymer can be employed to improve mechanical properties. Alginate is an example of a naturally occurring polymer with a well-noted history for improving wound healing due to its excellent ability to swell and maintain a moist microenvironment, which aids healing (Aderibigbe and Buyana, 2018). However, alginate alone does not possess ideal attributes for electrospinning due to its low chain entanglement (Nie et al., 2008). Poly (vinyl alcohol) (PVA) is a reputable polymer for electrospinning and as a result is frequently selected as a copolymer. Indeed, PVA is extensively used on an industrial scale and is favored in the medical industry due to excellent physical properties, processability, and biocompatibility. Tarun et al. developed an electrospun matrix composed of PVA/ sodium alginate (Tarun and Gobi, 2012). It was demonstrated that the matrix displayed excellent water vapor transmission rates, thus maintaining a moist wound microenvironment. Furthermore, *in vivo* studies using the full-thickness wound model in rats exhibited seemingly new epithelium development, void of any local adverse reactions. Indeed, the movement of epithelial cells across the surface of a wound is enabled in a wound that is kept moist, and in turn, promotes efficient healing (Field and Kerstein, 1994). Wounds that are kept moist typically present with less scar tissue formation (Atiyeh et al., 2003).

A further example of a natural polymer includes chitosan, which has noted antibacterial and antifungal properties, which would be highly beneficial for a wound dressing. It was suggested by Ignatova et al. that the crosslinking of PVA/Q-chitosan (a chitosan derivative) through the photo-crosslinking electrospinning procedure, would have antimicrobial effects on both Gram-positive and Gram-negative bacteria (Ignatova et al., 2006). The author's results showed that the matrix had exceptional resistance to the growth of bacteria exhibiting activity against *E. coli* and *S. aureus*. However, it is important to note that with polymers like chitosan there are drawbacks. Chitosan, as an example, is poorly soluble (Shete et al., 2012), and so tends to be dissolved in acidic conditions, namely using acetic acid or trifluoroacetic acid for example (Geng et al., 2005; Bazmandeh et al., 2019; Gu et al., 2019). The toxicity and cost associated with such solvents can imped the potential of chitosan in wound and anti-scarring therapies (Mengistu Lemma et al., 2016), however, during the electrospinning process much of the solvent evaporates under ideal conditions, and so could help alleviate these unwanted side effects when harsher solvents are required (Golecki et al., 2014; Haider et al., 2015).

Another natural polymer of noted potency as a wound-healing material is silk fibroin, a protein produced by some insects (e.g., silkworm). Fibroin makes for an excellent wound repair candidate as it is highly biocompatible, contains anti-inflammatory properties, and has notable anti-scarring potential. As such, much attention has turned to the electrospinning of silk to fabricate bioactive wound dressings. For example, Ju et al. developed electrospun silk fibroin nanofibers as a dressing material for the treatment of burn wounds. The authors found that the expression of IL-1α, which is pro-inflammatory, had significantly lower expression levels in silk fibroin treated skin compared to a gauze control treatment in the skin of male Sprague-Dawley rats where second degree burn wounds were induced on the backs. Further to this, the expression profile of TGF-β1 peaked at Day 21 post-wounding before declining, compared to at in gauze treated wounds which crested at Day 7. It was also noted that the silk fibroin nanofibers induced rapid collagen formation, which organized within the wound in a similar fashion to that of normal skin as opposed to a scarring composition (Ju et al., 2016).

ELECTROSPUN POLYMERS WITH ADDED THERAPEUTICS FOR SCAR TREATMENT

With the variety of production avenues for electrospinning nanofibers (blending, core/shell, attachment), there lays the opportunity for the incorporation and delivery of a variety of anti-scaring therapeutics. As discussed, alginate offers an excellent polymer choice for wound dressings as it promotes a moist wound environment, and hence reduces the extent of scarring. In a study by Shalumon et al. the use of electrospun sodium alginate/PVA nanofibers loaded with ZnO nanoparticles (via the blending method) as an antibacterial wound dressing was explored. The study concluded that a concentration of between 0.5 and 5% is required for the fibers to have antibacterial activity as tested with *S. aureus* and *E. coli*, with minimal cytotoxic effects (using L929 murine fibroblast cells) (Shalumon et al., 2011). These nanofibers were tested *in vivo* using C57BL/6J mice, where UVB irradiation was employed to produce visible skin lesions, and scar formation was evident within 48–96 h. When these lesions where treated with the nanofiber dressings it was reported that no burn marks were detectible after 24 h post-injury. This rapid recovery was further confirmed by the downregulation of inflammatory cytokines IL-6, IL-1B, and TNF-a after 24 h compared to untreated controls. Taken together this electrospun device shows excellent potential for the reduction of scar tissue formation in a burn wound model (Hajiali et al., 2016).

A historic but still pertinent avenue for the treatment of wounds and scars is the use of essential oils (Sequeira et al., 2019). Previous research as developed electrospun nanofibers composed of alginate/polyethylene glycol (PEO) infused with lavender essential oil, for the treatment of UV-induced skin burns. These fibers showed antibacterial efficacy *in vitro* against *S. aureus*, and furthermore reduced the production of pro-inflammatory cytokines both *in vitro* and *in vivo* (Hajiali et al., 2016). The authors found that the burns of mice treated with the lavender-infused nanofibers healed faster compared to the untreated group. Karami et al. developed electrospun fibers of PCL and polylactic acid (PLA) which encapsulated thymol from thyme essential oil for the treatment of skin infections, with a focus on *E. coli* and *S. aureus* (Karami et al., 2013). Application of these nanofibers *in vivo* using a full-thickness wound model in Male Wistar rats resulted in an enhancement in granulation tissue formation and re-epithelialization at 14 days post-wounding (92.3%) compared to gauze (68%) and commercial (Comfeel Plus) (87%) controls. Histologically, the wounds treated with the commercial dressing exhibited some epidermal tissue at day 14, but this was more extensive in the nanofiber treated wounds (Karami et al., 2013). These results demonstrate the power of essential oils as efficient wound healing therapeutics, which could be employed for the reduction in scar tissue formation.

In another study conducted by Gao et al., endothelial progenitor cells were cultured on composite fibers consisting of PCL/collagen and bioactive glass nanoparticles *in vitro* (Gao et al., 2017). *In vivo* wound healing studies using specific pathogen-free male Sprague-Dawley rats revealed evident blood vessel formation, as well as upregulation of angiogenic markers such as hypoxia-inducible factor−1 alpha (HIF-1α) and vascular endothelial growth factor (VEGF). Throughout the *in vivo* study, wound healing potential was superior in wounds treated with nanofibers containing the bioglass nanoparticles. These bioglass-loaded nanofibers achieved 60% wound closure in the first week and ~90% closure with 2 weeks, compared to nanofibers containing no bioglass beads which achieved only 50 and 80% closure within week 1 and week 2, respectively. The total area of scar tissue in wounds treated with the bioactive glass-loaded nanofibers was significantly smaller and with highly organized collagen deposition compared to treatment with unloaded nanofibers (Gao et al., 2017).

Many studies have explored the use of electrospun nanomaterials in the treatment of diabetic foot ulcers (DFU). DFU are categorized as a major complication of diabetes mellitus,

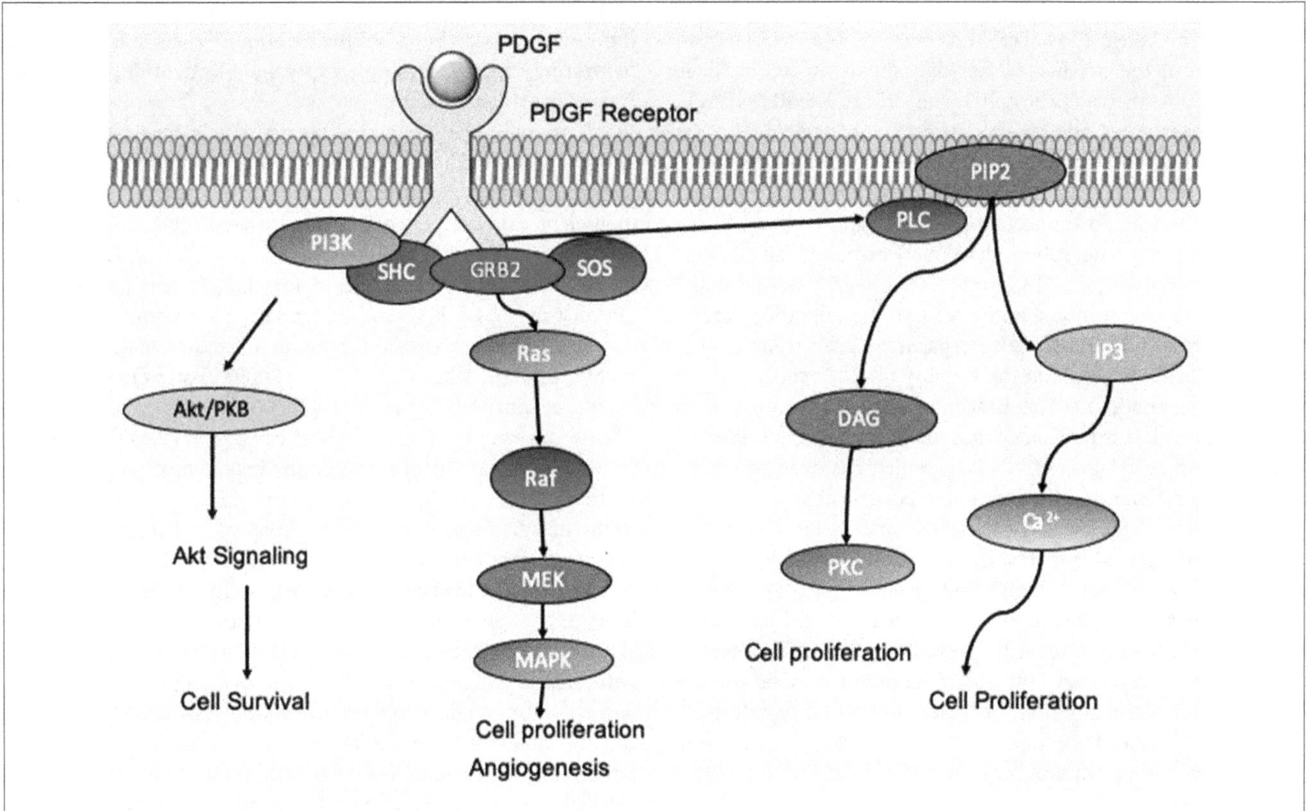

FIGURE 4 | Schematic showing the molecular pathways associated with PDGF. PDGF activation gives rise to an increase in cell proliferation, migration, and angiogenesis through AkT, MAPK, and calcium pathways for example. PDGF is essential for efficient wound repair and minimization of potential scar tissue. Commercial product REGRANEX® utilizes recombinant human PDGF for the treatment of diabetic foot ulcers.

and typically present on the feet, toes, and heels. DFU result from peripheral neuropathy, poor circulation, and impaired immune function, or a combination of these foundations. Of diabetic patients in the USA, 20% of foot ulcer cases displayed insufficiencies in peripheral atrial supply. Moreover, 50% of patients primarily displayed peripheral neuropathy, and ~30% presented with a combination of these conditions (Reiber et al., 1999)[4] As such, with a wide-reaching cohort of diabetic patients suffering from chronic wounds, there is a continuous need for efficient wound healing options which result in rapid and scar-free results. Indeed, Yang et al. developed an electrospun dressing composed of poly(dl-lactide)-poly(ethylene glycol) (PDLLA-PEG) fibers which had polyethyleneimine (PEI)/pbFGF polyplexes incorporated by the emulsion loading technique, advantageous for the integration of fragile genetic material. PEG was also added to the shell portion of the fibers to aid in smooth release of the cargo. The authors found that the structure was able to sustain release of the polyplexes over a 4-week period, and successful transfection was observed that ensued for over 28 days, enhancing the proliferative capacity of the mouse embryo fibroblast cells *in vitro*. The efficacy of the fibers *in vivo* was tested in skin wounds generated on the dorsal area of diabetic male Sprague Dawley (SD) rats. The fibers containing PEI/pbFGF complexes resulted in a significantly higher wound recovery rate compared to untreated wounds, exhibiting improved vascularization and completed re-epithelialization (Yang et al., 2012). These are important outcomes as the more rapid and efficient cell migration corresponds to a reduction in scar tissue formation (Hadjizadeh et al., 2017). Yuan et al. also explored the combination of growth factors and electrospun materials for skin regeneration. The authors utilized a dual-spinneret electrospinner to manufacture fibers composed of chitosan- PEO and fibrinogen, loading the polymers with PDGF via blending directly before electrospinning (Yuan et al., 2018). PDGF is a critical player in wound repair initiation and progression, acting as a chemotactic instrument for neutrophils, monocytes, and fibroblasts (Sá et al., 2018). Furthermore, PDGF can block fibroblast differentiation into myofibroblasts thus decreasing scar formation (Yuan et al., 2018). Indeed, a therapy option of wound repair termed Regranex® is the only growth factor wound treatment for diabetic ulcers currently FDA approved, utilizing recombinant human PDGF (**Figure 4**) (Fang and Galiano, 2008). A single daily application of Regranex® has been shown to enhance wound closure, with a 30% faster healing time observed. It must also be noted that in the case of Regranex® it was previously suggested that it increased the rate of mortality related to malignancy development in patients treated with

[4]https://www.niddk.nih.gov/about-niddk/strategic-plans-reports/diabetes-in-america-2nd-edition

>3 tubes of the product, as concluded from a post-marketing retrospective study. However, this warning has since been removed from the product packaging, and many studies have disproved this theory (Ziyadeh et al., 2011; REGRANEX®, 2018). Nevertheless, daily application is considered to be inconvenient for the patient, impacting the quality of life. Thus, the delivery of this growth factor in a controlled manner could be of great benefit. In the instance of Yuan and authors, it was observed that the nanofibers developed exhibited an average fiber diameter of 202.3 ± 113.2 nm, PDGF integrity was retained, and upon release promoted an increase in the migration rate of human dermal fibroblasts. With regards to cytotoxicity, there was a significant decrease in the viability of cells exposed to the nanofibers (unloaded) at 72 h post-incubation compared to a no scaffold control. It is postulated that this decrease is the result of the degree of acetylation of chitosan, which has been shown to elicit strong cellular interactions due to positive charges (Aranaz et al., 2009). Indeed, other groups have observed a decrease in cell viability after 24 h in bladder carcinoma cells exposed to chitosan with a degree of acetylation greater than 50% (Younes et al., 2016). This is an interesting observation, and so should be factored into the rational for novel wound healing devices. However, it is suggested that this observation may be unique to *in vitro* experimentation, as prior studies using chitosan observed negligible toxic effect *in vivo*, linked with metabolic clearance of biodegradation products (Kean and Thanou, 2010; Jeong et al., 2017).

CELL DELIVERY VIA ELECTROSPUN POLYMERS FOR SCAR TREATMENT

The use of cells in regenerative medicine is widely explored and considered by many to hold great promise[5]. For example, mononuclear umbilical cord cells are easily available and have few associated ethical issues. Furthermore, it has been previously demonstrated that these cell types can be cultured on electrospun nanofibers (Chua et al., 2006).

In light of the advantageous potential of cell therapies for regenerative purposes, they are not without limitations. Therapies of this nature would require a large number of donors, these cells would not survive past low passage numbers, and there is the potential risk of rejection from the host (Venkat et al., 2018). A further example of potential cell therapies includes allogeneic bone marrow cells, which are easily available but carry the risk of rejection and would require specialized techniques for cell harvest and separation. Martinello et al. used allogenic mesenchymal stem cells to treat wounds in a large animal study using female Bergamasca sheep. It was found that at 15 Days post-injury, when compared to a control group, sheep treated with allogeneic bone marrow cells presented with a higher degree of wound closure, reepithelialization, as well as a reduction in inflammation. The latter of which the authors postulate may result in a decreased myofibroblast development and thus scar formation (Martinello et al., 2018).

[5]https://www.mayoclinic.org/tests-procedures/bone-marrow-transplant/in-depth/stem-cells/art-20048117

In saying this, autologous cells helps mitigate the problem of immune rejection, but nevertheless require the same specialized harvesting and separation expertise (Venkat et al., 2018; Ramotowski et al., 2019).

Many studies have explored the use of cells for wound healing and scar tissue minimization. However, the most typical route for this exploration is the direct injection of cells, which can be highly inefficient, and incurs substantial cell death due to shear forces through the injection needle (Burdick et al., 2016). Electrospun nanofibers may be the solution for the efficient and effective delivery of cells for skin regeneration. Electrospun nanofibers have high surface areas, and therefore have the capacity to retain many cultured cells (Chen et al., 2009). For example, it was shown by Zhao et al. that electrospun nanofibers composed of silk fibroin could successfully host cardiomyocytes (Zhao et al., 2019). This capability of electrospun fibers to host cells is thought by many to be owed to the likeness to the natural ECM, fitting to the fibrous nature of collagen, thereby facilitating the natural proliferation of cells (Ramakrishna et al., 2006).

The disadvantage of using these nanofibers for this purpose, however, is the restricted control over pore structure. The pore size in this instance is proportional to the fiber diameters, with smaller diameters resulting in smaller pore sizes, which consequently can decrease cell infiltration (Wu and Hong, 2016). In some cases, cells only infiltrate the uppermost portion of the nanofibers, which reduces the advantages of three-dimensional cell culture. When nanofibers are compared to microfibers in this regard, it has been shown that larger pore sizes, inherent to macrofibers, promote stem cell differentiation, coupled with improved cellular permeation, however nanofibers are associated with higher cell attachment (Wu and Hong, 2016).

Mahjour et al. developed a skin substitute composed of electrospun PCL/collagen fibers for the treatment of burn wounds. The fibers in question were layered in a composite manner, with different layers infused with keratinocytes (top layer) and fibroblasts (bottom layer). The electrospun fibers were applied in an *in vivo* mouse model of wound healing. Data collected from the study showed that the cell incorporated composite fibers integrated into the wound bed in a highly effective way, becoming unrecognizable after Day 21 post-implantation. This was in comparison to blank fiber scaffolds which received the lowest score of integration. Furthermore, at Day 21, wounds treated with the cell-incorporated composite fibers had 7% remaining non-reepithelialized skin and 45% wound contraction, whereas the blank composite fibers had only 21% re-epithelialization and 56% wound contraction (Mahjour et al., 2015).

Mesenchymal stem cells (MSCs) are multipotent stem cells typically isolated from bone marrow, adipose tissues, and the dermis (Orbay et al., 2012). MSCs have shown avid potential in skin repair, promoting angiogenesis, reducing inflammation, and facilitating the establishment of an ECM (Jackson et al., 2012). When MSCs enter an inflammatory environment a switch to an immunomodulatory phenotype is initiated by Interferon-gamma (IFNγ), Tumor Necrosis Factor-alpha (TNFα) and IL-1β (Ren et al., 2008). When this phenotype is active; there is evidence suggesting that MSCs can suppress the proliferation of B cells as well as natural killer cells (Corcione et al., 2006; Sotiropoulou et al., 2006). This suppression enhances the acute immune response to damage and can reduce a pro-fibrotic response that can result from sustained inflammation (Redd et al., 2004). Williams et al. tried to reduce scar sizes in ischemic cardiomyopathy through injection of allogeneic MSCs (Williams et al., 2013). The authors suggested that MSCs could reverse ventricular remodeling, and, indeed, it was shown that MSCs stimulate endogenous cardiac stem cells to proliferate and differentiate. The resulting mature cardiomyocytes exhibited therapeutic effect by secretion of growth factors and cytokines.

Similarly, Li et al. showed that MSCs loaded into a 3D graphene foam decreased scar tissue formation. The foam resulted in upregulation of VEGF as well as bFGF leading to enhanced neovascularization, as well as heightening levels of TGF-β3, which prevents scarring. The MSC loaded foams were tested *in vivo* in a full-thickness wound model using wild-type rats. The use of MSCs in the foam resulted in a significant closure of the wound from day 3 post-wounding compared to controls of untreated and unloaded foam, this trend was observed consistently until endpoint at 14 Days post-wounding (Li et al., 2015).

With such obvious potential, it is not surprising that many researchers have explored the incorporation of stem cells like MSCs into electrospun nanofibers for wound and scar treatments. For example, Ma et al. integrated bone marrow-derived MSCs (BM-MSCs) into nanofibers comprised of collagen and PLGA. The device demonstrated enhanced healing profiles in a full-thickness wound model *in vivo* using rats. The wounds treated with the BM-MSCs loaded nanofibers resulted in faster closure times compared to the untreated control, closing 8 days earlier (Ma et al., 2011). Furthermore, it was observed that localized treatment with the BM-MSCs resulted in a decrease in myofibroblast numbers. The authors postulated this may be due to MSCs ability to express hepatocyte growth factor 8 which inhibits myofibroblastic differentiation (Ma et al., 2011). These results suggest that this device would reduce scar tissue formation whilst allowing rapid and efficient wound repair.

In another study, Machula et al. electrospun nanofiber membranes of tropoelastin seeded with adipose-derived stem cells for wound healing applications (Machula et al., 2014). The authors found that the stem cells rapidly proliferated on the nanofibers and partook in efficient ECM establishment, covering the entire scaffold *in vitro*. Application of the cell-nanofiber device in an *in vivo* excisional wound model with female SCID mice showed an enhancement in wound closure and restoration of normal epithelium compared to control wounds treated with petrolatum jelly-impregnated gauze. The average thickness of re-epithelized skin tissue for the control and stem cell-nanofiber treated groups was $27.7 \pm 7.8\,\mu m$ and $51.9 \pm 11.27\,\mu m$, respectively ($p = 0.001$). It is postulated by the authors that the electrospun tropoelastin device may persist within the scar tissue of healed skin and in doing so enhance the tensile strength of any resultant scar tissue.

A limitation associated with stem cell culture on electrospun nanofibers is that small pore size may result in a blockage in nutrient diffusion and cellular infiltration. If this problem can be mitigated, it could lead to a highly potent regenerative device.

CONCLUSIONS AND FUTURE DIRECTIONS

As detailed in this review, the use of electrospun nanofibers for scar treatment has substantial potential. With a plethora of polymers being "*electrospinnable*" alone or in conjunction with therapeutic agents or cells, the problem of scar management could be significantly improved. However, much work is still required to get such therapies into the clinic. Indeed, there are currently 5 clinical trials exploring the use of electrospun nanofibers[6]; yet, none of these are scar tissue-specific, and no current trials are recruiting. Conversely, there are 760 clinical trials listed for skin scarring[7], 140 of which are recruiting[8]. This suggests that much research is focusing on novel therapies for scar treatment and prevention, which is a favorable scenario, and indeed these therapies if approved could in future be incorporated into electrospun nanofibers. Recent results have been notably discouraging. Metelimumab, for example, a TGF-β1 targeting antibody, exhibited no improvement in the treatment of systemic sclerosis compared to a placebo control[9]. In saying this, an RNAi-based inhibitor of connective tissue growth factor (CTGF) termed RXI 109 has completed phase I trials and is now in phase II trials for hypertrophic scar treatment[10]. With promising therapies in the pipeline, it is exciting to hypothesize the efficiency of their delivery via electrospun nanofibers.

Encouragingly, electrospun nanofibers can be manufactured on an industrial scale, with the production of continuous nanofibers from a variety of polymers already proven (Ramachandran and Gouma, 2008; Zhang et al., 2012; Ma et al., 2015; Wang et al., 2018). Translating nanofiber production from laboratory to commercial scale is readily accommodated through the application of multi-jet nozzle electrospinners, which have been reported to process as much as 6.5 kg/h of polymer to produce fibers (Persano et al., 2013). Current commercial examples include the Zeus Bioweb™ composites, composed of electrospun polytetrafluoroethylene (PTFE). The Bioweb™ exhibits a high surface area and possesses an advantageously minute pore size, typically in the range of 1–4 μm. Zeus boasts a variety of Bioweb™ applications including scaffold potential and implantable structures in the body[11]. A further commercial example of an electrospinning product is the SpinCare™ system by Nicast. SpinCare™ is a handheld device that fabricates nanofibers from polymers directly for tailored wound healing

[6]https://clinicaltrials.gov/ct2/results?cond=&term=electrospinning&cntry=&state=&city=&dist=&Search=Search (Date visited November 15, 2019).
[7]https://clinicaltrials.gov/ct2/results?cond=Skin+Scarring&term=&cntry=&state=&city=&dist= (Date visited November 15, 2019).
[8]https://clinicaltrials.gov/ct2/results?cond=Skin+Scarring&Search=Apply&recrs=a&age_v=&gndr=&type=&rslt= (Date visited November 15, 2019).
[9]https://clinicaltrials.gov/ct2/show/NCT00432328
[10]https://clinicaltrials.gov/ct2/show/NCT02246465
[11]https://www.zeusinc.com/products/biomaterials/bioweb-composites

applications. These nanofibers provide a semi-permeable coverage facilitating excellent moisture regulation. The fibers are also comfortable as they are made to fit the shape of the patient's wound[12].

It is well-believed that the combination of gene therapies with biomaterials hold great potential as future generation therapeutic devices (Bleiziffer et al., 2007; Goker et al., 2019). Although promising, gene therapy is not without limitations. For example, therapies of this nature are historically challenging to deliver into cells, due to similarities in charges between nucleic acids and cell membranes. Viral gene delivery is the most common form of gene therapy due to its high efficiency. These vectors, however, are met with numerous trepidations as they can result in mutagenesis and have a restricted capacity for genetic material (Mingozzi and High, 2013). Non-viral options for gene therapy also exist and include cationic polymers (Olden et al., 2018), liposomes (Balazs and Godbey, 2011), and peptides (McCarthy et al., 2014; Cole et al., 2019). Indeed, recent literature published by Mulholland et al. explored the delivery of an siRNA complexed with a cell penetrating peptide termed RALA from an electrospun bilayer wound patch. The use of the RALA peptide significantly enhanced the transfection efficient of the nucleic acids *in vitro* using HMEC-1 endothelial cells, downregulating expression anti-angiogenic FK506-binding protein-like FKBPL. This high efficiency translated to significant upsurge in angiogenic activity *in vivo* in wounds on the backs of C57BL/6 mice, resulting in an increase in blood vessel density of 326% compared to untreated wounds (Mulholland et al., 2019). This technology holds excellent potential for scar tissue treatment as a vast array of nucleic acids could be delivered in this manner.

Taken together, with the literature and the state-of-the-art technology discussed in this review, it can be rationalized that electrospinning shows great promise for the development of next generation devices for the treatment and management of scars.

[12]http://nicast.com/spincare/product-description/

AUTHOR'S NOTE

This manuscript was an invited paper for the article collection on Biomaterials for Skin Wound Repair: Tissue Engineering, Guided Regeneration, and Wound Scarring Prevention.

AUTHOR CONTRIBUTIONS

EM wrote the manuscript and produced all figures and tables with the aid of SMART Servier Medical Art.

ACKNOWLEDGMENTS

I would like to thank Dr. James Illingworth for his constant support in the writing of this article.

REFERENCES

Acevedo, C. A., Sánchez, E., Orellana, N., Morales, P., Olguín, Y., Brown, D. I., et al. (2019). Re-epithelialization appraisal of skin wound in a porcine model using a salmon-gelatin based biomaterial as wound dressing. *Pharmaceutics* 11:196. doi: 10.3390/pharmaceutics11050196

Aderibigbe, B. A., and Buyana, B. (2018). Alginate in wound dressings. *Pharmaceutics* 10:42. doi: 10.3390/pharmaceutics10020042

Anjum, F., Agabalyan, N. A., Sparks, H. D., Rosin, N. L., Kallos, M. S., and Biernaskie, J. (2017). Biocomposite nanofiber matrices to support ECM remodeling by human dermal progenitors and enhanced wound closure. *Sci. Rep.* 7:10291. doi: 10.1038/s41598-017-10735-x

Aranaz, I., Mengibar, M., Harris, R., Panos, I., Miralles, B., Acosta, N., et al. (2009). Functional characterization of chitin and chitosan. *Curr. Chem. Biol.* 3, 203–230. doi: 10.2174/187231309788166415

Atiyeh, B. S., Amm, C. A., and El Musa, K. A. (2003). Improved scar quality following primary and secondary healing of cutaneous wounds. *Aesthetic Plast. Surg.* 27, 411–417. doi: 10.1007/s00266-003-3049-3

Atkinson, J.-A. M., McKenna, K. T., Barnett, A. G., McGrath, D. J., and Rudd, M. (2005). A randomized, controlled trial to determine the efficacy of paper tape in preventing hypertrophic scar formation in surgical incisions that traverse Langer's skin tension lines. *Plast. Reconstr. Surg.* 116, 1648–1656; discussion 1657–1658. doi: 10.1097/01.prs.0000187147.73963.a5

Baker, S. C., Atkin, N., Gunning, P. A., Granville, N., Wilson, K., Wilson, D., et al. (2006). Characterisation of electrospun polystyrene scaffolds for three-dimensional *in vitro* biological studies. *Biomaterials* 27, 3136–3146. doi: 10.1016/j.biomaterials.2006.01.026

Balazs, D. A., and Godbey, W. (2011). Liposomes for use in gene delivery. *J. Drug Deliv.* 2011, 1–12. doi: 10.1155/2011/326497

Barnes, L. A., Marshall, C. D., Leavitt, T., Hu, M. S., Moore, A. L., Gonzalez, J. G., et al. (2018). Mechanical forces in cutaneous wound healing: emerging therapies to minimize scar formation. *Adv. Wound Care* 7, 47–56. doi: 10.1089/wound.2016.0709

Basar, A. O., Castro, S., Torres-Giner, S., Lagaron, J. M., and Turkoglu Sasmazel, H. (2017). Novel poly(ε-caprolactone)/gelatin wound dressings prepared by emulsion electrospinning with controlled release capacity of Ketoprofen anti-inflammatory drug. *Mater. Sci. Eng. C* 81, 459–468. doi: 10.1016/j.msec.2017.08.025

Bazmandeh, A. Z., Mirzaei, E., Ghasemi, Y., and Kouhbanani, M. A. J. (2019). Hyaluronic acid coated electrospun chitosan-based nanofibers prepared by simultaneous stabilizing and coating. *Int. J. Biol. Macromol.* 138, 403–411. doi: 10.1016/j.ijbiomac.2019.07.107

Berman, B., Maderal, A., and Raphael, B. (2017). Keloids and hypertrophic scars: pathophysiology, classification, and treatment. *Dermatol. Surg.* 43(Suppl. 1), S3–S18. doi: 10.1097/DSS.0000000000000819

Bhardwaj, N., and Kundu, S. C. (2010). Electrospinning: a fascinating fiber fabrication technique. *Biotechnol. Adv.* 28, 325–347. doi: 10.1016/j.biotechadv.2010.01.004

Bleiziffer, O., Eriksson, E., Yao, F., Horch, R. E., and Kneser, U. (2007). Gene transfer strategies in tissue engineering. *J. Cell. Mol. Med.* 11, 206–223. doi: 10.1111/j.1582-4934.2007.00027.x

Bonvallet, P. P., Culpepper, B. K., Bain, J. L., Schultz, M. J., Thomas, S. J., and Bellis, S. L. (2014). Microporous dermal-like electrospun scaffolds promote accelerated skin regeneration. *Tissue Eng. Part A* 20, 2434–2445. doi: 10.1089/ten.tea.2013.0645

Broughton, G., Janis, J. E., and Attinger, C. E. (2006). Wound healing: an overview. *Plast. Reconstr. Surg.* 117(7 Suppl.), 1e-S–32e-S. doi: 10.1097/01.prs.0000222562.60260.f9

Burdick, J. A., Mauck, R. L., and Gerecht, S. (2016). To serve and protect: hydrogels to improve stem cell-based therapies. *Cell Stem Cell* 18, 13–15. doi: 10.1016/j.stem.2015.12.004

Caley, M. P., Martins, V. L. C., and O'Toole, E. A. (2015). Metalloproteinases and wound healing. *Adv. Wound Care* 4, 225–234. doi: 10.1089/wound.2014.0581

Campos, P. M. B. G. M., Ricci, G., Semprini, M., and Lopes, R. A. (1999). Histopathological, morphometric, and stereologic studies of dermocosmetic skin formulations containing vitamin a and/or glycolic acid. *J. Cosmet. Sci.* 50, 159–70.

Carswell, L., and Borger, J. (2019). Hypertrophic scarring keloids. *StatPearls*.

Chen, M., Patra, P. K., Lovett, M. L., Kaplan, D. L., and Bhowmick, S. (2009). Role of electrospun fibre diameter and corresponding specific surface area (SSA) on cell attachment. *J. Tissue Eng. Regen. Med.* 3, 269–279. doi: 10.1002/term.163

Cheng, G., Yin, C., Tu, H., Jiang, S., Wang, Q., Zhou, X., et al. (2019). Controlled co-delivery of growth factors through layer-by-layer assembly of core–shell nanofibers for improving bone regeneration. *ACS Nano* 13, 6372–6382. doi: 10.1021/acsnano.8b06032

Chua, K.-N., Chai, C., Lee, P.-C., Tang, Y.-N., Ramakrishna, S., Leong, K. W., et al. (2006). Surface-aminated electrospun nanofibers enhance adhesion and expansion of human umbilical cord blood hematopoietic stem/progenitor cells. *Biomaterials* 27, 6043–6051. doi: 10.1016/j.biomaterials.2006.06.017

Cole, G., Ali, A. A., McErlean, E., Mulholland, E. J., Short, A., McCrudden, C. M., et al. (2019). DNA vaccination via RALA nanoparticles in a microneedle delivery system induces a potent immune response against the endogenous prostate cancer stem cell antigen. *Acta Biomater.* 96, 480–490. doi: 10.1016/j.actbio.2019.07.003

Commander, S., Chamata, E., Cox, J., Dickey, R., and Lee, E. (2016). Update on postsurgical scar management. *Semin. Plast. Surg.* 30, 122–128. doi: 10.1055/s-0036-1584824

Corcione, A., Benvenuto, F., Ferretti, E., Giunti, D., Cappiello, V., Cazzanti, F., et al. (2006). Human mesenchymal stem cells modulate B-cell functions. *Blood* 107, 367–372. doi: 10.1182/blood-2005-07-2657

Corr, D. T., Gallant-Behm, C. L., Shrive, N. G., and Hart, D. A. (2009). Biomechanical behavior of scar tissue and uninjured skin in a porcine model. *Wound Repair Regen.* 17, 250–259. doi: 10.1111/j.1524-475X.2009.00463.x

Cui, W., Li, X., Zhou, S., and Weng, J. (2007). Investigation on process parameters of electrospinning system through orthogonal experimental design. *J. Appl. Polym. Sci.* 103, 3105–3112. doi: 10.1002/app.25464

Darby, I. A., Laverdet, B., Bonté, F., and Desmoulière, A. (2014). Fibroblasts and myofibroblasts in wound healing. *Clin. Cosmet. Investig. Dermatol.* 7, 301–311. doi: 10.2147/CCID.S50046

Deng, A., Yang, Y., Du, S., and Yang, S. (2018). Electrospinning of *in situ* crosslinked recombinant human collagen peptide/chitosan nanofibers for wound healing. *Biomater. Sci.* 6, 2197–2208. doi: 10.1039/C8BM00492G

Desmoulière, A., Chaponnier, C., and Gabbiani, G. (2005). Tissue repair, contraction, and the myofibroblast. *Wound Repair Regen.* 13, 7–12. doi: 10.1111/j.1067-1927.2005.130102.x

Dunn, L., Prosser, H. C. G., Tan, J. T. M., Vanags, L. Z., Ng, M. K. C., Bursill, C. A. (2013). Murine Model of Wound Healing. *J. Vis. Exp.* e50265. doi: 10.3791/50265

Ehrlich, H. P., Desmoulière, A., Diegelmann, R. F., Cohen, I. K., Compton, C. C., Garner, W. L., et al. (1994). Morphological and immunochemical differences between keloid and hypertrophic scar. *Am. J. Pathol.* 145, 105–113.

Fang, R. C., and Galiano, R. D. (2008). A review of becaplermin gel in the treatment of diabetic neuropathic foot ulcers. *Biologics* 2, 1–12. doi: 10.2147/BTT.S1338

Field, C. K., and Kerstein, M. D. (1994). Overview of wound healing in a moist environment. *Am. J. Surg.* 167, S2–S6. doi: 10.1016/0002-9610(94)90002-7

Fu, X.-B., Sun, T.-Z., Li, X.-K., and Sheng, Z.-Y. (2005). Morphological and distribution characteristics of sweat glands in hypertrophic scar and their possible effects on sweat gland regeneration. *Chin. Med. J.* 118, 186–191.

Gao, W., Jin, W., Li, Y., Wan, L., Wang, C., Lin, C., et al. (2017). A highly bioactive bone extracellular matrix-biomimetic nanofibrous system with rapid angiogenesis promotes diabetic wound healing. *J. Mater. Chem. B* 5, 7285–7296. doi: 10.1039/C7TB01484H

Gassner, H. G., Sherris, D. A., and Otley, C. C. (2000). Treatment of facial wounds with botulinum toxin A improves cosmetic outcome in primates. *Plast. Reconstr. Surg.* 105, 1948–1953. doi: 10.1097/00006534-200005000-00005

Geng, X., Kwon, O., and Jang, J. (2005). Electrospinning of chitosan dissolved in concentrated acetic acid solution. *Biomaterials* 26, 5427–5432. doi: 10.1016/j.biomaterials.2005.01.066

Ghosh, P., Han, G., De, M., Kim, C. K., and Rotello, V. M. (2008). Gold nanoparticles in delivery applications. *Adv. Drug Deliv. Rev.* 60, 1307–1315. doi: 10.1016/j.addr.2008.03.016

Goker, F., Larsson, L., Del Fabbro, M., and Asa'ad, F. (2019). Gene delivery therapeutics in the treatment of periodontitis and peri-implantitis: a state of the art review. *Int. J. Mol. Sci.* 20:3551. doi: 10.3390/ijms20143551

Golecki, H. M., Yuan, H., Glavin, C., Potter, B., Badrossamay, M. R., Goss, J. A., et al. (2014). Effect of solvent evaporation on fiber morphology in rotary jet spinning. *Langmuir* 30, 13369–13374. doi: 10.1021/la5023104

Grove, G. L., and Kligman, A. M. (1983). Age-associated changes in human epidermal cell renewal. *J. Gerontol.* 38, 137–142. doi: 10.1093/geronj/38.2.137

Gu, X., Cao, R., Li, Y., Liu, S., Wang, Z., Feng, S., et al. (2019). Three-component antibacterial membrane of poly(butylene carbonate), poly(lactic acid) and chitosan prepared by electrospinning. *Mater. Technol.* 34, 463–470. doi: 10.1080/10667857.2019.1576822

Hadjizadeh, A., Ghasemkhah, F., and Ghasemzaie, N. (2017). Polymeric scaffold based gene delivery strategies to improve angiogenesis in tissue engineering: a review. *Polym. Rev.* 57, 505–556. doi: 10.1080/15583724.2017.1292402

Haider, A., Haider, S., and Kang, I.-K. (2015). A comprehensive review summarizing the effect of electrospinning parameters and potential applications of nanofibers in biomedical and biotechnology. *Arab. J. Chem.* 11, 1165–1188. doi: 10.1016/j.arabjc.2015.11.015

Hajiali, H., Summa, M., Russo, D., Armirotti, A., Brunetti, V., Bertorelli, R., et al. (2016). Alginate–lavender nanofibers with antibacterial and anti-inflammatory activity to effectively promote burn healing. *J. Mater. Chem. B* 4, 1686–1695. doi: 10.1039/C5TB02174J

He, C.-L., Huang, Z.-M., and Han, X.-J. (2009). Fabrication of drug-loaded electrospun aligned fibrous threads for suture applications. *J. Biomed. Mater. Res. Part A* 89A, 80–95. doi: 10.1002/jbm.a.32004

He, S., Xia, T., Wang, H., Wei, L., Luo, X., and Li, X. (2012). Multiple release of polyplexes of plasmids VEGF and bFGF from electrospun fibrous scaffolds towards regeneration of mature blood vessels. *Acta Biomater.* 8, 2659–2669. doi: 10.1016/j.actbio.2012.03.044

He, W., Ma, Z., Yong, T., Teo, W. E., and Ramakrishna, S. (2005). Fabrication of collagen-coated biodegradable polymer nanofiber mesh and its potential for endothelial cells growth. *Biomaterials* 26, 7606–7615. doi: 10.1016/j.biomaterials.2005.05.049

Hsieh, J. Y., Smith, T. D., Meli, V. S., Tran, T. N., Botvinick, E. L., and Liu, W. F. (2017). Differential regulation of macrophage inflammatory activation by fibrin and fibrinogen. *Acta Biomater.* 47, 14–24. doi: 10.1016/j.actbio.2016.09.024

Hu, M. S., Cheng, J., Borrelli, M. R., Leavitt, T., Walmsley, G. G., Zielins, E. R., et al. (2018). An improved humanized mouse model for excisional wound healing using double transgenic mice. *Adv. Wound Care* 7, 11–17. doi: 10.1089/wound.2017.0772

Ignatova, M., Starbova, K., Markova, N., Manolova, N., and Rashkov, I. (2006). Electrospun nano-fibre mats with antibacterial properties from quaternised chitosan and poly(vinyl alcohol). *Carbohydr. Res.* 341, 2098–2107. doi: 10.1016/j.carres.2006.05.006

Im, J. S., Yun, J., Lim, Y.-M., Kim, H.-I., and Lee, Y.-S. (2010). Fluorination of electrospun hydrogel fibers for a controlled release drug delivery system. *Acta Biomater.* 6, 102–109. doi: 10.1016/j.actbio.2009.06.017

Jackson, B. A., and Shelton, A. J. (1999). Pilot study evaluating topical onion extract as treatment for postsurgical scars. *Dermatol. Surg.* 25, 267–269. doi: 10.1046/j.1524-4725.1999.08240.x

Jackson, W. M., Nesti, L. J., and Tuan, R. S. (2012). Mesenchymal stem cell therapy for attenuation of scar formation during wound healing. *Stem Cell Res. Ther.* 3:20. doi: 10.1186/scrt111

Jeong, K.-J., Song, Y., Shin, H.-R., Kim, J. E., Kim, J., Sun, F., et al. (2017). *In vivo* study on the biocompatibility of chitosan-hydroxyapatite film depending on degree of deacetylation. *J. Biomed. Mater. Res. Part A* 105, 1637–1645. doi: 10.1002/jbm.a.35993

Jiang, H., Wang, L., and Zhu, K. (2014). Coaxial electrospinning for encapsulation and controlled release of fragile water-soluble bioactive agents. *J. Control Release* 193, 296–303. doi: 10.1016/j.jconrel.2014.04.025

Ju, H. W., Lee, O. J., Lee, J. M., Moon, B. M., Park, H. J., Park, Y. R., et al. (2016). Wound healing effect of electrospun silk fibroin nanomatrix in burn-model. *Int. J. Biol. Macromol.* 85, 29–39. doi: 10.1016/j.ijbiomac.2015.12.055

Karami, Z., Rezaeian, I., Zahedi, P., and Abdollahi, M. (2013). Preparation and performance evaluations of electrospun poly(ε-caprolactone), poly(lactic acid), and their hybrid (50/50) nanofibrous mats containing thymol as an herbal drug for effective wound healing. *J. Appl. Polym. Sci.* 129, 756–766. doi: 10.1002/app.38683

Kean, T., and Thanou, M. (2010). Biodegradation, biodistribution and toxicity of chitosan. *Adv. Drug Deliv. Rev.* 62, 3–11. doi: 10.1016/j.addr.2009.09.004

Kiani, M. T., Higgins, C. A., and Almquist, B. D. (2018). The Hair follicle: an underutilized source of cells and materials for regenerative medicine. *ACS Biomater. Sci. Eng.* 4, 1193–1207. doi: 10.1021/acsbiomaterials.7b00072

Koh, H. S., Yong, T., Chan, C. K., and Ramakrishna, S. (2008). Enhancement of neurite outgrowth using nano-structured scaffolds coupled with laminin. *Biomaterials* 29, 3574–3582. doi: 10.1016/j.biomaterials.2008.05.014

Kordestani, S. S. (2019). "Wound care management," in *Atlas of Wound Healing* (Elsevier), 31–47. Available online at: https://linkinghub.elsevier.com/retrieve/pii/B9780323679688000057

Krafts, K. P. (2010). Tissue repair: the hidden drama. *Organogenesis* 6, 225–233. doi: 10.4161/org.6.4.12555

Kryczka, J., and Boncela, J. (2015). Leukocytes: the double-edged sword in fibrosis. *Mediators Inflamm.* 2015, 1–10. doi: 10.1155/2015/652035

Lagaron, J. M., Solouk, A., Castro, S., and Echegoyen, Y. (2017). "Biomedical applications of electrospinning, innovations, and products," in *Electrospun Materials for Tissue Engineering and Biomedical Applications*, eds T. Uyar and E. Kny (Elsevier; Woodhead Publishing), 57–72. doi: 10.1016/B978-0-08-101022-8.00010-7

Li, B., and Wang, J. H.-C. (2011). Fibroblasts and myofibroblasts in wound healing: force generation and measurement. *J. Tissue Viability* 20, 108–120. doi: 10.1016/j.jtv.2009.11.004

Li, Z., Wang, H., Yang, B., Sun, Y., and Huo, R. (2015). Three-dimensional graphene foams loaded with bone marrow derived mesenchymal stem cells promote skin wound healing with reduced scarring. *Mater. Sci. Eng. C* 57, 181–188. doi: 10.1016/j.msec.2015.07.062

Liao, Y., Zhang, L., Gao, Y., Zhu, Z.-T., and Fong, H. (2009). Preparation, characterization, and encapsulation/release studies of a composite nanofiber mat electrospun from an emulsion containing poly (lactic-co-glycolic acid). *Polymer* 49, 5294–5299. doi: 10.1016/j.polymer.2008.09.045

Lim, X., Tateya, I., Tateya, T., Muñoz-Del-Río, A., and Bless, D. M. (2006). Immediate inflammatory response and scar formation in wounded vocal folds. *Ann. Otol. Rhinol. Laryngol.* 115, 21–929. doi: 10.1177/000348940611 501212

Longaker, M. T., Gurtner, G. C., Werner, S., and Barrandon, Y. (2008). Wound repair and regeneration. *Nature* 453, 314–321. doi: 10.1038/nature07039

Ma, K., Liao, S., He, L., Lu, J., Ramakrishna, S., and Chan, C. K. (2011). Effects of nanofiber/stem cell composite on wound healing in acute full-thickness skin wounds. *Tissue Eng. Part A* 17, 1413–1424. doi: 10.1089/ten.tea.2010.0373

Ma, L., Yang, G., Wang, N., Zhang, P., Guo, F., Meng, J., et al. (2015). Trap effect of three-dimensional fibers network for high efficient cancer-cell capture. *Adv. Healthc. Mater.* 4, 838–843. doi: 10.1002/adhm.201400650

Machula, H., Ensley, B., and Kellar, R. (2014). Electrospun tropoelastin for delivery of therapeutic adipose-derived stem cells to full-thickness dermal wounds. *Adv. Wound Care* 3, 367–375. doi: 10.1089/wound.2013.0513

Mackool, R. J., Gittes, G. K., and Longaker, M. T. (1998). Scarless healing. The fetal wound. *Clin. Plast. Surg.* 25, 357–365.

Mahjour, S. B., Fu, X., Yang, X., Fong, J., Sefat, F., and Wang, H. (2015). Rapid creation of skin substitutes from human skin cells and biomimetic nanofibers for acute full-thickness wound repair. *Burns* 41, 1764–1774. doi: 10.1016/j.burns.2015.06.011

Marshall, C. D., Hu, M. S., Leavitt, T., Barnes, L. A., Lorenz, H. P., and Longaker, M. T. (2018). Cutaneous scarring: basic science, current treatments, and future directions. *Adv. Wound Care* 7, 29–45. doi: 10.1089/wound.2016.0696

Martinello, T., Gomiero, C., Perazzi, A., Iacopetti, I., Gemignani, F., DeBenedictis, G. M., et al. (2018). Allogeneic mesenchymal stem cells improve the wound healing process of sheep skin. *BMC Vet. Res.* 14:202. doi: 10.1186/s12917-018-1527-8

Mashhadi, S. A., and Loh, C. Y. Y. (2011). A knotless method of securing the subcuticular suture. *Aesthetic Surg. J.* 31, 594–595. doi: 10.1177/1090820X11411080

McCarthy, H. O., McCaffrey, J., McCrudden, C. M., Zholobenko, A., Ali, A. A., McBride, J. W., et al. (2014). Development and characterization of self-assembling nanoparticles using a bio-inspired amphipathic peptide for gene delivery. *J. Control Release* 189, 141–149. doi: 10.1016/j.jconrel.2014.06.048

Mengistu Lemma, S., Bossard, F., and Rinaudo, M. (2016). Preparation of pure and stable chitosan nanofibers by electrospinning in the presence of poly(ethylene oxide). *Int. J. Mol. Sci.* 17:1790. doi: 10.3390/ijms17111790

Mingozzi, F., and High, K. A. (2013). Immune responses to AAV vectors: overcoming barriers to successful gene therapy. *Blood* 122, 23–36. doi: 10.1182/blood-2013-01-306647

Mirastschijski, U., Sander, J. T., Zier, U., Rennekampff, H. O., Weyand, B., and Vogt, P. M. (2015). The cost of post-burn scarring. *Ann. Burns Fire Disasters* 28, 215–222.

Monaco, J. L., and Lawrence, W. T. (2003). Acute wound healing an overview. *Clin. Plast. Surg.* 30, 1–12. doi: 10.1016/S0094-1298(02)00070-6

Montagna, W., and Yun, J. S. (1964). The skin of the domestic pig. *J. Invest. Dermatol.* 42, 11–21. doi: 10.1038/jid.1964.110

Mulholland, E. J., Ali, A., Robson, T., Dunne, N. J., and McCarthy, H. O. (2019). Delivery of RALA/siFKBPL nanoparticles via electrospun bilayer nanofibres: an innovative angiogenic therapy for wound repair. *J. Control Release.* 316, 53–65. doi: 10.1016/j.jconrel.2019.10.050

Nie, H., He, A., Zheng, J., Xu, S., Li, J., and Han, C. C. (2008). Effects of chain conformation and entanglement on the electrospinning of pure alginate. *Biomacromolecules* 9, 1362–1365. doi: 10.1021/bm701349j

Olden, B. R., Cheng, Y., Yu, J. L., and Pun, S. H. (2018). Cationic polymers for non-viral gene delivery to human T cells. *J. Control Release* 282, 140–147 doi: 10.1016/j.jconrel.2018.02.043

Orbay, H., Tobita, M., and Mizuno, H. (2012). Mesenchymal stem cells isolated from adipose and other tissues: basic biological properties and clinical applications. *Stem Cells Int.* 2012:461718. doi: 10.1155/2012/461718

Park, K., Ju, Y. M., Son, J. S., Ahn, K.-D., and Han, D. K. (2007). Surface modification of biodegradable electrospun nanofiber scaffolds and their interaction with fibroblasts. *J. Biomater. Sci. Polym. Ed.* 18, 369–382. doi: 10.1163/156856207780424997

Persano, L., Camposeo, A., Tekmen, C., and Pisignano, D. (2013). Industrial upscaling of electrospinning and applications of polymer nanofibers: a review. *Macromol. Mater. Eng.* 298, 504–520. doi: 10.1002/mame.201200290

Prabhakaran, M. P., Venugopal, J., Chan, C. K., and Ramakrishna, S. (2008). Surface modified electrospun nanofibrous scaffolds for nerve tissue engineering. *Nanotechnology* 19:455102. doi: 10.1088/0957-4484/19/45/455102

Qin, Y. (2016). (Ed.). "Functional wound dressings," in *Woodhead Publishing Series in Textiles, Medical Textile Materials* (Elsevier; Woodhead Publishing), 89–107. doi: 10.1016/B978-0-08-100618-4.00007-8

Quinn, J. A., Yang, Y., Buffington, A. N., Romero, F. N., and Green, M. D. (2018). Preparation and characterization of crosslinked electrospun poly(vinyl alcohol) nanofibrous membranes. *Polymer* 134, 275–281. doi: 10.1016/j.polymer.2017.11.023

Ramachandran, K., and Gouma, P.-I. (2008). Electrospinning for bone tissue engineering. *Recent Pat. Nanotechnol.* 2, 1–7. doi: 10.2174/187221008783478608

Ramakrishna, S., Fujihara, K., Teo, W.-E., Yong, T., Ma, Z., and Ramaseshan, R. (2006). Electrospun nanofibers: solving global issues. *Mater. Today* 9, 40–50. doi: 10.1016/S1369-7021(06)71389-X

Ramirez, H., Patel, S. B., and Pastar, I. (2014). The role of TGFβ signaling in wound epithelialization. *Adv. Wound Care* 3, 482–491. doi: 10.1089/wound.2013.0466

Ramotowski, C., Qu, X., and Villa-Diaz, L. G. (2019). Progress in the use of induced pluripotent stem cell-derived neural cells for traumatic spinal cord injuries in animal populations: meta-analysis and review. *Stem Cells Transl. Med.* 8, 681–693. doi: 10.1002/sctm.18-0225

Redd, M. J., Cooper, L., Wood, W., Stramer, B., and Martin, P. (2004). Wound healing and inflammation: embryos reveal the way to perfect repair. *Philos. Trans. R. Soc. Lond. B Biol. Sci.* 359, 777–784. doi: 10.1098/rstb.2004.1466

REGRANEX® (2018). *REGRANEX® (Becaplermin) Gel for Topical Use. Highlights of Prescribing Information.*

Reiber, G. E., Vileikyte, L., Boyko, E. J., del Aguila, M., Smith, D. G., Lavery, L. A., et al. (1999). Causal pathways for incident lower-extremity ulcers in patients with diabetes from two settings. *Diabetes Care* 22, 157–162. doi: 10.2337/diacare.22.1.157

Ren, G., Zhang, L., Zhao, X., Xu, G., Zhang, Y., Roberts, A. I., et al. (2008). Mesenchymal stem cell-mediated immunosuppression occurs via concerted action of chemokines and nitric oxide. *Cell Stem Cell* 2, 141–150. doi: 10.1016/j.stem.2007.11.014

Sá, O., Lopes, N., Alves, M., and Caran, E. (2018). Effects of glycine on collagen, PDGF, and EGF expression in model of oral mucositis. *Nutrients* 10:1485. doi: 10.3390/nu10101485

Sarrazy, V., Billet, F., Micallef, L., Coulomb, B., and Desmoulière, A. (2011). Mechanisms of pathological scarring: role of myofibroblasts and current developments. *Wound Repair Regen.* 19(Suppl. 1), s10–s15. doi: 10.1111/j.1524-475X.2011.00708.x

Schilling, J. A. (1976). Wound healing. *Surg. Clin. North Am.* 56, 859–874. doi: 10.1016/S0039-6109(16)40983-7

Seaton, M., Hocking, A., and Gibran, N. S. (2015). Porcine models of cutaneous wound healing. *ILAR J.* 56, 127–138. doi: 10.1093/ilar/ilv016

Sencadas, V., Ribeiro, C., Nunes-Pereira, J., Correia, V., and Lanceros-Méndez, S. (2012). Fiber average size and distribution dependence on the electrospinning parameters of poly(vinylidene fluoride–trifluoroethylene) membranes for biomedical applications. *Appl. Phys. A* 109, 685–691. doi: 10.1007/s00339-012-7101-5

Sequeira, R. S., Miguel, S. P., Cabral, C. S. D., Moreira, A. F., Ferreira, P., and Correia, I. J. (2019). Development of a Poly(vinyl alcohol)/Lysine electrospun membrane-based drug delivery system for improved skin regeneration. *Int. J. Pharm.* 570:118640. doi: 10.1016/j.ijpharm.2019.118640

Shalumon, K. T., Anulekha, K. H., Nair, S. V., Nair, S. V., Chennazhi, K. P., and Jayakumar, R. (2011). Sodium alginate/poly(vinyl alcohol)/nano ZnO composite nanofibers for antibacterial wound dressings. *Int. J. Biol. Macromol.* 49, 247–254. doi: 10.1016/j.ijbiomac.2011.04.005

Shan, Y.-H., Peng, L.-H., Liu, X., Chen, X., Xiong, J., and Gao, J.-Q. (2015). Silk fibroin/gelatin electrospun nanofibrous dressing functionalized with astragaloside IV induces healing and anti-scar effects on burn wound. *Int. J. Pharm.* 479, 291–301. doi: 10.1016/j.ijpharm.2014.12.067

Shete, A. S., Yadav, A. V., and Murthy, S. M. (2012). Chitosan and chitosan chlorhydrate based various approaches for enhancement of dissolution rate of carvedilol. *Daru* 20:93. doi: 10.1186/2008-2231-20-93

Singer, A. J., and Clark, R. A. F. (1999). Cutaneous wound healing. *N. Engl. J. Med.* 341, 738–746. doi: 10.1056/NEJM199909023411006

Sotiropoulou, P. A., Perez, S. A., Gritzapis, A. D., Baxevanis, C. N., and Papamichail, M. (2006). Interactions between human mesenchymal stem cells and natural killer cells. *Stem Cells* 24, 74–85. doi: 10.1634/stemcells.2004-0359

Storch, J. E., and Rice, J. (eds.). (2005). *Reconstructive Plastic Surgical Nursing.* Oxford: Blackwell Publishing Ltd. doi: 10.1002/9780470774656

Tanaka, A., Hatoko, M., Tada, H., Iioka, H., Niitsuma, K., and Miyagawa, S. (2004). Expression of p53 family in scars. *J. Dermatol. Sci.* 34, 17–24. doi: 10.1016/j.jdermsci.2003.09.005

Tarun, K., and Gobi, N. (2012). Calcium alginate/PVA blended nano fibre matrix for wound dressing. *Indian J. Fibre Text Res.* 37, 127–132.

Thomas, J. R., and Somenek, M. (2012). Scar revision review. *Arch. Facial Plast. Surg.* 14:162. doi: 10.1001/archfacial.2012.223

van Zuijlen, P. P. M., Ruurda, J. J. B., van Veen, H. A., van Marle, J., van Trier, A. J. M., Groenevelt, F., et al. (2003). Collagen morphology in human skin and scar tissue: no adaptations in response to mechanical loading at joints. *Burns* 29, 423–431. doi: 10.1016/S0305-4179(03)00052-4

Venkat, P., Shen, Y., Chopp, M., and Chen, J. (2018). Cell-based and pharmacological neurorestorative therapies for ischemic stroke. *Neuropharmacology* 134, 310–322. doi: 10.1016/j.neuropharm.2017.08.036

Wakuda, Y., Nishimoto, S., Suye, S., and Fujita, S. (2018). Native collagen hydrogel nanofibres with anisotropic structure using core-shell electrospinning. *Sci. Rep.* 8:6248. doi: 10.1038/s41598-018-24700-9

Wang, L., Yang, J., Ran, B., Yang, X., Zheng, W., Long, Y., et al. (2017). Small molecular TGF-β1-inhibitor-loaded electrospun fibrous scaffolds for preventing hypertrophic scars. *ACS Appl. Mater. Interfaces* 9, 32545–32553. doi: 10.1021/acsami.7b09796

Wang, M., Xiao, Y., Lin, L., Zhu, X., Du, L., and Shi, X. (2018). A microfluidic chip integrated with hyaluronic acid-functionalized electrospun chitosan nanofibers for specific capture and nondestructive release of CD44-overexpressing circulating tumor cells. *Bioconjug. Chem.* 29, 1081–1090. doi: 10.1021/acs.bioconjchem.7b00747

Wang, X., Ge, J., Tredget, E. E., and Wu, Y. (2013). The mouse excisional wound splinting model, including applications for stem cell transplantation. *Nat. Protoc.* 8, 302–309. doi: 10.1038/nprot.2013.002

Wei, Q., Xu, F., Xu, X., Geng, X., Ye, L., Zhang, A., et al. (2016). The multifunctional wound dressing with core-shell structured fibers prepared by coaxial electrospinning. *Front. Mater. Sci.* 10, 113–121. doi: 10.1007/s11706-016-0339-7

Werner, S., and Grose, R. (2003). Regulation of wound healing by growth factors and cytokines. *Physiol. Rev.* 83, 835–870. doi: 10.1152/physrev.2003.83.3.835

White, W., Brody, G. S., Glaser, A. A., Marangoni, R. D., Beckwith, T. G., Must, J. S., et al. (1971). Tensiometric studies of unwounded and wounded skin. *Ann. Surg.* 173, 19–25. doi: 10.1097/00000658-197101000-00003

Williams, A. R., Suncion, V. Y., McCall, F., Guerra, D., Mather, J., Zambrano, J. P., et al. (2013). Durable scar size reduction due to allogeneic mesenchymal stem cell therapy regulates whole-chamber remodeling. *J. Am. Heart Assoc.* 2:e000140. doi: 10.1161/JAHA.113.000140

Wu, J., and Hong, Y. (2016). Enhancing cell infiltration of electrospun fibrous scaffolds in tissue regeneration. *Bioact. Mater.* 1, 56–64. doi: 10.1016/j.bioactmat.2016.07.001

Xie, Q., Jia, L., Xu, H., Hu, X., Wang, W., and Jia, J. (2016). Fabrication of core-shell PEI/pBMP2-PLGA electrospun scaffold for gene delivery to periodontal ligament stem cells. *Stem Cells Int.* 2016, 1–11. doi: 10.1155/2016/5385137

Yan, D., Jones, J., Yuan, X., Xu, X., Sheng, J., Lee, J. C. M., et al. (2013). Plasma treatment of random and aligned electrospun PCL nanofibers. *J. Med. Biol. Eng.* 33, 171–178. doi: 10.5405/jmbe.1072

Yang, X., Yang, J., Wang, L., Ran, B., Jia, Y., Zhang, L., et al. (2017). Pharmaceutical intermediate-modified gold nanoparticles: against multidrug-resistant bacteria and wound-healing application via an electrospun scaffold. *ACS Nano* 11, 5737–5745. doi: 10.1021/acsnano.7b01240

Yang, X. H., Xiao, Y. Y., Tan, T. X., Luo, J. J., Fan, P. J., and Lei, S. R. (2016). C-jun is increased in hypertrophic scar and inhibits apoptosis in fibroblasts. *Int. J. Clin. Exp. Med.* 9, 3132–3138.

Yang, Y., Xia, T., Chen, F., Wei, W., Liu, C., He, S., et al. (2012). Electrospun fibers with plasmid bFGF polyplex loadings promote skin wound healing in diabetic rats. *Mol. Pharm.* 9, 48–58. doi: 10.1021/mp200246b

Younes, I., Frachet, V., Rinaudo, M., Jellouli, K., and Nasri, M. (2016). Cytotoxicity of chitosans with different acetylation degrees and molecular weights on bladder carcinoma cells. *Int. J. Biol. Macromol.* 84, 200–207. doi: 10.1016/j.ijbiomac.2015.09.031

Yuan, T. T., DiGeorge Foushee, A. M., Johnson, M. C., Jockheck-Clark, A. R., and Stahl, J. M. (2018). Development of electrospun chitosan-polyethylene oxide/fibrinogen biocomposite for potential wound healing applications. *Nanoscale Res. Lett.* 13:88. doi: 10.1186/s11671-018-2491-8

Zamani, M., Prabhakaran, M. P., and Ramakrishna, S. (2013). Advances in drug delivery via electrospun and electrosprayed nanomaterials. *Int. J. Nanomedicine* 8, 2997–3017. doi: 10.2147/IJN.S43575

Zhang, N., Deng, Y., Tai, Q., Cheng, B., Zhao, L., Shen, Q., et al. (2012). Electrospun TiO_2 nanofiber-based cell capture assay for detecting circulating tumor cells from colorectal and gastric cancer patients. *Adv. Mater.* 24, 2756–2760. doi: 10.1002/adma.201200155

Zhao, G., Bao, X., Huang, G., Xu, F., and Zhang, X. (2019). Differential effects of directional cyclic stretching on the functionalities of engineered cardiac tissues. *ACS Appl. Biol. Mater.* 2, 3508–3519. doi: 10.1021/acsabm.9b00414

Ziade, M., Domergue, S., Batifol, D., Jreige, R., Sebbane, M., Goudot, P., et al. (2013). Use of botulinum toxin type A to improve treatment of facial wounds: a prospective randomised study. *J. Plast. Reconstr. Aesthet. Surg.* 66, 209–214. doi: 10.1016/j.bjps.2012.09.012

Ziyadeh, N., Fife, D., Walker, A. M., Wilkinson, G. S., and Seeger, J. D. (2011). A matched cohort study of the risk of cancer in users of becaplermin. *Adv. Skin Wound Care* 24, 31–39. doi: 10.1097/01.ASW.0000392922.30229.b3

14

Parameter-Dependency of Low-Intensity Vibration for Wound Healing in Diabetic Mice

*Rita E. Roberts[1,2,3], Onur Bilgen[4], Rhonda D. Kineman[3,5] and Timothy J. Koh[1,2,3]**

[1] Department of Kinesiology and Nutrition, University of Illinois at Chicago, Chicago, IL, United States, [2] Center for Tissue Repair and Regeneration, University of Illinois at Chicago, Chicago, IL, United States, [3] Jesse Brown VA Medical Center, Chicago, IL, United States, [4] Department of Mechanical and Aerospace Engineering, Rutgers University, Piscataway, NJ, United States, [5] Department of Medicine, Section of Endocrinology, Diabetes and Metabolism, University of Illinois at Chicago, Chicago, IL, United States

***Correspondence:**
Timothy J. Koh
tjkoh@uic.edu

Chronic wounds in diabetic patients represent an escalating health problem, leading to significant morbidity and mortality. Our group previously reported that whole body low-intensity vibration (LIV) can improve angiogenesis and wound healing in diabetic mice. The purpose of the current study was to determine whether effects of LIV on wound healing are frequency and/or amplitude dependent. Wound healing was assessed in diabetic (db/db) mice exposed to one of four LIV protocols with different combinations of two acceleration magnitudes (0.3 and 0.6 g) and two frequencies (45 and 90 Hz) or in non-vibration sham controls. The low acceleration, low frequency protocol (0.3 g and 45 Hz) was the only one that improved wound healing, increasing angiogenesis and granulation tissue formation, leading to accelerated re-epithelialization and wound closure. Other protocols had little to no impact on healing with some evidence that 0.6 g accelerations negatively affected wound closure. The 0.3 g, 45 Hz protocol also increased levels of insulin-like growth factor-1 and tended to increase levels of vascular endothelial growth factor in wounds, but had no effect on levels of basic fibroblast growth factor or platelet derived growth factor-bb, indicating that this LIV protocol induces specific growth factors during wound healing. Our findings demonstrate parameter-dependent effects of LIV for improving wound healing that can be exploited for future mechanistic and therapeutic studies.

Keywords: low-intensity vibration, wound healing, angiogenesis, growth factors, diabetes

INTRODUCTION

Chronic wounds represent an escalating health problem around the world, especially in diabetic patients. Over 415 million people (8.3% of the world's adult population) are afflicted with diabetes and associated complications, including chronic wounds (Chatterjee et al., 2017). People with diabetes incur a 25% lifetime risk of developing chronic wounds, which often lead to amputation, resulting in decreased quality of life, high morbidity and mortality (Ramsey et al., 1999; Jeffcoate and Harding, 2003; Hoffstad et al., 2015). Wound healing typically occurs through overlapping phases of inflammation, proliferation and remodeling (Koh and DiPietro, 2011; Eming et al., 2014). Although chronic wounds are known to exhibit defects in each phase of healing, including dysregulated inflammation, impaired perfusion and neovascularization, and poor tissue maturation (Blakytny and Jude, 2006), few therapies are available to improve healing of diabetic wounds.

Energy-based modalities are often used in conjunction with standard treatments for hard to heal chronic wounds. These treatments use laser, electrical, or mechanical stimulation, in an attempt to modify the cellular and biochemical environment to improve angiogenesis and healing (Ennis et al., 2016; Game et al., 2016; Sousa and Batista Kde, 2016). Recently, our group demonstrated that whole body low-intensity vibration (LIV) can improve angiogenesis and wound healing in diabetic mice, potentially by increasing growth factors such as insulin-like growth factor (IGF)-1 and vascular endothelial growth factor (VEGF) in the wound (Weinheimer-Haus et al., 2014). In addition, we and others have demonstrated that LIV can rapidly increase systemic and regional (i.e., skin) blood flow (Nakagami et al., 2007; Maloney-Hinds et al., 2008; Tzen et al., 2018; Zhu et al., 2020) and can inhibit progression of pressure ulcers (Arashi et al., 2010; Sari et al., 2015). However, much remains to be learned about how LIV signals influence different aspects of wound healing.

The purpose of the current study was to identify LIV amplitudes and frequencies that promote healing in diabetic mice. The hypothesis of this study was that effects of LIV on wound healing are frequency and amplitude dependent.

MATERIALS AND METHODS

Animals

Diabetic db/db mice (BKS.Cg-Dock7m+/+Leprdb/J) were obtained from the Jackson Laboratory. Experiments were performed on 12–16 weeks-old male mice. Only mice with fasting blood glucose >250 mg/dl were included in the study. Mice were housed in environmentally controlled conditions with a 12-h light/dark cycle. Water and food were available *ad libitum*. Two wounds from each of four mice were analyzed for each assay (N = 8 total for each assay). To minimize bias, mice were randomly assigned to experimental groups and resulting samples were coded and analyzed in a blinded fashion. All procedures involving animals were approved by the Animal Care Committee at the Jesse Brown Veterans' Affairs Medical Center [OLAW Assurance number D16-00722 (A4456-01)].

Excisional Wounding

Mice were subjected to excisional wounding as described previously (Weinheimer-Haus et al., 2014). Briefly, mice were anesthetized with isoflurane and their dorsum was shaved and cleaned with alcohol. Four 8 mm wounds were made on the back of each mouse with a dermal biopsy punch and covered with Tegaderm (3M, Minneapolis, MN, United States) to keep the wounds moist and maintain consistency with treatment of human wounds.

Low-Intensity Vibration

Following wounding, mice were randomly assigned to one of four whole-body LIV treatment groups or to a non-vibration sham (control) group. LIV treatment groups utilized different combinations of low (45 Hz) and high (90 Hz) frequencies and low (0.3 g) and high (0.6 g) peak accelerations. Harmonic LIV signals were calibrated using an accelerometer attached directly to top surface of the vibrating plate (Weinheimer-Haus et al., 2014). For LIV treatment, mice were placed in an empty cage directly on a vibrating plate, and LIV was applied for 30 min per day for 7 days/week starting on the day of wounding [cf (Weinheimer-Haus et al., 2014) for image of set-up]. Non-vibrated sham controls were similarly placed in a separate empty cage but were not subjected to LIV.

Wound Closure

Wound closure was assessed in digital images of the external wound surface taken immediately after injury and on days 3, 6, and 10 post-injury. Wound area was measured using Fiji Image J and expressed as a percentage of the area immediately after injury.

Wound Histology

Skin wounds were collected from the pelt of each animal on day 10 post-injury, followed by embedding in tissue freezing medium and freezing in isopentane cooled with dry ice. Each wound was cryosectioned from one edge to well past the center and 10-μm sections were selected from the center of the wound for staining and analysis of re-epithelialization, granulation tissue formation, angiogenesis and collagen deposition (Weinheimer-Haus et al., 2014). For all wound healing analyses, digital images were obtained using a Keyence BZ-X710 microscope with 2×/0.10 or 20×/0.75 Nikon objectives and BZ-X Analyzer software.

Re-Epithelialization and Granulation Tissue Area

Wound re-epithelialization and granulation tissue area were assessed by morphometric analysis of hematoxylin and eosin stained cryosections from the wound center (Weinheimer-Haus et al., 2014). The distance between the wound edges, defined by the distance between the first hair follicle encountered at each end of the wound, and the distance that the epithelium had traversed into the wound, were measured using image analysis software. Re-epithelialization was then calculated as: [(distance traversed by epithelium)/(distance between wound edges) × 100]. Granulation tissue area was measured as the area of new tissue formation between wound edges. Re-epithelialization and granulation tissue area were measured in three sections per wound and was averaged over sections to provide a representative value for each wound.

Angiogenesis and Collagen Deposition

Dermal healing was assessed using immunohistochemical staining for platelet-derived endothelial cell adhesion molecule-1 (also called CD31) for angiogenesis and Masson's trichrome stain for collagen deposition (Weinheimer-Haus et al., 2014). For angiogenesis assessment, sections were first air-dried, fixed in cold acetone, washed with PBS, quenched with 0.3% hydrogen peroxide, then washed again with PBS. Sections were blocked with buffer containing 3% bovine serum albumin and then incubated overnight with CD31 antibody (1:100, Biolegend, San Diego, CA, United States). Sections were then washed with PBS and incubated with biotinylated anti-rat secondary antibody (1:200, Vector Laboratories, Burlingame, CA, United States). After a wash with PBS, sections were incubated with avidin D-horseradish peroxidase (1:1000) and developed with a 3-amino-9-ethylcarbazole kit (Vector Laboratories). Image J was used to quantify the percentage of CD31-stained area relative to the total area of the wound bed. For each assay, digital images covering the majority of the wound bed (usually three images at ×20 magnification) were first obtained. The percent area stained in each image was then quantified by counting the number of pixels staining above a threshold intensity and normalizing to the total number of pixels. Threshold intensity was set such that only clearly stained pixels were counted. The software allowed the observer to exclude staining identified as artifact, large vessels, and areas deemed to be outside the wound bed. For trichrome analysis, staining was performed according to the manufacturer's directions (IMEB, San Marcos, CA, United States), and Image J was used to quantify the percentage of blue collagen-stained area relative to the total area of the wound bed. For both trichrome and CD31 staining, three sections per wound were analyzed, and data were averaged over sections to provide a representative value for each wound.

ELISA

Wounds were snap frozen and stored in LN2 and then homogenized in cold PBS (10 μl of PBS per mg wound tissue) supplemented with protease inhibitor cocktail (Sigma Aldrich, St. Louis, MO, United States) using a dounce homogenizer and then centrifuged. Supernatants were used for enzyme-linked immunoassay of IGF-1, VEGF, basic fibroblast growth factor (bFGF) and platelet derived growth factor (PDGF)-bb (R&D Systems, Minneapolis, MN, United States).

Statistics

Values are reported as means $\pm$ standard deviation. Measurements of wound healing or wound growth factors were compared between treatment groups using one-way ANOVA. Dunnett's multiple comparisons test was used when ANOVAs demonstrated significance. Differences between groups were considered significant if $P \leq 0.05$.

RESULTS

LIV Promotes Wound Closure in a Parameter Dependent Fashion

Mice were treated with one of four LIV protocols: low (45 Hz) frequency, low (0.3 g) acceleration (LL), high (90 Hz) frequency, high (0.6 g) acceleration (HH), low frequency, high acceleration (LH) or high frequency, low acceleration (HL) (**Table 1**). Consistent with our previous study (Weinheimer-Haus et al., 2014), none of the protocols in the current study altered blood glucose levels of the diabetic db/db mice (data not shown). The LL protocol was the only one to increase external measurements of wound closure on days 6 and 10 post-injury compared to sham control, whereas the LH and HH protocols decreased wound closure at all time points (**Figure 1**). Similarly, the LL protocol was the only one to increase histological measurements of re-epithelialization on day 10 post-injury compared to sham control, whereas the LH and HH protocols decreased re-epithelialization (**Figure 1**). In short, the LL protocol improved wound closure in diabetic mice, whereas the LH and HH protocols impaired wound closure.

TABLE 1 | LIV protocols.

	LL	LH	HL	HH
Acceleration (g)	0.3	0.6	0.3	0.6
Frequency (Hz)	45	45	90	90

LL, low acceleration, low frequency; LH, low acceleration, high frequency; HL, high acceleration, low frequency; HH, high acceleration, high frequency.

LIV Promotes Wound Angiogenesis and Granulation Tissue Formation in a Parameter Dependent Fashion

Similar to the wound closure measurements, the LL protocol was the only LIV protocol to increase granulation tissue area on day 10 post-injury compared to sham controls (bar graph in **Figure 2**, example images in **Figure 1**). The other protocols produced no significant change in granulation tissue area. In addition, only the LL protocol induced a robust increase in angiogenesis on day 10 as assessed by CD31 staining compared to sham controls (**Figure 2**). The other protocols produced no significant change in angiogenesis. In short, the LL protocol improved angiogenesis and granulation tissue formation in diabetic mice, whereas the other protocols had no effect.

LIV Enhances Wound IGF-1 Levels in a Parameter Dependent Fashion

Associated with the accelerated re-epithelialization and dermal healing, the LL protocol significantly increased levels of IGF-1 and tended to increase levels of VEGF in wounds on day 10 post-injury compared to sham controls (**Figure 3**). The other protocols did not alter wound levels of IGF-1 or VEGF. In addition, none of the LIV protocols altered wound levels of either bFGF or PDGF-bb. Thus, LIV induces specific growth factors during wound healing in a parameter dependent fashion.

DISCUSSION

Despite the escalating socioeconomic impact of diabetic wounds, effective treatments remain elusive. In this study, we sought to determine the parameter dependency of a novel therapeutic approach to improve diabetic wound healing using whole-body LIV. The major finding of this study is that only LIV with relatively low frequency (45 Hz) and low acceleration levels (0.3 g) improve wound healing in diabetic mice. Compared to non-vibrated control mice, such LIV treatment increased

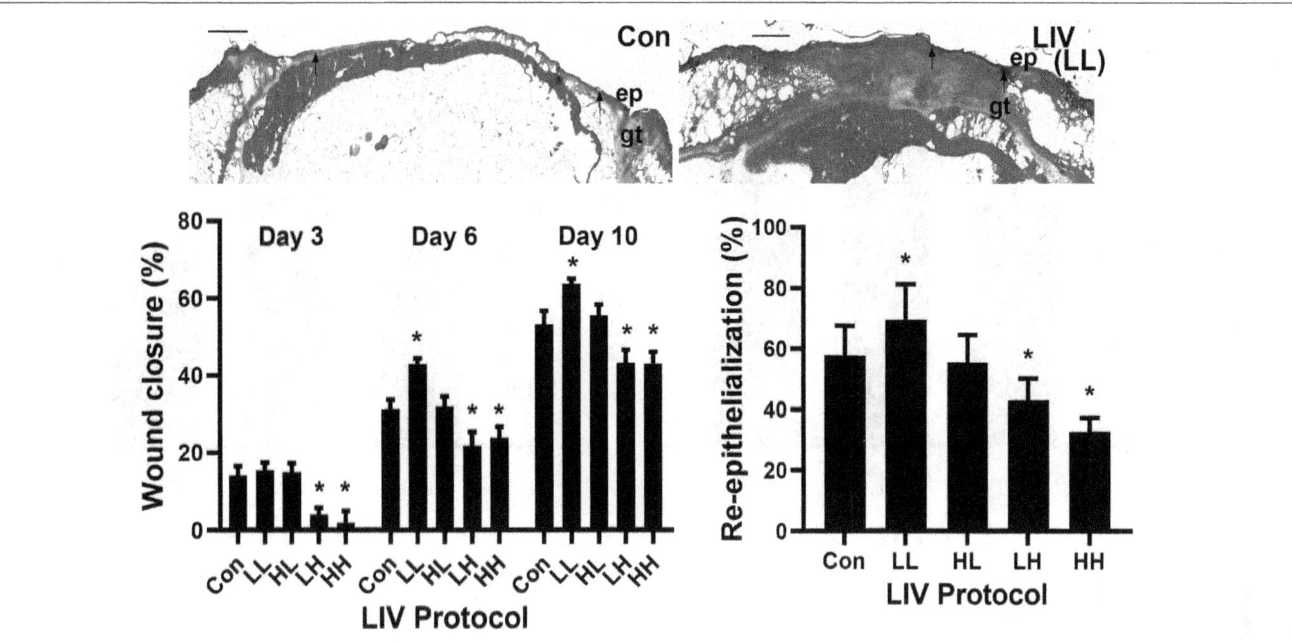

FIGURE 1 | Parameter dependency of low-intensity vibration (LIV) for improving wound closure. Mice either received one of four protocols of whole-body LIV: 0.3 g at 45 Hz (LL), 0.3 g at 90 Hz (LH), 1.0 g at 45 Hz (HL), 1.0 g at 90 Hz (HH) or sham control treatment (Con) for 30 min per day, starting the day of wounding for 5 days per week. Left: Wound closure was measured in digital images of wound surface on days 3, 6, and 10 post-injury. Right: Re-epithelialization was measured in hematoxylin and eosin stained sections from center of day 10 wounds. Top: Representative images of hematoxylin and eosin stained sections; arrows mark ends of epithelial tongues growing into wound, ep = epithelium, gt = granulation tissue, scale bar = 500 μm. Two wounds from each of four mice were analyzed for each assay (N = 8 total for each assay). *Mean value significantly different from that of Con for same time point, $P \leq 0.05$.

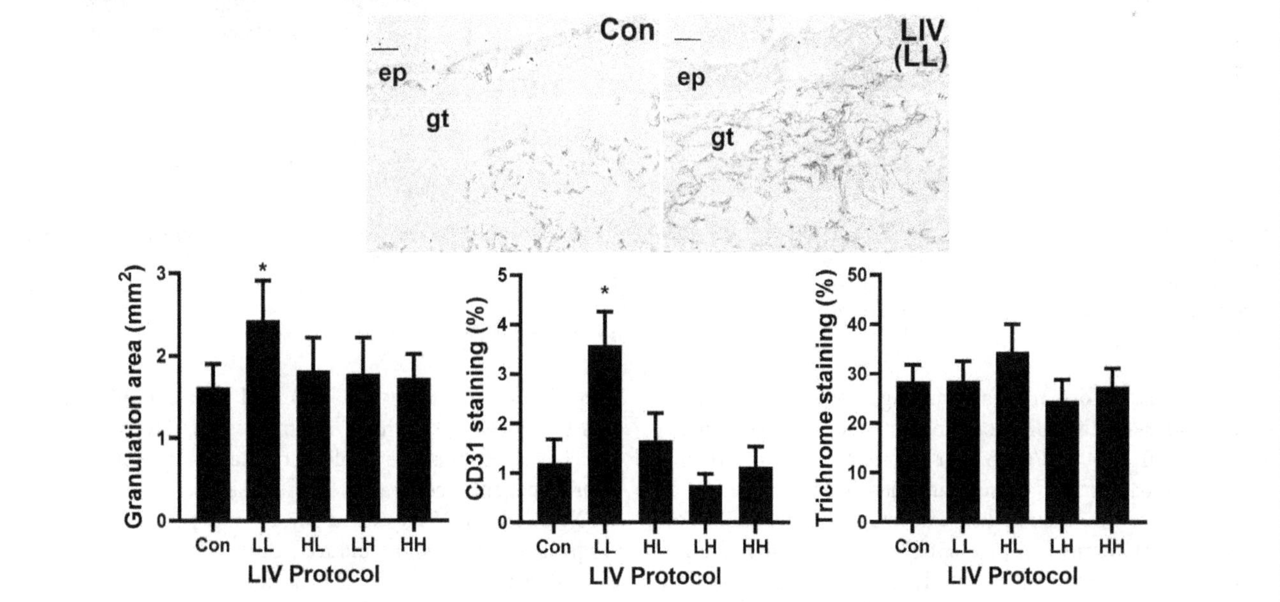

FIGURE 2 | Parameter dependency of low-intensity vibration (LIV) for improving granulation and angiogenesis. Mice either received one of four protocols of whole-body LIV: 0.3 g at 45 Hz (LL), 0.3 g at 90 Hz (LH), 1.0 g at 45 Hz (HL), 1.0 g at 90 Hz (HH) or sham control treatment (Con) for 30 min per day, starting the day of wounding for 5 days per week. Left: Granulation tissue thickness was measured as the area of granulation tissue divided by the distance between wound edges in hematoxylin and eosin stained sections from center of day 10 wounds. Center: Angiogenesis was measured as percent area stained with antibody against CD31 in sections from center of day 10 wounds. Top: Representative images of CD31 stained sections; ep, epithelium; gt, granulation tissue; scale bar = 50 μm. Right: Collagen deposition assessed as percent area stained blue in Trichrome stained sections of center of day 10 wounds. Two wounds from each of four mice were analyzed for each assay (N = 8 total for each assay). *Mean value significantly different from that of Con, $P \leq 0.05$.

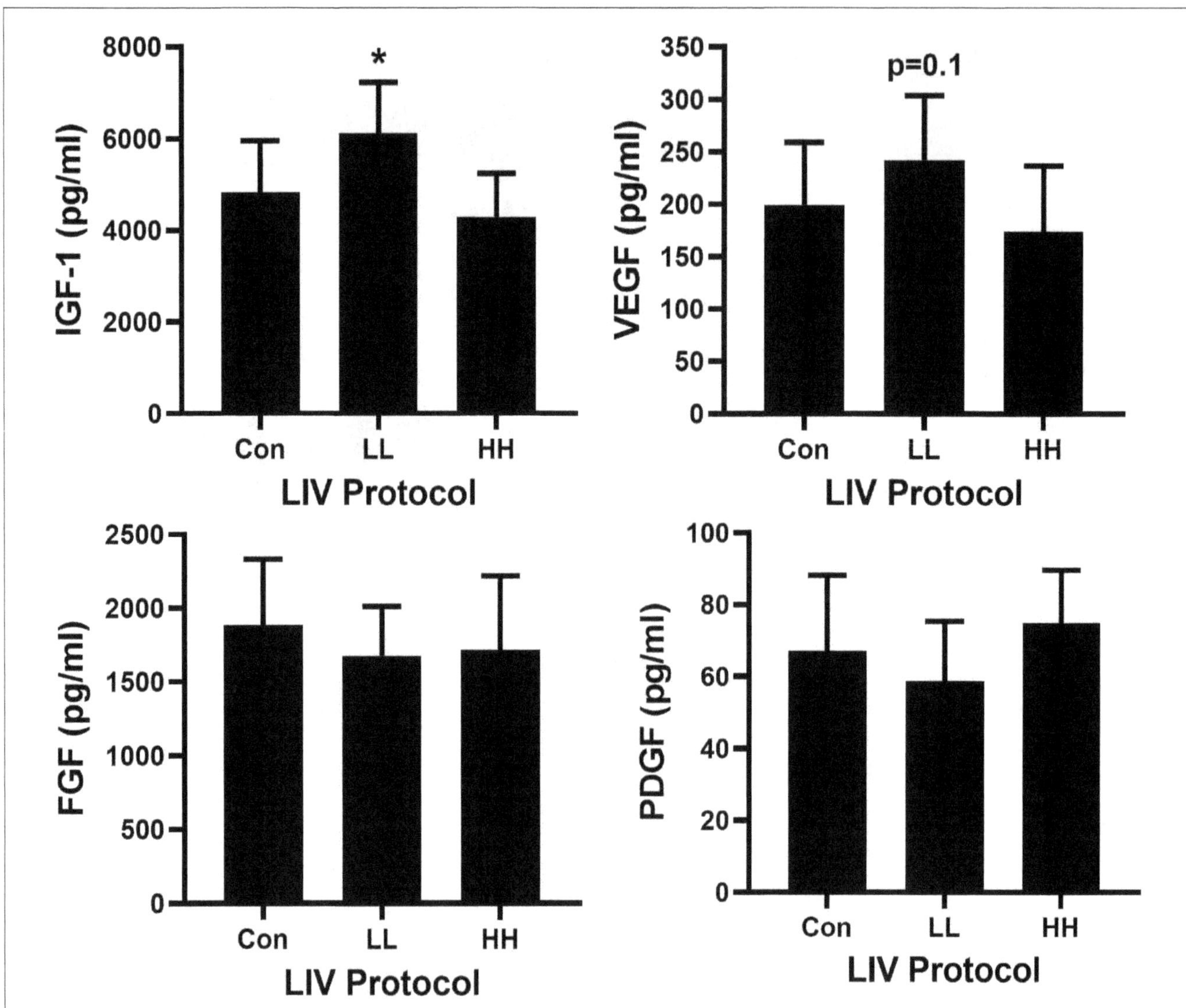

FIGURE 3 | Parameter dependency of low-intensity vibration (LIV) for increasing IGF-1 in wounds. Mice either received one of two protocols of whole-body LIV: 0.3 *g* at 45 Hz (LL), 1.0 g at 90 Hz (HH) or sham control treatment (Con) for 30 min per day, starting the day of wounding for 5 days per week. Protein levels of IGF-1, VEGF, FGF-b, and PDGF-bb measured in homogenates of day 10 wounds using ELISA. Two wounds from each of four mice were analyzed for each assay ($N = 8$ total for each assay). *Mean value significantly different from that of Con, $P \leq 0.05$.

granulation tissue formation and angiogenesis, and accelerated closure and re-epithelialization. In contrast, LIV with higher frequency (90 Hz) and/or higher acceleration levels (0.6 g) tended to impair wound closure and had little to no effect on angiogenesis or granulation tissue formation. Thus, LIV does indeed exhibit parameter-dependent effects on wound healing.

The results of the current study are consistent with our previous study, in which we reported that LIV with 45 Hz frequency and 0.4 g acceleration increased angiogenesis, granulation tissue formation, and re-epithelialization (Weinheimer-Haus et al., 2014). This protocol was similar to our LL protocol (45 Hz frequency, 0.3 g acceleration). In addition, data in the present study demonstrates that protocols with higher frequency and/or acceleration do not improve skin healing. Related studies on the effect of LIV with similar frequency (47 Hz) and acceleration (0.2 g) on pressure ulcers (3.15 min treatments per day) demonstrated that LIV can improve healing of stage I pressure ulcers in elderly patients compared to standard care (Arashi et al., 2010). Similar LIV treatment for 15 min per day also reduced progression of pressure induced deep tissue injury associated with downregulation of matrix metalloproteinase-2 and -9 activity in rats (Sari et al., 2015).

A number of studies have focused on the effects of vibrations on skin blood flow in both rodents and humans, which could influence wound healing along with other physiological processes. LIV with frequency of 47 Hz and unknown acceleration increased skin blood flow measured by intravital microscopy of the mouse ear in what appears to be a nitric oxide dependent manner (Nakagami et al., 2007;

Ichioka et al., 2011). A series of studies has also shown that vibrations can increase skin blood flow as measured by laser Doppler flowmetry when vibrations were applied to the forearm or lower leg in healthy human participants or diabetic patients (Lohman et al., 2007; Maloney-Hinds et al., 2009; Johnson et al., 2014). These latter studies used frequencies between 30 and 50 Hz and accelerations between 6 and 7 g, and found no difference in skin blood flow response between 30 and 50 Hz protocols (Maloney-Hinds et al., 2008). These protocols may be considered high-intensity vibration, since LIV is typically considered to utilize accelerations <1.0 g. We performed a similar experiment using LIV with frequency of 30 Hz and accelerations of 0.4 g and found that LIV signals also increase lower leg skin blood flow in healthy human participants but this effect only lasts while LIV is applied (Tzen et al., 2018). A recent study compared LIV protocols with frequencies of 35 and 100 Hz and an amplitude of 1 mm and found that the 100 Hz protocol produced larger increase in skin blood flow over the first metatarsal head (Zhu et al., 2020). Finally, recent systematic reviews have provided additional evidence that vibration can increase blood flow in the lower extremities in diabetic patients (Sa-Caputo et al., 2017; Gomes-Neto et al., 2019). These studies support the translation of LIV into a treatment that can improve wound healing in human patients.

Limitations of this study include the small number of parameters tested; two frequencies and two accelerations. However, our finding that only the 45 Hz, 0.3 g protocol improved wound healing narrows the solution space for pro-healing parameters. The parameters were measured at the surface of the vibrating plate; the actual vibrations experienced by the wound could be different and would be extremely difficult to measure. In addition, although we have identified growth factors that are increased by LIV and are associated with angiogenesis, granulation tissue formation and closure, the precise mechanisms involved remain to be elucidated. Along the same lines, although we assessed effects of LIV on re-epithelialization, granulation and angiogenesis, more detailed analysis of the effects of LIV on wound cells, including keratinocytes, fibroblasts, endothelial cells and inflammatory cells awaits further study.

In summary, our findings demonstrate parameter-dependent effects of LIV for improving wound healing and only LIV with 45 Hz frequency and 0.3 g acceleration levels increased angiogenesis, granulation tissue formation and re-epithelialization associated with increased wound levels of IGF-1. Importantly, the LIV protocol could easily be translated to clinical trials for diabetic patients with chronic wounds.

AUTHOR CONTRIBUTIONS

RR helped design the study, performed experiments, and wrote the manuscript. OB, RK, and TK helped design the study and write the manuscript. All authors contributed to the article and approved the submitted version.

REFERENCES

Arashi, M., Sugama, J., Sanada, H., Konya, C., Okuwa, M., Nakagami, G., et al. (2010). Vibration therapy accelerates healing of Stage I pressure ulcers in older adult patients. *Adv. Skin Wound Care* 23, 321–327. doi: 10.1097/01.ASW.0000383752.39220.fb

Blakytny, R., and Jude, E. (2006). The molecular biology of chronic wounds and delayed healing in diabetes. *Diabet Med.* 23, 594–608. doi: 10.1111/j.1464-5491.2006.01773.x

Chatterjee, S., Khunti, K., and Davies, M. J. (2017). Type 2 diabetes. *Lancet* 389, 2239–2251. doi: 10.1016/S0140-6736(17)30058-2

Eming, S. A., Martin, P., and Tomic-Canic, M. (2014). Wound repair and regeneration: mechanisms, signaling, and translation. *Sci. Transl. Med.* 6:265sr6. doi: 10.1126/scitranslmed.3009337

Ennis, W. J., Lee, C., Gellada, K., Corbiere, T. F., and Koh, T. J. (2016). Advanced Technologies to Improve Wound Healing: Electrical Stimulation, Vibration Therapy, and Ultrasound-What Is the Evidence? *Plast Reconstr. Surg.* 138(3 Suppl.), 94S–104S. doi: 10.1097/PRS.0000000000002680

Game, F. L., Apelqvist, J., Attinger, C., Hartemann, A., Hinchliffe, R. J., Londahl, M., et al. (2016). Effectiveness of interventions to enhance healing of chronic ulcers of the foot in diabetes: a systematic review. *Diabetes Metab. Res. Rev.* 32(Suppl. 1), 154–168. doi: 10.1002/dmrr.2707

Gomes-Neto, M., de Sa-Caputo, D. D. C., Paineiras-Domingos, L. L., Brandao, A. A., Neves, M. F., Marin, P. J., et al. (2019). Effects of Whole-Body Vibration in Older Adult Patients With Type 2 Diabetes Mellitus: A Systematic Review and Meta-Analysis. *Can. J. Diabetes* 43, 524–529e2. doi: 10.1016/j.jcjd.2019.03.008

Hoffstad, O., Mitra, N., Walsh, J., and Margolis, D. J. (2015). Diabetes, lower-extremity amputation, and death. *Diabetes Care* 38, 1852–1857. doi: 10.2337/dc15-0536

Ichioka, S., Yokogawa, H., Nakagami, G., Sekiya, N., and Sanada, H. (2011). In vivo analysis of skin microcirculation and the role of nitric oxide during vibration. *Ostomy Wound Manag.* 57, 40–47.

Jeffcoate, W. J., and Harding, K. G. (2003). Diabetic foot ulcers. *Lancet* 361, 1545–1551. doi: 10.1016/S0140-6736(03)13169-8

Johnson, P. K., Feland, J. B., Johnson, A. W., Mack, G. W., and Mitchell, U. H. (2014). Effect of whole body vibration on skin blood flow and nitric oxide production. *J. Diabetes. Sci. Technol.* 8, 889–894. doi: 10.1177/1932296814536289

Koh, T. J., and DiPietro, L. A. (2011). Inflammation and wound healing: the role of the macrophage. *Exp. Rev. Mol. Med.* 13:e23. doi: 10.1017/S1462399411001943

Lohman, E. B. III, Petrofsky, J. S., Maloney-Hinds, C., Betts-Schwab, H., and Thorpe, D. (2007). The effect of whole body vibration on lower extremity skin blood flow in normal subjects. *Med. Sci. Monit.* 13, CR71–CR76.

Maloney-Hinds, C., Petrofsky, J. S., and Zimmerman, G. (2008). The effect of 30 Hz vs. 50 Hz passive vibration and duration of vibration on skin blood flow in the arm. *Med. Sci. Monit* 14, CR112–CR116.

Maloney-Hinds, C., Petrofsky, J. S., Zimmerman, G., and Hessinger, D. A. (2009). The role of nitric oxide in skin blood flow increases due to vibration in healthy adults and adults with type 2 diabetes. *Diabetes Technol. Ther.* 11, 39–43. doi: 10.1089/dia.2008.0011

Nakagami, G., Sanada, H., Matsui, N., Kitagawa, A., Yokogawa, H., Sekiya, N., et al. (2007). Effect of vibration on skin blood flow in an in vivo microcirculatory model. *Biosci. Trends* 1, 161–166.

Ramsey, S. D., Newton, K., Blough, D., McCulloch, D. K., Sandhu, N., Reiber, G. E., et al. (1999). Incidence, outcomes, and cost of foot ulcers in patients with diabetes. *Diabetes Care* 22, 382–387.

Sa-Caputo, D., Paineiras-Domingos, L., Carvalho-Lima, R., Dias-Costa, G., de Paiva, P. C., de Azeredo, C. F., et al. (2017). Potential Effects of Whole-Body Vibration Exercises on Blood Flow Kinetics of Different Populations: A Systematic Review with a Suitable Approach. *Afr. J. Tradit Complement Altern Med.* 14(4 Suppl.), 41–51. doi: 10.21010/ajtcam.v14i4S.6

Sari, Y., Sanada, H., Minematsu, T., Nakagami, G., Nagase, T., Huang, L., et al. (2015). Vibration inhibits deterioration in rat deep-tissue injury through HIF1-MMP axis. *Wound Repair Regen* 23, 386–393. doi: 10.1111/wrr.12286

Sousa, R. G., and Batista Kde, N. (2016). Laser therapy in wound healing associated with diabetes mellitus - Review. *An Bras. Dermatol.* 91, 489–493. doi: 10.1590/abd1806-4841.20163778

Tzen, Y. T., Weinheimer-Haus, E. M., Corbiere, T. F., and Koh, T. J. (2018). Increased skin blood flow during low intensity vibration in human participants: Analysis of control mechanisms using short-time Fourier transform. *PLoS One* 13:e0200247. doi: 10.1371/journal.pone.0200247

Weinheimer-Haus, E. M., Judex, S., Ennis, W. J., and Koh, T. J. (2014). Low-intensity vibration improves angiogenesis and wound healing in diabetic mice. *PLoS One* 9:e91355. doi: 10.1371/journal.pone.0091355

Zhu, T., Wang, Y., Yang, J., Liao, F., Wang, S., and Jan, Y. K. (2020). Wavelet-based analysis of plantar skin blood flow response to different frequencies of local vibration. *Physiol. Meas* 41, 025004. doi: 10.1088/1361-6579/ab6e56

15

Thermal Analysis of Blood Flow Alterations in Human Hand and Foot based on Vascular-Porous Media Model

Yue-Ping Wang, Rui-Hao Cheng, Ying He and Li-Zhong Mu*

School of Energy and Power Engineering, Dalian University of Technology, Dalian, China

***Correspondence:**
Ying He
heying@dlut.edu.cn

Microvascular and Macrovascular diseases are serious complications of diabetic mellitus, which significantly affect the life quality of diabetic patients. Quantitative description of the relationship between temperature and blood flow is considerably important for non-invasive detection of blood vessel structural and functional lesions. In this study, thermal analysis has been employed to predict blood flow alterations in a foot and a cubic skin model successively by using a discrete vessel-porous media model and further compared the blood flows in 31 diabetic patients. The tissue is regarded as porous media whose liquid phase represents the blood flow in capillaries and solid phase refers to the tissue part. Discrete vascular segments composed of arteries, arterioles, veins, and venules were embedded in the foot model. In the foot thermal analysis, the temperature distributions with different inlet vascular stenosis were simulated. The local temperature area sensitive to the reduction of perfusion was obtained under different inlet blood flow conditions. The discrete vascular-porous media model was further applied in the assessment of the skin blood flow by coupling the measured skin temperatures of diabetic patients and an inverse method. In comparison with the estimated blood flows among the diabetic patients, delayed blood flow regulation was found in some of diabetic patients, implying that there may be some vascular disorders in these patients. The conclusion confirms the one in our previous experiment on diabetic rats. Most of the patients predicted to be with vascular disorders were diagnosed as vascular complication in clinical settings as well, suggesting the potential applications of the vascular-porous media model in health management of diabetic patients.

Keywords: thermal analysis, vascular disorder, blood flow estimation, diabetic foot, porous media model

INTRODUCTION

Due to lifestyle changes, reduced physical activity, and increased obesity, the prevalence of diabetes has increased from 4.7% in 1980 to 8.5% in 2014. It is estimated that there will be more than 629 million adult diabetic patients in 2045 (Glovaci et al., 2019). Diabetic foot is one of the common and dangerous complications of diabetes mellitus, with an incidence rate of 6.3% worldwide (Zhang et al., 2017). All layers of tissues from the skin to bones will be affected by ulcers. In severe cases, amputations are required and even contralateral foot wound or repeated amputations may be induced, which not only reduces the life qualities of patients but also causes huge medical pressure and economic losses. Therefore, early detection of diabetic foot is of vital importance. Diabetic complications are always accompanied with structural and functional disorders of the peripheral vascular system. Orchard and Strandness, (1993) found that calcification occurs in the posterior tibial artery, anterior tibial artery, and the arteries at the plantar level among diabetic patients through X-ray. The atherosclerotic plaque leads to occlusion of blood vessels. The vascular occlusion may reduce blood flow and further obstruct the transport of active substances which induce the onset of foot ulceration. Additionally, abnormal hemodynamic and metabolic dysfunctions contribute to the autoregulation of vasomotion disorders and eventually result in ischemia which would intensify ulceration. Therefore, the key factor of early diagnosis of diabetic foot is to detect the dysfunctions of macro/microvasculature as early as possible.

The methods for clinical evaluation of the lower extremity arterial disease include intermittent claudication observation, foot arterial pulsation measurement, ankle-brachial blood pressure index measurement, and so on. Among them, the ankle-brachial index (ankle-brachial index, ABI) is a proven reproducible inspection method. A hand-held Doppler probe can be used to measure the systolic blood pressure of the ankle and arms, and then calculate the ratio of the two. This operation is simple and non-invasive, and the results have been verified in the lesions confirmed by angiography. However, in some elderly patients, calcium deposition in the middle arteries and poor vascular compressibility may occur, resulting in an increase in the ABI, leading to false normals. The mainstream non-invasive methods for detecting the microcirculation blood perfusion rate include the Doppler effect–based laser Doppler flowmetry (laser Doppler flowmetry, LDF) direct detection and the transcutaneous oxygen content that indirectly reflects the perfusion rate through the partial pressure of oxygen. The high price of the abovementioned instruments and poor portability limit their wide application. On the other hand, plethysmograph (Schürmann et al., 2001), laser speckle imager (Briers, 1996), and other blood perfusion rate detection methods based on mechanical and ultrasound technology are still immature. Therefore, effective methods for non-invasive detection of vascular disease in diabetic patients still need further study.

Skin temperature variation is closely associated with the blood perfusion rate, suggesting that monitoring temperature alterations may be employed to study vascular reactivity. Through wavelet cross-correlation analysis of laser Doppler flowmetry (LDF) and skin temperature signal in healthy subjects, Frick et al. pointed out skin temperature monitoring can be used as a tracer of microvessel tone (Frick et al., 2015). The response to the cold pressor test in patients with type 2 diabetes differs essentially from that of healthy subjects in the endothelial frequency range (Smirnova et al., 2013). Podtaev et al. analyzed the correlation degree and phase shift between skin temperature fluctuations and periodic changes of the blood flow caused by oscillations in vasomotor smooth muscle tone (Podtaev et al., 2008). Thermography can be conveniently transformed into skin blood flow through a new developed spectral filter approach (Sagaidachnyi et al., 2017). Nieuwenhoff et al. (2016) also found the time constant expressing skin temperature variation rate can reflect the blood flow of the skin through the skin temperature heating test and heat transfer modeling. Reproducibility was confirmed in the assessment of axon reflex-related vasodilation. Coupling with thermography of tongue and bioheat transfer analysis, the state of the lingual circulation system can be assessed, which provides evidence for the traditional diagnosis method *via* observing the tongue surface state in Chinese medicine (Zhang and Zhu, 2010).

In the past 2 decades, various medical instruments for detecting pathological conditions in the circulatory system have been developed based on the correlation between temperature and blood flow, some of which are listed in **Table 1** showing the devices, experimental thermal environment, experimental subjects, and analytical models. Haga et al. (2012) developed an instrument and algorithm for estimation of blood perfusion from the measured skin temperature. A similar fingertip temperature measurement instrument has been also designed, which can record the temperature change within 75 s after the fingertip touches the sensor (Nagata et al., 2009). The developed heat transfer model was in analogy with the circuit where the thermal conductivity corresponds to the electrical resistance. As blood flow of capillaries affect the effective thermal conductivity of the skin, blood perfusion could be further inferred from the resistance value in the circuit model. In Wang et al.'s heating experiments on diabetic rats implemented by a microtest device, the blood perfusion before and after heating was evaluated by coupling a 1D bioheat transfer model and genetic algorithm (Wang et al., 2020). Apart from the conventional genetic algorithm, the Box–Kanemasu method (Ricketts et al., 2008) was also employed for prediction of blood perfusion from measured temperatures in Rickettes et al.'s study. It is seen a common feature from the abovementioned studies that various optimization algorithms have been used to estimate the blood perfusion rate or thermophysical parameters based on the surface temperature. This approach can be categorized as inverse analysis which is distinguished from the forward one to compute the surface and depth temperature distributions by using the given boundary conditions. In order to estimate these parameters, choosing a suitable heat transfer model for matching the added surface heating source is a key factor as well.

With the development of thermal imaging technology, a lot of research practices have been carried out around computer-aid diagnosis of diabetic foot by infrared thermography (Hernandez-Contreras et al., 2016; Muhammad et al., 2017). Comparing with other imaging modalities such as MRI, CT, and ultrasound, infrared thermal imaging is safer and more convenient (Bandalakunta Gururajarao et al., 2019). In the circumstance of critical ischemia, as a non-invasive method, thermal imaging is more effective than the toe brachial pressure index (Kevin et al., 2019). Sivanandam et al. (2012) collected the infrared thermal image of plantar among healthy people and diabetic patients with and without early signs of ulceration. It is found that the foot temperature of a diabetic subject without the complication of ulceration was 2°C lower than that of the healthy subjects. The average foot skin temperature in diabetic patients with early signs

TABLE 1 | Experimental study on the thermal method of vasomotor function.

Experimental device	Thermal environment	Experimental subject	Analytical method	References
Holdable heat-stimulated blood flow test instrument	Temperature measurement with local heating and recovery	Healthy people's hand	2-D cylindrical tissue model in a cylindrical coordinate system	Haga et al. (2012)
Fingertip temperature dual sensor	No external thermal stimulation	Healthy people's finger tip	0-D parametric model analogous to a circuit	Nagata et al. (2009)
Microtest	Temperature measurement with local heating and recovery	Healthy and diabetic SD rats' paw	1-D vascular-porous media bioheat transfer model	Wang et al. (2020)
A laminated flat thermocouple sensor	No external thermal stimulation	Healthy rats' liver tissue	2-D finite difference tissue heat transfer model	Ricketts et al. (2008)
14-node thermal mapping sensors	Temperature measurement with local heating and recovery	Healthy people's arm	2-D finite element bioheat transfer model	Webb et al. (2015)
Coupling of the optical probe with the Peltier element	Temperature measurement with local heating and recovery	Healthy and diabetic people's lower limb	Spectral analysis by using a wavelet transform	Mizeva et al. (2018)
Infrared thermography and photoplethysmography	No external thermal stimulation	Healthy people's fingertip	Morelet wavelet transfrom	Sagaidachnyi et al. (2014)
Temperature sensorHRTS-5760, Honeywell International, Inc., United States	Temperature measurement with local heating and recovery	Healthy and diabetic people's palm	Wavelet analysis of temperature	Podtaev et al. (2014)
Microtest	Temperature measurement with local heating and recovery	Healthy people's/ diabetic patients' finger tip	Wavelet analysis of temperature	Zubareva et al. (2019), Parshakov et al. (2016), Parshakov et al. (2017), Antonova et al. (2016)

of ulceration decreased by 0.5°C when compared with control subjects. The results suggest that diabetic patients with vascular complications and early signs of ulceration present different variation mechanisms in temperature distribution, of which one is mainly due to blood flow rate decreasing, but another may be caused by the occurrence of inflammation. Bagavathiappan et al. (2008) observed temperature gradients in the influenced regions of patients with vascular disorders and ischemic gangrene from thermal imaging. It was also displayed that diabetic subjects with neuropathy had higher mean foot temperature than non-neuropathic subjects (Bagavathiappan et al., 2010). The thermal imaging analyses show that there is usually a rapid rise about 0.7°C in skin temperature when a local wound occurs. If an inflammation occurs, the skin temperature will increase by 2.2°C (Chen et al., 2021). Van Netten et al. (2013) explored the applicability of infrared thermal imaging for detection of signs of diabetic foot by comparing the mean temperature between the lateral and the contralateral foot and found that the mean temperature difference of the feet in diabetic patients with diffusive complications is larger than 3°C.

Astasio et al. obtained thermograms of the sole in 277 diabetics and analyzed the temperature distribution patterns in four areas of the soles (Astasio et al., 2018) Additionally, they found a much lower mean temperature of soles in diabetics by further comparisons of the thermal maps with those of nondiabetics (Astasio-Picado et al., 2020). Using combined discrete wavelet transform and higher order spectra techniques (Muhammad et al., 2018a) or double density-dual tree-complex wavelet transform (Muhammad et al., 2018b), original foot thermal images can be decomposed for providing various valuable information in the diagnosis of the diabetic foot. The application of machine learning into infrared image processing can improve the accuracy and speed for classification of diabetic foot thermograms (He et al., 2021). In the future, a neural network model can be inserted into mobile phones for early detection of diabetic ulcers after training by using numerous foot temperature data for diabetic ulcer patients and healthy subjects (Serlina et al., 2020) (Amith et al., 2021). New techniques continuously appear to help identifying risk zones of diabetic foot, such as using a retrained MASK-R-CNN mode (Maldonado et al., 2020). In choosing the training data, it is pointed out that the temperatures of toes and the upper half of foot are better than those in other regions (Carlos Padierna et al., 2020) Although average skin temperature is a meaningful index for early diagnosis of diabetic foot in diabetic patients, it is rather insufficient to distinguish different stages of early signs. The foot temperature of diabetic patients with only vascular disease is frequently lower than that of healthy people. However, when it further develops into neuropathy, there will be an increase in the local foot temperature, which is associated with early inflammation in some places. Moreover, multiple vascular stenoses will have varying degrees of impact on each local foot temperature. Therefore, spatial variations of skin temperature should be more concerned. It is without doubt to see that the thermography-based diagnosis technique is powerful for detection of early stages of diabetic foot. However, few research studies concern with the underlying mechanisms associated with diabetic foot, such as the coherence between the altered foot vasculatures and tissue wound or the influence of arterial occlusion on blood perfusion in tissues. It has been known that skin temperature variations are closely associated with the variations of blood perfusion. Despite that detailed temperature changes can be detected using current thermography-based techniques, it is still difficult to define the serious degrees of the diseased vascular system simply based on thermal images.

In this regard, bio-heat transfer modeling is helpful for establishment of a quantitative relationship between blood flow rates and temperature distribution. This kind of work has been extensively explored in numerous available literature reports. Ma et al. (2015) simplified foot tissue as a three-layer structure of skin, fat, and a core zone and gave an analytical mathematical solution for the simplified one-dimensional case. In Copetti et al.'s study (Copetti et al., 2017), thermal analysis on the foot was carried out by using a two-dimensional finite element model. However, dimensionality reduction results in the loss of complete three-dimensional (3D) temperature information. Rafael et al. (2016) presented a 3D-finite element simulation to predict the temperature variations of the foot with 5 ulcers at the depth of 5 mm away from the sole of the foot. Although the remarkably higher temperatures in ulcers have been achieved, the influence of altered blood flow and vasculatures on tissue temperatures has not been taken into account. No matter the above 2D or 3D heat transfer computation, they were all performed by using a one Pennes equation, and the thermal effect of blood phase is reflected in the blood perfusion term (Pennes, 1998). Due to the simplicity of the Pennes equation, it has been widely used in macroscale bio-heat transfer computation such as hand (Shao et al., 2014) and even thermal characteristics of the whole body (Tang et al., 2016) which has clinical significance such as the treatment of breast tumor by using hyperthermia therapy (Barrios et al., 2019). However, determination of the local blood perfusion rate in the tissue is always a challenging work, especially in pathological conditions when the blood perfusion rate becomes non-uniform. Another limitation of the Pennes equation is that the influence of blood flow directions is neglected, resulting in over or under estimations of blood perfusion in some conditions. The discrete vascular bioheat transfer model provides an alternative method to compute the non-uniform local blood perfusion.

The important feature of the discrete vascular bioheat transfer model is to consider the vessels as a separate domain and calculate the heat exchange between the surrounding tissues. Among them, embedded 1D/3D multiscale modeling has been extensively employed to deal with heat transfer between vessels and tissues. By using this kind of model, Tang et al. (2020) computed the distribution of oxygen and temperature distribution in microcirculation. The influence of the red blood cell on oxygen transport can be further addressed in the work of Wang et al. (2021). He and Liu, (2017) proposed a coupled continuum-discrete model (CCD) for thermal analysis. They classified the blood vessels as visible vessels and invisible vessels. The thermal effect of visible vessels includes blood heat transfer and the conduction between the blood vessel and the surrounding tissue. The effect of invisible vessels was converted to the blood perfusion term corresponding to the continuum parts. The CCD model can well capture a richer and complex thermal interaction of the vascular network and solid tissue compared to the conventional bioheat transfer model. Stephen studied the effect of surface cooling on the internal temperature of the brain by inserting a one-dimensional vascular structure into the brain region (Blowers, 2018; Blowers et al., 2018). The 1D vascular model contains the arteries, arterioles, veins, and venules. The capillaries were represented by the liquid phase of porous media whose solid phase corresponds to the white or gray matter of the brain. It is found from their study that due to the inclusion of the directional flow, scalp cooling has a larger impact on cerebral temperatures than the predictions by previous bioheat transfer models. Although the discrete vascular-porous media model is more complex than the Pennes equation, it can describe the biological heat transfer process more realistically, and the inversion of the blood flow is more reliable. Image-based voxel mesh generation provides an easy-implemented way to apply the discrete vascular-porous media model in the analysis of the real geometric structure.

In this study, the discrete vascular-porous media bioheat transfer model has been applied in thermal analysis on a cubic tissue model and a foot to evaluate the influence of the blood flow with various vasculatures. The tissue is regarded as a porous media, while the embedded vasculature includes arteries, arterioles, venules, and veins. The conductive and convective effects of blood flow in multi-scaled blood vessels on tissue temperature are well-addressed in the model. The temperature distributions for various degrees of foot vascular stenosis were simulated, and the relationship between the foot temperature distribution and blood flow was quantitatively correlated. A cubic porous media model embedded with the vessel network was also coupled with the measured skin temperature data for analysis of blood flow regulation in diabetic patients. The blood flow in the conditions of skin heating and power off were estimated according to the test setting, and comparisons of the predicted blood flow were made between healthy people and diabetic patients.

METHODS

The Developed Portable Thermal Sensor for Skin Temperature Measurement

In order to compare the automatic regulation of the blood flow between diabetic patients and healthy people, a programmable heating and temperature measurement device using a flexible material has been developed which is named by the superficial perfusion assessment system (SPAS). As shown in **Figure 1A**, the substrate of the SPAS is made of a double-layer flexible printed circuit (FPC) board, which is formed by 3 layers of polyimide, 2 layers of copper foil, and 4 layers of adhesive bonding. The top layer is welded with a high-precision temperature sensor chip si7051 and FPC connector. The circuit that is coiled into a loop near the center of the bottom layer generates heat when energized, which thermally stimulates the surface of the skin. The detailed content about the production and debugging of the film can be obtained from Cheng's master thesis (Cheng, 2020).

In the measurement, a medical tape was used to fix the SPAS on the skin of a hand, as shown in **Figure 1B**. Since the movement of a hand may cause the deviation of the flexible sensor, the

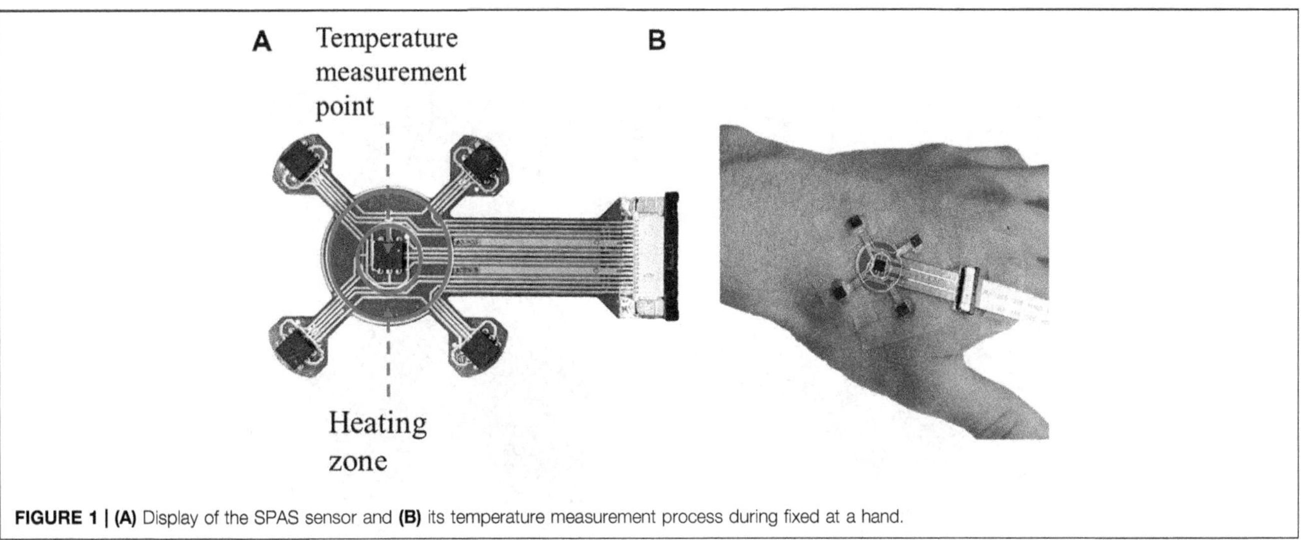

FIGURE 1 | (A) Display of the SPAS sensor and **(B)** its temperature measurement process during fixed at a hand.

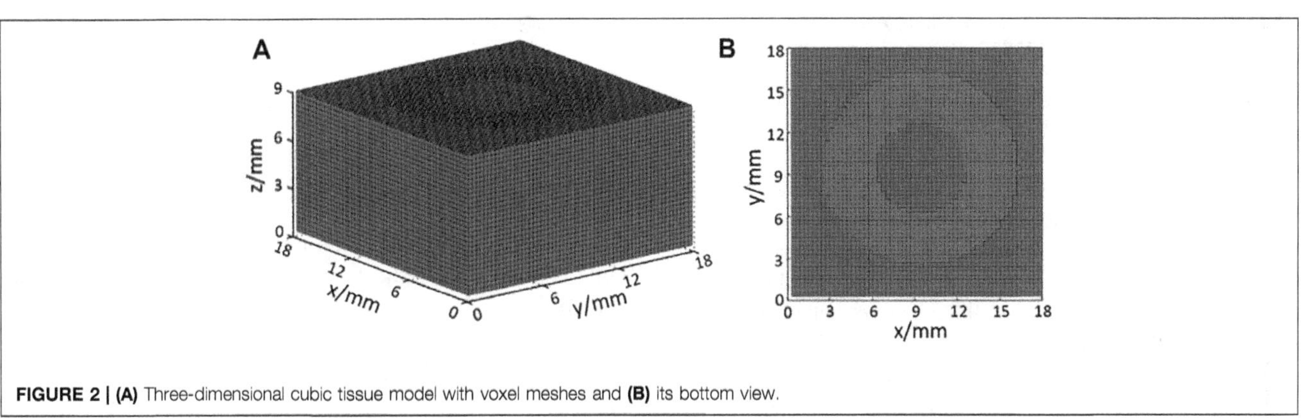

FIGURE 2 | (A) Three-dimensional cubic tissue model with voxel meshes and **(B)** its bottom view.

subject should remain as stable as possible during the test. After manually turning on the device, the measurement will start and end automatically when the setting period is reached. The duration of an experiment is set to 2,750 s including 3 stages. In the first 750 s, the heating power is 0 W/m2, which is called the resting phase. Then, it comes to the heating phase by heating the skin with a power of 150 W/m^2 for 1,000 s. After the power is switched off, the SPAS continues to record the temperature for another 1,000 s referring to the recovery phase.

Geometric Models and Mathematical Descriptions of the Vascular Porous Media Model

According to the shape and size of the SPAS equipment, a cubic tissue model was designed, as shown in **Figure 2A** which could describe the heat exchange between the skin surface and deeper tissue. The volume of the tissue model is 1.8 × 1.8 × 0.9 cm^3, and the voxel size is set as 0.3 mm. The upper surface of the model is the skin and conducts convective heat exchange with the surrounding environment. As shown in **Figure 2B**, the red area corresponds to the heating ring of the SPAS whose inner radius is 3.5 mm, and the outer one is 6.9 mm. An input heat flux as 150 W/m^2 is imposed on the red region at the heating phase, and zero is set in resting and recovery phases.

The subcutaneous tissue includes a large number of blood vessels to satisfy material and energy transport. As it is difficult to determine the specific structure of the blood vessels under the skin, an angiogenesis algorithm was used to generate blood vessels to fill the tissue area. In this tissue model, an inlet artery and an outlet vein were assumed inside the tissue model, as shown in **Figure 3A**. Then, the rapidly exploring random tree (RRT) algorithm was implemented as that in the work by Blowers et al. (Blowers, 2018) where it was used to generate brain vasculature. The procedures of the algorithm are as follows:

1) A new node is generated randomly inside the target tissue space.
2) Previous nodes are searched completely to find the closest segment or node.
3) A new segment is created by linking the created node with the closest point or with the nearest node of the nearest segment.
4) If the generated segment is connected to an existing segment (not at a node), a new node will be generated on the existing segment and will be divided in two segments.

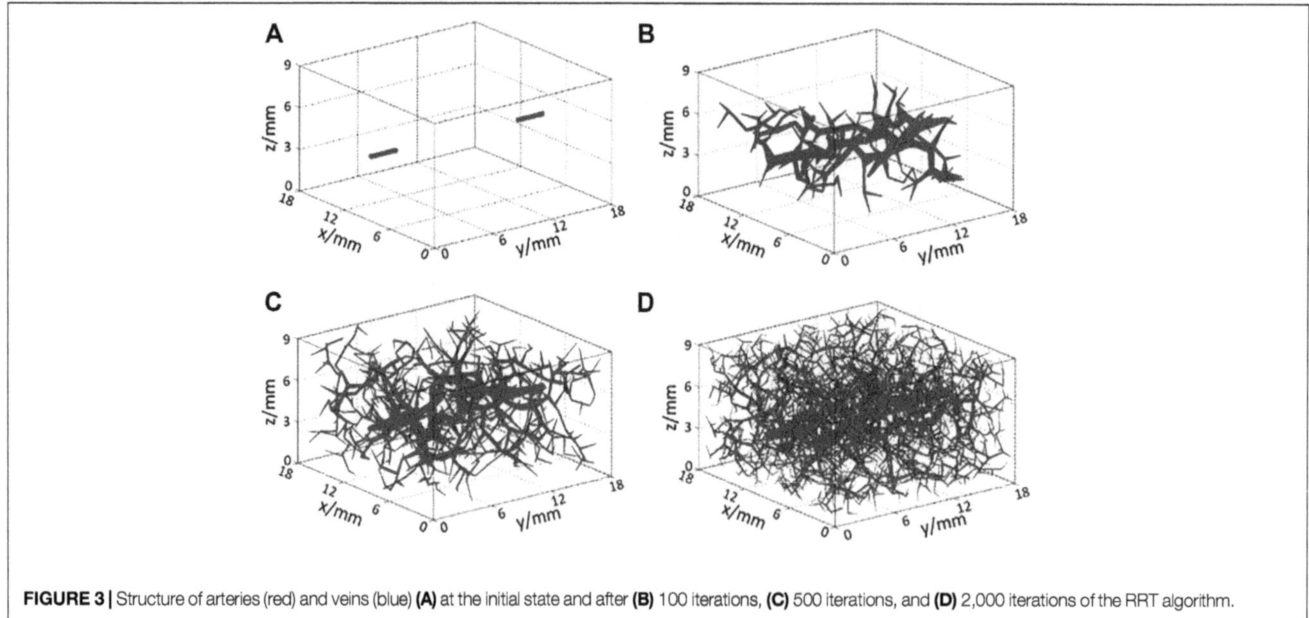

FIGURE 3 | Structure of arteries (red) and veins (blue) **(A)** at the initial state and after **(B)** 100 iterations, **(C)** 500 iterations, and **(D)** 2,000 iterations of the RRT algorithm.

5) The procedures 1–4 are repeated until the set number of iterations is completed.

The structures of the generated vessels after 100, 500, and 2,000 iterations of the RRT algorithm are shown in **Figures 3B–D**, respectively, where red lines represent arteries and arterioles, and blue lines represent veins and venules. As the number of iterations increased, blood vessels filled the entire space gradually so that blood could be perfused adequately to each part of the target tissue. In the generation of smaller vessels from the main arteries, two iteration criteria were set to end the RRT computation. If the numbers of vessels have no significant changes and the blood flow rate in the smallest vessel equals to a known value in the arteriole or venule, the computation will stop. In **Figure 3D**, the diameter of the smallest size of the vessel is 34 μm, which matches the size of the smallest arteriole. Additionally, to incorporate the thermal effects of capillaries, the voxel volume is regarded as a porous medium, whereby the liquid phase represents the blood in capillaries and the solid phase represents the solid tissue. Using this method, a complete multi-scale vascular and porous media model is formed. In the work, a cubic tissue and real geometric foot model have been constructed for the applications of the vascular porous media model.

Computation of Flow Rates in the 1D Vessel Network

Blood flow in 1D vessels is described by Poiseuille's law. The relationship between blood velocity and pressure is described by **Eq. 1**:

$$\boldsymbol{u}_b = -\frac{R^2}{8\mu}\frac{\partial P_b}{\partial \boldsymbol{s}}, \tag{1}$$

where R is the vessel radius, P_b is the blood pressure, $\boldsymbol{s}$ is the direction of the blood flow, μ is the blood viscosity, and $\boldsymbol{u}_b$ is the blood velocity. The continuity equation of blood in 1D blood vessels is:

$$\pi R^2 \nabla \cdot \boldsymbol{u}_b = -q_a + q_v, \tag{2}$$

where q_a and q_v denote the arterial outflow and venous inflow of blood. As blood can flow across the vessel wall and exchange with tissue at the capillary scale, q_a and q_v are set as 0 for non-terminal branches and assigned some values according to actual situations for terminal branches.

Computation of Flow Rates in Porous Media

In porous media, the capillary blood flow is assumed to occur *via* several thin capillaries. As such, the momentum equation can be simplified as the Darcy equation, which can be expressed as follows:

$$\nabla P = -\frac{\mu}{K}\boldsymbol{V}_{Darcy}, \tag{3}$$

where K is the permeability of porous media, and V_{Darcy} is the Darcy velocity. The Darcy velocity is related to the actual velocity V by: $V_{\mathrm{Darcy}} = \varepsilon V$ and ε represents the liquid volume fraction in the porous media. The continuity equation for the porous media is given as follows:

$$\rho_b \nabla \cdot \boldsymbol{V}_{Darcy} = Q_a - Q_v, \tag{4}$$

where Q_a and Q_v are the exchanged blood flows between tissue and arteries/veins, respectively. There is no velocity perpendicular to the skin. Therefore, the boundary pressure for skin can be given as:

$$\left.\frac{\partial P}{\partial n}\right|_{skin} = 0. \tag{5}$$

The blood flow at the interconnection between the discrete vascular and porous media are determined by the outflow of the arteries (q_a) and the inflow of veins (q_v) into the total ones into the tissue (Q_a) and out of the tissue (Q_v). The relationship between them could be written as:

$$q_a = Q_a/n;\ qv = Q_v/m,$$

where n and m are the number of nodes that the peripheral arteries and peripheral veins intersect with a voxel. Outflow or inflow from the surrounding blood vessels are evenly distributed to each coupling node in this study.

Computation of Blood and Tissue Temperature

For simplicity, the 1D arterial vessel network, the 3D solid tissue phase, the 3D capillary phase, and the 1D venous vessel structure are denoted 1, 2, 3, and 4, respectively. The heat transfer processes in these four regions are expressed as follows:

$$V_1\rho_b c_b\frac{\partial T_1}{\partial t} = V_1K_b(\nabla^2T_1) - V_1\rho_b c_b \boldsymbol{U}_1(\nabla T_1) + \beta_{1-2}(T_2 - T_1) + \beta_{1-3}(T_3 - T_1), \tag{6}$$

$$V_2\varepsilon_2\rho c\frac{\partial T_2}{\partial t} = V_2\varepsilon_2K_c(\nabla^2T_2) + \beta_{1-2}(T_1 - T_2) + \beta_{2-3}(T_3 - T_2) + \beta_{2-3}(T_3 - T_2) + \beta_{2-4}(T_4 - T_2) + V_2Q_{gen}, \tag{7}$$

$$V_3\varepsilon_3\rho_b c_b\frac{\partial T_3}{\partial t} = V_3\varepsilon_3K_b(\nabla^2T_3) - V_3\rho_b c_b \boldsymbol{U}_3(\nabla T_3) + \beta_{1-3}(T_1 - T_3) + \beta_{2-3}(T_2 - T_3) + \beta_{3-4}(T_4 - T_3) + c_bM_{1-3}(T_3 - T_1), \tag{8}$$

$$V_4\rho_b c_b\frac{\partial T_4}{\partial t} = V_4K_b(\nabla^2T_4) - V_4\rho_b c_b \boldsymbol{U}_4(\nabla T_4) + \beta_{2-4}(T_2 - T_4) + \beta_{3-4}(T_3 - T_4) + c_bM_{3-4}(T_4 - T_3), \tag{9}$$

where V_{1-4} denotes the volume of the domain, and $U_{1,\,2,\,4}$ are the blood velocities in different regions. As the soft tissue is the solid phase in the porous media, U_3 does not exist. ε_2 is the volume fraction of the tissue within the porous domain, and ε_3 is the volume fraction of the blood; therefore, $\varepsilon_2 + \varepsilon_3 = 1$. K and K_b are the conduction coefficients for the tissue and blood phases, respectively. c_b and c are the heat capacities for blood and tissue. The tissue parameters include two components which are the soft tissue and bone. M_{1-3} and M_{3-4} represent the mass exchange from domain 3 to domain 1 and from domain 3 to domain 4, reflecting convective heat transfer from arteries to voxels and from voxels to veins, respectively. Q_{gen} represents tissue metabolic heat generation. Heat exchange between the blood and the surrounding tissue through the vessel wall is described by the heat exchange coefficient $\beta_{x\text{-}y}$ which is defined as follows:

$$\beta_{x-y} = \varepsilon hA_{surf}, \tag{10}$$

where h is the convection coefficient of the blood and vessel wall, and A_{surf} is the surface area of the blood vessels. Vascular blood flow can be approximated as the laminar flow in a rigid pipe, so this convection coefficient can be deduced from the Nusselt number:

$$Nu = \frac{hD_v}{2K_b}. \tag{11}$$

It is well established that for a laminar flow in a pipe, Nu can be approximated to be a constant with the value of 4 (Blowers, 2018). At the surface of the foot model and the top surface of the cubic model, there is heat exchange with the environment and a Robin boundary condition can be prescribed as:

$$-K_c\frac{\partial T}{\partial n} = h(T - T_\infty), \tag{12}$$

where T_∞ is the environment temperature, and h is the convective heat transfer coefficient. The adiabatic boundary condition was set for the plane connecting the foot to the leg in the foot model and the other surface of the cubic model:

$$-K_c\frac{\partial T}{\partial n} = 0. \tag{13}$$

Having set the boundary conditions for the heat and mass transfer equations, the temperatures of the four domains could be solved with the given flow rates within domains 1, 3, and 4. A MATLAB program was developed based on an open-source code on GitHub [https://github.com/sblowers/VaPor] for the implementation of numerical computation. The physical parameters used in this computation are described in **Table 2**.

In this model, $\boldsymbol{u_b}$ represents the velocities in blood vessels including the velocities in arteries ($\boldsymbol{U_1}$) and veins ($\boldsymbol{U_4}$) which are solved by **Eqs 1** and **2**. The vessel network model used in this work is a 1-dimensional one with the information of radii and lengths. In the computation of the blood flow of the 1D model, the velocity in every segment is computed by **Eq. 1**, while the velocities at the bifurcation nodes should be computed by combining **Eqs 1, 2** to satisfy the continuity condition of mass flow at these points. The direction of the blood flow in every segment depends on the known position of every vessel segment generated by the RRT algorithm. The direction of vector $\boldsymbol{u_b}$ refers to the one in the 3D information of the network. Similar implementation can be found in the works of Pozrikidis (Pozrikidis, 2009) and Blowers, (2018) for blood flow simulation through vascular networks. On the other hand, $\boldsymbol{U_3}$ can be obtained by solving **Eqs 3, 4**. $\boldsymbol{V_{\mathrm{Darcy}}}$ represents the Darcy velocity in the porous medium model which is related to the velocity of the blood flow in a capillary ($\boldsymbol{U_3}$).

Since voxel-based meshes are employed, the finite difference method (FDM) can be easily employed for the discretization of **Eqs 6–9**. The real geometric 3D model reconstructed from medical images can also be directly transformed into a voxel mesh for the computation by the FDM. Currently, the steady-state temperature is considered; thus, the discretization of the time derivative term is not needed. The convection term is discretized using the first-order upwind difference scheme. The diffusion terms of the equations are discretized using the central difference scheme. The discrete governing equation can be then written as a stiffness-matrix form as:

TABLE 2 | Physical parameters used in the foot model.

Physical parameter	Value	Unit	References
Blood viscosity, μ	3.5	mPa s	Bagavathiappan et al. (2008)
Permeability of porous media, K	1.5×10^{-13}	m^2	Bagavathiappan et al. (2008)
Blood density, ρ_b	1,050	kg/m^3	Bagavathiappan et al. (2008)
Specific heat capacity of blood, c_b	3,800	J/(kg K)	Bagavathiappan et al. (2008)
Thermal conductivity of blood, K_b	0.50	W/m^3	Bagavathiappan et al. (2008)
Tissue density, $\rho_{soft\ tissue}$	1,270	kg/m^3	Antonova et al. (2016)
Specific heat capacity of the soft tissue, $c_{soft\ tissue}$	3,768	J/(kg K)	Antonova et al. (2016)
Thermal conductivity of the soft tissue, $K_{soft\ tissue}$	0.35	W/m^3	Antonova et al. (2016)
Bone density, ρ_{bone}	1,418	kg/m^3	Antonova et al. (2016)
Specific heat capacity of the bone, c_{bone}	2,409	J/(kg K)	Antonova et al. (2016)
Thermal conductivity of the bone, K_{bone}	2.21	W/m^3	Antonova et al. (2016)
Metabolism, Q_{gen}	368	W/m^3	Antonova et al. (2016)

$$\boldsymbol{Ax} = \boldsymbol{B}, \tag{14}$$

where $\boldsymbol{x}$ is the temperature matrix, A is the coefficient matrix of temperature, and B is the loading term derived from the known terms in the governing equations. Through the built-in Gaussian elimination algorithm in MATLAB, the above algebraic equation can be solved. It takes about 10 min in MATLAB on a PC with an Intel i7 6700k QuadCore processor and 32 GB of RAM for a foot model with a 1.5 mm-voxel size and 50,000 generated vessels.

RESULTS

The process of the thermal analysis on the cubic tissue and foot model are basically the same, among which the heating source should be taken into account for the cubic model. Since the measurement period is sufficiently long, the stable heating and power-off instance were chosen for the analysis in the cubic tissue model. The blood temperature of the inlet artery is constant at 37°C. The convective and radiative boundary condition is assigned at the skin of which the total heat transfer coefficient was set to be 8.0 W/m^2 K. The environmental temperature was set as 23°C, following the same environmental condition of Sivanandam et al. (2012). The results of the heat transfer computation in the two models are presented in *Tissue Temperature Distributions Under Heating and Power-Off Condition and Temperature Distributions for Different Vasculatures on Foot* sections, respectively. The inversion of blood flow for healthy people and diabetic patients is illustrated in *Inverse Analysis of Skin Blood Flow in Healthy People and Diabetic Patients* section.

Tissue Temperature Distributions Under Heating and Power-Off Condition

When there is no external heat stimulation on the skin (resting and recovery stage), the computed tissue temperature distribution is shown in **Figure 4A**, and the temperature distribution of internal tissue sections coupling with vessels is displayed in **Figure 4B**. In this phase, blood flow is the heat source; thus the highest temperature is located at the arterial entrance. As illustrated in **Figure 4B**, the temperatures of blood vessels gradually decrease along the flow direction due to the heat exchange between the blood vessel and the surrounding tissue. At the skin surface, it is seen that the skin temperature in the upstream is slightly higher than that in the downstream position.

When the skin surface is heated by the SPAS (heating stage), the temperature of the heated ring zone at the skin surface increases significantly, as shown in **Figure 4C**. At this time, blood plays a role of heat dissipation; thus, the coolest area is located at the arterial inlet. **Figure 4D** shows the temperature distribution of the inner section and blood vessels. As the blood is heated during flowing, the temperature of blood at the downstream is increasing; thus, the cooling effect of the blood flow in the downstream is weaker than that in the upstream of the blood flow. This effect is also reflected in the skin surface that the surface skin temperature in the downstream area of the heating ring is higher than that in other areas.

Temperature Distributions for Different Vasculatures on the Foot

The vascular—porous media model has been applied in the thermal analysis on the foot and for establishing a quantitative relationship between the blood flow and temperature distribution. The foot model in this study was reconstructed from sequential medical images. Simpleware software (Exeter, United Kingdom) was used to identify the bone and soft tissue automatically from CT images. The structure of the basic blood vessel of this foot model was obtained from the available website (https://human.biodigital.com). and further developed by using the RRT algorithm. **Figure 5** shows the foot skin temperature distribution from a dorsal, side, and plantar view. The temperature ranges from 24.28°C to 32.12°C. In **Figure 5A**, it can be observed that the temperature of the skin near the large blood vessels is higher, and it decreases gradually to the distal end. In **Figure 5C**, the computed average temperature of the foot plantar region is 29.42°C, which is 0.5°C higher than the experimental data (Sivanandam et al., 2012). In addition, the computed temperature distribution shows the temperature of the arch is higher than that of the sole and heel, and the toes are the coldest area of the whole foot. Specifically, the 1st and 5th toes are warmer than the 2nd, 3rd, and 4th toes. The computed temperature values closely approach the experimental data, and the abovementioned characteristics for the temperature distribution are consistent with the standard thermographic

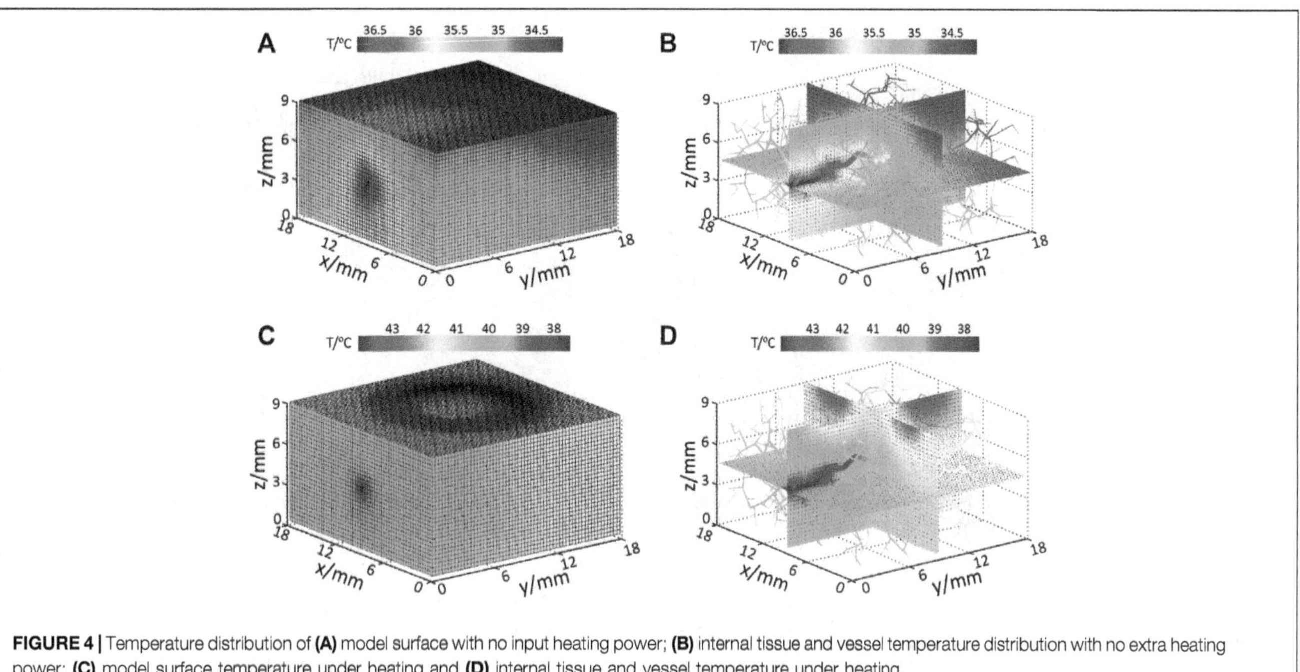

FIGURE 4 | Temperature distribution of **(A)** model surface with no input heating power; **(B)** internal tissue and vessel temperature distribution with no extra heating power; **(C)** model surface temperature under heating and **(D)** internal tissue and vessel temperature under heating.

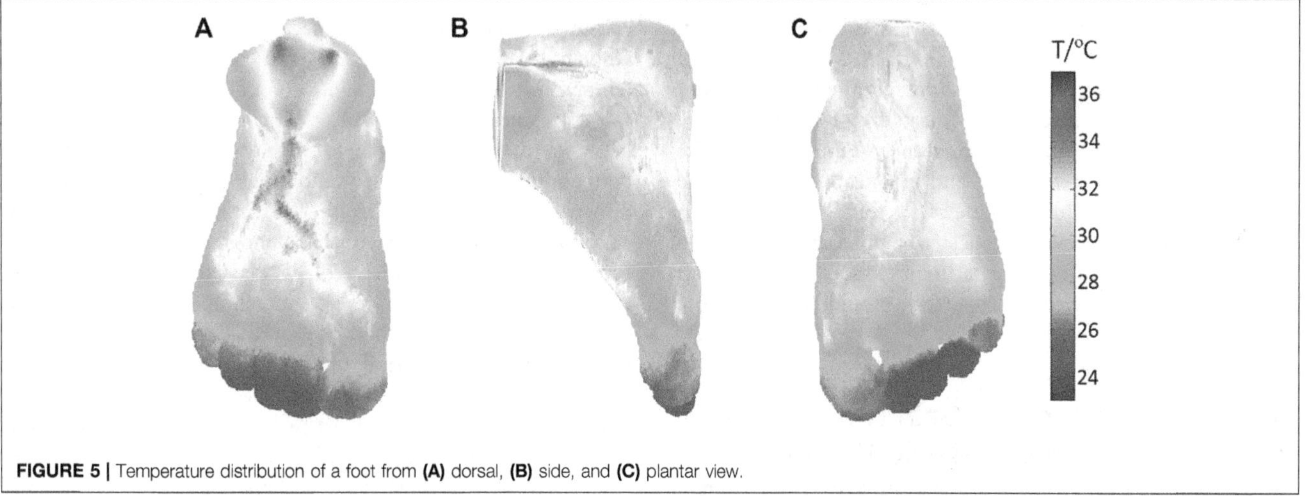

FIGURE 5 | Temperature distribution of a foot from **(A)** dorsal, **(B)** side, and **(C)** plantar view.

patterns of feet (Alfred et al., 2015), confirming the validity of the vascular porous media model.

Figures 6A–C show the distribution of arterial blood flow when occlusion occurs in the anterior tibial artery, posterior tibial artery, and peroneal artery, respectively. The occlusion positions in the three inlet arteries were specifically marked, wherein the anterior tibial artery supplies blood to the dorsal part of the foot, the posterior tibial artery supplies blood to the plantar region, and the peroneal artery supplies blood to the lateral areas. The vasculature in the foot model can be also seen clearly. As the total number of vessels is more than 1×10^6, it is difficult to visualize all vessels concurrently; only the vessels with diameter >100 μm are displayed. It is observed that the blood flow in the non-blocked inlet vessels and its downstream vessels gradually decreases along with the bifurcation generations. Apart from the blood flow in the major blood vessels, the arteriole and venule flow rates are <0.01 ml/s, indicating that the blood had been perfused to all parts of the foot. In contrast, no blood flows through the downstream area of the blocked vessel which will affect the distribution of the foot temperature.

The temperature distributions on the surface of the foot when the three inlet vessels are blocked, as shown in **Figure 7**, where the rows indexed (a–c), (d–f), and (g–i) correspond to the temperature contours for the occlusion of the anterior tibial artery, posterior tibial artery, and peroneal artery, respectively. When the anterior tibial artery is occluded, the temperature of the upper surface of the foot decreases considerably, especially in the

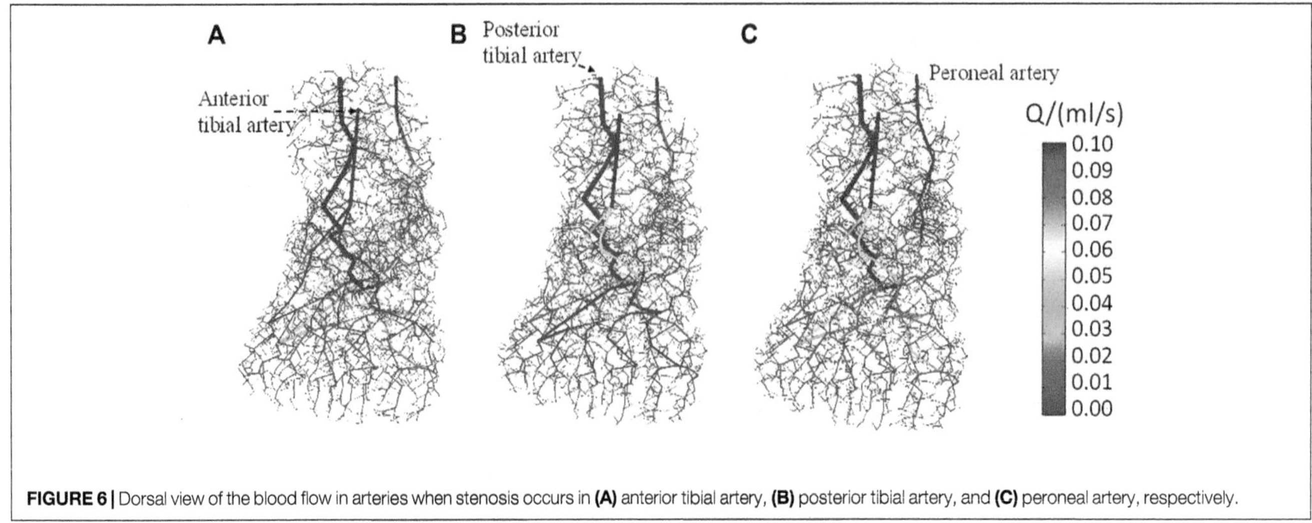

FIGURE 6 | Dorsal view of the blood flow in arteries when stenosis occurs in **(A)** anterior tibial artery, **(B)** posterior tibial artery, and **(C)** peroneal artery, respectively.

central region more influenced by the occluded feeding artery. If observed from the lateral side and foot sole, as shown in **Figures 7B,C**, there are no remarkable changes in the temperature compared to the healthy case. As the blood flow in the peroneal artery is at the normal state, the temperature decreases in the heel are small. This means when occlusion occurs in the anterior tibial artery, the most affected area in the skin temperature is the plantar surface. Moreover, in the middle and lower part of the foot, especially the toes, the lower temperature areas are enlarged which can even be seen from the dorsal and side view. Similarly, as seen in **Figures 7D–I**, the occlusions of the posterior tibial and peroneal artery have the impacts on the sole and lateral side of the foot. Meanwhile, it is noted that the occlusion in the posterior tibial artery seems to result in the largest lower temperature area, suggesting that the occlusion in the posterior tibial artery should be paid more attention to.

Inverse Analysis of the Skin Blood Flow in Healthy People and Diabetic Patients

The vascular porous media model has applied in the thermal analysis of blood flow regulation in the SPAS test. The measurements by using the SPAS were implemented on five healthy people denoted by N1~N5 and 31 diabetic patients denoted by DM1~DM31. The experiments have been approved by the Biological and Medical Ethics Committee of Dalian University of Technology. The data collection of diabetic patients was performed in the First Affiliated Hospital of Anhui Medical University. The ages, BMI indices, and blood glucose levels of the subjects are shown in **Table A1** as an **Appendix**. The temperature curves of a typical diabetic patient (DM1) and healthy people (N2) are shown in **Figure 8**. In each phase, the temperature of the diabetic patient is higher than that of the healthy person. In the heating phase, both the temperature rises rapidly and then stabilizes for a sufficiently long period. However, after heating is over, the temperature of the healthy person returns to the level before heating, but the temperature of the diabetic patient has not declined to the resting stage range.

The ambient temperature varies slightly in different tests, as shown in **Figure 8**, since the tests were carried out during a short period of several days. In order to estimate the blood flow in each test, the temperature distributions of the cubic tissue model were computed for various inlet flow rates from 0 to 0.01 ml/s, and the ambient temperature was set to 20 to 24°C, respectively. The skin temperature at the center point surrounded by the heating ring was subsequently extracted. A set of curves for the relationships between the skin temperature, blood flow, and ambient temperature were achieved and could be fitted as a two-dimensional graph by using the surface fitting tool toolbox in MATLAB. **Figures 9A,B** give the temperature variations at the recovery and heating phase. It is clear to see that the skin temperature increases with the input blood flow rate without external heating; meanwhile, the increase of the environmental temperature can also lead to the slight increase of the skin temperature. If an external constant heat is added, the center-point skin temperature decreases with the input blood flow rate. Temperature varies significantly when the input blood flow changes from 0 to 0.002 ml/s and then tends to vary slowly when the blood flow is further increased. Having the set of fitted curves, the input arterial blood flow rate could be determined from the measured environmental and skin temperatures.

In order to analyze the blood flow during the stable period of each stage, the measured temperature data of the last 100 s in each stage were extracted to evaluate the average blood flow during resting, heating, and recovery stages. The obtained results for the healthy people are displayed in **Figure 10**. The typical blood flow variation pattern for the healthy subjects is the blood flow rates at the resting and recovery phases, which are distinctly lower than that at the heating stage although there are slight differences among the healthy subjects. The blood flow increases at the heating stage since the blood vessels dilate for heat dissipation when the skin is heated. The smallest blood flow at the heating phase is 0.32 ml/s which is larger than the largest blood flow rate of 0.23 ml/s at the resting phase among healthy people. At the

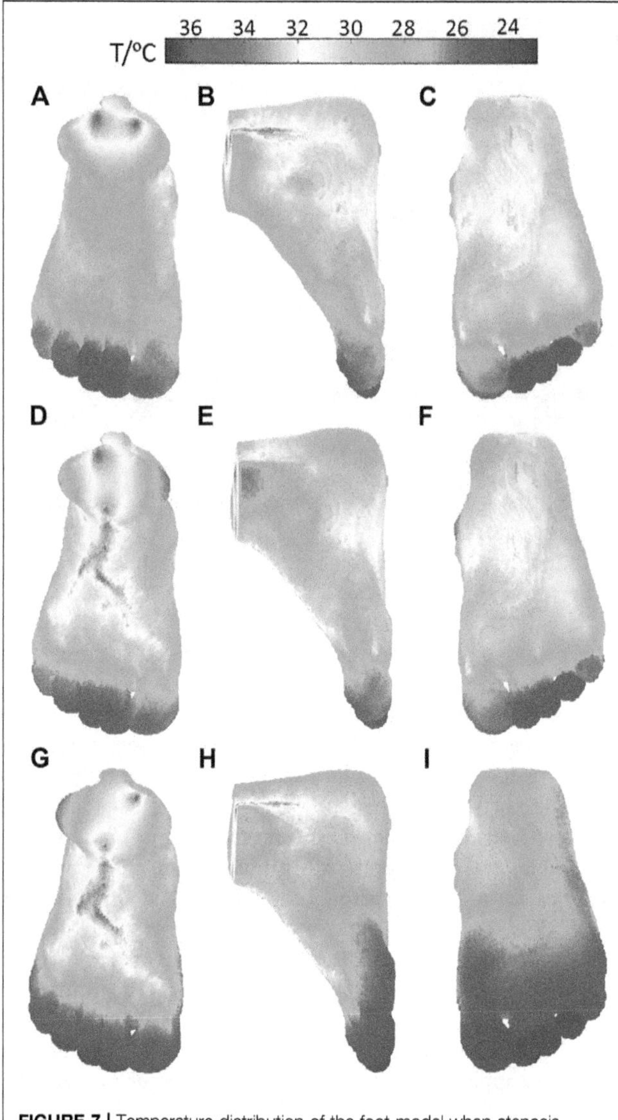

FIGURE 7 | Temperature distribution of the foot model when stenosis occurs in **(A–C)** anterior tibial artery occlusion, **(D–F)** posterior tibial artery, and **(G–I)** peroneal artery.

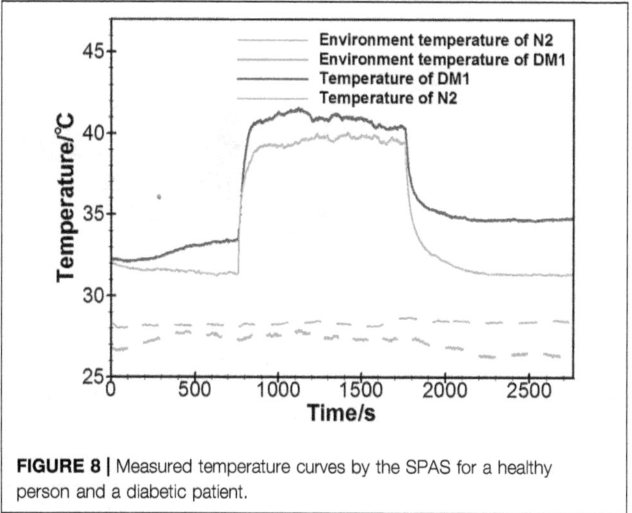

FIGURE 8 | Measured temperature curves by the SPAS for a healthy person and a diabetic patient.

recovery phase after the power is off, the blood flow returns to the resting level before heating with the difference of less than 10%.

However, the blood flow variation patterns of individuals with diabetes vary greatly, especially at the recovery stage. According to the blood flow alteration patterns at the resting and recovery stage, the estimated results can be classified into three groups shown in **Figures 11A–C**, respectively. In **Figure 11A**, the blood flow rate during heating is greater than that of the resting phase, but the increment is smaller compared to that of healthy people. It is noticeable that the blood flow rate at the recovery stage is even larger than that at the heating stage. In **Figure 11B**, the variation pattern of the blood flow rate at the resting and heating stage is close to that of healthy subjects; however, the blood flow rate at the recovery stage is only slightly reduced from the value at the heating stage, whose value is close to the average one of the resting and heating stage. Seven sets of data in the third group are shown in **Figure 11C**. The pattern of the blood flow variation for the group of diabetic patients is similar to that of healthy subjects that the blood flow rate at the resting and recovery stage are remarkably lower than the one at the heating stage.

DISCUSSION

In this study, thermal analysis of blood flow was performed in a cubic tissue and a real geometric foot model by using a discrete vascular-porous media model. The discrete vascular-porous media model was first put forward by Blowers et al. in analyzing the effect of therapeutic hypothermia of the human brain. It is our opinion that the advantage of the model is to take into account the influence of the vasculature more precisely. Hence, a MATLAB program was further extended to allow the model to calculate more complex conditions with a ring-mounted vessel structure and a vascular stenosis. The blood flow rates in vasculatures and temperature distributions have been achieved under various thermal conditions, providing the possibilities to analyze blood flow conditions in the tissue from the surface temperature.

In analyzing the thermal responses measured by the SPAS, the inlet arterial blood flow of the three stages was estimated and compared between healthy subjects and diabetic patients. It is seen that the blood flow rate at the recovery phase fell back to the level at the resting phase for healthy subjects. However, in the diabetic group, the blood flow in the recovery phase is close to the blood flow rate at the heating phase and even larger than it, which manifests that the vasodilation under a thermal stimulation is delayed in some of the diabetic patients. The results further support our previous studies (Wang et al., 2020) on SD rats that the blood flow drops rapidly after thermal stimulation for all healthy rats, but the delay of the declination occurs in some diabetic rats. Compared to the 2nd blood flow variation pattern in diabetic patients, the 1st blood flow variation pattern suggests more delayed time to thermal response. It is implied that the diabetes with delayed autoregulated vasomotion may be suffering

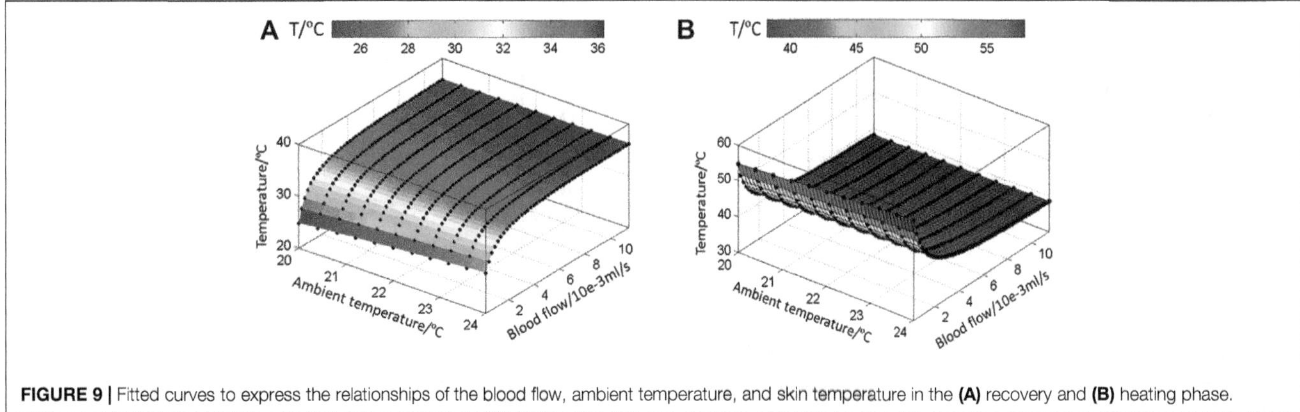

FIGURE 9 | Fitted curves to express the relationships of the blood flow, ambient temperature, and skin temperature in the **(A)** recovery and **(B)** heating phase.

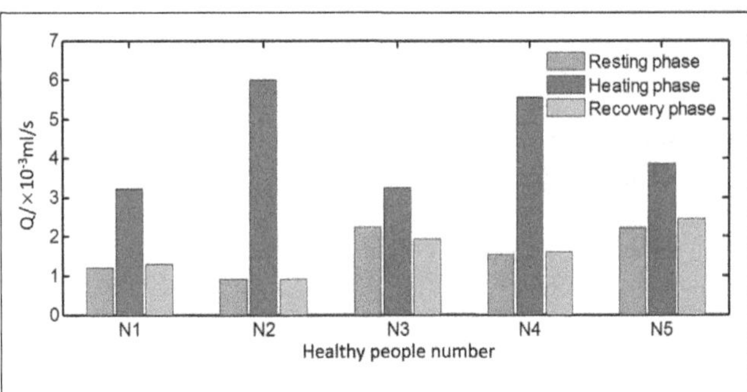

FIGURE 10 | Average blood flow rate of healthy subjects during rest, heating, and recovery phases.

from peripheral vascular diseases and needs to be more concerned. By comparing the analytical results to the clinical diagnoses by the First Affiliated Hospital of Anhui Medical University for the 15 diabetic subjects, it is found that except one patient, the other patients are suffering different kinds of complications, including hypertension, peripheral vascular disease, or peripheral neuropathy.

Both the skin temperature variation in diabetic patients and rats in our experiments show the similar pattern that the severe the diabetic mellitus is, the faster the skin temperature increases. Although constant thermal conductivity and the same vasculature were assigned in the work, it will not affect the estimated blood flow pattern in healthy and diabetic patients. Nonetheless, the possibility still exists that some estimated healthy blood flow patterns may have some abnormalities due to neglecting the impacts of aging and fat thickness.

Aging may cause the decrease of the microvasculature density and increase of vessel stiffness, leading to the increase of peripheral resistance. This kind of alteration can be also reflected in the change of effective conductivity. If microvasculature density decreases, the effective thermal resistance will increase. Similarly, fat thickness increasing will increase the thermal resistance as well. These factors can lead to faster temperature increasing in the heating stage of the test and reinforce the predicted blood flow variation pattern, which is with a higher ratio of the blood flow in the recovery phase to that in the heating phase. In addition, the increase of thermal resistance can result in a damping of the magnitude of the skin temperature oscillation and a larger phase lag to the blood flow (Tang et al., 2017).

It is commonly known that the foot temperature of diabetic patients is lower which is caused by the lower blood perfusion rate (Uraiwan et al., 2018). **Equations 6–9** have the similar form of the Pennes equation, but they describe the heat transfer process of arteries, tissue, capillaries, and veins more in detail rather than using a lumped source/sink term in the Pennes equation. The vascular-porous media model captures the thermal effect of heat conduction and convection within their regions and between blood vessels and their surrounding tissues. The alterations of blood vessel structures could also be explored. The Pennes equation could be applied in thermal analysis of foot, but it needs more assumptions for blood perfusion. The computed temperature of the foot *via* the vascular-porous media model is in a favorable agreement with thermography, showing the prospective applications in the assessment of vascular alterations for a diabetic foot.

With the development of medical imaging technology such as laser speckle flowmetry or thermography, it has been possible to directly obtain structural lesions of the blood vessels of body parts. However, early detection of the diabetic foot needs to be performed at a high frequency. Medical imaging testing is not yet suitable for daily inspections due to the high cost. Thermography is a prospective way for screening the microvasculature, but a more reliable algorithm for converting the temperature to blood flow is needed. The voxel-based vascular-porous media model provides a useful way for the conversion. Additionally, the medical image could only reflect the structural lesions but not functional lesions. It is found that the diabetic vascular functional lesions may appear before structural lesions through rat experiments (Wei et al., 2021). Coupling with thermography and the porous media model, the stenosis degree of peripheral vessels, vascular density variation, or vasodilation dysfunction may be detected, which are meaningful for the early diagnosis of a diabetic foot.

In our previous study, we measured the foot and finger temperature simultaneously and found that the foot skin

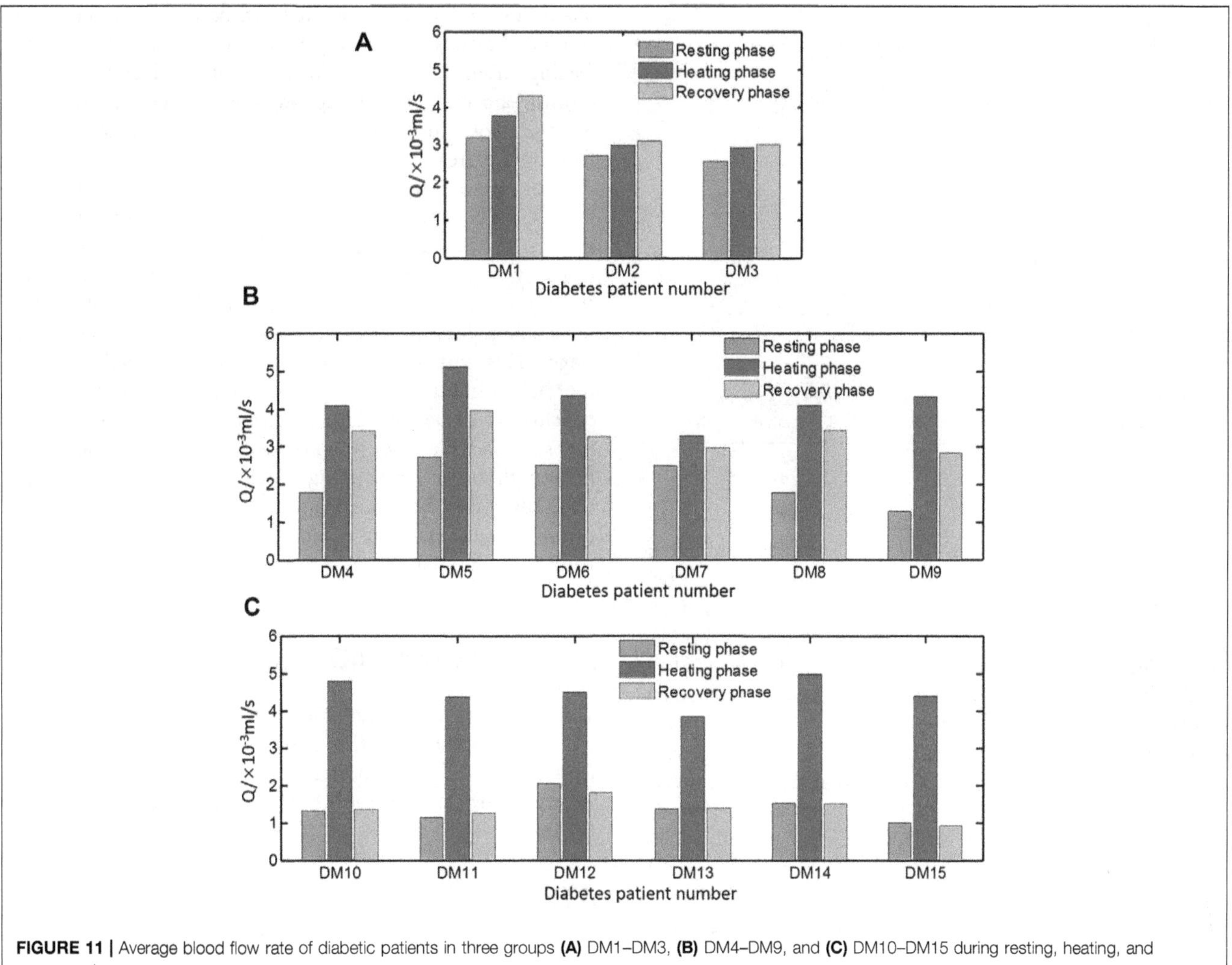

FIGURE 11 | Average blood flow rate of diabetic patients in three groups **(A)** DM1–DM3, **(B)** DM4–DM9, and **(C)** DM10–DM15 during resting, heating, and recovery phases.

temperature is more sensitive to reflect the endothelial dysfunction, but finger temperature can also give the same information (Tang, 2017). Since vascular abnormalities frequently occur in a similar fashion (Abularrage et al., 2005), abnormal vasomotion of hand could reflect the foot vascular disease to a certain extent. Compared to foot, hand is more accessible for measurement. Despite that, we did not focus on the coherence between the data in the hand and foot; there are three patients suffering peripheral neuropathy among the screened abnormal blood flow patients through the thermal analysis of SPAS data. This reveals that the hand skin temperature can also be a tracer for the early detection of the diabetic foot. More data from hand and foot should be collected simultaneously and compared for showing the coherence between them in detecting the endothelial dysfunction.

Additionally, although the relationship between the temperature and blood flow distribution was established in the foot model, the inversion of the blood flow of inlet arteries of the foot is not as simple as the process in the cubic model. Different inlet blood vessels or intermediated blood vessels own their respective temperature influencing areas, and the abnormal temperature distribution is a combined result of multiple blood flow under different degrees of stenosis. Therefore, in the future, it is necessary to divide the foot into several areas and apply available optimization methods to comprehensively investigate the coupling effect of various vascular disorders on temperature.

In generation of the foot vasculature, the nodes of the main blood vessels of the foot were manually set with reference to the physiological model obtained from the website, where the distance between the vessel and bone can be determined from the slices of the foot. After setting the arterial and venous nodes, the vessel network was compared to the physiological model again. Although the website provides the detailed structure of the foot including all tissues, the specific data could not be obtained. Thus, we manually made a vessel network according to the relative distance and size of the physiological model and inserted into the voxel-based model. The names and positions of the foot blood vessels in our model are also in agreement with the ones in the literature (Manzi et al., 2011).

The RRT algorithm was implemented to generate the blood vessels so that the blood is perfused into various regions of the tissue. **Figure 12** shows the number of vessel elements and relative

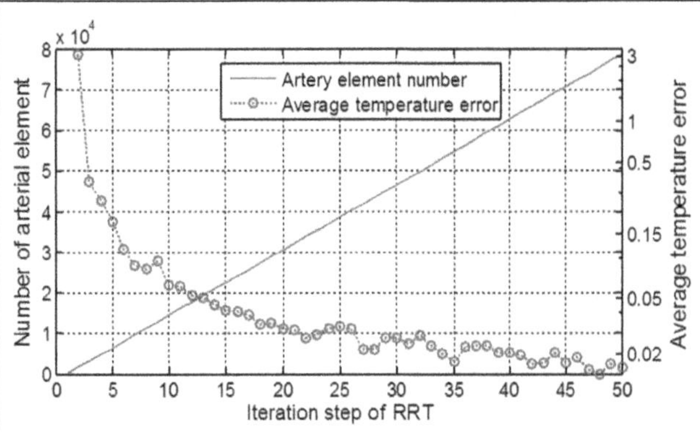

FIGURE 12 | Artery element number and average temperature error along with the increment of iteration steps in the RRT algorithm.

temperature errors along with the increasing RRT iterations. The number of iteration steps increases by 1,000 step each time, and the mean square error of the surface temperature between the newly computed temperature and original one was computed. The initial average error reached 3°C and gradually reduced as the iteration number increases. It is seen that the more iteration steps are used, the smaller blood vessels can be included and larger computational burden is resulted in. At the 50,000 s′ step, the average temperature error has been reduced to 0.01°C, and temperature distribution has hardly changed even with more iteration steps. Therefore, the iteration of this foot model is set as 50,000. In the computation for the cubic tissue model, the iteration step is set as 2,000 due to the smaller model size.

Despite of the reasonable structure and sizes of the vessels, it should be noted that the model has not reflected the individual differences in the foot structure. Our rat experimental study has shown that the microvasculature alteration occurs after the endothelial dysfunction (Wei et al., 2021). In the current study, it is assumed that the microvasculature has not been changed since the blood flow alterations due to the change of vasodilation is the first aim of the work. On the other hand, the iteration number of the RRT algorithm may give an impact on the structure of the vascular network and further influence the blood flow in a one-dimensional straight tube model. In the future we may optimize the RRT algorithm in the setting of the bifurcation angle of blood vessels and fractional dimensions so that various altered vasculatures in pathological conditions can be generated. Using MR angiography for showing the main vessels is an alternative way as well.

CONCLUSION

In this study, a vascular-porous media model has been applied in the thermal analysis of foot and a cubic tissue. Since the blood flow and the heat exchange within tissues during the flow process was considered by using a multiscale model, the temperature distributions under various thermal and blood flow conditions can be achieved so that the non-linear relationship between the blood flow and skin temperature can be further deduced. The computed results in the foot model reveals that the stenosis of feeding arteries can lead to temperature decreases in the downstream for different degrees, among which the occlusion of the posterior tibial artery has the largest lower-temperature area.

Then, analysis of the thermal response test imposed on type 2 diabetic patients and healthy subjects show that for a healthy subject, the blood flow rate after heating power is off at the recovery stage decreases to the level as that of the resting condition, whereas in some diabetic patients, the blood flow rates solely decrease slightly or even increase further at this stage. This implies that the vasodilation function to the thermal stimulus is delayed in the subject, which verifies the conclusions in our previous studies on diabetic rats. Most of the screened diabetic patients with peripheral vascular or neuropath disease are in agreement with those diagnosed clinically. It is believed that the discrete vascular-porous media model may have more applications, especially to studies of the diabetic foot by coupling with thermography imaging.

AUTHOR CONTRIBUTIONS

Y-PW drafted the manuscript and analyzed the data of this work. YH made substantial contributions to the design of this work and revised it critically for important intellectual content. R-HC made efforts in the data acquisition. L-ZM collected the raw data of foot CT images.

REFERENCES

Abularrage, C. J., Sidawy, A. N., Aidinian, G., Singh, N., Weiswasser, J. M., and Arora, S. (2005). Evaluation of the Microcirculation in Vascular Disease. *J. Vasc. Surg.* 42 (3), 574–581. doi:10.1016/j.jvs.2005.05.019

Alfred, G., Cynthia, F., Kevin, C., Camilleri, K. P., Raffaele, C. D., Mizzi, A., et al. (2015). Thermographic Patterns of the Upper and Lower Limbs: Baseline Data. *Int. J. Vasc. Med.* 2015, 831369. doi:10.1155/2015/831369

Amith, K., Muhammad, E. H. C., Mamun, B. I. R., Sawal, H. M. A., Md, A. H., Serkan, K., et al. (2021). A Machine Learning Model for Early Detection of Diabetic Foot Using Thermogram Images. *Comput. Biol. Med.* 137, 104838. doi:10.1016/j.compbiomed.2021.104838

Antonova, N., Tsiberkin, K., Podtaev, S., Paskova, V., Velcheva, I., and Chaushev, N. (2016). Comparative Study between Microvascular Tone Regulation and Rheological Properties of Blood in Patients with Type 2 Diabetes Mellitus. *Clin. Hemorheol. Microcirc.* 64, 837–844. doi:10.3233/CH-168000

Astasio, A., Escamilla, M. E., Martínez, N., Sánchez Rodríguez, R., and Gómez-Martín, B. (2018). Thermal Map of the Diabetic Foot Using Infrared Thermography. *Infrared Phys. Techn.* 93, S1350449518302512. doi:10.1016/j.infrared.2018.07.008

Astasio-Picado, Á., Escamilla Martínez, E., and Gómez-Martín, B. (2020). Comparative thermal Map of the Foot between Patients with and without Diabetes through the Use of Infrared Thermography. *Enfermería Clínica (English Edition)* 30 (2), 119–123. doi:10.1016/j.enfcle.2018.11.004

Bagavathiappan, S., Philip, J., Jayakumar, T., Raj, B., Rao, P. N. S., Varalakshmi, M., et al. (2010). Correlation between Plantar Foot Temperature and Diabetic Neuropathy: A Case Study by Using an Infrared Thermal Imaging Technique. *J. Diabetes Sci. Technol.* 4 (6), 1386–1392. doi:10.1177/193229681000400613

Bagavathiappan, S., Saravanan, T., Philip, J., Jayakumar, T., Raj, B., Karunanithi, R., et al. (2008). Investigation of Peripheral Vascular Disorders Using thermal Imaging. *Diabetes Vasc. Dis.* 8 (2), 102–104. doi:10.1177/1474651408008008020901

Bandalakunta Gururajarao, S., Venkatappa, U., Shivaram, J. M., Sikkandar, M. Y., and Al Amoudi, A. (2019). Infrared Thermography and Soft Computing for Diabetic Foot Assessment. *Infrared Thermography Soft Comput. Diabetic Foot Assess.*, 73–97. doi:10.1016/b978-0-12-816086-2.00004-7

Barrios, A., Debnath, O. B., Ito, K., Saito, K., and Uesaka, M. (2019). "Blood Flow Effect in Combination of Hyperthermia with Radiation Therapy for Treatment in Breast Tumor," in 2019 URSI Asia-Pacific Radio Science Conference (AP-RASC), New Delhi, India, 9-15 March 2019.

Blowers, S. J. (2018). *Modelling Brain Temperatures in Healthy Patients and Those with Induced Hypothermia* Edinburgh: The University of Edinburgh.

Blowers, S., Marshall, I., Thrippleton, M., Andrews, P., Harris, B., Bethune, I., et al. (2018). How Does Blood Regulate Cerebral Temperatures during Hypothermia. *Sci. Rep.* 8 (1), 7877. doi:10.1038/s41598-018-26063-7

Briers, J. D. (1996). Laser Speckle Contrast Analysis (LASCA): a Nonscanning, Full-Field Technique for Monitoring Capillary Blood Flow. *J. Biomed. Opt.* 1 (2), 174–179. doi:10.1117/12.231359

Carlos Padierna, L., Fabián Amador-Medina, L., Olivia Murillo-Ortiz, B., and Villaseñor-Mora, C. (2020). Classification Method of Peripheral Arterial Disease in Patients with Type 2 Diabetes Mellitus by Infrared Thermography and Machine Learning. *Infrared Phys. Techn.* 111, 103531. doi:10.1016/j.infrared.2020.103531

Chen, Z. Z., Gao, M. J., and Zhang, W. Z. (2021). Analytic Strategies for Early Diagnosis of Diabetic Foot Using Infrared thermal Imaging Technology. *China J. Traditional Chin. Med. Pharm.* 36 (2), 963–967.

Cheng, R. H. (2020). *Development of Thermal Response Measuring System for Assessing Blood Perfusion in Microcirculation.* Dalian: Dalian University of Technology.

Copetti, M. I. M., Durany, J., Fernández, J. R., and Poceiro, L. (2017). Numerical Analysis and Simulation of a Bio-thermal Model for the Human Foot. *Appl. Maths. Comput.* 305, 103–116. doi:10.1016/j.amc.2017.01.067

Frick, P., Mizeva, I., and Podtaev, S. (2015). Skin Temperature Variations as a Tracer of Microvessel Tone. *Biomed. Signal Process. Control.* 21, 1–7. doi:10.1016/j.bspc.2015.04.014

Glovaci, D., Fan, W., and Wong, N. D. (2019). Epidemiology of Diabetes Mellitus and Cardiovascular Disease. *Curr. Cardiol. Rep.* 21 (4), 21–28. doi:10.1007/s11886-019-1107-y

Haga, T., Ibe, A., Aso, Y., Ishizawa, M., Miyajima, M., and Takeda, K. (2012). Development of Methodology for Estimation of Skin Blood Perfusion by Applying Inverse Analysis of Skin Model. *Biomed. Eng.* 50 (4), 317–328. doi:10.11239/jsmbe.50.317

He, Y., Deng, B., Wang, H., Cheng, L., Zhou, K., Cai, S., et al. (2021). Infrared Machine Vision and Infrared Thermography with Deep Learning: A Review. *Infrared Phys. Techn.* 116 (2), 103754. doi:10.1016/j.infrared.2021.103754

He, Z.-Z., and Liu, J. (2017). A Coupled Continuum-Discrete Bioheat Transfer Model for Vascularized Tissue. *Int. J. Heat Mass Transfer* 107, 544–556. doi:10.1016/j.ijheatmasstransfer.2016.11.053

Hernandez-Contreras, D., Peregrina-Barreto, H., Rangel-Magdaleno, J., and Gonzalez-Bernal, J. (2016). Narrative Review: Diabetic Foot and Infrared Thermography. *Infrared Phys. Techn.* 78, 105–117. doi:10.1016/j.infrared.2016.07.013

Kevin, C., Falzon, O., and Sturgeon, C. (2019). Thermography to Assess Success of Lower Limb Endovascular Revascularisation in Diabetics with Critical Ischaemia. *Eur. J. Vasc. Endovascular Surg.* 58 (6), e36. doi:10.1016/j.ejvs.2019.06.545

Ma, W., Liu, W., and Li, M. (2015). Modeling Heat Transfer from Warm Water to Foot: Analytical Solution and Experimental Validation. *Int. J. Therm. Sci.* 98, 364–373. doi:10.1016/j.ijthermalsci.2015.07.030

Maldonado, H., Bayareh, R., Torres, I. A., Vera, A., Gutiérrez, J., and Leija, L. (2020). Automatic Detection of Risk Zones in Diabetic Foot Soles by Processing Thermographic Images Taken in an Uncontrolled Environment. *Infrared Phys. Techn.* 105, 103187. doi:10.1016/j.infrared.2020.103187

Manzi, M., Cester, G., Palena, L. M., Alek, J., Candeo, A., and Ferraresi, R. (2011). Vascular Imaging of the Foot: The First Step toward Endovascular Recanalization. *Radiographics* 31 (6), 1623–1636. doi:10.1148/rg.316115511

Mizeva, I., Zharkikh, E., Dremin, V., Zherebtsov, E., Makovik, I., Potapova, E., et al. (2018). Spectral Analysis of the Blood Flow in the Foot Microvascular Bed during thermal Testing in Patients with Diabetes Mellitus. *Microvasc. Res.* 120, 13 20. doi:10.1016/j.mvr.2018.05.005

Muhammad, A., Eddie, Ng., and Shu, Oh. (2018a). Automated Characterization of Diabetic Foot Using Nonlinear Features Extracted from Thermograms. *Infrared Phys. Techn.* 89, 325–337. doi:10.1016/j.infrared.2018.01.022

Muhammad, A., Eddie, Ng., Shu, Oh., Heng, M. L., Hagiwara, Y., Tan, J. H., et al. (2018b). Automated Detection of Diabetic Foot with and without Neuropathy Using Double Density-Dual Tree-Complex Wavelet Transform on Foot Thermograms. *Infrared Phys. Techn.* 92, 270–279. doi:10.1016/j.infrared.2018.06.010

Muhammad, A., Eddie, N. G., Tan, J. H., Heng, M. L., Tong, J. W. K., and Rajendra Acharya, U. (2017). Computer Aided Diagnosis of Diabetic Foot Using Infrared Thermography: A Review. *Comput. Biol. Med.* 91, 326. doi:10.1016/j.compbiomed.2017.10.030

Nagata, K., Hattori, H., Sato, N., Ichige, Y., and Kiguchi, M. (2009). Heat Transfer Analysis for Peripheral Blood Flow Measurement System. *Rev. Scientific Instr.* 80 (6), 064902. doi:10.1063/1.3155458

Nieuwenhoff, M. D., Wu, Y., Huygen, F. J. P. M., Schouten, A. C., van der Helm, F. C. T., and Niehof, S. P. (2016). Reproducibility of Axon Reflex-Related Vasodilation Assessed by Dynamic thermal Imaging in Healthy Subjects. *Microvasc. Res.* 106, 1–7. doi:10.1016/j.mvr.2016.03.001

Orchard, T. J., and Strandness, D. E. (1993). Assessment of Peripheral Vascular Disease in Diabetes. Report and Recommendations of an International Workshop Sponsored by the American Heart Association and the American Diabetes Association 18-20 September 1992, New Orleans, Louisiana. *J. Am. Podiatr Med. Assoc.* 83 (2), 685–695. doi:10.7547/87507315-83-12-685

Parshakov, A., Zubareva, N., and Frick, S. P. (2016). Detection of Endothelial Dysfunction Using Skin Temperature Oscillations Analysis during Local Heating in Patients with Peripheral Arterial Disease. *Microcirculation* 23 (6), 406–415. doi:10.1111/micc.12283

Parshakov, A., Zubareva, N., Podtaev, S., and Frick, P. (2017). Local Heating Test for Detection of Microcirculation Abnormalities in Patients with Diabetes-Related Foot Complications. *Adv. Skin Wound Care* 30 (4), 158–166. doi:10.1097/01.asw.0000508635.06240.c9

Pennes, H. H. (1998). Analysis of Tissue and Arterial Blood Temperatures in the Resting Human Forearm. *J. Appl. Physiol.* 85 (1), 5–34. doi:10.1152/jappl.1998.85.1.5

Podtaev, S., Stepanov, R., Smirnova, E., and Loran, E. (2014). Wavelet-analysis of Skin Temperature Oscillations during Local Heating for Revealing Endothelial Dysfunction. *Microvasc. Res.* 97, 109–114. doi:10.1016/j.mvr.2014.10.003

Podtaev, S., Morozov, M., and Frick, P. (2008). Wavelet-based Correlations of Skin Temperature and Blood Flow Oscillations. *Cardiovasc. Eng.* 8 (3), 185–189. doi:10.1007/s10558-008-9055-y

Pozrikidis, C. (2009). Numerical Simulation of Blood Flow through Microvascular Capillary Networks. *Bull. Math. Biol.* 71 (6), 1520–1541. doi:10.1007/s11538-009-9412-z

Rafael, B., Arturo, V., Lorenzo, L., and Gutierrez, M. I. (2016). "Simulation of the Temperature Distribution on a Diabetic Foot Model: A First Approximation," in 13th International Conference on Electrical Engineering, Computing Science and Automatic Control (CCE), IEEE, Mexico City, Mexico, 24 November 2016, 1–5.

Ricketts, P. L., Mudaliar, A. V., Ellis, B. E., Pullins, C. A., Meyers, L. A., Lanz, O. I., et al. (2008). Non-invasive Blood Perfusion Measurements Using a Combined Temperature and Heat Flux Surface Probe. *Int. J. Heat Mass. Transf* 51 (23-24), 5740–5748. doi:10.1016/j.ijheatmasstransfer.2008.04.051

Sagaidachnyi, A. A., Skripal, A. V., Fomin, A. V., and Usanov, D. A. (2014). Determination of the Amplitude and Phase Relationships between Oscillations in Skin Temperature and Photoplethysmography-Measured Blood Flow in Fingertips. *Physiol. Meas.* 35 (2), 153–166. doi:10.1088/0967-3334/35/2/153

Sagaidachnyi, A. A., Fomin, A. V., Usanov, D. A., and Skripal, A. V. (2017). Thermography-based Blood Flow Imaging in Human Skin of the Hands and Feet: a Spectral Filtering Approach. *Physiol. Meas.* 38 (2), 272–288. doi:10.1088/1361-6579/aa4eaf

Schürmann, M., Zaspel, J., Gradl, G., Wipfel, A., and Christ, F. (2001). Assessment of the Peripheral Microcirculation Using Computer-Assisted Venous Congestion Plethysmography in Post-Traumatic Complex Regional Pain Syndrome Type I. *J. Vasc. Res.* 38 (5), 453–461. doi:10.1159/000051078

Serlina, S., Saldy, Y., Cahyono, K., and Mukhtar, M. (2020). Evaluation Risk of Diabetic Foot Ulcers (DFUs) Using Infrared Thermography Based on mobile Phone as Advanced Risk Assessment Tool in the Community Setting: A Multisite Cross-Sectional Study. *Enfermería Clínica* 30, 453–457. doi:10.1016/j.enfcli.2019.07.136

Shao, H., He, Y., and Mu, L. (2014). Numerical Analysis of Dynamic Temperature in Response to Different Levels of Reactive Hyperaemia in a Three-Dimensional Image-Based Hand Model. *Comput. Methods Biomech. Biomed. Engin* 17 (5-8), 865–874. doi:10.1080/10255842.2012.723698

Sivanandam, S., Anburajan, M., Venkatraman, B., Menaka, M., and Sharath, D. (2012). Medical Thermography: a Diagnostic Approach for Type 2 Diabetes Based on Non-contact Infrared thermal Imaging. *Endocrine* 42 (2), 343–351. doi:10.1007/s12020-012-9645-8

Smirnova, E., Podtaev, S., Mizeva, I., and Loran, E. (2013). Assessment of Endothelial Dysfunction in Patients with Impaired Glucose Tolerance during a Cold Pressor Test. *Diabetes Vasc. Dis. Res.* 10 (6), 489–497. doi:10.1177/1479164113494881

Tang, Y., He, Y., Shao, H., and Ji, C. (2016). Assessment of Comfortable Clothing thermal Resistance Using a Multi-Scale Human Thermoregulatory Model. *Int. J. Heat Mass Transfer* 98, 568–583. doi:10.1016/j.ijheatmasstransfer.2016.03.030

Tang, Y. L. (2017). *Mechanism Study of Thermal Methods for the Detection of Diabetic Microvascular Dysfunction* (Dalian: Dalian University of Technology). PhD thesis.

Tang, Y. L., Mizeva, I., and He, Y. (2017). A Modeling Method on the Influence of Blood Flow Regulation on Skin Temperature Pulsations. *Proc. SPIE* 10337, 1–6. doi:10.1117/12.2267952

Tang, Y., Mu, L., and He, Y. (2020). Numerical Simulation of Fluid and Heat Transfer in a Biological Tissue Using an Immersed Boundary Method Mimicking the Exact Structure of the Microvascular Network. *Fluid Dyn. Mater. Process.* 16 (2), 281–296. doi:10.32604/fdmp.2020.06760

Uraiwan, C., Patsakorn, N., Tanchanok, D., and Yamauchi, J. (2018). An Exploration of the Relationship between Foot Skin Temperature and Blood Flow in Type 2 Diabetes Mellitus Patients: a Cross-Sectional Study. *J. Phys. Ther. Sci.* 30 (11), 1359–1363. doi:10.1589/jpts.30.1359

Van Netten, J. J., Van Baal, J. G., Liu, C., van der Heijden, F., and Bus, S. A. (2013). Infrared thermal Imaging for Automated Detection of Diabetic Foot Complications. *J. Diabetes Sci. Technol.* 7 (5), 1122–1129. doi:10.1177/193229681300700504

Wang, Y.-P., Tang, Y.-L., and He, Y. (2021). Numerical Analysis of the Influence of RBCs on Oxygen Transport within a Tissue with an Embedded Capillary Network. *Proc. Inst. Mech. Eng. C: J. Mech. Eng. Sci.* 235 (2), 412–427. doi:10.1177/0954406220954482

Wang, Y., Mu, L., He, Y., Tang, Y., Liu, C., Lu, Y., et al. (2020). Heat Transfer Analysis of Blood Perfusion in Diabetic Rats Using a Genetic Algorithm. *Microvasc. Res.* 131, 104013. doi:10.1016/j.mvr.2020.104013

Webb, R. C., Ma, Y., Krishnan, S., Li, Y., Yoon, S., Guo, X., et al. (2015). Epidermal Devices for Noninvasive, Precise, and Continuous Mapping of Macrovascular and Microvascular Blood Flow. *Sci. Adv.* 1 (9), e1500701. doi:10.1126/sciadv.1500701

Wei, Y., Chen, H., Chi, Q., He, Y., Mu, L., Liu, C., et al. (2021). Synchronized Research on Endothelial Dysfunction and Microcirculation Structure in Dorsal Skin of Rats with Type 2 Diabetes Mellitus. *Med. Biol. Eng. Comput.* 59 (5), 1151–1166. doi:10.1007/s11517-021-02363-5

Zhang, P., Lu, J., Jing, Y., Tang, S., Zhu, D., and Bi, Y. (2017). Global Epidemiology of Diabetic Foot Ulceration: a Systematic Review and Meta-Analysis. *Ann. Med.* 49 (2), 106–116. doi:10.1080/07853890.2016.1231932

Zhang, Y., and Zhu, K. (2010). Relationship between Tongue Temperature and Lingual Circulation System in Blood Stasis Syndrome and Blood Deficiency Syndrome. *Space Med. Med. Eng.* 23 (4), 267–273.

Zubareva, N., Parshakov, A., Podtaev, S., Frick, P., and Mizeva, I. (2019). "Recovery of Endothelial Function in Microvessels in Patients with Peripheral Artery Disease (PAD) after Conservative and Surgery Treatment," in Saratov Fall Meeting 2018: Computations and Data Analysis: from Nanoscale Tools to Brain Functions.

APPENDIX

TABLE A1 | Information on healthy people and diabetic patients in the experiments.

Number of subject	Age	BMI
N1	52	22.0
N2	23	20.55
N3	23	18.21
N4	25	25.09
N5	28	28.34
DM1	35	20.99
DM2	48	33.14
DM3	44	25.0
DM4	32	25.69
DM5	57	28.88
DM6	64	28.7
DM7	47	26.85
DM8	49	29.39
DM9	50	30.0
DM10	34	28.53
DM11	37	32.57
DM12	50	26.9
DM13	51	22.14
DM14	66	27.9
DM15	57	25.25

16

Electrospun Nanofibrous Poly (Lactic Acid)/Titanium Dioxide Nanocomposite Membranes for Cutaneous Scar Minimization

Teresa C. O. Marsi[1†], Ritchelli Ricci[1†], Tatiane V. Toniato[1], Luana M. R. Vasconcellos[2], Conceição de Maria Vaz Elias[3], Andre D. R. Silva[4], Andre S. A. Furtado[5], Leila S. S. M. Magalhães[5], Edson C. Silva-Filho[5], Fernanda R. Marciano[6], Andrea Zille[7], Thomas J. Webster[8] and Anderson O. Lobo[5]*

[1] *Institute of Research and Development, University of Vale Do Paraiba, São José dos Campos, Brazil,* [2] *Department of Bioscience and Oral Diagnosis, Institute of Science and Technology, São Paulo State University, São Paulo, Brazil,* [3] *Scientific and Technological Institute, Brasil University, São Paulo, Brazil,* [4] *Air Force Academy, Brazilian Air Force, Pirassununga, Brazil,* [5] *LIMAV - Interdisciplinary Laboratory for Advanced Materials, Materials Science & Engineering Graduate Program, UFPI-Federal University of Piaui, Teresina, Brazil,* [6] *Department of Physics, Federal University of Piaui, Teresina, Brazil,* [7] *Department of Textile Engineering, Centre for Textile Science and Technology, University of Minho, Guimarães, Portugal,* [8] *Department of Chemical Engineering, Northeastern University, Boston, MA, United States*

***Correspondence:**
Anderson O. Lobo
lobo@ufpi.edu.br

[†] *These authors have contributed equally to this work*

Poly (lactic acid) (PLA) has been increasingly used in cutaneous tissue engineering due to its low cost, ease of handling, biodegradability, and biocompatibility, as well as its ability to form composites. However, these polymers possess a structure with nanoporous that mimic the cellular environment. In this study, nanocomposites are prepared using PLA and titanium dioxide (TiO_2) (10 and 35%—w/w) nanoparticles that also function as an active anti-scarring agent. The nanocomposites were prepared using an electrospinning technique. Three different solutions were prepared as follows: PLA, 10% PLA/TiO_2, and 35% PLA/TiO_2 (w/w%). Electrospun PLA and PLA/TiO_2 nanocomposites were characterized morphologically, structurally, and chemically using electron scanning microscopy, transmission electron microscopy, goniometry, and X-ray diffraction. L929 fibroblast cells were used for *in vitro* tests. The cytotoxic effect was evaluated using 3-(4,5-dimethylthiazol-2-yl)-2,5-diphenyltetrazolium bromide assays. Versicam (VCAN), biglicam (BIG), interleukin-6 (IL6), interleukin-10 (IL-10), and type-1 collagen (COL1A1) genes were evaluated by RT-qPCR. *In vivo* tests using Wistar rats were conducted for up to 15 days. Nanofibrous fibers were obtained for all groups that did not contain residual solvents. No cytotoxic effects were observed for up to 168 h. The genes expressed showed the highest values of versican and collagen-1 ($p < 0.05$) for PLA/TiO_2 nanocomposite scaffolds when compared to the control group (cells). Histological images showed that PLA at 10 and 35% w/w led to a discrete inflammatory infiltration and expression of many newly formed vessels, indicating increased metabolic activity of this tissue. To summarize, this study supported the potential of PLA/TiO_2 nanocomposites ability to reduce cutaneous scarring in scaffolds.

Keywords: PLA, nanocomposites, electrospinning, cutaneous scarring, gene expression, *in vivo*

INTRODUCTION

The standard treatment for skin lesions uses dressings that come in direct contact with the injured region. By replacing these dressings with scaffolds, this treatment becomes non-invasive to minimally invasive along with other positive outcomes such as a reduction in patient recovery times, medical costs and consumption of scarce and valuable health-care resources around the world for treatment of large-scale musculoskeletal injuries with traumatic lesions, birth defects and surgical excisions (Bardosova and Wagner, 2015; Beyth et al., 2015; Walmsley et al., 2015; Ghannadian et al., 2018). Bioabsorbable and biodegradable polymers have been shown enough mechanical properties that accelerate the cell proliferation process while providing antimicrobial protection. This makes them promising materials for biomedical applications as they have been shown to optimize the tissue repair process which in turn speeds up patient recovery times (Simoes, 2011; Wang et al., 2014; Fonseca et al., 2015). Among the various polymers, poly (lactic acid) (PLA) has proven to be an ideal candidate material due to its mechanical properties, good biocompatibility, low cost, and the adjustable degradation profile with CO_2, H_2O (Hidalgo et al., 2013; Tawakkal et al., 2014; Annunziata et al., 2015; Toniatto et al., 2017) and polyester as by-products, either from the esterification of lactic acid and its fermentation (Toniatto et al., 2017).

PLA-based nanofibrous fibers have large surface areas, allowing them to interact with large volumes of other substances in their environment. This is a distinguishing feature of this material (Bayon et al., 2016; Toniatto et al., 2017; Salles et al., 2018). The fiber surfaces have several characteristics that make them similar to the extracellular matrices (ECMs) used in biomedical applications. In addition, the interaction of the cells and the substrate influences their morphology, proliferation, and viability (Braunger et al., 2017). ECMs have been assumed to be inert structures that consist of proteins and polysaccharides that are synthesized and secreted by cells. Their sole purpose was once considered to fill up extracellular space. However, recent research indicates that ECMs perform other key roles. They function as scaffolds, aid in cell binding, allow for tissue formation, and play an important role in the control of cell growth, differentiation, adhesion, migration, proliferation, and angiogenesis (Villarreal-Gómez et al., 2016; Saldin et al., 2017).

Studies have shown that titanium dioxide (TiO_2) nanoparticles are highly biocompatible and have good physical, chemical, mechanical, and biological properties. These nanoparticles have a variety of uses in many biomedical applications. One study found that they help increase protein absorption and reduce infections caused by both Gram-positive and Gram-negative bacteria (Roy et al., 2007; Liou and Chang, 2012; Kandiah et al., 2014; Wu et al., 2014; Toniatto et al., 2017).

Electrospinning of polymers can be used to generate three-dimensional fibrous structures and is therefore used to produce mats with these polymers. The electrospun mats closely resemble natural ECM (Villarreal-Gómez et al., 2016; Toniatto et al., 2017) and are capable of supporting cell adhesion and proliferation. Due to their inherent material properties, these mats not only provide a three-dimensional structure but are also biocompatible, bioabsorbable, and have antibacterial properties, making them extremely desirable for use in scaffolds and medical devices (Roux et al., 2013; Stocco et al., 2018). PLA/TiO_2–nanofibrous fibers produced by electrospinning are being studied in order to evaluate their potential in dressing and wound healing applications (Bayon et al., 2016; Toniatto et al., 2017; Ghosal et al., 2018; Salles et al., 2018).

In prior studies, we have shown that PLA/TiO_2-based scaffolds have bactericidal properties and do not exhibit cytotoxicity (Toniatto et al., 2017). Here, we further evaluated the toxicity of electrospun PLA in fibroblast cells and rats (skin model) and compare the results when the material is embedded two different concentrations of TiO_2 nanoparticles PLA/TiO_2−10% w/w (PLA—A) and PLA/TiO_2−35% w/w (PLA—B). We also investigated their potential to upregulate specific genes related to the regenerative process. These electrospun scaffolds are biocompatible and showed no inflammations in rats. They were also found to have upregulated the versicam and type-1 collagen genes. These results provide a strong rationale to use PLA/TiO_2 scaffolds as dressings for skin lesion applications.

MATERIALS AND METHODS

Materials

Chloroform, N, N-diethylformamide (DMF), ethyl alcohol, Dulbecco's MEM (DMEM), Fetal Bovine Serum (FBS), 3-4,5-dimethylthiazol-2-yl-2,5-diphenyltetrazolol bromide, neutral buffered Formalin, Hematoxilin and Eosin were purchased from Sigma-Aldrich® (USA). PLA (2003D, with 4.30% of D-lactic acid monomer) was donated by NatureWorks (Minnetonka, Minnesota, United States). TiO_2 nanoparticles were donated by Evonik Degussa (AEROXIDE® TiO_2 P25, Essen, North Rhine-Westphalia, Germany). NCTC clone 929 (L CELL, L-929) cells were purchased from a bank cell in Rio de Janeiro, Brazil. 24-wells plates were purchased from Ciencor®. RNAeasyTM mini kit was purchased from Qiagen (São Paulo, Brazil). Versicam, biglicam, interleukins-6, interleukins-10, collagen-1 genes, complementary DNA (cDNA), RNA, and GoTaq® qPCR Master Mix amplifier kit were purchased from Promega (São Paulo, Brazil).

Electrospinning of PLA/TiO_2 Nanocomposite Membranes

Three types of solutions were prepared: PLA, PLA with 10% TiO_2 by weight, and PLA with 35% TiO_2 by weight. In the first step, 0.09 g of PLA was dissolved in 0.6 mL of chloroform at room temperature for about 150 min in closed system. Three sets of these PLA solution compositions were prepared. Afterwards in two separate containers, TiO_2 nanoparticles (0.01 and 0.05 g, respectively) were dispersed in 0.4 mL DMF using a tip ultrasound (Sonics, VCX 500) for ~90 min. A third container with 0.4 mL DMF was also prepared without the addition of TiO_2. Subsequently, each of the three DMF solutions (two of them containing TiO_2 of different concentrations, and one without TiO_2) was added to each of the three PLA solutions in chloroform and then stirred magnetically for 20 h in an enclosed system at

TABLE 1 | Description of produced solutions prior electrospinning process.

Scaffolds	PLA (g)	TiO_2 (g)	Chloroform (mL)	DMF (mL)
PLA	0.09	–	0.6	0.4
PLA–A	0.09	0.01	0.6	0.4
PLA–B	0.09	0.05	0.6	0.4

room temperature. **Table 1** summarizes the masses and volumes of three prepared solutions. The electrospinning process was performed under a temperature and humidity-controlled exhaust hood (at a temperature of 25 ± 2°C and relative humidity of 30–40%). The electrospinning parameters/apparatus used were: 12 kV (Bertan 203R), syringe (5 mL, BD®), metal needle (23G, Inbras), infusion rate (0.05 mL/h), on a collector covered with aluminum foil (100 × 100 × 1 mm, at a distance of 10 cm) and total time of 30 min.

Characterization of Structural, Physical, and Chemical Properties

The samples were characterized after 24 h under vacuum. Scanning electron microscope (SEM, Zeiss EVO MA10) was used to analyze the morphology and determine the diameters of the fibers. To aid the analysis, a thin layer of gold (~10 nm thickness) was deposited using sputtering under an Argon plasma at a pressure of 0.2 mbar under an applied current of 30 mA for 2 min. The micrographs were obtained using magnifications of 500x, 1,000x, and 5,000x. Images were obtained using the SEM and analyzed using ImageJ software to establish the mean diameters for the fibers, and the mean and standard deviations of the data were calculated. Transmission electron microscopy (TEM, Philips CM120) was used to evaluate the homogeneity of the TiO_2 nanoparticles incorporated into the fibers. To perform the analysis, the fibers were collected for 5 s onto a copper transmission grid of 3.05 mm in diameter. The grid was positioned at a working distance of 10 cm, and the material was deposited for a few seconds, until a thin layer was formed on the grid.

A goniometer (Krüss DSA 100) operating in dynamic mode was used to measure the angle between the scaffolds and air using water and diiodomethane. Two microliters of deionized water was dropped on each scaffold and images were recorded after 1 min. This test was performed on 5 samples, and the mean and standard deviations for the results were calculated.

TGA measurements were carried out in a STA 7200 Hitachi (Tokyo, Japan). TGA plots were obtained within the range of 25–900°C under nitrogen atmosphere (200 $mL{\cdot}min^{-1}$) at $10°C{\cdot}min^{-1}$. Specimens were left at room temperature (25°C) until equilibrium was reached and placed in an aluminum pan. Data was plotted as weight loss percentage vs. temperature, and the mass of dried residues was calculated for each case. The derivative thermogravimetric (DTG) analysis was also performed to identify the maximum peaks of the thermal transformation events.

DSC analyses were carried out in a Mettler-Toledo DSC822 instrument (Giessen, Germany). Analyses were carried out in an aluminum sample pan under nitrogen atmosphere with a flow rate of 20 mL min^{-1} and heating rate of 10°C min^{-1}. In order to eliminate the thermal history of the material, the first heating cycle was obtained in the range of 0–110°C, afterwards it was cooled down to 0°C and heated again up to 500°C. The graph was plotted as heat flow vs. temperature.

The tensile strength, elongation at break and fracture strain of the nanofibers were measured using a texture analyzer (TA.XT plus, Stable Micro Systems Ltd., Vienna, UK). Rectangular samples of the polymeric scaffolds were specifically cut to have dimensions of 10.00 × 30.00 × 0.10 mm and fixed with the probe provided by instrumentation attached to a 5 kg load cell. Measurements were recorded at 25°C with a strain rate of 1 $mm.min^{-1}$ ($N = 3$).

X-ray diffraction (XRD) (PANalytical X'Pert Pro diffractometer) using a monochromatic X-Ray CuKα radiation, was used to study the crystalline structure of the samples. Data were collected over a range of 10–80° using a scanning speed of 0.08 degrees per minute. Data was analyzed using HighScore 3.0a software (PaNalytical, Almelo, Netherlands) for phase identification. The crystalline index was calculated as the ratio of the crystalline scattering fraction to the total crystalline and amorphous scattering.

Biomedical Characterizations of PLA/TiO_2 Nanocomposite Membranes

Prior to performing any biological assay, the samples were vacuum dried. For the biological assays, L929 fibroblasts cells were cultured in Dulbecco's Modified Eagle's Medium supplemented with fetal bovine serum (90:10 v/v) and kept in a 5% CO_2 atmosphere at 37°C for 7 days to obtain a confluence layer. The polymer sheets were sterilized in ultraviolet radiation and then placed in 70% ethyl alcohol, washed with phosphate-buffered saline, and hydrated with the DMEM/FBS medium prior to use in the biological assays (Lobo et al., 2008).

A 3-(4,5-dimethylthiazol-2-yl)-2,5-diphenyltetrazolium bromide (MTT) assay was used to analyze the scaffold (PLA only, PLA—A, and PLA—B) scaffolds for cytotoxicity. Twenty thousand cells were plated in a 24-well plate. After 24 h, a 10 × 10 mm square piece of each of the scaffold types was placed on separate plates. After both 24 and 168 h, 100 μL MTT (1 mg/mL) was added to the culture medium in each well. The plate was then covered with an aluminum foil and incubated for 2 h in an oven with a consistent a 5% CO_2 atmosphere and 37°C temperature (Lobo et al., 2008). The MTT was then removed and 100 μL of dimethyl sulfoxide (DMSO) was added in each sample. The absorbance was then measured using a spectrophotometer (570 nm wavelength; instrumentation by AsysHitech GmbH, Eugendorf, Austria). Cells were used as negative controls and latex fragments (10 × 10 mm) as positive controls for cytotoxicity tests. To normalize the results, the absorbance of a blank sample and DMSO were also measured. Gene expression analysis by RT-qPCR, and extraction of total RNA from adhered cells on scaffolds were performed after 7, 14, and 21 days. Versicam, Biglicam, interleukins-6, interleukins-10, and collagen-1 (COL1A1) genes were expressed upon performing RT-qPCR. The integrity of the RNA was evaluated using agarose

TABLE 2 | Description of the gene used in RT-qPCR.

Gene	Gene name	Primer sequences	Ref. Fast Pubmed
VCAN	Versicam	5′-CAAACCCTGCCTCAACGGAGG-3′ 5′-CCTTCAGCAGCATCCCATGTGCGT-3′	NM_001101
BGN	Biglycan	5′-GATGGCCTGAAGCTCAA-3′ 5′- GGTTGTTGAAGAGGCTG-3′	NM_199173
COL1A1	Type I Collagen alpha 1	5′-CCCTGGAAAGAATGGAGATGAT-3′ 5′-ACTGAAACCTCTGTGTCCCTTCA-3′	NM_000088.3
IL6	Interleukin 6	5′-AGCCAGAGCTGTGCAGATGA-3′ 5′-GCAGGCTGGCATTTGTGGTT-3′	NM_031168.2
IL-10	Interleukin 10	5′-AGCCAGCAGCTCTCAAGTC-3′ 5′-GTGTTCAGTGTGGTCCTGGAT-3′	NM_010548.2

gel electrophoresis (1.5%) and analyzed using the 18S and 28S bands. Thereafter, the outer diameter was measured (at 260 and 280 nm wavelengths using Nano Drop 2000 manufactured by Thermo Fisher) and the concentration and purity of the RNA sample was determined. Values A260/A280 between 1.8 and 2.0 were accepted. For the synthesis of deoxyribonucleic acid (cDNA), 2.0 μg of RNA obtained via reverse transcription was used following the manufacturer's instructions. The cDNA was amplified and an ABI PRISM 7500 sequence detector (Applied Biosystems, USA) was used for quantitative analysis of the gene expression. The primers analyzed are listed in **Table 2**. The conditions/parameters applied during this analysis were 95°C (for 5 min), 40 cycles of 15 min each at 95°C, 60°C (for 1 min), and a final cycle of 5 min at 72°C. Each experiment was repeated three times and the data was normalized according to the expression of the reference gene using the selection of the most appropriate endogenous control. Three reference genes were used: Glyceraldehyde 3-phosphate dehydrogenase (GAPDH), ribosomal 18S RNA (18SrRNA), and beta-beta smooth muscle (β-actin); β-actin was the preferred reference gene. The ΔΔCt method acquires average cycle limit values (Cts) of the target genes and compares them with the Cts of the average reference gene. Relative gene expression was calculated using the $2^{-\Delta\Delta Ct}$ method (Livak and Schmittgen, 2001).

The RNA samples were analyzed using the NanoDrop ND-1000 spectrophotometer (Thermo Fisher Scientific, USA) at wavelengths of 260 nm for RNA and 280 nm for the protein.

The primers were designed with the aid of the RTD program (Integrated DNA Technologies, www.idtdna.com) and Primer 3 software (frodo.wi.mit.edu/cgi-bin/primer3/primer3_www.cgi).

Experimental Model—*in-vivo*

All *in-vivo* procedures were performed in accordance with ethical standards. The testing protocol was approved by the Brazilian committee (10/2015-CEUA/ICT/CJSC-UNESP). Six male Wistar rats (*Rattus norvegicus*) aged 90 days and weighing between 350 and 400 g were used. The animals were provided with food and water *ad libitum*. The PLA, PLA—A, and PLA—B samples were implanted in the rat dorsal subcutaneous tissue ($n = 2$). The apparatus was cleaned using 70% ethanol and sterilized for 2 h using UV radiation and surgically inserted using procedures described in Camargo et al. (2010). The rats were euthanized 15 days after the surgery.

For histological analysis, a 10% neutral buffered formalin was applied on the surgical sites. After 48 h, the specimens were processed using paraffin embedding. The paraffin block was oriented parallel to the long axis of the material, and serial sections of 5 μm thickness were cut. Theses sections were then stained with hematoxylin and eosin. Histological qualitative evaluation was conducted using microscopic analysis.

Statistical Analysis

A sample size of 5 has been used in this study. The data was analyzed using two-way analysis of variance (ANOVA) followed by a Tukey's test (GraphPad Prism software, v. 5.01). A value of $p < 0.05$ was considered statistically significant.

RESULTS

Characterization of the Electrospun Scaffolds

Figures 1A–C shows SEM micrographs of PLA, PLA—A, and PLA—B nanofibrous scaffolds, respectively. The homogeneity of the nanofibers can be observed; the diameters of the nanofibers appear to be similar and they no obvious deformation and free of beads. The mean values of the diameters of the nanofibers in the samples of PLA with 10 and 35% TiO_2 were 332 ± 108 and 332 ± 95 nm, respectively—slightly larger than that observed in the PLA sample without TiO_2 (315 ± 87 nm). The images obtained by TEM showed that TiO_2 nanoparticles were homogeneously dispersed within the PLA fibers at both the concentration levels of 10 and 35%—w/w (**Figures 1B.1,C.1**). **Figure 1D** shows contact angle measurement using water. It can be observed that incorporation of TiO_2 nanoparticles causes an observable decrease in the contact angle. The PLA, PLA—A, and PLA—B samples had contact angles of 160.0 ± 3.0, 140.0 ± 2.1, 130.0 ± 2.2°, respectively. XRD measurements showed that TiO_2 has a different growth process in the single crystalline phase corresponding to the anatase phase (**Figure 1E**). The preferred orientation plane is the crystalline plane (101) around of $2\theta = 25°$, which is typical of the anatase phase and the rutile phase, indicating a high purity of the material. This is confirmed by the peaks, $2\theta = 37$, 49, 54, 56, 63, 70, and 76° at the corresponding crystallographic planes (1 0 3), (2 0 0), (2 1 1), (2 1 1), (2 0 4), (1 1 6), and (2 1 5) (Dinari and Haghighi, 2017; Pava-Gómez et al., 2018). The peaks at 25, 37, and 49° are characteristic of TiO_2 and are clearly observed when they are part in the fibers. The intensity of the XRD peaks was lower in the samples that contained the TiO_2 than in those without TiO_2 (**Figures 2A.1–A.3**). The measured crystalline index was 89, 87, and 82% for PLA, PLA—A, and PLA—B samples, respectively.

Figure 2 shows deconvolutions obtained from XRD, as shown in **Figure 1E**. The amplitude of the peak found between 16.45 and 16.80° was used to determine the proportion of pure PLA scaffold area. It was found that for the PLA membranes (**Figure 2A.1**), PLA—A membranes (**Figure 2A.2**), and PLA—B membranes (**Figure 2A.3**) had 60.2, 51.45, and 44.38% of

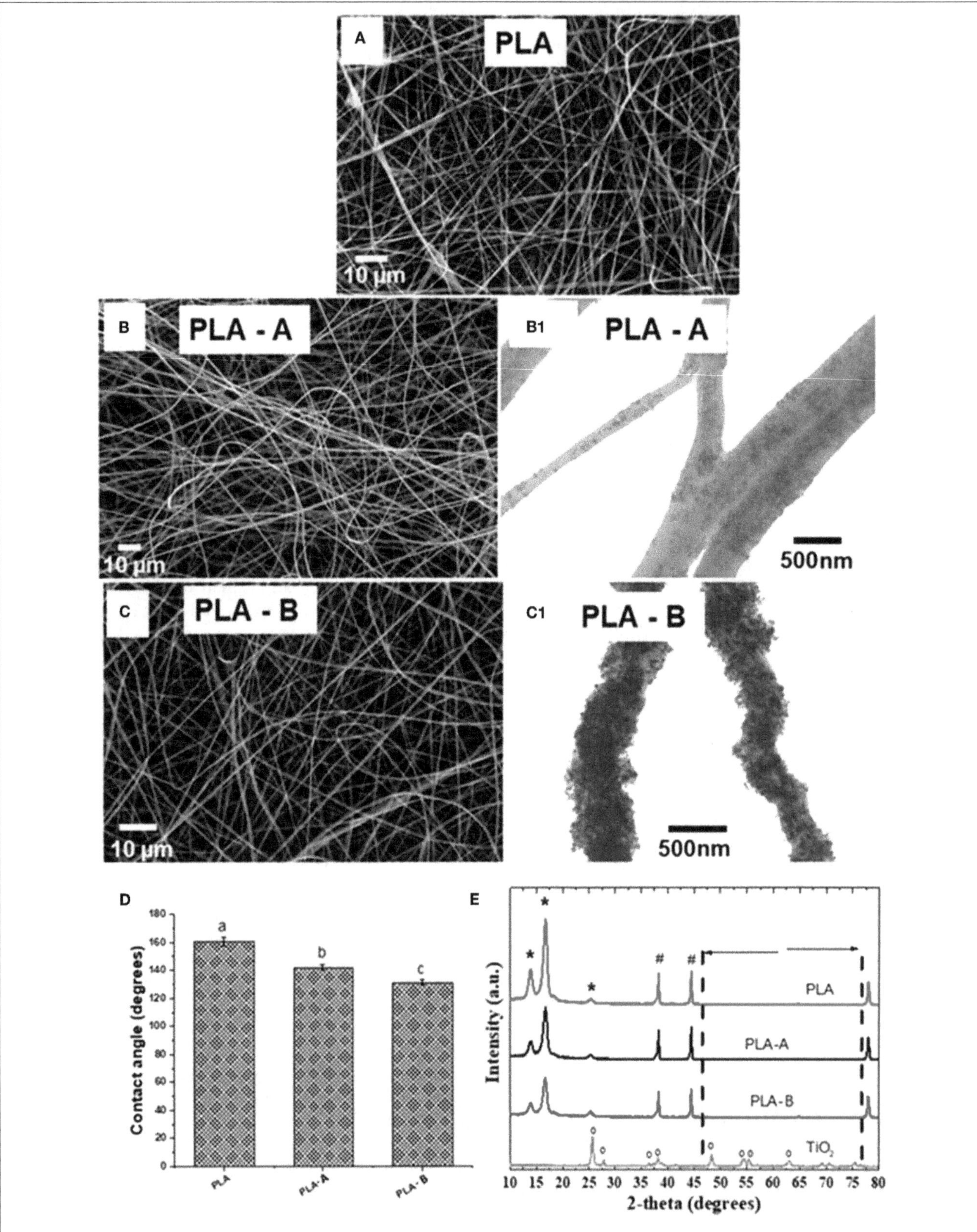

FIGURE 1 | (A) Micrograph for PLA fiber without TiO_2 addition; micrographs of polymer solutions with **(B)** PLA—A; **(C)** PLA—B. **(D)** Contact angles measured. **(E)** XRD of the developed membrane. Images obtained by TEM **(B.1)** PLA—A, **(C.1)** PLA—B. * and # referred to typical PLA crystalline planes. ° referred to typical TiO_2 crystaliine planes.

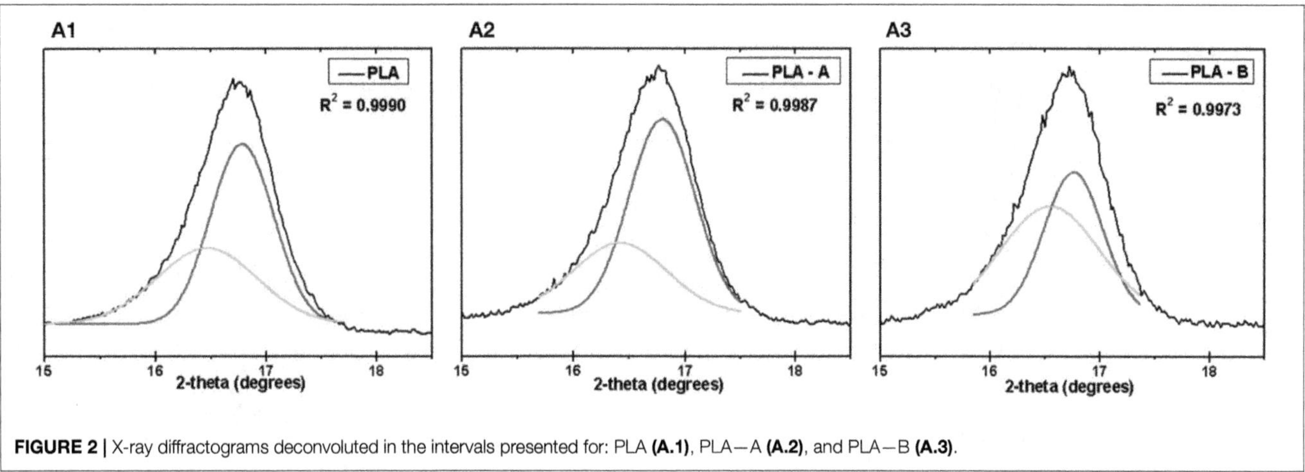

FIGURE 2 | X-ray diffractograms deconvoluted in the intervals presented for: PLA **(A.1)**, PLA—A **(A.2)**, and PLA—B **(A.3)**.

TABLE 3 | Main DSC thermal transitions ($n = 3$; S.D. < 1%), TGA mass loss temperature peaks and residual weight (R_w) at 900°C of samples ($n = 3$; ± S.D).

Sample	T_{Onset} (°C)	T_{Peak} (°C)	T_{Endset} (°C)	ΔH (J g^{-1})	T_g (°C)	DTG T_{Max} (°C)	R_w 900°C (%)	R_w 900°C (mg/mg)
PLA	132.8	154.9	170.1	57.7	55.3	326.6 ± 2.6	0	7.2/0
PLA—A (1st peak)	146.6	157.4	163.3	44.8	61.8	354.8 ± 5.6	5.0 ± 0.6	8.95/0.45
PLA—A (2nd peak)	308.1	350.5	364.4	638.8				
PLA—B (1st peak)	148.6	157.6	162.9	35.6	65.8	354.9 ± 2.2	28.2 ± 0.4	8.15/2.30
PLA—B (2nd peak)	330.8	356.8	368.8	540.2				

pure PLA membranes area respectively. Diffractogram fitting was performed in order to quantify the percentage of area formed under the curve where the characteristic PLA peaks are identified. For this, the deconvolution method with Gaussian function was used in a software Origin 8.0, obtaining curves with $R^2 = 0.99$. The study of this device has been used as a tool in several works of our research group (Silva et al., 2018, 2019a,b).

Table 3 and **Figure 3** display the result of the thermal characterization of the sample containing TiO_2 nanoparticles. The TGA result shows that the degradation temperature of the composite nanofiber (peak around 355°C against the peak at 326.6°C of the pure PLA) is significantly affected by the presence of TiO_2 but not by its concentrations in the polymer matrix (Laske et al., 2015; Wacharawichanant et al., 2017; AnŽlovar et al., 2018). It is clear from **Table 3** that the residual weight expressed in mg/mg is proportional to the TiO_2 content on the PLA electrospun nanofibers.

The DSC results display a glass transition temperature (Tg) and two endothermic peaks in the second heating cycle. The Tg (**Figure 3B** inset) increase with the amount of TiO_2 in the PLA matrix from the 55.4°C of pure PLA to the 61.8°C of PLA-A and 65.8°C of PLA-B. The first peak, attributed to the melting point of PLA, is slightly affected by the presence of the nanoparticles (peak around 157.5°C against the peak at 154.9°C of the pure PLA). The second one, attributed to the PLA degradation, has sharper peaks and shifts to a higher temperature in the presence of TiO_2. The introduction of higher concentration of TiO_2 in the PLA structure significantly decreases the melting enthalpy of both peaks.

The **Figure 4** illustrates the mechanical properties (FS, EM, and TS) of PLA/TiO_2 nanofibers with different TiO_2 contents. As can be seen, the mechanical properties of the scaffolds were affected by the addition of TiO_2. There is an increase in the value of these properties for PLA—A and subsequently a reduction for PLA—B. The changes in evaluated values are summarized in **Table 4**.

Cytotoxicity and Gene Expression Analyses

Cytotoxicity studies were performed at two different time points (24 and 168 h) and the analyzed groups were compared to a positive control (latex, **Figure 5A**). The expression of the genes of interest was studied using RT-qPCR from cDNA obtained by the reverse transcription of mRNA obtained from the fibroblast lineage. Before initiating the RT-qPCR reactions, expression of these genes was analyzed by semi-quantitative or end-point RT-PCR to ensure they were expressed (data not shown). The expression of extracellular matrix Versicam, Biglicam type 1 collagen, interleukins-6, and interleukins-10 were analyzed. It was observed that the expression of Versicam increased when L929 fibroblast cells were cultivated on PLA and PLA—A and PLA—B when compared to the control (only cells, $p < 0.05$, **Figure 5B**). Meanwhile, over expression of type I collagen (COL-1) occurred in the fibroblastic cells in contact when cultivated on PLA and PLA—A and PLA—B ($p < 0.05$, **Figure 5C**). No statistical differences were observed when the expressions of interleukins-6 and—10 were analyzed (**Figure 5D**).

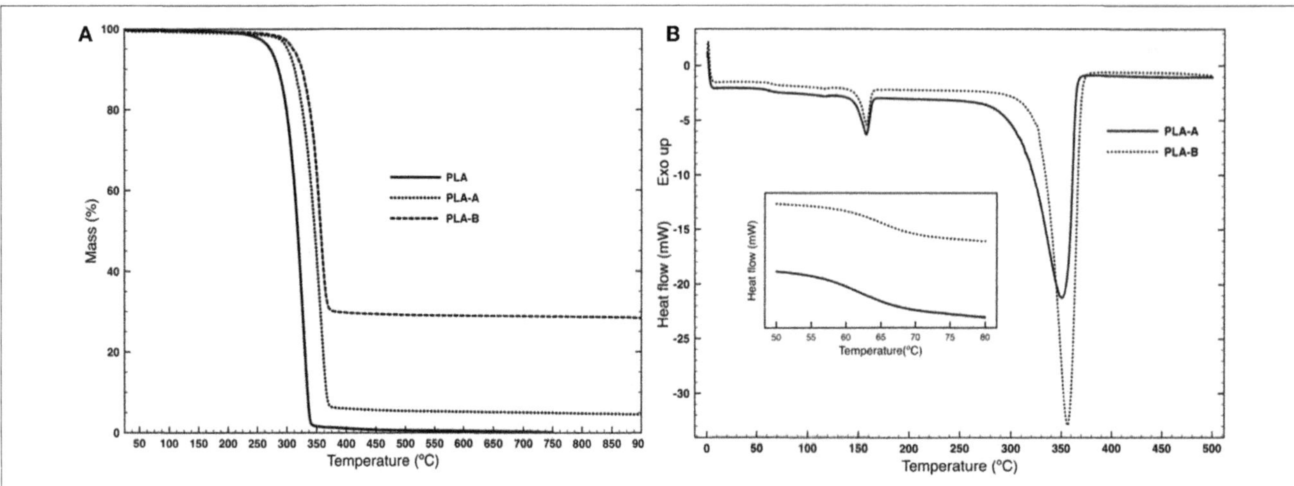

FIGURE 3 | (A) TGA curves from 25 to 900°C performed at a heating rate of 10°C min^{-1} under nitrogen atmosphere with a flow rate of 20 mL min^{-1} and **(B)** DSC thermogram from 0 to 500°C and the glass transition region between 40 and 80°C (inset) performed at a heating rate of 10°C min^{-1} under nitrogen atmosphere with a flow rate of 20 mL min^{-1} of the of PLA/TiO_2 samples.

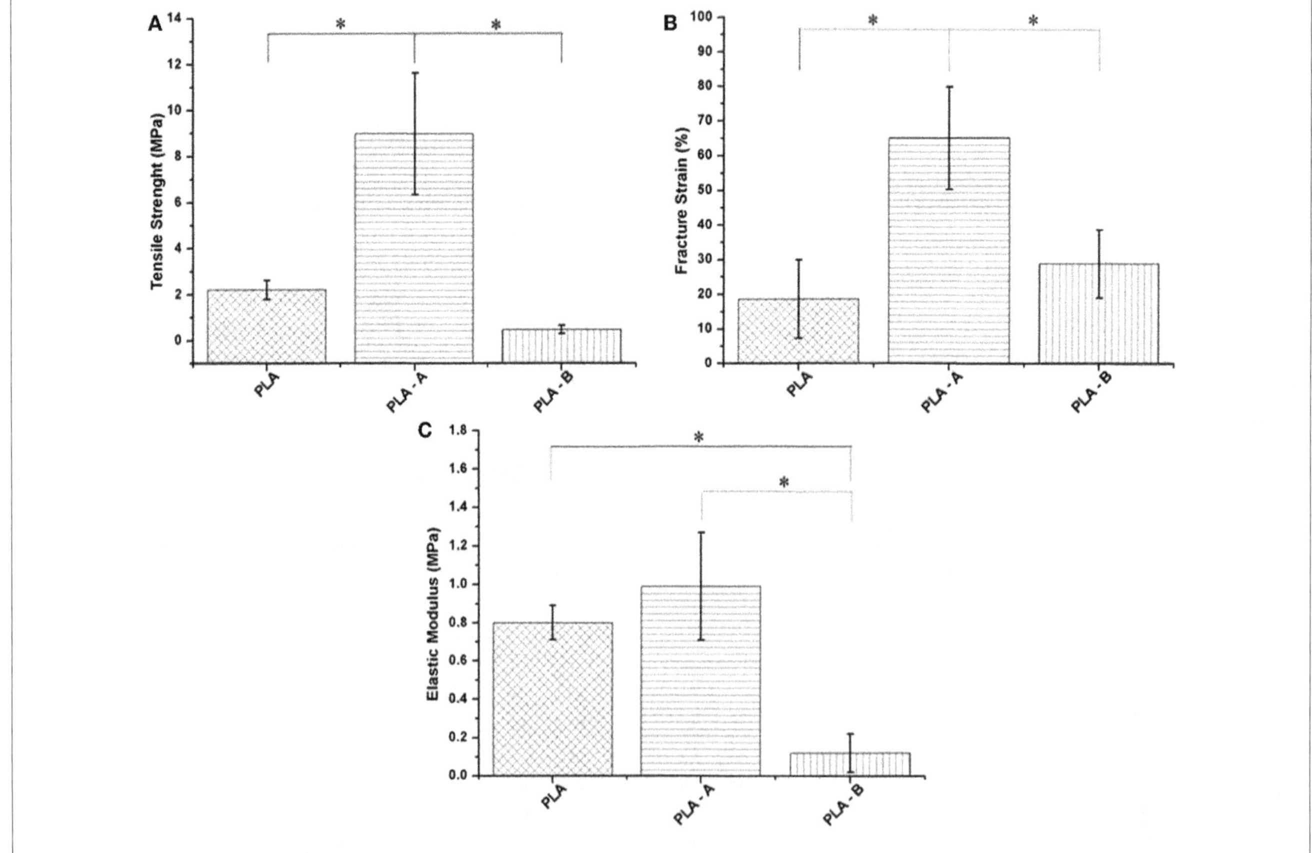

FIGURE 4 | (A) Variation in tensile strength (TS), **(B)** fracture strain (FS), and **(C)** elastic modulus (EM) of PLA nanofibers. Statistical test: One-way ANOVA followed by post-test multiple Tukey comparisons $^*P < 0.05$.

Histological Analysis

The groups were compared qualitatively to check for similar histological aspects. The figures show an overview of the control material and nanocomposites.

Clinically, the animals showed no signs of infection, and no foreign body reaction was observed under a microscope (**Figures 6–8**). A capsule of connective tissue was observed around the membranes of all the three types, indicating a close

TABLE 4 | Mechanical properties analysis of PLA—A and PLA—B over neat PLA scaffolds.

Scaffolds	Fracture strain (%)	Elastic modulus (MPa)	Tensile strength (MPa)
PLA	18.59	0.80	2.20
PLA—A	+250%	+23%	+308%
PLA—B	+55%	−85%	−78%

contact between the material and the surrounding connective tissue. The presence of discrete inflammatory infiltrate was also observed. However, the histological sections of PLA—A (**Figure 7**) and PLA—B (**Figure 8**) showed the newly formed vessels, suggesting a higher rate of metabolic activity in this tissue (compared to control, **Figure 6**). These observed differences are positive events that occurred in the regenerative process, influenced by presence of PLA/TiO_2 membranes.

DISCUSSION

None of the electrospun membranes showed beads formation, indicating that the work distances and applied voltage were appropriately chosen (Schuster et al., 2003). It was also observed that the solvents had completely evaporated during the electrospinning process, resulting in fiber diameters with little variation (Schuster et al., 2003; Efron and Moldawer, 2004; Zhang and An, 2007). The decision to keep the membranes for 15 h in a vacuum chamber resulted in the elimination of any residual liquid present in the nanofibers (Efron and Moldawer, 2004; Zhang and An, 2007). The incorporation of TiO_2 nanoparticles also did not promote bead formation, as seen in **Figures 1A–C**, indicating that our strategy to disperse these particles using ultrasound resulted in homogeneous dispersion of TiO_2 nanoparticles inside PLA fibers—as seen in **Figures 1B.1,C.1**—without inhibiting the PLA behavior—as shown by the XRD images (**Figure 1E**). A discrete reduction in contact angle was observed while using water when TiO_2 nanoparticles were incorporated into the PLA (**Figure 1D**). The XRD deconvolution analysis showed that the addition of TiO_2 interrupted the arrangement in the PLA polymer backbone by modifying its crystallinity (Baskaran et al., 2006). This intensity was assessed by deconvolutions of the XRD of **Figure 2A**. Crystallinity plays a very important role in the physical properties of biodegradable polymers—especially the thermal and mechanical behavior—and also affects their biodegradability (D'amico et al., 2016). The addition of 10 and 35% w/w of TiO_2 on the PLA matrix resulted in a significant decrease of crystallinity index of about 2 and 8%, respectively. Electrospun PLA exhibited two α crystal reflection peaks at 14.0 and 16.8° and a small phase peak at 25.0° due to the high degree of deformation that the electrospinning process causes to the material (**Figure 1E**). The positive shift of higher values of 2θ and the high degree of crystallinity of the of the electrospun nanofibers of PLA compared to the PLA films can be ascribed to the higher stretching of the polymer chains resulting in higher degree of molecular organization (Oliveira et al., 2013; Farid et al., 2018).

Thermogravimetric analysis (**Figure 3A**) showed that the degradation of PLA containing TiO_2 nanoparticles takes place in a well-defined single step with a derivative thermogravimetric (DTG) temperature peak at around 355°C (**Table 3**) with significant differences between nanoparticles content and pure PLA that showed a lower degradation peak at around 327°C in accordance with the DSC results (Mofokeng and Luyt, 2015; Zhang et al., 2015). After degradation, the weight remained constant until 900°C and leading to a residue content in function of the TiO_2 concentration (**Table 3**). PLA lead to a 0% residue at this temperature as previously observed (Virovska et al., 2014). With an increase of TiO_2 on the PLA nanofibers, there was an increase in residue produced which supports the presence of the nanoparticles in the nanospun fibers structure (Costa et al., 2013).

During the cooling cycle in the DSC analysis, no crystalline structures or other transitions appeared (data not shown). The DSC thermogram during the second heating shows two endothermic peaks at 157 and 350°C, indicating the melting and degradation peaks of PLA, respectively (Gupta et al., 2007). The inclusion of TiO_2 showed small differences in the melting peak (157°C) compared to the pure PLA (155°C). However, comparing the 10 and 35% TiO_2 containing PLA nanofibers, the degradation peak displayed a slight increase (from 351 to 357°C) and a large positive shift of around 20°C in the onset temperature (from 308 to 331°C). The Tg of PLA nanofibers showed a significant increase with the addition of TiO_2 in the polymer matrix (**Table 3**). This suggests an interaction between TiO_2 and PLA matrix (Zdraveva et al., 2018; Kaseem et al., 2019). These interactions restrict the mobility of the molecular chains in the PLA amorphous segments enhancing the cooperative motions of the chains which require much more activation energy to occur (Gasmi et al., 2019).

Moreover, the significant increase in decomposition onset temperature and the decrease in both enthalpy and crystallinity of the PLA composite with higher TiO_2 nanoparticles reinforce the hypothesis that there was an efficient inclusion of intermolecular bonding with the PLA matrix due to the anti-plasticizing effect of TiO_2 nanoparticles (El-Sayed et al., 2011; Amin et al., 2019).

Several researches have studied how addition of nanoparticles can improve mechanical properties in ultra-thin polymeric fibers. It has been proven that, the improvement in mechanical properties of PLA—A over neat PLA in this study was attributed to the favorable interactions between the polymer matrix and the homogeneous distribution of TiO_2 nanoparticles (as augmented in the internal friction) within the fibers as a filler, showed in the **Figure 1C.1**, making it toughest and most flexible (Ramier et al., 2014; Sadeghi and Shahedi, 2016; Feng et al., 2019). The reduction of TS, FS, and EM in PLA—B (**Figure 4** and **Table 4**) can be attributed to an anti-plasticizing effect, in which nano-TiO_2 might play the part of an anti-plasticizer due to increased interaction, a decreased the free volume between chains, a reduction in film flexibility and reduction in crystallinity, showed in **Figure 1E**, making it less tough (Shaili et al., 2015; Feng et al., 2019).

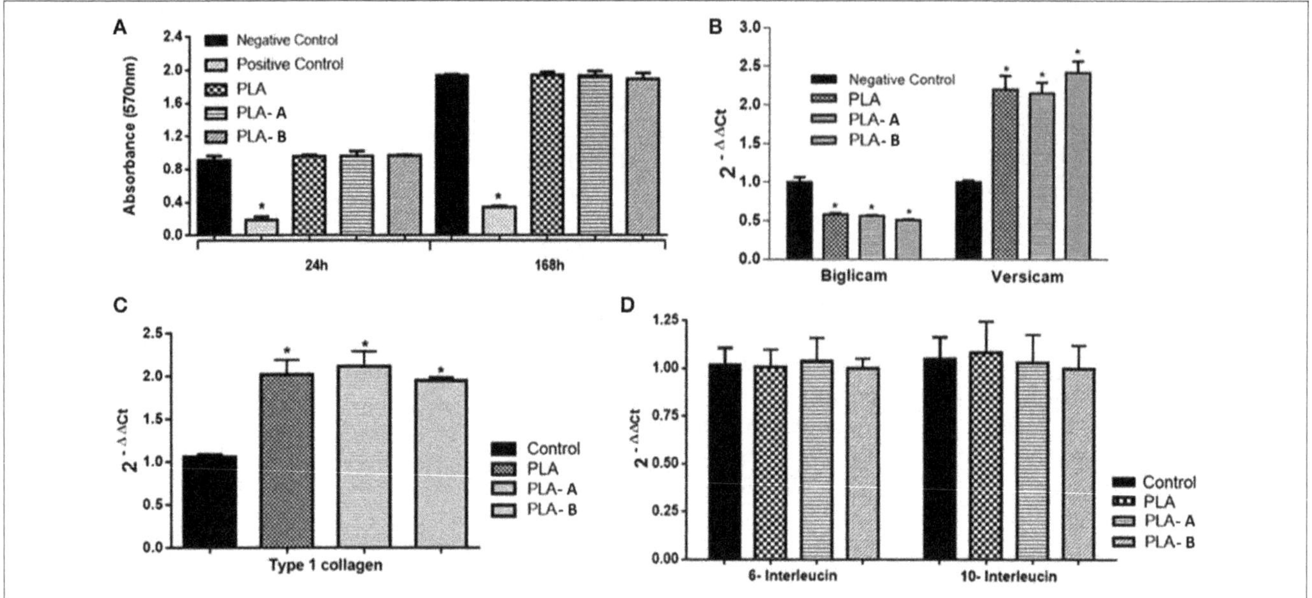

FIGURE 5 | (A) Cell viability assay performed by the MTT assay (PLA, PLA—A, and PLA—B). One-way statistical analysis ANOVA and post-test of Tukey Multiple Comparison **P* < 0.05 (compared to cells); **(B)** mRNA expression of the versicam and biglicam genes in L929 cells in the control groups and in the PLA, PLA—A, and PLA—B groups. **(C)** mRNA expression of the versicam and biglicam genes in the L929 cells in the control groups and in the PLA, PLA—A, and PLA—B groups. All groups were compared to the control group (cells only). **(D)** Expression of the interleukin-6 and–10 mRNA in L929 cells in the control groups and in the PLA, PLA—A, and PLA—B groups. Statistical test: One-way ANOVA followed by post-test multiple Tukey comparisons **P* < 0.05 (compared to control).

The membranes did not cause any decrease in the number of cells when compared to the control group in the cytotoxicity assay (**Figure 5A**). Cytotoxicity or evaluation of toxicity in cell culture is a complex *in-vivo* phenomenon that manifests a broad spectrum of effects, from cell death to metabolic aberrations—i.e., no cell death but functional changes (Kao et al., 2007). All groups of materials (PLA—A, and PLA—B) caused an over expression of the versicam mRNA in fibroblasts when compared to the control group. On the other hand, the biglicam showed a decrease in expression in the fibroblasts (down expression) when in contact with the studied nanocomposites in all three groups (**Figure 5B**). Type-I collagen was upregulated in all the membranes (**Figure 5C**). The electrospun membranes, however, did not show differences from control when analyzed for 6- and 10-interleukins (**Figure 5D**).

Type-I collagen plays an important role in maintaining the integrity of the extracellular matrix. Type-I collagen has a fibrillar type structure and is the most investigated type of collagen due to its abundance and the fact that it is the main structural element of several tissues. It is expressed in almost all connective tissues and plays a key role in the skin repair processes (Wong et al., 2013). Versicam is present in the dermis (Ruoslahti, 1989) and has important biological functions in the regulation of skin behavior (Bianco et al., 1990; Kinsella et al., 2004). Recent studies have shown that versicam interacts with leukocytes, promoting their adhesion. In addition, the incorporation of versicam into the ECM blocks monocyte adhesion and attenuates the inflammatory response. When binding to hyaluronic acid, versicam influences the T lymphocytes, aiding these cells to synthesize and secrete cytokines that assist the immune response. Versicam is emerging as a potential target in the treatment of inflammation, promising broad therapeutic benefits in the future due to the fact that it is an ECM molecule that plays a central role in the inflammatory process (Wight et al., 2014). The upregulation of versicam and type-1 collagen can be attributed to the activation of connective tissue formation, presumed to be related to repair of wounds and fibrotic diseases of the skin (Wahab et al., 1996).

A study conducted in 2001 compared down regulation of the decorin gene mRNA expression in post-surgical regenerated fibroblast cells in comparison to healthy human gingiva. The expression of mRNA for the versicam presented increased expression (upregulation) in this study (Ivanovski et al., 2001). In this study, the expression of versicam and biglicam genes corroborate with observations by Ivanovski. In our study, it was observed that all of the three groups of membranes (PLA, PLA—A, and PLA—B) caused over expression of the versicam in the fibroblasts when compared to the control group (**Figure 5B**). These findings are also in agreement with previous studies where the downregulation of decorin mRNA and upregulation of versicam in gingival cells and periodontal ligament cells were also observed (Haase et al., 1998). Other studies also report the correlation between exposure of growth factors, rates of cell proliferation, and synthesis of proteoglycans in other cell lines (Kähäri et al., 1991; Mauviel et al., 1995).

The gene expression findings of interleukins in the present study demonstrate that there is no change between the control and nanomaterials groups. The cited references support the idea that the developed membranes do not cause an inflammatory

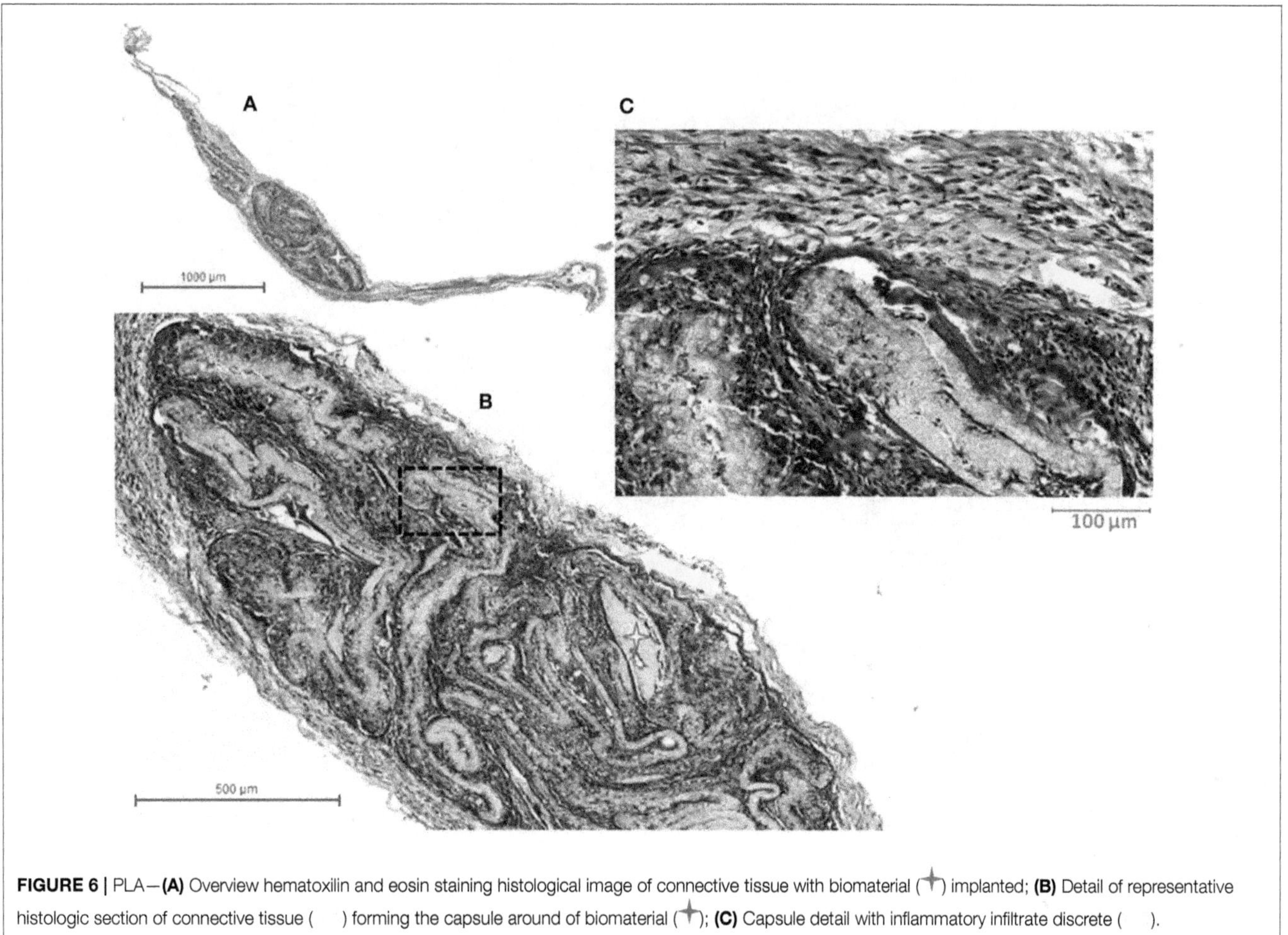

FIGURE 6 | PLA—**(A)** Overview hematoxilin and eosin staining histological image of connective tissue with biomaterial (✝) implanted; **(B)** Detail of representative histologic section of connective tissue ( ) forming the capsule around of biomaterial (✝); **(C)** Capsule detail with inflammatory infiltrate discrete ( ).

response in the cells of the fibroblast line used. This is an important property of a material that can be used in dressings in the future, since it would avoid problems related to scarring—such as excessive inflammatory response—that would delay the regenerative process (Kopf et al., 2010; Scheller et al., 2011).

TiO_2 has been proven to be a nanoparticle that can to modulate the immune functions, it is dependent to concentration, dose or route of administration (Lappas, 2015). The ability of TiO_2 nanoparticles in prove reactive oxygen species (ROS) and increase membrane permeability maximize antibacterial activity and improve the wound healing as was observed previously (Sankar et al., 2014). Moreover, the TiO_2 nanoparticles could cause enhanced blood coagulation, which is an important first step in the wound healing process (Seisenbaeva et al., 2017). Our *in vivo* results were (**Figures 4–6**) similar to Seisenbaeva et al. (2017) and in the study, it was observed that TiO_2 improved wound healing. We confirmed that the electrospun membranes with TiO_2 can stimulate and modulate inflammation, which is very important for human health, since there is bigger formation of blood vessels (Babelova et al., 2009; Moreth et al., 2014).

Various biological and synthetic skin replacements are available commercially available. Although there are over 3,000 types of dressings on the market, there is no product that is effective for treatment of chronic wounds such as venous leg ulcers, diabetic wounds, and pressure ulcers and burns. The membranes discussed in this study are ideal candidates for curative materials in the care of difficult-to-treat wounds and aiding the healing process and helping patients and health care professionals (Dhivya et al., 2015).

SUMMARY AND CONCLUSIONS

Three different membranes types were evaluated: One with PLA nanofibers but without TiO_2 content, and two with PLA and varying concentrations of TiO_2 (10% and 35%—w/w). A higher concentration of TiO_2 in the PLA structure significantly decreases the melting enthalpy of PLA. PLA with 10% of TiO_2 improved in more than 300% the tensile strain compared to PLA. All three membranes were found to be non-toxic against fibroblast L929 cells. The membranes also increased mRNA expression in Versicam and type-1 collagen, which are both important for the tissue repair

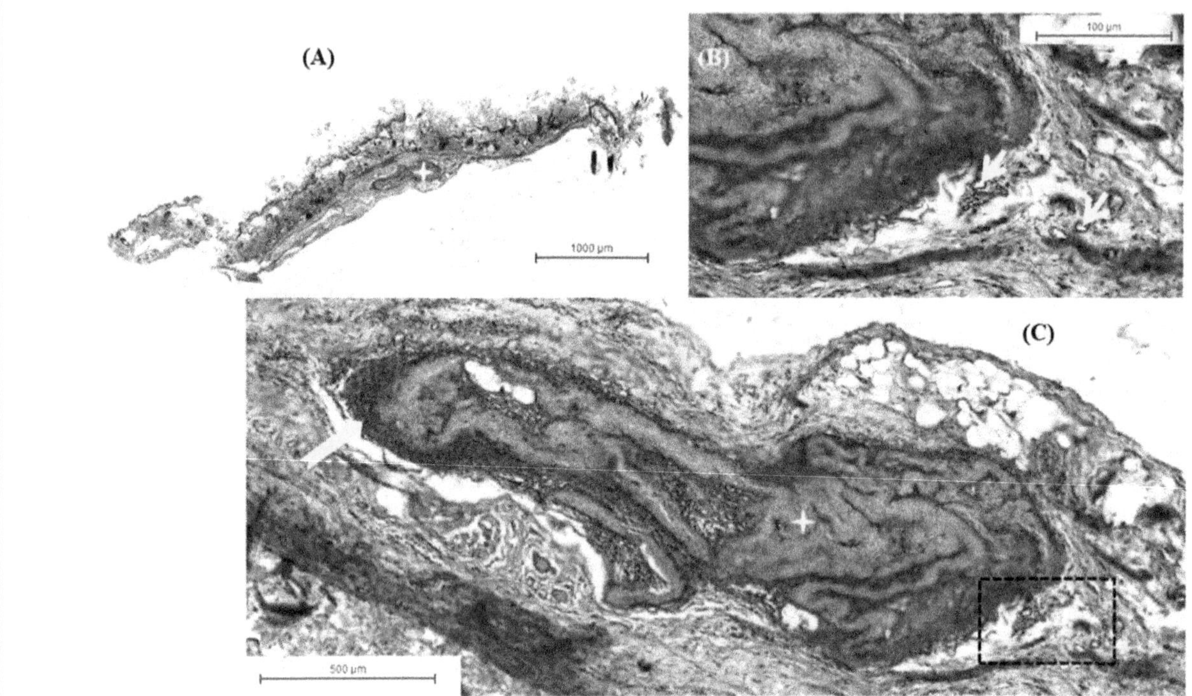

FIGURE 7 | PLA—**(A)** Overview hematoxilin and eosin staining histological image of connective tissue with biomaterial ( ) implanted; **(B)** Detail of representative histologic section of connective tissue ( ) forming the capsule around of biomaterial ( ) with inflammatory infiltrate discrete; **(C)** Capsule reveals details of neoformed blood vessels ( ).

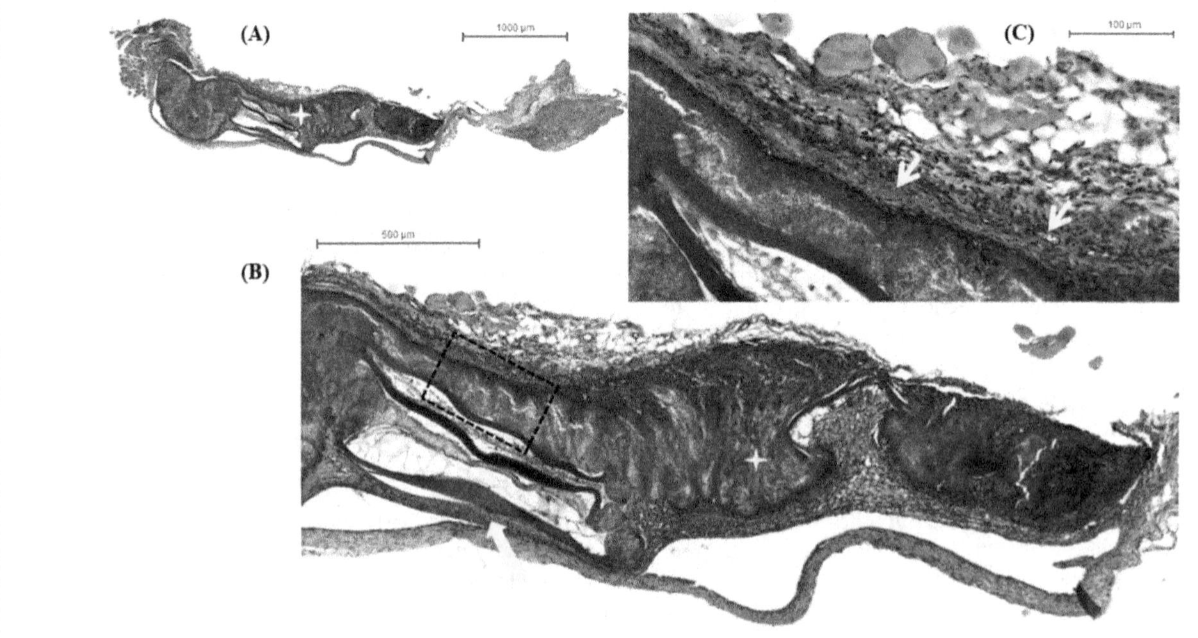

FIGURE 8 | PLA—**(A)** Overview hematoxylin and eosin staining histological image of connective tissue with biomaterial ( ) implanted; **(B)** Detail of representative histologic section of connective tissue ( ) forming the capsule around of biomaterial ( ) with inflammatory infiltrate discrete; **(C)** Capsule reveals details of neoformed blood vessels ( ).

process. It was also observed that the membranes did cause inflammations as demonstrated by the absence of alterations in the expression of interleukins-6 and−10. *In vivo* analysis indicated that our membranes can be used as materials for wound healing applications, as there were no inflammations observed, and the formation of blood vessels was identified.

AUTHOR CONTRIBUTIONS

All authors contributed to the design of the study, writing of the manuscript, and read and approved the final manuscript. TM and RR performed the biological *in vitro* and *in vivo* tests. TT, CE, AS, AF, AZ, and LM produced and characterized all membranes. LV, ES-F, FM, TW, and AL supervised all students.

FUNDING

This work was supported by the National Council for Scientific and Technological Development (CNPq, #303752/2017-3 and #404683/2018-5 to AL and #304133/2017-5 and #424163/2016-0 to FM). AZ acknowledges financial support of the FCT through UID/CTM/00264/2019 and Investigator FCT Research contract (IF/00071/2015) and the project PTDC/CTM—TEX/28295/2017 financed by FCT, FEDER, and POCI.

REFERENCES

Amin, M. R., Chowdhury, M. A., and Kowser, M. A. (2019). Characterization and performance analysis of composite bioplastics synthesized using titanium dioxide nanoparticles with corn starch. *Heliyon* 5:e02009. doi: 10.1016/j.heliyon.2019.e02009

Annunziata, M., Nastri, L., Borgonovo, A., Benigni, M., and Poli, P. P. (2015). Poly-DL-lactic acid membranes for bone regeneration. *J. Craniofacial Surg.* 26, 1691–1696. doi: 10.1097/SCS.0000000000001786

AnŽlovar, A., KrŽan, A., and Žagar, E. (2018). Degradation of PLA/ZnO and PHBV/ZnO composites prepared by melt processing. *Arab. J. Chem.* 11, 343–352. doi: 10.1016/j.arabjc.2017.07.001

Babelova, A., Moreth, K., Tsalastra-Greul, W., Zeng-Brouwers, J., Eickelberg, O., Young, M. F., et al. (2009). Biglycan, a danger signal that activates the NLRP3 inflammasome via toll-like and P2X receptors. *J. Biol. Chem.* 284, 24035–24048. doi: 10.1074/jbc.M109.014266

Bardosova, M., and Wagner, T. (2015). *Nanomaterials and Nanoarchitectures: A Complex Review of Current Hot Topics and their Applications*. Springer. doi: 10.1007/978-94-017-9921-8

Baskaran, R., Selvasekarapandian, S., Kuwata, N., Kawamura, J., and Hattori, T. (2006). Conductivity and thermal studies of blend polymer electrolytes based on PVAc-PMMA. *Solid State Ionics* 177, 2679–2682. doi: 10.1016/j.ssi.2006.04.013

Bayon, Y., Bohner, M., Eglin, D., Procter, P., Richards, R., Weber, J., et al. (2016). Innovating in the medical device industry - challenges & opportunities ESB 2015 translational research symposium. *J. Mater. Sci.: Mater. Med.* 27, 144. doi: 10.1007/s10856-016-5759-5

Beyth, N., Houri-Haddad, Y., Domb, A., Khan, W., and Hazan, R. (2015). Alternative antimicrobial approach: nano-antimicrobial materials. *Evid Based Complement Alternat Med.* 2015:246012. doi: 10.1155/2015/246012

Bianco, P., Fisher, L. W., Young, M. F., Termine, J. D., and Robey, P. G. (1990). Expression and localization of the two small proteoglycans biglycan and decorin in developing human skeletal and non-skeletal tissues. *J. Histochem. Cytochem.* 38, 1549–1563. doi: 10.1177/38.11.2212616

Braunger, J. A., Björnmalm, M., Isles, N. A., Cui, J., Henderson, T. M., O'Connor, A. J., et al. (2017). Interactions between circulating nanoengineered polymer particles and extracellular matrix components *in vitro*. *Biomater. Sci.* 5, 267–273. doi: 10.1039/C6BM00726K

Camargo, S. E., Rode Sde, M., do Prado, R. F., Carvalho, Y. R., and Camargo, C. H. (2010). Subcutaneous tissue reaction to castor oil bean and calcium hydroxide in rats. *J. Appl. Oral Sci.* 18, 273–278. doi: 10.1590/S1678-77572010000300014

Costa, R. G., Ribeiro, C., and Mattoso, L. H. (2013). Study of the effect of rutile/anatase TiO2 nanoparticles synthesized by hydrothermal route in electrospun PVA/TiO2 nanocomposites. *J. Appl. Polymer Sci.* 127, 4463–4469. doi: 10.1002/app.38031

D'amico, D. A., Montes, M. I., Manfredi, L. B., and Cyras, V. P. (2016). Fully bio-based and biodegradable polylactic acid/poly (3-hydroxybutirate) blends: use of a common plasticizer as performance improvement strategy. *Polymer Testing* 49, 22–28. doi: 10.1016/j.polymertesting.2015.11.004

Dhivya, S., Padma, V. V., and Santhini, E. (2015). Wound dressings–a review. *BioMedicine* 5:22. doi: 10.7603/s40681-015-0022-9

Dinari, M., and Haghighi, A. J. P. C. (2017). Surface modification of TiO2 nanoparticle by three dimensional silane coupling agent and preparation of polyamide/modified-TiO2 nanocomposites for removal of Cr (VI) from aqueous solutions. *Prog. Organ. Coatings.* 110, 24–34. doi: 10.1016/j.porgcoat.2017.04.044

Efron, P. A., and Moldawer, L. L. (2004). Cytokines and wound healing: the role of cytokine and anticytokine therapy in the repair response. *J. Burn Care Rehabil.* 25, 149–160. doi: 10.1097/01.BCR.0000111766.97335.34

El-Sayed, S., Mahmoud, K., Fatah, A., and Hassen, A. (2011). DSC, TGA and dielectric properties of carboxymethyl cellulose/polyvinyl alcohol blends. *Phys. B Condens. Matter.* 406, 4068–4076. doi: 10.1016/j.physb.2011.07.050

Farid, T., Herrera, V., and Kristiina, O. (2018). "Investigation of crystalline structure of plasticized poly (lactic acid)/Banana nanofibers composites," in *IOP Conference Series: Materials Science and Engineering* (Kitakyushu: IOP Publishing), 012031. doi: 10.1088/1757-899X/369/1/012031

Feng, S., Zhang, F., Ahmed, S., and Liu, Y. (2019). Physico-mechanical and antibacterial properties of PLA/TiO2 composite materials synthesized via electrospinning and solution casting processes. *Coatings* 9:525. doi: 10.3390/coatings9080525

Fonseca, C., Ochoa, A., Ulloa, M. T., Alvarez, E., Canales, D., and Zapata, P. A. (2015). Poly (lactic acid)/TiO2 nanocomposites as alternative biocidal and antifungal materials. *Mater. Sci. Eng.* 57, 314–320. doi: 10.1016/j.msec.2015.07.069

Gasmi, S., Hassan, M. K., and Luyt, A. S. (2019). Crystallization and dielectric behaviour of PLA and PHBV in PLA/PHBV blends and PLA/PHBV/TiO2 nanocomposites. *Express Polymer Lett.* 13, 199–212. doi: 10.3144/expresspolymlett.2019.16

Ghannadian, P., Moxley Jr, J. W., Machado de Paula, M. M., Lobo, A. O., and Webster, T. J. (2018). Micro-nanofibrillar polycaprolactone scaffolds as translatable osteoconductive grafts for the treatment of musculoskeletal defects without infection. *ACS Appl. Bio Mater.* 1, 1566–1578. doi: 10.1021/acsabm.8b00453

Ghosal, K., Agatemor, C., Špitálsky, Z., Thomas, S., and Kny, E. (2018). Electrospinning tissue engineering and wound dressing scaffolds from polymer–titanium dioxide nanocomposites. *Chem. Eng. J.* 358, 1262–1278. doi: 10.1016/j.cej.2018.10.117

Gupta, B., Revagade, N., and Hilborn, J. (2007). Poly (lactic acid) fiber: an overview. *Prog. Polym. Sci.* 32, 455–482. doi: 10.1016/j.progpolymsci.2007.01.005

Haase, H. R., Clarkson, R. W., Waters, M. J., and Bartold, P. M. (1998). Growth factor modulation of mitogenic responses and proteoglycan synthesis by human periodontal fibroblasts. *J. Cell. Physiol.* 174, 353–361.

Hidalgo, I., Sojot, F., Arvelo, F., Sabino, M. A. (2013). Functional electrospun poly (lactic acid) scaffolds for biomedical applications: experimental conditions, degradation and biocompatibility study. *Mol. Cell Biomech.* 10, 85–105. doi: 10.3970/mcb.2013.010.085

Ivanovski, S., Haase, H., and Bartold, P. (2001). Isolation and characterization of fibroblasts derived from regenerating human periodontal defects. *Arch. Oral Biol.* 46, 679–688. doi: 10.1016/S0003-9969(01)00036-X

Kähäri, V., Larjava, H., and Uitto, J. (1991). Differential regulation of extracellular matrix proteoglycan (PG) gene expression. Transforming growth factor-beta 1 up-regulates biglycan (PGI), and versican (large fibroblast PG) but down-regulates decorin (PGII) mRNA levels in human fibroblasts in culture. *J. Biol. Chem.* 266, 10608–10615.

Kandiah, K., Muthusamy, P., Mohan, S., and Venkatachalam, R. (2014). TiO2–graphene nanocomposites for enhanced osteocalcin induction. *Mater. Sci. Eng.* 38, 252–262. doi: 10.1016/j.msec.2014.02.010

Kao, C.-T., Ding, S.-J., Min, Y., Hsu, T. C., Chou, M.-Y., and Huang, T.-H. (2007). The cytotoxicity of orthodontic metal bracket immersion media. *Eur. J. Orthodontics* 29, 198–203. doi: 10.1093/ejo/cjl083

Kaseem, M., Hamad, K., and Ur Rehman, Z. (2019). Review of recent advances in polylactic acid/TiO2 composites. *Materials* 12:3659. doi: 10.3390/ma12223659

Kinsella, M. G., Bressler, S. L., and Wight, T. N. (2004). The regulated synthesis of versican, decorin, and biglycan: extracellular matrix proteoglycans that influence cellular phenotype. *Crit. Rev. Eukaryot. Gene Expr.* 14, 32. doi: 10.1615/CritRevEukaryotGeneExpr.v14.i3.40.

Kopf, M., Bachmann, M. F., and Marsland, B. J. (2010). Averting inflammation by targeting the cytokine environment. *Nat. Rev. Drug Discov.* 9:703. doi: 10.1038/nrd2805

Lappas, C. M. (2015). The immunomodulatory effects of titanium dioxide and silver nanoparticles. *Food Chem. Toxicol.* 85, 78–83. doi: 10.1016/j.fct.2015.05.015

Laske, S., Ziegler, W., Kainer, M., Wuerfel, J., and Holzer, C. (2015). Enhancing the temperature stability of PLA by compounding strategies. *Polymer Eng. Sci.* 55, 2849–2858. doi: 10.1002/pen.24176

Liou, J.-W., and Chang, H.-H. (2012). Bactericidal effects and mechanisms of visible light-responsive titanium dioxide photocatalysts on pathogenic bacteria. *Arch. Immunol. Ther. Exp.* 60, 267–275. doi: 10.1007/s00005-012-0178-x

Livak, K. J., and Schmittgen, T. D. (2001). Analysis of relative gene expression data using real-time quantitative PCR and the 2- ΔΔCT method. *Methods* 25, 402–408. doi: 10.1006/meth.2001.1262

Lobo, A. O., Antunes, E. F., Machado, A. H. A., Pacheco-Soares, C., Trava-Airoldi, V. J., and Corat, E. J. (2008). Cell viability and adhesion on as grown multi-wall carbon nanotube films. *Mater. Sci. Eng.* 28, 264–269. doi: 10.1016/j.msec.2007.01.003

Mauviel, A., Santra, M., Chen, Y. Q., Uitto, J., and Iozzo, R. V. (1995). Transcriptional regulation of decorin gene expression. Induction by quiescence and repression by tumor necrosis factor-alpha. *J. Biol. Chem.* 270, 11692–11700. doi: 10.1074/jbc.270.19.11692

Mofokeng, J., and Luyt, A. (2015). Morphology and thermal degradation studies of melt-mixed poly (lactic acid)(PLA)/poly (ε-caprolactone)(PCL) biodegradable polymer blend nanocomposites with TiO2 as filler. *Polymer Testing* 45, 93–100. doi: 10.1016/j.polymertesting.2015.05.007

Moreth, K., Frey, H., Hubo, M., Zeng-Brouwers, J., Nastase, M.-V., Hsieh, L. T.-H., et al. (2014). Biglycan-triggered TLR-2-and TLR-4-signaling exacerbates the pathophysiology of ischemic acute kidney injury. *Matrix Biol.* 35, 143–151. doi: 10.1016/j.matbio.2014.01.010

Oliveira, J. E., Mattoso, L. H., Orts, W. J., and Medeiros, E. S. (2013). Structural and morphological characterization of micro and nanofibers produced by electrospinning and solution blow spinning: a comparative study. *Adv. Mater. Sci. Eng.* 2013:409572. doi: 10.1155/2013/409572

Pava-Gómez, B., Vargas-Ramírez, X., Díaz-Uribe, C. J. J., and Chemistry, P. A. (2018). Physicochemical study of adsorption and photodegradation processes of methylene blue on copper-doped TiO2 films. *J. Photochem. Photobiol. Chem.* 360, 13–25. doi: 10.1016/j.jphotochem.2018.04.022

Ramier, J., Bouderlique, T., Stoilova, O., Manolova, N., Rashkov, I., Langlois, V., et al. (2014). Biocomposite scaffolds based on electrospun poly (3-hydroxybutyrate) nanofibers and electrosprayed hydroxyapatite nanoparticles for bone tissue engineering applications. *Mater. Sci. Eng.* 38, 161–169. doi: 10.1016/j.msec.2014.01.046

Roux, R., Ladavière, C., Montembault, A., and Delair, T. (2013). Particle assemblies: toward new tools for regenerative medicine. *Mater. Sci. Eng.* 33, 997–1007. doi: 10.1016/j.msec.2012.12.002

Roy, S. C., Paulose, M., and Grimes, C. A. J. B. (2007). The effect of TiO_2 nanotubes in the enhancement of blood clotting for the control of hemorrhage. *Biomaterials* 28, 4667–4672. doi: 10.1016/j.biomaterials.2007.07.045

Ruoslahti, E. (1989). Proteoglycans in cell regulation. *J. Biol. Chem.* 264, 13369–13372.

Sadeghi, K., and Shahedi, M. (2016). Physical, mechanical, and antimicrobial properties of ethylene vinyl alcohol copolymer/chitosan/nano-ZnO (ECNZn) nanocomposite films incorporating glycerol plasticizer. *J. Food Measur. Charact.* 10, 137–147. doi: 10.1007/s11694-015-9287-7

Saldin, L. T., Cramer, M. C., Velankar, S. S., White, L. J., and Badylak, S. F. (2017). Extracellular matrix hydrogels from decellularized tissues: structure and function. *Acta Biomater.* 49, 1–15. doi: 10.1016/j.actbio.2016.11.068

Salles, G. N., Calió, M. L., Afewerki, S., Pacheco-Soares, C., Porcionatto, M., and Hölscher, C. (2018). Prolonged drug-releasing fibers attenuate Alzheimer's Disease-like pathogenesis. *Appl Mater. Interfaces* 10, 36693–36702. doi: 10.1021/acsami.8b12649

Sankar, R., Dhivya, R., Shivashangari, K. S., and Ravikumar, V. (2014). Wound healing activity of Origanum vulgare engineered titanium dioxide nanoparticles in Wistar Albino rats. *J. Mater. Sci.* 25, 1701–1708. doi: 10.1007/s10856-014-5193-5

Scheller, J., Chalaris, A., Schmidt-Arras, D., and Rose-John, S. (2011). The pro-and anti-inflammatory properties of the cytokine interleukin-6. *Biochim. Biophys. Acta.* 1813, 878–888. doi: 10.1016/j.bbamcr.2011.01.034

Schuster, B., Kovaleva, M., Sun, Y., Regenhard, P., Matthews, V., Grötzinger, J., et al. (2003). Signaling of human ciliary neurotrophic factor (CNTF) revisited the interleukin-6 receptor can serve as an α-receptor for CNTF. *J. Biol. Chem.* 278, 9528–9535. doi: 10.1074/jbc.M210044200

Seisenbaeva, G. A., Fromell, K., Vinogradov, V. V., Terekhov, A. N., Pakhomov, A. V., Nilsson, B., et al. (2017). Dispersion of TiO 2 nanoparticles improves burn wound healing and tissue regeneration through specific interaction with blood serum proteins. *Sci. Rep.* 7:15448. doi: 10.1038/s41598-017-15792-w

Shaili, T., Abdorreza, M. N., and Fariborz, N. (2015). Functional, thermal, and antimicrobial properties of soluble soybean polysaccharide biocomposites reinforced by nano TiO2. *Carbohydr. Polymers* 134, 726–731. doi: 10.1016/j.carbpol.2015.08.073

Silva, A. D. R., Pallone, E. M. J. A., and Lobo, A. O. (2019a). Modification of surfaces of alumina-zirconia porous ceramics with $Sr2^{+}$ after SBF. *J. Austr. Ceramic Soc.* 55, 1–8. doi: 10.1007/s41779-019-00360-4.

Silva, A. D. R., Rigoli, W. R., Mello, D. C. R., Vasconcellos, L. M. R., Pallone, E. M. J. A., and Lobo, A. O. (2019b). Porous alumina scaffolds chemically modified by calcium phosphate minerals and their application in bone grafts. *Appl. Ceramic Teachnol.* 16, 562–573. doi: 10.1111/ijac.13153

Silva, A. D. R., Rigoli, W. R., Osiro, D., Mello, D. C. R., Vasconcellos, L. M. R., Lobo, A. O., et al. (2018). Surface modification using the biomimetic method in alumina-zirconia porous ceramics obtained by the replica method. *J. Biomed. Mater. Res. Part B.* 106, 2615–2624. doi: 10.1002/jbm.b.34078

Simoes, M. (2011). Antimicrobial strategies effective against infectious bacterial biofilms. *Curr. Med. Chem.* 18, 2129–2145. doi: 10.2174/092986711795656216

Stocco, T. D., Bassous, N. J., Zhao, S., Granato, A. E., Webster, T. J., and Lobo, A. O. (2018). Nanofibrous scaffolds for biomedical applications. *Nanoscale* 10, 12228–12255. doi: 10.1039/C8NR02002G

Tawakkal, I. S., Cran, M. J., Miltz, J., and Bigger, S. W. J. J. (2014). A review of poly (lactic acid)-based materials for antimicrobial packaging. *Food Sci.* 79, R1477–R1490. doi: 10.1111/1750-3841.12534

Toniatto, T., Rodrigues, B., Marsi, T., Ricci, R., Marciano, F., Webster, T., et al. (2017). Nanostructured poly (lactic acid) electrospun fiber with high loadings of TiO2 nanoparticles: insights into bactericidal activity and cell viability. *Mater. Sci. Eng.* 71, 381–385. doi: 10.1016/j.msec.2016.10.026

Villarreal-Gómez, L. J., Cornejo-Bravo, J. M., Vera-Graziano, R., and Grande, D. (2016). Electrospinning as a powerful technique for biomedical applications: a critically selected survey. *J. Biomater. Sci. Polymer* 27, 157–176. doi: 10.1080/09205063.2015.1116885

Virovska, D., Paneva, D., Manolova, N., Rashkov, I., and Karashanova, D. (2014). Electrospinning/electrospraying vs. electrospinning: a comparative study on the design of poly (l-lactide)/zinc oxide non-woven textile. *Appl. Surface Sci.* 311, 842–850. doi: 10.1016/j.apsusc.2014.05.192

Wacharawichanant, S., Ounyai, C., and Rassamee, P. (2017). Effects of organoclay to miscibility, mechanical and thermal properties of poly(lactic acid) and propylene-ethylene copolymer blends. *IOP Conf. Series Mater. Sci. Eng.* 223:012016. doi: 10.1088/1757-899X/223/1/012016

Wahab, N. A., Harper, K., and Mason, R. M. (1996). Expression of extracellular matrix molecules in human mesangial cells in response to prolonged hyperglycaemia. *Biochem. J.* 316, 985–992. doi: 10.1042/bj3160985

Walmsley, G. G., McArdle, A., Tevlin, R., Momeni, A., Atashroo, D., Hu, M. S., et al. (2015). Nanotechnology in bone tissue engineering. *Nanomedicine* 11, 1253–1263. doi: 10.1016/j.nano.2015.02.013

Wang, B., Lilja, M., Ma, T., Sörensen, J., Steckel, H., Ahuja, R., et al. (2014). Theoretical and experimental study of the incorporation of tobramycin and strontium-ions into hydroxyapatite by means of co-precipitation. *Appl. Surface Sci.* 314, 376–383. doi: 10.1016/j.apsusc.2014.06.193

Wight, T. N., Kang, I., and Merrilees, M. J. (2014). Versican and the control of inflammation. *Matrix Biol.* 35, 152–161. doi: 10.1016/j.matbio.2014.01.015

Wong, V. W., Gurtner, G. C., and Longaker, M. T. (2013). "Wound healing: a paradigm for regeneration," in *Mayo Clinic Proceedings* (Elsevier), 1022–1031. doi: 10.1016/j.mayocp.2013.04.012

Wu, S., Weng, Z., Liu, X., Yeung, K., and Chu, P. K. (2014). Functionalized TiO2 based nanomaterials for biomedical applications. *Adv. Funct. Mater.* 24, 5464–5481. doi: 10.1002/adfm.201400706

Zdraveva, E., Mijovic, B., Govorcin Bajsic, E., and Grozdanic, V. (2018). The efficacy of electrospun polyurethane fibers with TiO2 in a real time weathering condition. *Textile Res. J.* 88, 2445–2453. doi: 10.1177/00405175177 23025

Zhang, H., Huang, J., Yang, L., Chen, R., Zou, W., Lin, X., et al. (2015). Preparation, characterization and properties of PLA/TiO 2 nanocomposites based on a novel vane extruder. *RSC Adv.* 5, 4639–4647. doi: 10.1039/C4RA14538K

Zhang, J.-M., and An, J. (2007). Cytokines, inflammation and pain. *Int. Anesthesiol. Clin.* 45:27. doi: 10.1097/AIA.0b013e318034194e

17

An Exploratory Analysis of the Role of Adipose Characteristics in Fulltime Wheelchair Users' Pressure Injury History

Sharon Eve Sonenblum[1*], *Megan Measel*[2], *Stephen H. Sprigle*[1,3], *John Greenhalgh*[4] *and John McKay Cathcart*[5]

[1]*Rehabilitation Engineering and Applied Research Laboratory, The George W. Woodruff School of Mechanical Engineering, Georgia Institute of Technology, Atlanta, GA, United States,* [2]*Wallace H. Coulter Department of Biomedical Engineering, Georgia Institute of Technology, Atlanta, GA, United States,* [3]*College of Design, Georgia Institute of Technology, Atlanta, GA, United States,* [4]*FONAR Corporation, Melville, NY, United States,* [5]*School of Health Sciences, Ulster University, Northern Ireland, Coleraine, United Kingdom*

Correspondence:
Sharon Eve Sonenblum
ss427@gatech.edu

Aim: The goals of this study were 1) to identify the relationship between adipose (subcutaneous and intramuscular) characteristics and pressure injury (PrI) history in wheelchair users and 2) to identify subject characteristics, including biomechanical risk, that are related to adipose characteristics.

Materials and Methods: The buttocks of 43 full-time wheelchair users with and without a history of pelvic PrIs were scanned in a seated posture in a FONAR UPRIGHT® MRI. Intramuscular adipose (the relative difference in intensity between adipose and gluteus maximus) and the subcutaneous adipose characteristics (the relative difference in intensity between subcutaneous adipose under and surrounding the ischium) were compared to PrI history and subject characteristics.

Results: Participants with a history of PrIs had different subcutaneous fat (subQF) characteristics than participants without a history of PrIs. Specifically, they had significantly darker adipose under the ischium than surrounding the ischium (subQF effect size = 0.21) than participants without a history of PrIs (subQF effect size = 0.58). On the other hand, only when individuals with complete fat infiltration (n = 7) were excluded did individuals with PrI history have more fat infiltration than those without a PrI history. The presence of spasms (μ intramuscular adipose, 95% CI with spasms 0.642 [0.430, 0.855], without spasms 0.168 [−0.116, 0.452], $p = 0.01$) and fewer years using a wheelchair were associated with leaner muscle (Pearson Corr = −0.442, $p = 0.003$).

Conclusion: The results of the study suggest the hypothesis that changes in adipose tissue under the ischial tuberosity (presenting as darker SubQF) are associated with increased biomechanical risk for pressure injury. Further investigation of this hypothesis, and the role of intramuscular fat infiltration in PrI development, may help our understanding of PrI etiology. It may also lead to clinically useful diagnostic techniques that can identify changes in adipose and biomechanical risk to inform early preventative interventions.

Keywords: adipose, pressure injury, pressure ulcer, MRI, biomechanical risk, wheelchair, spinal cord injury

INTRODUCTION

Full-time wheelchair users are at a higher risk for pressure injuries (PrIs) due to continuous, high magnitude loading and lack of sensation (Bergstrom et al., 1995; Salzberg, et al., 1996). Disability categories with the highest PrI prevalence include paraplegia/quadriplegia, spina bifida, Alzheimer disease, hemiplegia, cerebral palsy, Parkinson disease, and multiple sclerosis (Sprigle et al., 2020). Previous research has identified many risk factors such as age, poor nutrition, and shearing, which significantly add to an individual's PrI risk (Braden and Bergstrom, 1987; European Pressure Ulcer Advisory Panel, National Pressure Injury Advisory Panel and Pan Pacific Pressure Injury Alliance, 2019). Investigation into the role of adipose and its relationship to tissue tolerance and PrI risk has been limited, despite considerable evidence on the effect of adipose on an individual's health (Garcia and Thomas 2006; Lemmer, Alvarado et al., 2019; Bogie, Schwartz et al., 2020).

There are multiple kinds of adipose depots, such as visceral, intramuscular, and subcutaneous, that differ in adipose characteristics. Intramuscular adipose tissue (IMAT) is the sum of the fat that lies underneath the fascia and between muscle groups and the fat that is infiltrated between and/or within the muscle fibers. Subcutaneous fat (SubQF), by definition, exists deep to the epidermis and dermis and represents the majority of body fat.

The majority of research about adipose is not focused on pressure injuries but on obesity, diabetes, and related disciplines. IMAT in obese and glucose-tolerant individuals has been found to be associated with decreased muscle quality and increased insulin resistance, which increases the risk for type 2 diabetes (Goodpaster, Thaete et al., 2000; Addison, Marcus et al., 2014). Like IMAT, previous research has shown that SubQF located in the abdominal region has been correlated with insulin resistance. However, in the gluteal–femoral region, the SubQF tissue has been shown to protect against metabolic dysregulation and insulin resistance (Patel and Abate 2013; Addison, Marcus et al., 2014). Additionally, lower body SubQF has been found to protect systemic glucose homeostasis and inhibit obesity-induced muscle pathophysiology (Booth, Magnuson et al., 2018). Previous research suggested that the protection might be due to fat storage capacity (Grundy 2015; Booth, Magnuson et al., 2018). As a result, this would increase blood flow, since an increased insulin resistance is correlated to decreased skin blood flow regulation (Snijder et al., 2005; Yim, Heshka et al., 2008; Liao, Burns et al., 2013; Bhattacharya and Mishra 2015; Lambadiari, Triantafyllou et al., 2015).

In early studies, IMAT has been found to be directly correlated with PrI history in individuals with a spinal cord injury (Ogawa, Lester et al., 2017; Lemmer, Alvarado et al., 2019). A follow-up study on individuals with spinal cord injuries found that IMAT was correlated with circulatory adipogenic and myogenic biomarkers (Bogie, Schwartz et al., 2020). Although IMAT is common, the mechanisms for its development and effects remain unknown. Therefore, understanding the individual characteristics that predict IMAT for a wheelchair user (e.g., age, years of immobility, spasticity, etc.) may inform the physiology behind the infiltration process. With this knowledge, future interventions may target improvement of muscle quality. Furthermore, it would be beneficial to confirm previous results regarding the relationship between IMAT and PrI development in a larger population of wheelchair users.

Contrary to the role of IMAT, a loss of subcutaneous fat (SubQF) has been shown to increase PrI risk (Garcia and Thomas 2006; Sonenblum, Seol et al., 2020). Obesity, exercise, and hypoxia can all change the characteristics of adipose (Alkhouli, Mansfield et al., 2013; Frayn and Karpe 2014; Lempesis et al., 2020). Furthermore, adipogenesis is a mechanosensitive process (Hara, Wakino et al., 2011; Levy, Enzer et al., 2012). Therefore, the constant loading experienced by wheelchair users who sit nearly 12 h/day (Sonenblum and Sprigle 2011; Sonenblum, Sprigle et al., 2012) has significant potential to change the characteristics of the SubQF of wheelchair users. To date, these changes have not been studied.

Biomechanical risk is an intrinsic characteristic of an individual's soft tissue to deform in response to extrinsic applied forces, and it is associated with PrI risk (Sonenblum, Seol et al., 2020). Understanding biomechanical risk is critical for assessing PrI risk and optimizing PrI prevention, but changes that occur in SubQF and how they influence biomechanical risk have not yet been studied. Furthermore, understanding what subject characteristics are associated with change in SubQF characteristics may help identify factors that assist in PrI prevention.

This study sought to accomplish two goals: (1) to identify the relationship between adipose (SubQF and IMAT) characteristics and PrI history in wheelchair users and 2) to identify subject characteristics, including biomechanical risk, that are related to adipose (SubQF and IMAT) characteristics. Because the changes in adipose are poorly understood, we also investigated whether IMAT was associated with SubQF characteristics.

METHODS

Subjects

Forty-three individuals who use wheelchairs as their primary mobility device were included in this exploratory secondary analysis. Participants were recruited from either the New York, Colorado, Georgia, or New Jersey area. This study was approved by institutional review boards at a primary research site and multiple clinical sites. All participants reviewed and signed the informed consent form as approved by their local institutional review board prior to participation in the study. Inclusion criteria required that the participants must have been using a wheelchair for at least 2 years and were able to remain stable while seated on flat foam in the MRI environment. If the participants had a current PrI, they could not be on restricted sitting time or be considered at risk from sitting on the test cushions or performing additional transfers. A subset of this population has been published previously in Sonenblum, Seol et al. (2020).

Study Protocol

Each subject had their characteristics, such as age, body mass index (BMI), PrI history, and presence of spasticity, collected *via* a self-reported health form. Participants reported a PrI history if they had experienced at least one prior PrI at an ischium or in the sacral/coccygeal region, and at which location(s) they had experienced the PrIs. Participants' buttocks were scanned while they sat in a FONAR UPRIGHT® MRI. Since these scans were originally taken for the purpose of measuring seated tissue deformation, a FONAR UPRIGHT® MRI was used, and T1-weighted (RF spoiled) 3D in-phase gradient echo scans were taken with participants seated. Scans had a 280-mm field of view with 3.0 mm contiguous slices in the sagittal plane. The field of view was centered on the right ischial tuberosity for most participants, unless participants had an active pressure ulcer on that side or any hardware that would cause an artifact in the MRI (such as a hip implant), in which case the left ischial tuberosity was the center of the field of view. Most participants were scanned while seated on an 18″ × 18″ cushion made with flat 3″ HR45 foam. However, five participants were not studied in this condition. Therefore, for this analysis, scans collected on a Matrx Vi (Invacare, n = 4), or Embrace (Permobil, n = 1) were used. Both the Embrace and Matrx Vi are contoured foam cushions, as opposed to flat foam, but they created a similar loaded condition to study the adipose characteristics of the buttocks.

Expert clinicians assisted with seating the subjects to have their pelvis in a neutral posture. The footrest was also adjusted to properly load the thighs and to keep the knees and hips close to 90° of flexion (Sonenblum, Seol et al., 2020).

An additional subject characteristic was measured with subjects seated on the same reference foam on which they were imaged. Compressible hip breadth was measured by measuring the bi-trochanteric distance twice: once with no tissue compression and once with maximum compression (i.e., until the tissue could not be compressed any farther), and the difference between the two was computed.

Data Processing

MRI Image Processing

The raw DICOM scans were imported into MRI analysis software, AnalyzePro (AnalyzeDirect, Overland Park, KS), for review and segmentation of the pelvis, gluteus maximus, and the subcutaneous fat of the side of the buttocks included in the MRI. Trained researchers under the supervision of an experienced radiographer (Cathcart) performed the segmentations for a single slice of the MRI scans located at the peak of the ischial tuberosity in the sagittal plane. Skin was included within the subcutaneous fat segmentation when visible since the scan resolution did not allow for separate segmentation of the two. The region pixel intensities and the coordinate location points from the adipose and gluteus maximus segmentations from the sagittal slice were extracted and interpreted using MATLAB R2020a (MathWorks, Natick, MA).

Measures associated with biomechanical risk included bulk tissue thickness and sagittal radius of curvature, and their calculations have been described previously (Sonenblum et al., 2020). Briefly, bulk tissue thickness is defined as the average tissue thickness under the ischial tuberosity measured in an oblique plane in a region 50 mm long. The radius of curvature is computed in a 50-mm region centered at the peak of the ischial tuberosity in the sagittal plane.

Because the scans were taken with a planar surface coil (Quad-Z Planar) located in the axial plane under the wheelchair cushion, there was an image intensity gradient along an axis orthogonal to the coil, i.e., in the superior–inferior direction. Therefore, it was necessary to correct for this gradient to allow for accurate comparison between the gluteus maximus and adipose intensities when calculating intramuscular fat infiltration.

To correct for the image intensity gradient, we used a control MRI scan of a basketball filled with dilute nickel chloride (to mimic human tissue) that was placed on top of the Quad-Z Planar coil at its center (**Figure 1**) with the same sequence parameters used to scan participants. Because the basketball was filled with a homogenous fluid, the smooth variation in pixel brightness from point to point (voxel to voxel) can be attributed to voxel distance from the conductive elements of the receiver coil. Therefore, a normalization curve was defined to represent the variation in intensity of the image using the power function through MATLAB's Curve Fitting Tool as a function of distance across the vertical axis of the scan (the superior–inferior direction). Sagittal voxel intensities in the buttocks scans were corrected by subtracting the normalization curve from the original scan intensities.

Intramuscular Adipose Tissue

To study the IMAT within the gluteus maximus, which resides predominantly posterior to the gluteus maximus (Sonenblum, Seol et al., 2020), adipose included in IMAT analysis was constrained to the region posterior to the ischial tuberosity and inferior to the gluteus maximus (**Figure 2**).

Several approaches were considered to quantify IMAT in the gluteus maximus. Methods like the midpoint method and the Otsu Method (Gorgey, Ogawa et al., 2017; Ogawa, Lester et al., 2017) rely on identifying adipose and gluteus intensities within the gluteus maximus and computing a cutoff threshold. While this is effective in many cases, for subjects with very lean gluteus

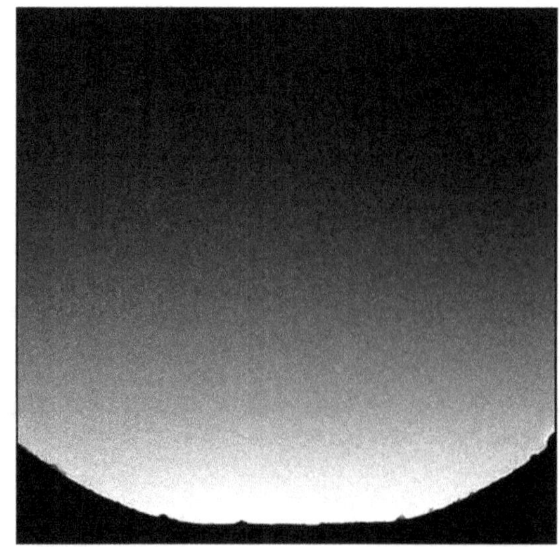

FIGURE 1 | The control scan of a basketball filled with dilute nickel chloride that was used to find the power function (i.e., normalization curve) for normalizing the intensity gradient in scans of the buttocks.

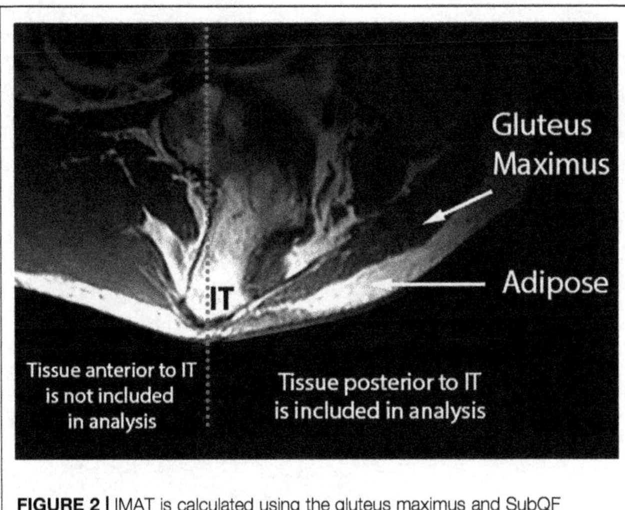

FIGURE 2 | IMAT is calculated using the gluteus maximus and SubQF intensities posterior to the ischial tuberosity.

maximi (i.e., no IMAT) or fully adipose infiltrated muscle (i.e., no discernable muscle tissue), identifying separate tissue types and therefore an intensity cutoff threshold is not effective.

Instead, we reported an effect size for each participant. The IMAT effect size is a standardized magnitude of difference between the corrected intensities of the gluteus maximus and the SubQF inferior to the gluteus (**Eq. 1**). Higher IMAT effect sizes indicated less IMAT within the gluteus maximus, while values closer to zero or even negative IMAT effect sizes indicate significant amounts of IMAT in the gluteus maximus.

Equation 1. IMAT effect size is the relative difference in intensity between adipose and gluteus maximus.

$$IMAT\ effect\ size = \frac{mean\ intensity\ of\ the\ adipose - mean\ intensity\ of\ the\ gluteus\ maximus}{pooled\ standard\ deviation\ of\ intensities\ in\ both\ tissues} \tag{1}$$

This approach was correlated (Pearson Corr = −0.601, p = 0.003) with the midpoint method for participants not at the extremes of low or high IMAT (e.g., the interquartile range). Furthermore, MRI scans were subjectively categorized based on who had low, medium, and high fat infiltration, and the effect size accurately predicted these categorizations.

Subcutaneous Adipose (SubQF) Tissue

Since the adipose under the pelvis is the most susceptible area to PrIs, we evaluated the SubQF under the ischium and compared it with the segmented SubQF surrounding the ischium in the sagittal plane (**Figure 3**). First, we located all SubQF inferior to a location 10 mm superior to the peak of the ischium. Then, we further divided this segment of SubQF into two regions: 1) under the ischium included 5 mm anterior and posterior of the ischium from 10 mm superior to the most inferior aspect of the ischial tuberosity, and 2) surrounding the ischium included regions anterior and posterior to the region under the ischium. This constrained the adipose included in analysis and avoided unintentional inclusion of visceral adipose. To describe the characteristics of the SubQF for each individual, we quantified the standardized magnitude of the difference in intensity under the ischium versus surrounding the ischium using the effect size (**Eq. 2**).

Equation 2. SubQF effect size is the relative difference in intensity between SubQF under and surrounding the ischium.

$$SubQF\ effect\ size = \frac{mean\ intensity\ of\ adipose\ surrounding\ the\ ischium - mean\ intensity\ of\ adipose\ under\ the\ ischium}{pooled\ standard\ deviation\ of\ intensities\ in\ both\ regions} \tag{2}$$

Data Analysis

The goals of this study were to identify the relationship between adipose characteristics and PrI history in wheelchair users and to identify subject characteristics that are related to adipose characteristics. To accomplish these goals, one-way ANOVA tests were run comparing adipose characteristics across individuals with and without a history of PrIs. Statistics were computed using Minitab 18.1. Four subject characteristics were considered: BMI, years using a wheelchair, presence of spasticity, and compressible hip breadth. All but hip breadth were assessed *via* self-report. The relationship between adipose characteristics

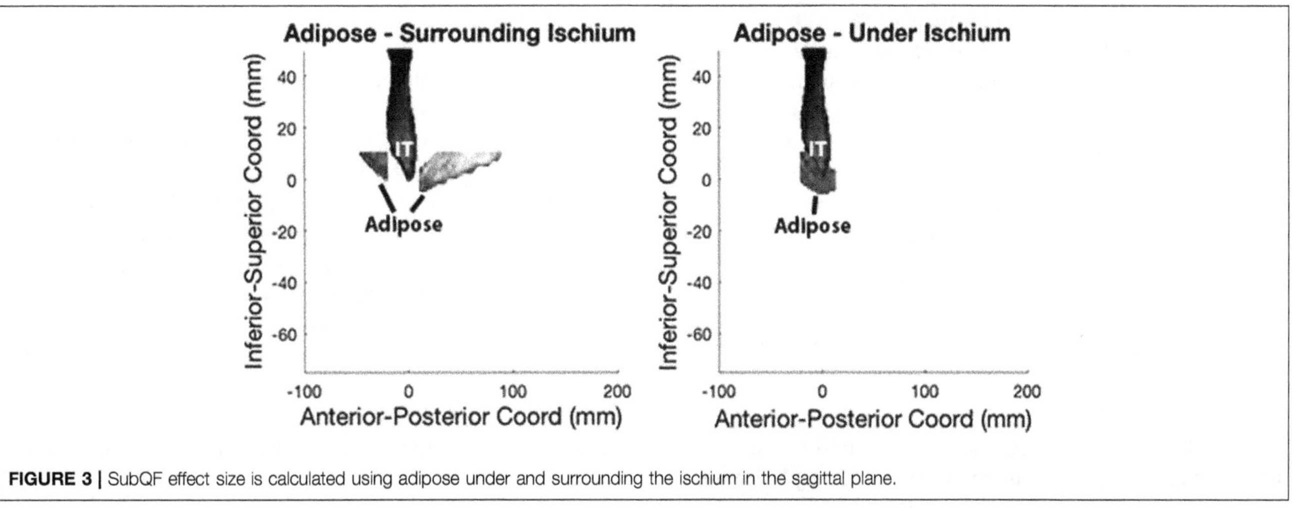

FIGURE 3 | SubQF effect size is calculated using adipose under and surrounding the ischium in the sagittal plane.

TABLE 1 | Participant characteristics.

	All		WC user No Hx (n = 21)		WC user PrI Hx (n = 22)	
	Mean (SD)	**Median (min–max)**	**Mean (SD)**	**Median (min–max)**	**Mean (SD)**	**Median (min–max)**
Age (years, n = 43)	46.8 (11.3)	47.0 (18.0–73.0)	44.8 (13.5)	46.0 (18.0–73.0)	48.8 (8.7)	48.5 (34.0–66.0)
BMI (n = 43)	23.9 (4.8)	23.1 (14.6–34.5)	24.5 (5.0)	23.9 (14.6–34.5)	23.3 (4.6)	21.5 (14.9–33.5)
Years using wheelchair (n = 43)	15.3 (12.2)	10.0 (2.0–46.0)	10.7 (9.3)	6.5 (2.0–37.0)	19.6 (13.3)	16.3 (3.0–46.0)
Compressible hip breadth (inches) (n = 39)	1.4 (0.8)	1.3 (0.3–3.0)	1.7 (0.8)	1.8 (0.5–3.0)	1.1 (0.8)	0.8 (0.3–3.0)
Sex	N	%	N	%	N	%
Female	8	19%	6	29%	2	9%
Male	35	81%	15	71%	20	91%
Diagnosis						
SCI	36	84%	17	81%	19	86%
Other	7	6%	4	19%	3	14%
Injury completeness (n = 41)						
Complete	22	54%	10	48%	12	60%
Incomplete	19	46%	11	52%	8	40%
Spasms (n = 38)						
Yes	24	63%	10	56%	14	70%
No	14	37%	8	44%	6	30%
Race						
Asian American	1	2%	1	5%		
Black/African American	2	5%	1	5%	1	5%
White	33	77%	16	76%	17	77%
Hispanic or Latino	5	12%	2	9%	3	14%
Two or More Races	1	2%			1	5%
Other	1	2%	1	5%	74">	86">

(SubQF effect size and IMAT effect size) and continuous characteristics—BMI, years using a wheelchair, and compressible hip breadth—were investigated with a correlation, while the presence of spasticity was studied with a one-way ANOVA.

To understand if adipose characteristics played a role in deformation of the seated buttocks, correlations were calculated between adipose characteristics (i.e., SubQF effect size and IMAT effect size) and bulk tissue thickness and sagittal radius of curvature. Finally, a correlation was calculated to investigate a relationship between subcutaneous adipose and intramuscular adipose characteristics.

RESULTS

Participants

Participants were predominantly men (81%) with spinal cord injuries (84%) (**Table 1**). The remaining participants had spinal cord disorders such as spinal bifida (n = 4) and spinal cord stroke (n = 1), while one participant had multiple sclerosis and one had fronto-temporal degeneration. They ranged in age from 18 to 73 years old and had between 2 and 46 years of experience using a wheelchair as their primary mobility device. Additional characteristics are presented in **Table 1** for all participants where responses and/or measurements were available.

Adipose Characteristics and Pressure Injuries

Subcutaneous Adipose

Characteristics of the adipose tissue underneath the ischium were different than the surrounding adipose in some people, leading to larger SubQF effect sizes. Larger, positive SubQF effect sizes indicate that the adipose under the ischium is darker than surrounding adipose (**Table 2**; **Figure 4**). Greater negative SubQF effect sizes indicate that the tissue under the ischium is brighter than the tissue surrounding the ischium.

Participants with a history of PrIs had a significantly greater SubQF effect size than participants without a history of PrIs (difference in effect size μ [95% CI] = −0.370 [−0.684, −0.555], p = 0.022).

A closer look at participants with a history of ischial PrIs (i.e., 12 of the overall 22 participants with pelvic PrIs, excluding the 10 that had sacral/coccygeal PrI) revealed darker tissue surrounding the ischium (**Figure 5**). Among participants with bright adipose surrounding the ischium (e.g., >2,200), only three had a history of ischial PrIs. Specifically, participants with a history of PrIs had darker adipose under the ischium relative to the surrounding ischium.

Intramuscular Adipose Tissue

Intramuscular adipose tissue varied, including very lean subjects with high effect sizes, such as the example on the left in **Figure 6** (IMAT effect size = 0.689, gluteus maximus intensity darker than SubQF intensity), subjects with some IMAT present in the gluteus maximus (IMAT effect sizes >0), and subjects with complete fat infiltration. For these subjects with no muscle visible given all the adipose infiltration, IMAT effect size varied from −0.275 to −1.059 because the gluteus maximus intensity was brighter than the SubQF intensity (e.g., **Figure 6**, right).

One-way ANOVA showed that there was no relationship between fat infiltration and PrI history (**Table 2**). However, when individuals with complete fat infiltration (n = 7)

TABLE 2 | Adipose characteristics.

Variable	All (n = 43)	No PrI (n = 21)	Yes PrI (n = 22)	p-value
	Mean (SD)	Mean (SD)	Mean (SD)	
Adipose intensity surrounding the ischium	2,022 (671)	2,019 (657)	2,026 (700)	0.974
Adipose intensity under the ischium	1,707 (783)	1,873 (842)	1,548 (704)	0.176
SubQF effect size	0.40 (0.53)	0.21 (0.56)	0.58 (0.45)	0.022
Adipose intensity posterior to the ischium	1,517 (387)	1,586 (388)	1,451 (383)	0.258
Gluteus Maximus Intensity	1,324 (306)	1,313 (239)	1,334 (364)	0.831
IMAT effect size	0.50 (0.55)	0.59 (0.60)	0.41 (0.51)	0.280
Average bulk thickness (mm)	14.8 (6.1)	17.1 (7.1)	12.5 (3.9)	0.012
Sagittal radius of curvature (mm)	83.7 (38.1)	93.9 (44.7)	73.6 (27.5)	0.085

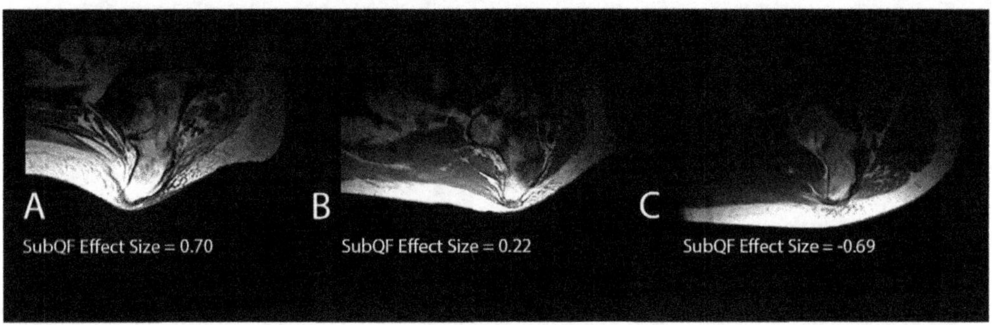

FIGURE 4 | Examples of subjects with different SubQF effect sizes. Subject A had a SubQF effect size of 0.7, indicating darker adipose under the ischium than surrounding the ischium, while subject B had a SubQF effect size of 0.22, indicating adipose under the ischium was only slightly darker than surrounding ischium. Subject C (SubQF effect size of −0.69) actually had brighter adipose under the ischium.

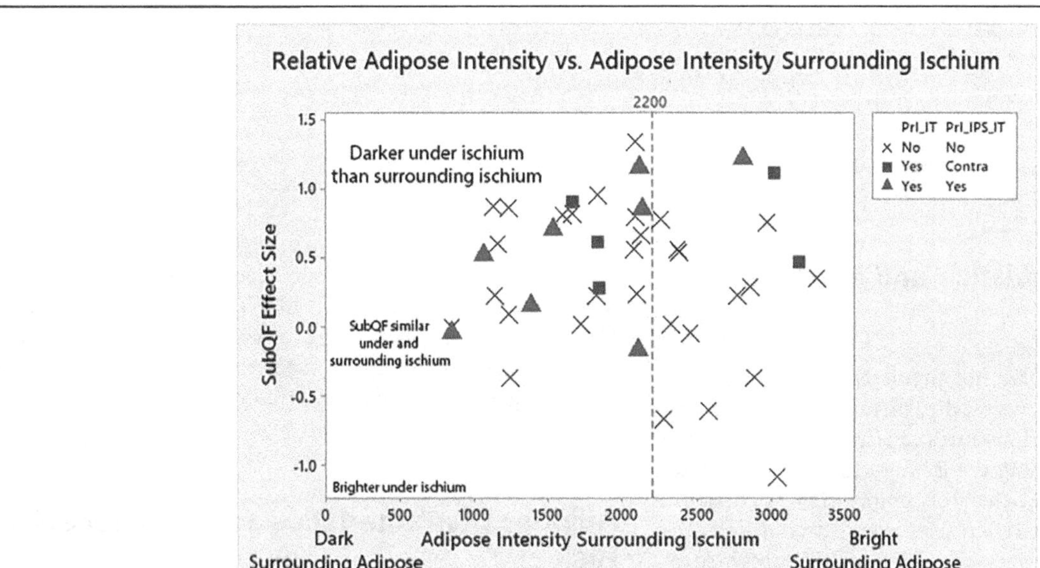

FIGURE 5 | Adipose under the ischium was darker than surrounding adipose (larger SubQF effect size) for people with a history of PrIs, indicating changes to adipose characteristics under the ischium. People with ischial PrIs were also less likely to have bright surrounding adipose.

(i.e., their muscle is indistinguishable from the adipose) were excluded, individuals with PrI history had more fat infiltration than those without a PrI history (IMAT effect size with PrIs n = 19 and μ, 95% CI = 0.56 [0.428, 0.693] vs. without n = 17 and μ = 0.86 [0.716, 0.997], difference in IMAT effect size μ, 95% CI = 0.29 [0.102, 0.471], p = 0.004).

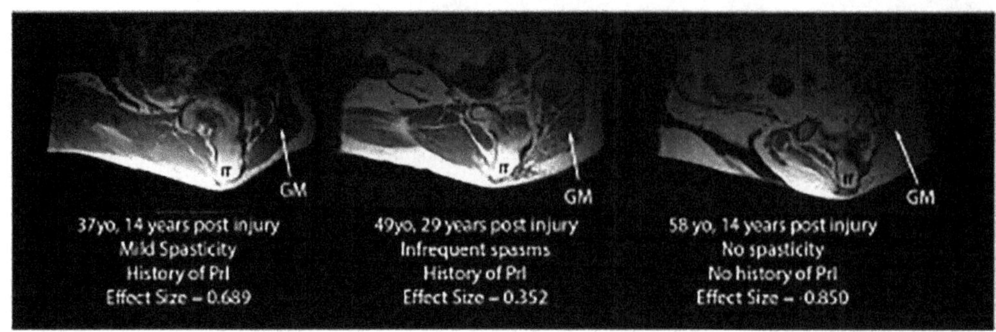

FIGURE 6 | Examples of IMAT effect sizes varying from lean (IMAT effect size = 0.689) to full fat infiltration (IMAT effect size = −0.850).

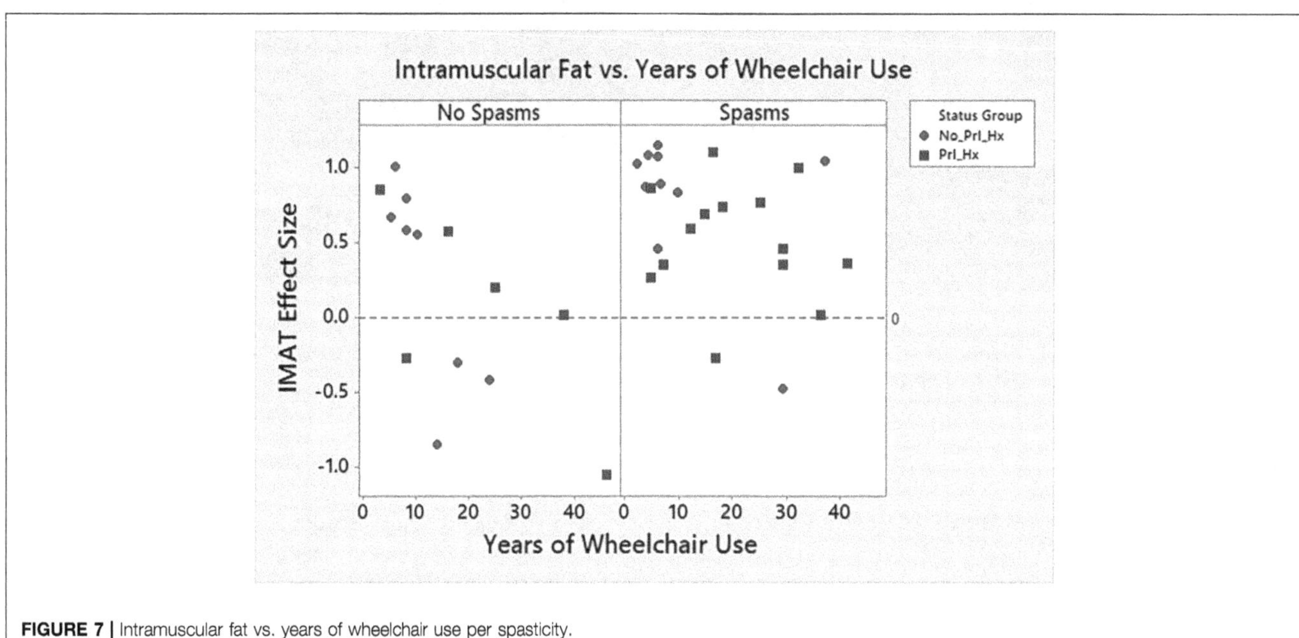

FIGURE 7 | Intramuscular fat vs. years of wheelchair use per spasticity.

Adipose Characteristics and Individual Characteristics

Subcutaneous Adipose

Patient characteristics were not predictive of subcutaneous adipose characteristics. Specifically, there was no significant correlation between the differences in adipose inferior to the ischium versus surrounding the ischium (SubQF effect size) and BMI, years using wheelchair, or compressible hip breadth. Furthermore, one-way ANOVA tests revealed no differences in subcutaneous effect sizes according to the presence of spasms.

Intramuscular Adipose Tissue

Some patient characteristics were associated with intramuscular adipose (**Figure 7**). Specifically, the presence of spasms was associated with a greater IMAT effect size, or leaner muscle (μ, 95% CI with spasms 0.642 [0.430, 0.855], without spasms 0.168 [−0.116, 0.452], p = 0.01). BMI was not associated with intramuscular adipose (Pearson Corr = −0.148, p = 0.339) nor was compressible hip breadth (Pearson Corr = −0.193, p = 0.239), but years using a wheelchair was negatively correlated with IMAT effect size (Pearson Corr = −0.442, p = 0.003), suggesting more fat infiltration with more years in the wheelchair.

Adipose Characteristics and Biomechanical Risk

Subcutaneous Adipose

Subcutaneous effect size was negatively correlated with tissue thickness (Pearson Corr = −0.489, $p < 0.01$) and sagittal radius of curvature = −0.564, $p < 0.01$). That is, as SubQF effect size goes up (darker adipose under IT), tissue thickness goes down, and the radius of curvature goes down or the shape becomes more peaked. In other words, darker adipose under the IT is associated with a higher biomechanical risk.

Intramuscular Adipose

Intramuscular adipose (IMAT effect size) was not related to either tissue thickness or radius of curvature of the seated buttocks (Pearson Corr = 0.092 and = −0.073 respectively).

Intramuscular Adipose vs. Subcutaneous Adipose

SubQF effect size was not related to IMAT effect size (Pearson Corr = −0.100).

DISCUSSION

This study is the first to integrate an assessment of both subcutaneous and intramuscular adipose in wheelchair users and to assess how adipose relates both to PrI risk and biomechanical risk (i.e., the tissue response to loading).

Tissue with darker subcutaneous adipose under the IT compared with surrounding adipose measured with an MRI was associated with a higher biomechanical risk when seated. These individuals were also more likely to have a history of PrIs, but not necessarily at the ipsilateral ischial tuberosity that was studied. The relationship between adipose and tissue tolerance likely evolves over time in response to load. Buttocks with good structural integrity and low biomechanical risk, such as the buttocks of an able-bodied adult, provide ample protection from development of PrIs.

There are a number of physiological reasons why changes to adipose characteristics might occur over time for wheelchair users and consequently influence tissue tolerance and biomechanical risk. Studies have shown that exposure to mild, prolonged hypoxia increases fat storage and decreases proinflammatory gene expression. In contrast, acute exposure to severe hypoxia decreases fat storage and increases proinflammatory expression (Lempesis et al., 2020). Loading over time will also bring about changes to the mechanical structure of the subcutaneous adipose (Edsberg, Cutway et al., 2000; Edsberg, Natiella et al., 2001). For example, omental adipose has a higher proportion of fibrous proteins than subcutaneous adipose (Alkhouli et al., 2013). Thus, if the tissue were to differentiate in response to load, the distribution of fibrous proteins might change. Additionally, the extracellular matrix of adipose is composed primarily of collagen, yet elastin provides greater distensibility (Alkhouli et al., 2013). Therefore, a change in the distribution of collagen and elastin would result in a change in mechanical properties and biomechanical risk. Finally, lipid formation is known to change in response to load (Hara et al., 2011), and this may also affect the mechanical properties and, thus, the biomechanical risk (Ben-Or Frank et al., 2015).

Clinically, the association between adipose characteristics and biomechanical risk presents an opportunity both for assessment and intervention. For years, clinicians have been assessing tissue quality *via* palpation. The results of this study suggest that palpation may be augmented with an objective assessment of SubQF adipose quality to understand biomechanical risk and tissue tolerance. As MRI is not practical for regular clinical use, this would require clinically viable tools to assess SubQF quality, whether *via* imaging, assessment of mechanical properties, or an alternative approach. Furthermore, if changes in mechanical structure of the adipose increases risk, improving the SubQF quality could be an interventional goal. Lastly, combined with the finding that there is little gluteus maximus coverage of the ischium while seated (Sonenblum et al., 2020), these results provide further evidence that adipose plays an important role in PrI development.

In terms of intramuscular adipose tissue, our results contrasted with the studies of Lemmer, Alvarado et al. (2019) and Wu and Bogie (2013). Our study found that there was no relationship between the amount of fat infiltration and PrI history, which was unanticipated. It is possible that when studying such small sample sizes as done in Lemmer, Alvarado et al. (2019) (n = 38, but only n = 11 did not have a PrI history) and Wu and Bogie (2013) (n = 10 wheelchair users), IMAT was serving as a proxy for other effects such as time since injury, or in the present study, time since injury could be confounding the effect of IMAT. It is also worth noting that the methodology used to measure IMAT was different between these studies. Lemmer, Alvarado et al., (2019) and Wu and Bogie (2013) used CT scans to measure IMAT, which allowed for a more precise calculation of the ratio of adipose and muscle than is possible using MRI. On the other hand, CT scans come with increased radiation exposure and a supine posture that was undesirable for the present data collection approach.

However, when the completely fat-infiltrated subjects (IMAT effect size <0, or gluteus maximus intensity > adipose intensity) were excluded in our study, subjects with a higher amount of fat infiltration were more likely to have a history of PrI. Fat infiltration increases insulin resistance (Kalyani et al., 2014), which may be associated with decreased microvascular flow to the skeletal muscle and could explain the increased risk in this subset of the population. The difference in findings between people with partial fat infiltration and full fat infiltration may indicate that people who are fully fat infiltrated may have a different pathology of fat infiltration, making fat infiltration contribute less to their risk for PrI. For example, one participant experienced fat infiltration secondary to chemotherapy. Another possibility is that the properties and oxygen demand of the fully infiltrated muscle are different than that of the partially infiltrated muscle. Previous research has shown that in the abdominal region, subcutaneous fat has been correlated with insulin resistance (Patel and Abate, 2013). However, in the gluteal–femoral region, subcutaneous adipose tissue has been shown to increase insulin, which would increase blood flow (Snijder et al., 2005; Yim et al., 2008; Lambadiari et al., 2015). If the IMAT properties conformed to properties similar to SubQF upon full fat infiltration, then this could explain a change in perfusion and risk. At the same time, oxygen requirements are lower with enlarged fat cells, which may be the phenotype present in a fully infiltrated muscle (Frayn and Karpe, 2014). However, additional research would need to be conducted to confirm these new hypotheses.

Since BMI is a common method used to measure an individual's body fat, one would expect that the amount of fat infiltration and BMI would be directly correlated. However, there was no relationship between fat infiltration and BMI. This is consistent with Bogie et al. (2020). Time since injury is a much stronger predictor of IMAT, suggesting that the process occurs at some point after injury, likely as a result of disuse and atrophy, in response to myogenic and adipogenic markers identified in (Bogie et al., 2020). BMI (i.e., body weight and height) was self-reported in this study, so the accuracy of BMI values is unknown. However, our findings were similar when analyzed as SCI-adjusted BMI category, which would be less sensitive to precise weight measurements.

Limitations

The MRI scans used in this study were not optimized for studying intramuscular or SubQF adipose. There are imaging protocols that would provide more detailed information about the adipose, such as a Dixon protocol. Furthermore, the characteristics and etiology of the darker presentation of SubQF observed would be more thoroughly investigated using histology and mechanical testing as opposed to MRI. However, we believe that the results of this investigation provide important preliminary results to drive future work, in which histology and mechanical testing will relate the imaging results to specific changes in adipose characteristics.

While this study explored a large group of individuals with and without PrI history, there was a difference in the years of wheelchair use between the two groups that may have impacted IMAT analysis. Additional factors and comorbidities, such as chemotherapy or diabetes, were also not analyzed but may have influenced IMAT. Further studies that will include longitudinal analysis and consideration of additional factors and comorbidities would be beneficial to better understand the natural history of fat infiltration.

The few participants who used a wheelchair for reasons other than a spinal cord injury may expect a different adipose and muscle presentation given the differences in autonomic nervous system function. However, variability in nervous system function among individuals with SCI also exists, and this is best addressed by studying a larger population.

CONCLUSION

The results of the study suggest a hypothesis that changes in adipose tissue under the ischial tuberosity are associated with increased biomechanical risk for pressure injury. Further investigation of this hypothesis is warranted, including histology to understand the specific changes in tissue characteristic associated with darker fat, mechanical testing to identify changes in mechanical properties, and measurement of blood flow responses in regions with dark adipose. Further investigation of this hypothesis may lead to clinically useful diagnostic techniques that can identify changes in adipose and biomechanical risk to inform early preventative interventions.

AUTHOR CONTRIBUTIONS

SES and SHS designed the original study methods including research questions and data collection approach, and secured funding. SES provided study oversight and the analysis plan for this manuscript. SES drafted, revised, and submitted the manuscript. MM conducted the data analysis for this manuscript and contributed significantly to the initial manuscript draft and revisions. SHS provided critical insights to data analysis and revised the draft manuscript. JG was instrumental in developing the MRI data collection protocols and the gradient correction approach, participated in data collection, and revised the manuscript. JC supervised MRI analysis, provided expertise as a radiographer, and revised the manuscript.

ACKNOWLEDGMENTS

The authors acknowledge and thank the clinical team, Kelly Waugh, PT, MAPT, ATP, Mary Shea, MA, OTR, ATP, and Trevor Dyson-Hudson, PhD for their efforts collecting high quality data for this study. Finally, the authors also acknowledge our research participants, who contributed their time, along with patience and enthusiasm, and without whom this work could not have been completed.

REFERENCES

Addison, O., Marcus, R. L., LaStayo, P. C., and Ryan, A. S. (20142014). Intermuscular Fat: A Review of the Consequences and Causes. *Int. J. Endocrinol.* 2014, 309570. doi:10.1155/2014/309570

Alkhouli, N., Mansfield, J., Green, E., Bell, J., Knight, B., Liversedge, N., et al. (2013). The Mechanical Properties of Human Adipose Tissues and Their Relationships to the Structure and Composition of the Extracellular Matrix. *Am. J. Physiology-Endocrinology Metab.* 305 (12), E1427–E1435. doi:10.1152/ajpendo.00111.2013

Ben-Or Frank, M., Shoham, N., Benayahu, D., and Gefen, A. (2015). Effects of Accumulation of Lipid Droplets on Load Transfer between and within Adipocytes. *Biomech. Model. Mechanobiol* 14 (1), 15–28. doi:10.1007/s10237-014-0582-8

Bergstrom, N., Braden, B., Boynton, P., and Bruch, S. (1995). Using a Research-Based Assessment Scale in Clinical Practice. *Nurs. Clin. North. Am.* 30 (3), 539–551.

Bhattacharya, S., and Mishra, R. K. (2015). Pressure Ulcers: Current Understanding and Newer Modalities of Treatment. *Indian J. Plast. Surg.* 48 (1), 4–16. doi:10.4103/0970-0358.155260

Bogie, K. M., Schwartz, K., Li, Y., Wang, S., Dai, W., and Sun, J. (2020). Exploring Adipogenic and Myogenic Circulatory Biomarkers of Recurrent Pressure Injury Risk for Persons with Spinal Cord Injury. *J. Circ. Biomark* 9, 1–7. doi:10.33393/jcb.2020.2121

Booth, A. D., Magnuson, A. M., Fouts, J., Wei, Y., Wang, D., Pagliassotti, M. J., et al. (2018). Subcutaneous Adipose Tissue Accumulation Protects Systemic Glucose Tolerance and Muscle Metabolism. *Adipocyte* 7 (4), 261–272. doi:10.1080/21623945.2018.1525252

Braden, B., and Bergstrom, N. (1987). A Conceptual Schema for the Study of the Etiology of Pressure Sores. *Rehabil. Nurs. J.* 12 (1). doi:10.1002/j.2048-7940.1987.tb00541.x

Edsberg, L. E., Cutway, R., Anain, S., and Natiella, J. R. (2000). Microstructural and Mechanical Characterization of Human Tissue at and Adjacent to Pressure Ulcers. *J. Rehabil. Res. Dev.* 37 (4), 463–471.

Edsberg, L. E., Natiella, J. R., Baier, R. E., and Earle, J. (2001). Microstructural Characteristics of Human Skin Subjected to Static versus Cyclic Pressures. *J. Rehabil. Res. Dev.* 38 (5), 477–486.

European Pressure Ulcer Advisory Panel, National Pressure Injury Advisory Panel and Pan Pacific Pressure Injury Alliance (2019). *Prevention and Treatment of Pressure Ulcers/Injuries: Clinical Practice Guideline.* Editor E. Haesler (EPUAP/NPIAP/PPPIA).

Frayn, K. N., and Karpe, F. (2014). Regulation of Human Subcutaneous Adipose Tissue Blood Flow. *Int. J. Obes.* 38 (8), 1019–1026. doi:10.1038/ijo.2013.200

Garcia, A. D., and Thomas, D. R. (2006). Assessment and Management of Chronic Pressure Ulcers in the Elderly. *Med. Clin. North America* 90 (5), 925–944. doi:10.1016/j.mcna.2006.05.018

Goodpaster, B. H., Thaete, F. L., and Kelley, D. E. (2000). Thigh Adipose Tissue Distribution Is Associated with Insulin Resistance in Obesity and in Type 2 Diabetes Mellitus. *Am. J. Clin. Nutr.* 71 (4), 885–892. doi:10.1093/ajcn/71.4.885

Gorgey, A., Ogawa, M., Lester, R., and Akima, H. (2017). Quantification of Intermuscular and Intramuscular Adipose Tissue Using Magnetic Resonance Imaging after Neurodegenerative Disorders. *Neural Regen. Res.* 12 (12), 2100. doi:10.4103/1673-5374.221170

Grundy, S. M. (2015). Adipose Tissue and Metabolic Syndrome: Too Much, Too Little or Neither. *Eur. J. Clin. Invest.* 45 (11), 1209–1217. doi:10.1111/eci.12519

Hara, Y., Wakino, S., Tanabe, Y., Saito, M., Tokuyama, H., Washida, N., et al. (2011). Rho and Rho-Kinase Activity in Adipocytes Contributes to a Vicious Cycle in Obesity that May Involve Mechanical Stretch. *Sci. Signal.* 4 (157), ra3. doi:10.1126/scisignal.2001227

Lambadiari, V., Triantafyllou, K., and Dimitriadis, G. D. (2015). Insulin Action in Muscle and Adipose Tissue in Type 2 Diabetes: The Significance of Blood Flow. *Wjd* 6 (4), 626–633. doi:10.4239/wjd.v6.i4.626

Lemmer, D. P., Alvarado, N., Henzel, K., Richmond, M. A., McDaniel, J., Graebert, J., et al. (2019). What Lies beneath: Why Some Pressure Injuries May Be Unpreventable for Individuals with Spinal Cord Injury. *Arch. Phys. Med. Rehabil.* 100 (6), 1042–1049. doi:10.1016/j.apmr.2018.11.006

Lempesis, I. G., van Meijel, R. L. J., Manolopoulos, K. N., and Goossens, G. H. (2020). Oxygenation of Adipose Tissue: A Human Perspective. *Acta Physiol. (Oxf)* 228 (1), e13298. doi:10.1111/apha.13298

Levy, A., Enzer, S., Shoham, N., Zaretsky, U., and Gefen, A. (2012). Large, but Not Small Sustained Tensile Strains Stimulate Adipogenesis in Culture. *Ann. Biomed. Eng.* 40 (5), 1052–1060. doi:10.1007/s10439-011-0496-x

Liao, F., Burns, S., and Jan, Y.-K. (2013). Skin Blood Flow Dynamics and its Role in Pressure Ulcers. *J. Tissue Viability* 22 (2), 25–36. doi:10.1016/j.jtv.2013.03.001

Ogawa, M., Lester, R., Akima, H., and Gorgey, A. S. (2017). Quantification of Intermuscular and Intramuscular Adipose Tissue Using Magnetic Resonance Imaging after Neurodegenerative Disorders. *Neural Regen. Res.* 12 (12), 2100–2105. doi:10.4103/1673-5374.221170

Patel, P., and Abate, N. (2013). Body Fat Distribution and Insulin Resistance. *Nutrients* 5 (6), 2019–2027. doi:10.3390/nu5062019

Salzberg, C. A., Byrne, D. W., Cayten, C. G., van Niewerburgh, P., Murphy, J. G., and Viehbeck, M. (1996). A New Pressure Ulcer Risk Assessment Scale for Individuals with Spinal Cord Injury1. *Am. J. Phys. Med. Rehabil.* 75 (2), 96–104. doi:10.1097/00002060-199603000-00004

Snijder, M. B., Visser, M., Visser, M., Dekker, J. M., Goodpaster, B. H., Harris, T. B., et al. (2005). Low Subcutaneous Thigh Fat Is a Risk Factor for Unfavourable Glucose and Lipid Levels, Independently of High Abdominal Fat. The Health ABC Study. *Diabetologia* 48 (2), 301–308. doi:10.1007/s00125-004-1637-7

Sonenblum, S. E., Sprigle, S., and Lopez, R. A. (2012). Manual Wheelchair Use: Bouts of Mobility in Everyday Life. *Rehabil. Res. Pract.* 2012, 753165. doi:10.1155/2012/753165

Sonenblum, S. E., Seol, D., Sprigle, S. H., and Cathcart, J. M. (2020). Seated Buttocks Anatomy and its Impact on Biomechanical Risk. *J. Tissue Viability* 29 (2), 69–75. doi:10.1016/j.jtv.2020.01.004

Sonenblum, S. E., and Sprigle, S. (2011). Distinct Tilting Behaviours with Power Tilt-In-Space Systems. *Disabil. Rehabil. Assistive Techn.* 6 (6), 526–535. doi:10.3109/17483107.2011.580900

Sprigle, S., McNair, D., and Sonenblum, S. (2020). Pressure Ulcer Risk Factors in Persons with Mobility-Related Disabilities. *Adv. Skin Wound Care* 33 (3), 146–154. doi:10.1097/01.asw.0000653152.36482.7d

Wu, G. A., and Bogie, K. M. (2013). Not just Quantity: Gluteus Maximus Muscle Characteristics in Able-Bodied and SCI Individuals - Implications for Tissue Viability. *J. Tissue Viability* 22 (3), 74–82. doi:10.1016/j.jtv.2013.03.003

18

Anatomical Characteristics of Cutaneous Branches Extending from the Second Dorsal Metacarpal Artery

Peng Liu†, Zhongyuan Deng†, Tao Zhang* and Xiaojian Li*

Department of Burn and Plastic, Guangzhou Red Cross Hospital, Medical College, Jinan University, Guangzhou, China

***Correspondence:**
Tao Zhang
z.t-1231@163.com
Xiaojian Li
lixj64@163.com

† These authors have contributed equally to this work

Background: A second dorsal metacarpal artery cutaneous branches flap is often used to repair skin defects in the hand. The location of the cutaneous branch of that artery is very critical for the removal of the flap. In this study, we quantitatively analyzed the origin of the cutaneous branches of the second dorsal metacarpalartery and the distribution characteristics of the radial and ulnar side to provide an anatomical basis for designing a flap.

Methods: Sixteen upper limb specimens were perfused with latex. Four specimens were infused with ethyl acetate plus plastic, and four specimens were perfused with red latex to create pellucid specimens. The origin, travel paths, and distribution of the cutaneous branches of the second dorsal metacarpal artery were anatomically observed, and we measured the length of the cutaneous branch from the midpoint of the second web space edge. We also measured the diameters and pedicle lengths of the radial and ulnar distributions of cutaneous branches of the second dorsal metacarpal artery.

Results: The cutaneous branches of the second dorsal metacarpal artery were mainly clustered at three positions, the second cluster point was at 43.9%, the fourth cluster point was at 61.2%, and the fifth cluster point was at 72.1%. The first cluster point was at 30.8% and the sixth cluster point was at 85.6%. The diameter and pedicle length of the sixth cluster point were the largest. There was no significant difference in the distribution of the diameters and pedicle lengths of the cutaneous branch between the radial and ulnar side. The second dorsal metacarpal artery sent out 1–2 cutaneous branches before the tendon joint, and formed a blood vessel anastomosis with other cutaneous branches located further from the tendon joint. The dorsal branch of the radial nerve in the hand extended a nerve branch at the wrist joint and traveled between the cutaneous branches of the second dorsal metacarpal artery to dominate the corresponding skin.

Conclusion: Three clusters in the distal second dorsal metacarpal artery were selected to be the flap pedicle containing a cutaneous nerve for use in repairing a skin defect in the hand and fingers.

Keywords: second dorsal metacarpal artery, cutaneous branches, cluster distribution, skin wound repair, anatomical characteristics

INTRODUCTION

The hand is the most commonly used appendage in daily life and the most vulnerable part of the body. An injured hand is likely to cause physical dysfunction, adversely affect a person's appearance, and produce apsychological burden (Masakatsu et al., 2018; Viktor and Max, 2018; Xu et al., 2018). Dorsal metacarpal artery flaps are used to repair hand tissue defects, and especially defects of the fingers. Some advantages of the dorsal metacarpal artery flap include a simple operation, convenient tissue transfer, and similarities in characteristics of tissue cortex, toughness, and elasticity (Isaraj, 2011; Schiefer et al., 2012).

The second dorsal metacarpal artery is relatively anatomically consistent and rarely absent. Therefore, a second dorsal metacarpal artery flap is usually used to cover a hand skin defect. Current research shows that the second dorsal metacarpal skin flap is usually designed so as to allow the second metacarpal dorsal artery to serve as the vascular pedicle when repairing small area skin defects in the hand. However, a disadvantage of that design is that it sacrifices the second dorsal metacarpal artery and injures a large amount of tissue (Wang et al., 2011; Chi et al., 2018; Webster and Saint-Cyr, 2020).

Recent studies have shown that the second dorsal metacarpal artery extends cutaneous branches that interconnect in the superficial fascia to form a rich reticular structure rich in blood vessels. The cutaneous branches arising from the dorsal metacarpal artery are mainly distributed in the distal 1/3 segment, and have a mean diameter > 0.2 mm. A cutaneous branch of the second dorsal metacarpal artery can be used as the vascular pedicle when repairing a small area defect in hand (Da-Ping and Morris, 2001; Guang-Rong et al., 2005; Zhang et al., 2009; Appleton and Morris, 2014). However, it is difficult to use ultrasound to verify the exact positions of the cutaneous branches before surgery due to their lack of distinction. Therefore, a quantitative analysis of the anatomical distribution of cutaneous branches is helpful for designing the flap.

Vascular perfusion is a common method to study vascular construction such as blood vessel traveling, distribution, and anastomosis. Different fillers can be used to perfuse blood vessels, and then the blood vessel travel can be displayed by anatomy, transparency, corrosion and radiography. These fillers are rubber, plastic, gelatin, and oil, etc. Latex is the emulsion before the rubber solidifies. The blood vessel specimens perfused with the red latex are elastic, easy to stretch and not easy to break. This method is suitable for microanatomy observation research. Ethyl acetate and plastic perfusion is a method to make cast specimens. The blood vessels are perfused with ethyl acetate and plastic mixed with staining agent. After ethyl acetate and plastic hardening, the specimens are corroded with acid to leave only the ethyl acetate and plastic model of blood vessels. Compared with the latex perfusion, the cast specimens made of ethyl acetate and plastic perfusion can show three-dimensional blood vessels traveling and distribution.

Although numerous studies have described using cutaneous branches flaps with the dorsal metacarpal artery serving as a pedicle, no quantitative analysis has been performed on the distribution patterns of the cutaneous branches, including their radial and ulnar distributions. This study used anatomical techniques such as vascular perfusion, casting, and transparency to study the distribution patterns of the cutaneous branches, including their radial and ulnar distributions, to provide ananatomical basis for designing a flap.

MATERIALS AND METHODS

A total of 24 upper limb specimens were legally obtained from the Human Anatomy Department of Southern Medical University in Guangzhou, China. 24 upper limb specimens were amputated at the human elbow joint and immediately the brachial artery was perfused with colored materials. These specimens were placed in a −18°C refrigerator for storage. We performed the anatomical experiments after 1 week. Next, 16 of the specimens were injected with latex for microanatomy examination, four specimens were embedded with ethyl acetate and plastic for use as cast specimens, and four specimens were injected with latex to create transparent specimens. The study protocol was approved by the Institutional Review Board of Guangzhou Red Cross Hospital.

Latex Specimens for Microanatomy

A glass catheter was carefully inserted into the brachial artery, which was filled with a certain amount of red latex. Next, a longitudinal incision was made between the second and third metacarpal bones on the dorsum of the hand, and the skin tissue was elevated from the deep fascia to expose cutaneous branches extending from the second dorsal metacarpal artery. The lengths, diameters, and positions of cutaneous branches extending from the second dorsal metacarpal artery were measured. The distance between the midpoint of the second web space edge and the midpoint of the second metacarpal bone was set as a unit, and

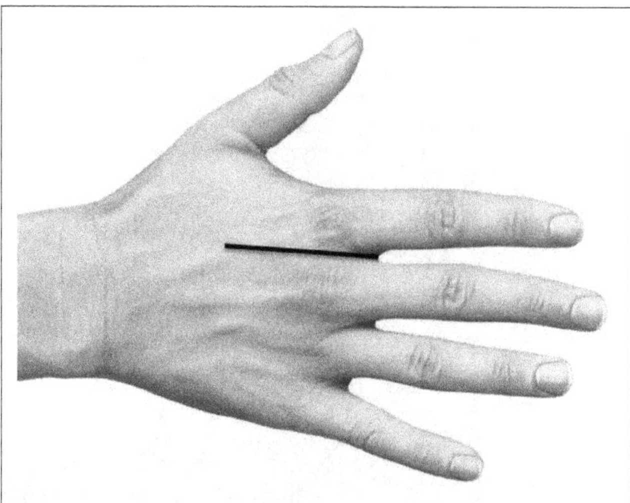

FIGURE 1 | The distance between the midpoint of the second web space edge and the midpoint of the second metacarpal bone was set as the standard unit length (100%).

we measured the distance of all branches to the midpoint of the second web space edge.

Cast Specimens

A glass catheter was carefully inserted into the brachial artery, which was then injected with 10 mL of an ethyl acetate and plastic solution enough to fill the blood vessel; the solution was replenished with a certain amount of ethyl acetate and plastic mixture every 2 h. The mixture was replenished five times in total. The brachial artery was filled with self-setting dental tray material during the final replenishment. After its preparation, the casting specimen was immersed in a 25% hydrochloric acid bath and allowed to slowly corrode in a week. The positions, distribution, and anastomotic connections of cutaneous branches extending from the second dorsal metacarpal artery were observed.

Transparent Specimens for Direct Observation

An appropriate amount of red latex was perfused into the brachial artery. After it solidified in the blood vessels, the specimen was soaked and subsequently fixed in 75% alcohol; after which, it was air-dried in a ventilated location. Finally, the specimen was soaked in glycerol to make it transparent.

Statistical Analysis

All data were analyzed using SPSS Statistics for Windows, Version 17.0 (SPSS, Inc., Chicago, IL, United States). The distance between the midpoint of the second web space edge and the midpoint of the second metacarpal bone was established as the standard unit length (100%) (**Figure 1**). The distance of each

TABLE 1 | The clusters distribution of cutaneous branches from the second dorsal metacarpal artery in 16 specimens.

Cluster	Cutaneous branches	Relative distance (%)*	Diameter (mm)	The length of pedicle (mm)
1	9	30.8	0.38 ± 0.15	5.93 ± 1.08
2	21	43.9	0.45 ± 0.13	5.62 ± 2.02
3	16	53.4	0.43 ± 0.13	5.57 ± 1.13
4	22	61.2	0.41 ± 0.11	6.47 ± 1.68
5	22	72.1	0.41 ± 0.17	6.46 ± 2.01
6	13	85.6	0.47 ± 0.20	7.41 ± 1.86

**The distance between the midpoint of the second web space edge and the midpoint of the second metacarpal bone was set as the standard unit length (100%). The relative distance is equal to the distance from each cutaneous branches to the midpoint of the second web space edge divided by the standard unit length.*

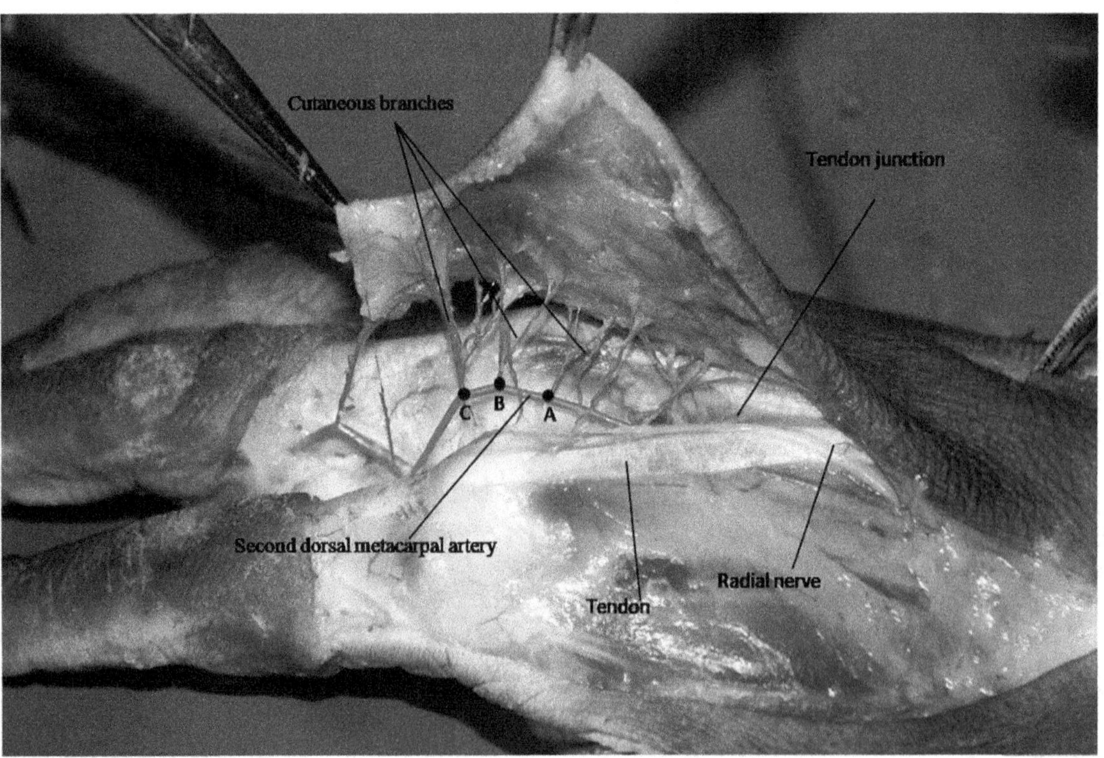

FIGURE 2 | The cutaneous branches from the second dorsal metacarpal artery are mainly clustered at three positions: the second cluster point is at 43.9% **(A)**, the fourth cluster point is at 61.2% **(B)**, and the fifth cluster point was at 72.1% **(C)**.

TABLE 2 | The distribution of the diameter and pedicle length of the cutaneous branches between the radial and ulnar side.

	Radial (n = 55)	Ulnar (n = 48)	t	*p
Diameter (mm)	0.42 ± 0.12	0.43 ± 0.17	−0.443	0.659
The length of pedicle (mm)	6.04 ± 1.64	6.44 ± 1.97	−1.121	0.265

*p was less than 0.05 means that it was significant difference in the distribution of the diameter and pedicle length of the cutaneous branch between the radial and ulnar side.

cutaneous branch to the midpoint of the second web space edge was recorded. The data were subjected to K-means clustering to quantitatively analyze the origin distribution of the cutaneous branches. The diameters and pedicle lengths of the radial and ulnar distributions of cutaneous branches extending from the second dorsal metacarpal artery were quantitatively analyzed by the independent t-test.

RESULTS

Origin Distribution of the Cutaneous Branches From the Second Dorsal Metacarpal Artery

All cutaneous branches extending from the second dorsal metacarpal artery were counted in 16 specimens, and a total of 103 branches were identified. The cutaneous branches were mainly clustered at three positions: the second cluster point was at 43.9%, and included 21 branches, the fourth cluster point was at 61.2%, and included 22 dermal branches, and the fifth cluster point was at 72.1%, and included 22 cutaneous branches. The first cluster point was at 30.8% and the sixth cluster point was at 85.6%. It was obvious that the cutaneous branches were less distributed at the second cluster point; however, the diameters and pedicle lengths of the branches at the sixth cluster point were the largest (**Table 1** and **Figure 2**).

Distribution Characteristics of the Diameters and Pedicle Lengths of the Radial and Ulnar Distributions of Cutaneous Branches Extending From the Second Dorsal Metacarpal Artery

A total of 55 branches were distributed in the radial side of the second dorsal metacarpal artery and 48 branches were distributed in the ulnar side. There were seven more branches in the radial side than in the ulnar side. The mean diameter of the radial branches was smaller than that of the ulnar cutaneous branches; however, there was no significant difference in the distribution of the diameter of the cutaneous branches in the radial and ulnar sides (p = 0.659). The mean pedicle length of the radial branches was significantly less than that of the ulnar branches (p = 0.265). Therefore, there was no significant difference in the distribution of the diameters and pedicle lengths of the cutaneous branches in the radial and ulnar side (**Table 2** and **Figure 3**).

The Anatomical Relationship Between Cutaneous Branches and the Dorsal Branches of the Radial Nerve

The second dorsal metacarpal artery travels between the second and third metacarpal bones, and emits numerous cutaneous branches along the way. The cutaneous branches are mainly concentrated in the distal parts of the second and third tendon

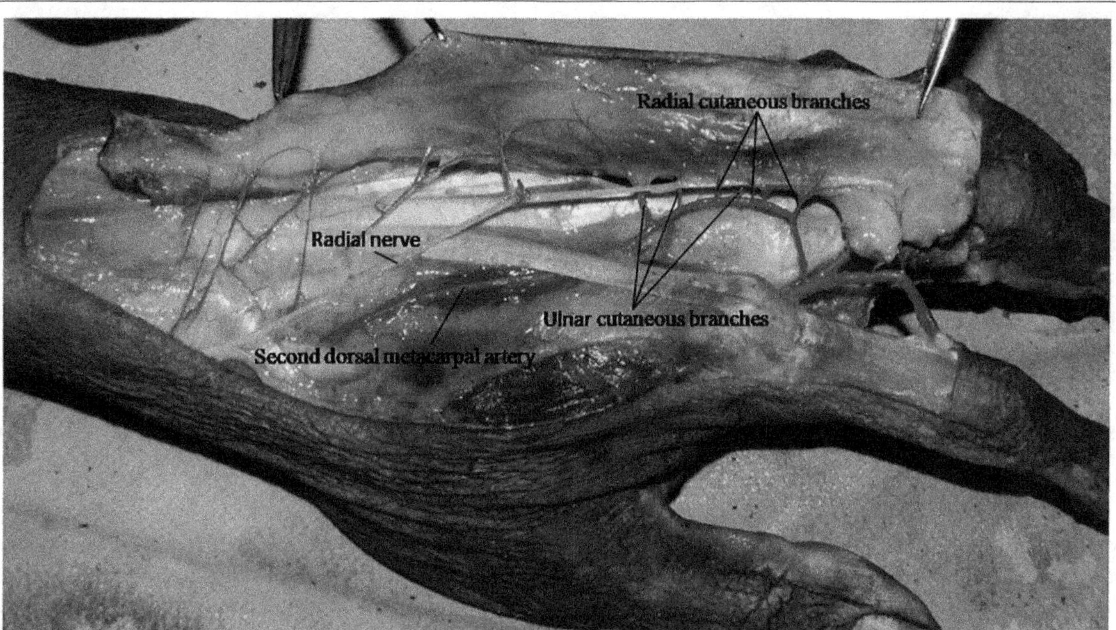

FIGURE 3 | The distribution of the diameter and pedicle length of the cutaneous branch between the radial and ulnar side was no significant difference.

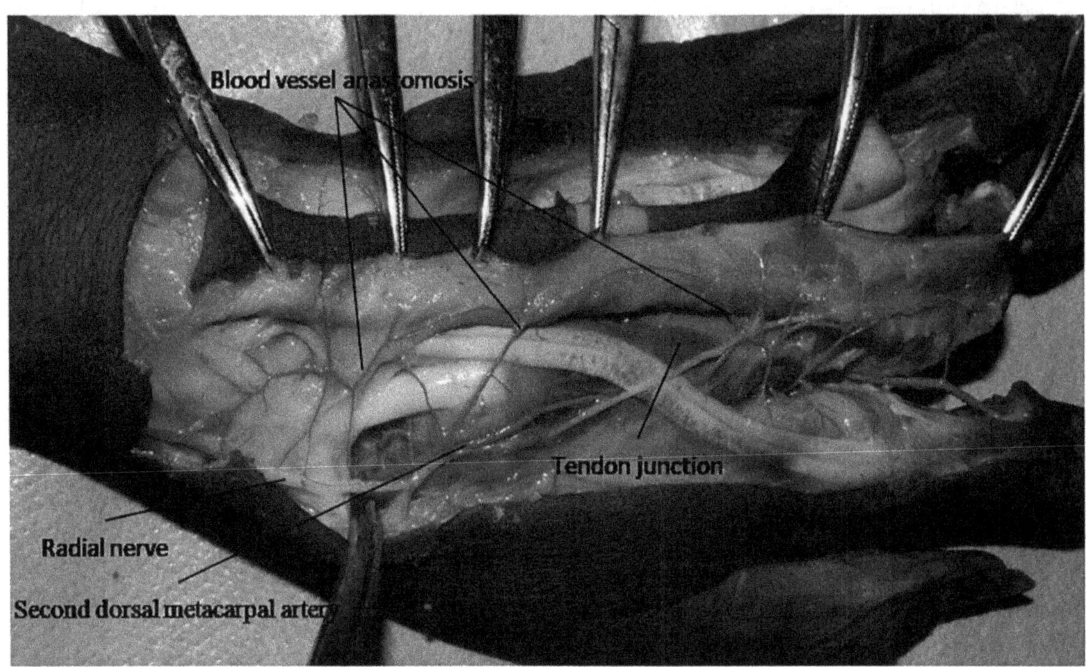

FIGURE 4 | The cutaneous branches extended in the proximal part of the tendon joint, and formed a blood vessel anastomosis with the cutaneous branches farther from the tendon joint.

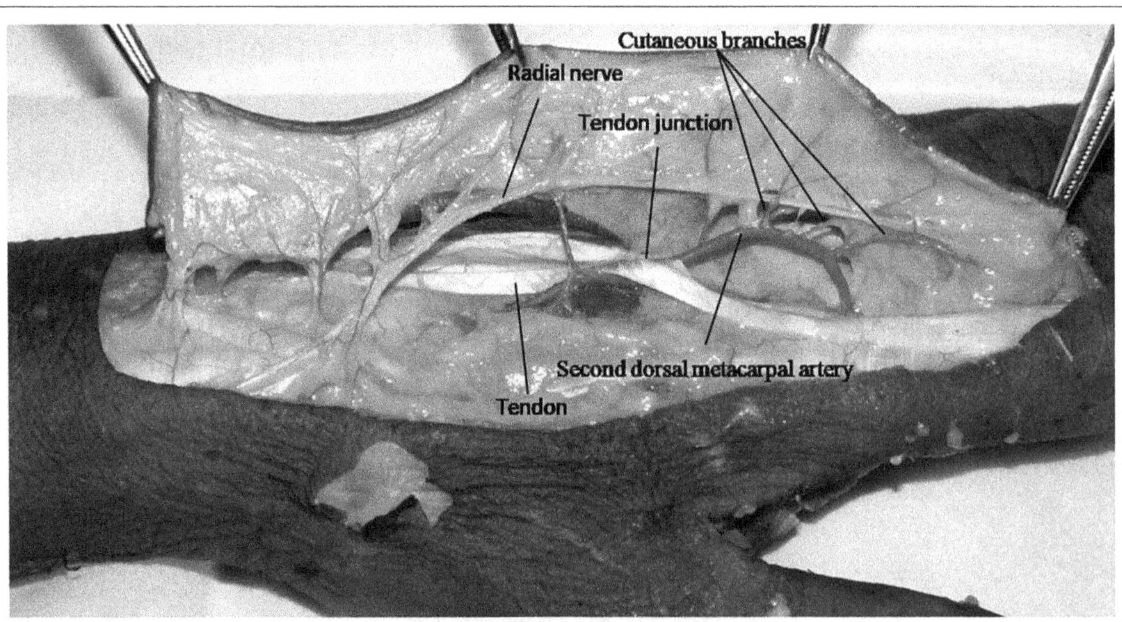

FIGURE 5 | The dorsal branch of the radial nerve in the hand extended a nerve branch at the wrist joint and traveled between the cutaneous branches of the second dorsal metacarpal artery.

joints. However, this anatomical study found that the second dorsal metacarpal artery also emitted 1–2 cutaneous branches prior to the tendon joint, and formed a blood vessel anastomosis with the cutaneous branches located further from the tendon joint. The diameter of the cutaneous branches ranged from 0.31 to 0.47 mm (**Figure 4**). The dorsal branch of the radial nerve in the hand extended a nerve branch at the wrist joint and traveled between the cutaneous branches of the second dorsal metacarpal artery to dominate the corresponding skin. This anatomical feature can provide an anatomical basis for designing the second dorsal metacarpal artery flap with a sensory nerve (**Figure 5**).

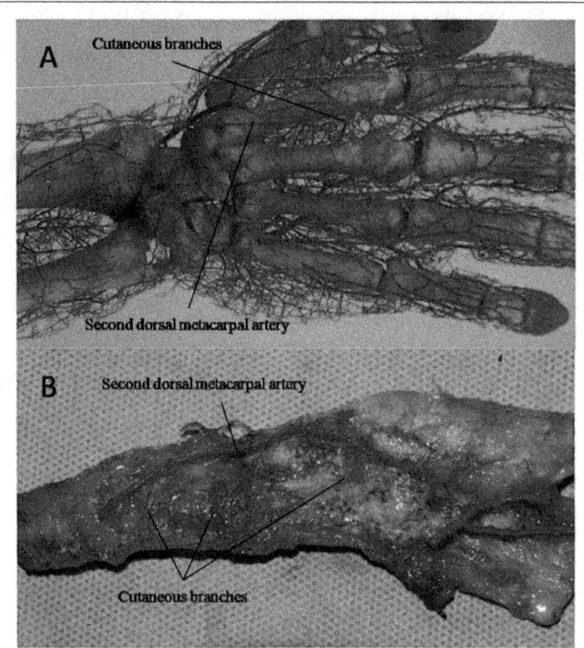

FIGURE 6 | The cast specimens **(A)** and transparent specimens **(B)** also showed no significant difference in the distribution of cutaneous branches on the radius and ulnar side.

DISCUSSION

The second dorsal metacarpal artery flap is an important flap commonly used to repair skin defects in the hand. Cutaneous branches of the dorsal metacarpal artery form a vascular chain that supplies blood for the second dorsal metacarpal artery flap. In this study, we analyzed the origin distribution of cutaneous branches and the diameters and pedicle lengths of the radial and ulnar distribution of cutaneous branches extending from the second dorsal metacarpal artery. The three locations of the clustered cutaneous branches were found to be used for clinicians to design cutaneous branches flap and perform operation. The anatomical adjacent relationship between the cutaneous branches and dorsal cutaneous nerve was also observed.

The second dorsal metacarpal artery originates from the radial artery or dorsal carpal artery network. It then travels on the superficial surface of the dorsal interosseous muscles, and emits numerous cutaneous branches along the way that nourish the corresponding skin tissue (Marx et al., 2001; De Rezende et al., 2004; Al-Baz et al., 2019). Our study found that the cutaneous branches of the second dorsal metacarpal artery were mainly distributed in six clusters, of which there were more cutaneous branches distributed at 43.9, 61.2, and 72.1% of the cluster points. A clinician can locate the vascular pedicle prior to surgery in this position. Our statistical analysis showed that an average of 6.4 branches originated from the second dorsal metacarpal artery. Therefore, we conducted a k-mean clustering analysis to establish six categories for better evaluating the cluster characteristics of cutaneous branches, and obtain more information than could be provided by a two-step cluster analysis (Liu et al., 2015).

Clinically, the second dorsal metacarpal artery flap is designed based on the principle of point, line and surface, and usually has a symmetrical design. However, many vascular branches are often anatomically dominant (Schaverien and Saint-Cyr, 2008; Saint-Cyr et al., 2010; Sun et al., 2013). A study of the radial and ulnar distribution of cutaneous branches is helpful for

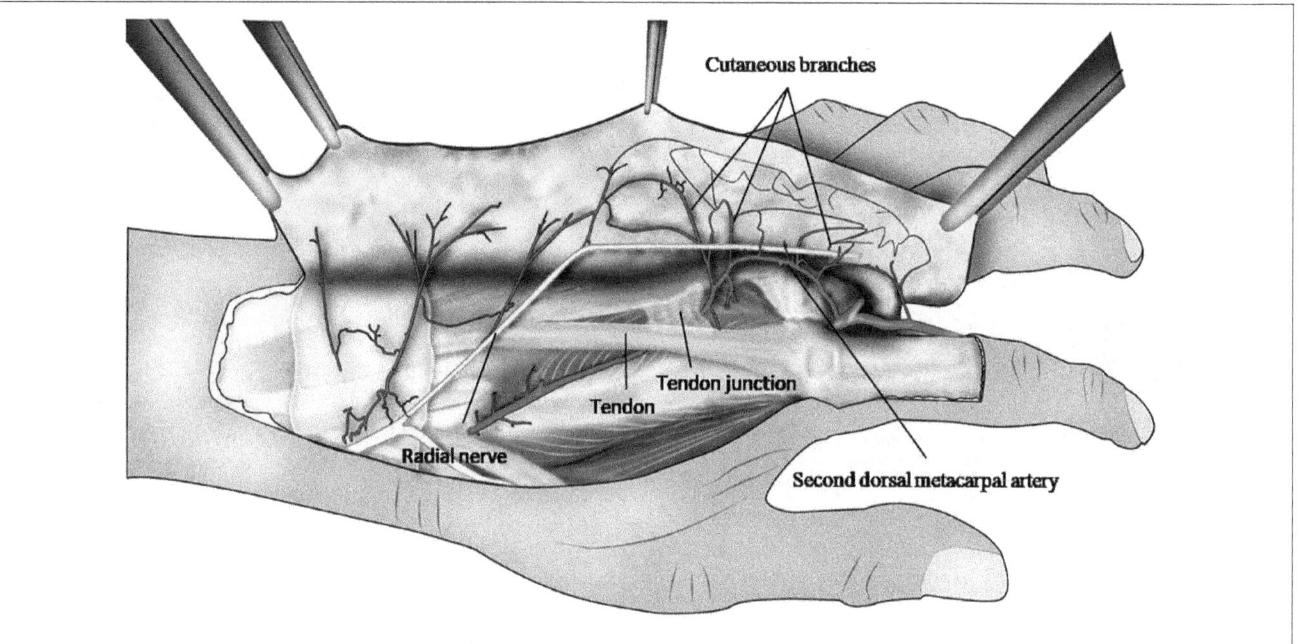

FIGURE 7 | This ideograph presents the anatomical angioarchitecture and the distribution among the cutaneous branches arising from the second dorsal metacarpal artery, and reveals the design of cutaneous branches flap with the second dorsal metacarpal artery pedicle.

determining the size and shape of a flap. This study found no significant difference in the distribution of the diameter and pedicle length of the cutaneous branch in the radial and ulnar side (**Figure 6**).

While most previous studies have focused on the cutaneous branches at the distal part from the tendon joint, there are usually 1–2 cutaneous branches with a diameter of 0.37 ± 0.11 mm before the tendon joint (Yoon et al., 2007; Zhu et al., 2013; Rozen et al., 2015; van Alphen et al., 2016). The cutaneous branches of the distal and proximal parts of the second dorsal metacarpal artery link with each other, which can increase the length of the vascular pedicle of the flap and enlarge its rotational coverage. The dorsal branch of the radial nerve travels between the radial and ulnar cutaneous branches. This anatomical feature can help clinicians to design the second dorsal metacarpal artery flap to include sensory nerves that restore the sensory function of the wound surface and improve the tactile function of the fingertips.

Based on our anatomical observations and statistical studies, the cutaneous branches near or in the cluster points of the second dorsal metacarpal artery were used as the flap pedicle, and the surface projection of the second dorsal metacarpal artery served as the flap axis. A cutaneous branches flap is designed to cut the plane between the shallow and deep fascia (**Figure 7**). During the surgical procedure, we preserved the fascial tissue around the pedicle as much as possible in order to avoid vascular spasm caused by excessive distortion or rotation of the cutaneous branches. During the process of lifting the flap, it was not necessary to cut the deep fascia so as to protect both the second dorsal metacarpal artery and the original root of the cutaneous branches. After the operation, the patient's index finger and middle finger movement was normal and finger sensory function was good, as judged by a 2 mm two-point discrimination (Delikonstantinou et al., 2011; **Figure 8**).

However, the diameters of cutaneous branches are small enough that naked branches extremely are prone to vasospasm.

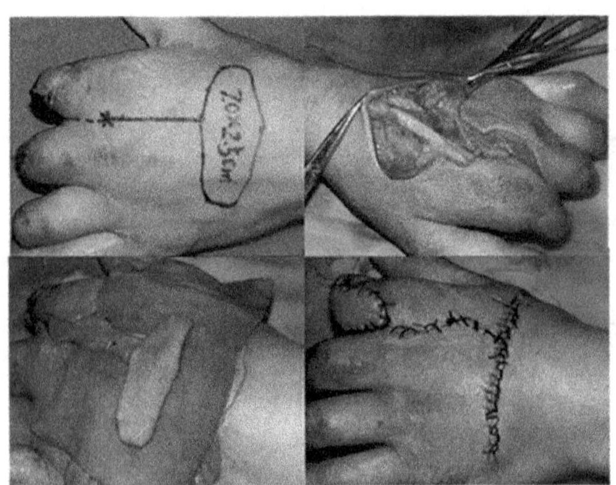

FIGURE 8 | The second dorsal metacarpal artery flap with cutaneous nerve was recovered to repair the skin defect of the hand. After the operation, the patient's finger movement was normal and finger sensory was good due to 2 mm two-point discrimination.

Before the operation it is very important to perform a Doppler exploration. During the operation, it is necessary to pay attention to the anastomosis of cutaneous branches, and to protect the anastomosis linking between the cutaneous branches as much as possible.

CONCLUSION

Cutaneous branches of the second dorsal metacarpal artery were mainly clustered at three positions: 43.9, 61.2, and 72.1% in the distal second dorsal metacarpal artery, which was chosen as the flap pedicle with a cutaneous nerve to repair the skin defect in the hand and fingers of a patient.

AUTHOR CONTRIBUTIONS

In the beginning of work, XL gave the idea to observe the anastomosis relationship and the distribution of the perforators arising from the second dorsal metacarpal artery. TZ, ZD, and PL dissected carefully the second dorsal metacarpal artery and its perforators, included the linking among the perforators in the superficial fascia and dermis. TZ made the pellucid specimen reveal the course of the perforators and anastomosis between the adjacent branches. In the same time, we measured the diameter and the length of pedicle of the perforators in the course of dissection, then ZD and PL conducted not only a chi-square test to compare the quantities of ulnar and radial branches from second dorsal metacarpal artery in two groups with SPSS 17.0, but also the cluster analysis which was a two-step clustering procedure to observe the integrated distribution of the perforators. ZD and PL design the flap to cover the defect of finger based on the anatomy of second dorsal metacarpal artery perforators. In the whole course, XL provided a great helping for us to complete this research. All authors contributed to the article and approved the submitted version.

FUNDING

This work was supported by research grant 20191A011015 (PL) from General Guidance Project of Guangzhou Municipal Health Committee, research grant A2019273 (PL) from Guangdong Medical Science and Technology Research Fund, research grant from Guangzhou high-level clinical key specialty construction fund (XL), research grant from 59-special technology project of Guangzhou (XL), research grant from 2019 Ph.D. Workstation Scientific Research Fund of Guangzhou Red Cross Hospital, and research grant from 2018 Project Funds of Guangzhou Red Cross Hospital.

REFERENCES

Al-Baz, T., Gad, S., and Keshk, T. (2019). Evaluation of dorsal metacarpal artery perforator flaps in the reconstruction of hand soft-tissue defects. *Menoufia Med. J.* 32, 1256–1261.

Appleton, S. E., and Morris, S. F. (2014). Anatomy and physiology of perforator flaps of the upper limb. *Hand Clin.* 30, 123–135. doi: 10.1016/j.hcl.2013.12.003

Chi, Z., Lin, D., and Chen, Y. (2018). Routine closure of the donor site with a second dorsal metacarpal artery flap to avoid the use of a skin graft after harvest of a first dorsal metacarpal artery flap. *J. Plastic Reconstruct. Aesthetic Surg.* 71, 870–875. doi: 10.1016/j.bjps.2018.01.031

Da-Ping, Y., and Morris, S. F. (2001). Reversed dorsal digital and metacarpal island flaps supplied by the dorsal cutaneous branches of the palmar digital artery. *Ann. Plastic Surg.* 46, 444–449. doi: 10.1097/00000637-200104000-00017

De Rezende, M. R., Mattar, J. R., and Cho, A. B. (2004). Anatomic study of the dorsal arterial system of the hand. *Rev. Hosp. Clin. Fac. Med. Sao Paulo* 59, 71–76. doi: 10.1590/s0041-87812004000200005

Delikonstantinou, I. P., Gravvanis, A. I., and Dimitriou, V. (2011). Foucher first dorsal metacarpal artery flap versus littler heterodigital neurovascular flap in resurfacing thumb pulp loss defects. *Ann. Plast. Surg.* 67, 119–122. doi: 10.1097/sap.0b013e3181ef6f6d

Guang-Rong, Y., Feng, Y., and Shi-Min, C. (2005). Microsurgical second dorsal metacarpal artery cutaneous and tenocutaneous flap for distal finger reconstruction: anatomic study and clinical application. *Microsurgery* 25, 30–35. doi: 10.1002/micr.20077

Isaraj, S. (2011). Use of dorsal metacarpal artery flaps in post burn reconstruction - two cases report. *Macedonian J. Med. Sci.* 4:11.

Liu, P., Qin, X., and Zhang, H. (2015). The second dorsal metacarpal artery chain-link flap: an anatomical study and a case report. *Surg. Radiol. Anat.* 37, 349–356. doi: 10.1007/s00276-014-1372-9

Marx, A., Preisser, P., and Peek, A. (2001). Anatomy of the dorsal mid-hand arteries–anatomic study and review of the literature. *Handchir. Mikrochir. Plast. Chir.* 33, 77–82.

Masakatsu, H., Takashi, M., and Yoshihito, T. (2018). Functional reconstruction of severely burned hand with osseous blood flow deficiency with immediate surgery using an abdominal bipediceled flap: a case report. *Eplasty* 18:11.

Rozen, W. M., Katz, T. L., and Hunter-Smith, D. J. (2015). Vascularization of the dorsal base of the second metacarpal bone: implications for a reverse second dorsal metacarpal artery flap. *Plast. Reconstr. Surg.* 135, 231–232.

Saint-Cyr, M., Mujadzic, M., and Wong, C. (2010). The radial artery pedicle perforator flap: vascular analysis and clinical implications. *Plast. Reconstr. Surg.* 125, 1469–1478. doi: 10.1097/prs.0b013e3181d511e7

Schaverien, M., and Saint-Cyr, M. (2008). Perforators of the lower leg: analysis of perforator locations and clinical application for pedicled perforator flaps. *Plast. Reconstr. Surg.* 122, 161–170. doi: 10.1097/prs.0b013e3181774386

Schiefer, J. L., Schaller, H., and Rahmanian-Schwarz, A. (2012). Dorsal metacarpal artery flaps with extensor indices tendons for reconstruction of digital defects. *J. Invest. Surg.* 25, 340–343. doi: 10.3109/08941939.2011.640384

Sun, C., Hou, Z. D., and Wang, B. (2013). An anatomical study on the characteristics of cutaneous branches-chain perforator flap with ulnar artery pedicle. *Plast. Reconstr. Surg.* 131, 329–336. doi: 10.1097/prs.0b013e318277884c

van Alphen, N. A., Laungani, A. T., and Christner, J. A. (2016). The distally based dorsal metatarsal artery perforator flap: vascular study and clinical implications. *J. Reconstr. Microsurg.* 32, 245–250. doi: 10.1055/s-0035-1554936

Viktor, M. G., and Max, G. (2018). Wrist scar contracture, hand deviation: anatomy and treatment with trapeze-flap plasty. *Plastic Reconstruct. Surg. Burns* 26, 235–242. doi: 10.1007/978-3-319-78714-5_26

Wang, P., Zhou, Z., and Dong, Q. (2011). Reverse second and third dorsal metacarpal artery fasciocutaneous flaps for repair of distal- and middle-segment finger soft tissue defects. *J. Reconstr. Microsurg.* 27, 495–502. doi: 10.1055/s-0031-1284235

Webster, N., and Saint-Cyr, M. (2020). Flaps based on the dorsal metacarpal artery. *Hand Clin.* 36, 75–83. doi: 10.1016/j.hcl.2019.09.001

Xu, G., Jianli, C., and Ziping, J. (2018). Risk factors for pedicled flap necrosis in hand soft tissue reconstruction: a multivariate logistic regression analysis. *ANZ J. Surg.* 88, 127–131.

Yoon, S. W., Rebecca, A. M., and Smith, A. A. (2007). Reverse second dorsal metacarpal artery flap for reconstruction of fourth-degree burn wounds of the hand. *J. Burn. Care Res.* 28, 521–523. doi: 10.1097/bcr.0b013e318053daab

Zhang, X., He, Y., and Shao, X. (2009). Second dorsal metacarpal artery flap from the dorsum of the middle finger for coverage of volar thumb defect. *J. Hand Surg. Am.* 34, 1467–1473. doi: 10.1016/j.jhsa.2009.04.040

Zhu, H., Zhang, X., and Yan, M. (2013). Treatment of complex soft-tissue defects at the metacarpophalangeal joint of the thumb using the bilobed second dorsal metacarpal artery-based island flap. *Plast. Reconstr. Surg.* 131, 1091–1097. doi: 10.1097/prs.0b013e3182865c26

19

Morphology and Mechanical Properties of Plantar Fascia in Flexible Flatfoot: A Noninvasive *In Vivo* Study

Zhihui Qian[1], Zhende Jiang[1], Jianan Wu[1], Fei Chang[2], Jing Liu[1], Lei Ren[1,3]* and Luquan Ren[1]*

[1]Key Laboratory of Bionic Engineering, Jilin University, Changchun, China, [2]Orthopaedic Medical Center, The Second Hospital of Jilin University, Changchun, China, [3]School of Mechanical, Aerospace and Civil Engineering, University of Manchester, Manchester, United Kingdom

***Correspondence:**
Lei Ren
lei.ren@manchester.ac.uk
Jing Liu
jingliu@jlu.edu.cn

Plantar fascia plays an important role in human foot biomechanics; however, the morphology and mechanical properties of plantar fascia in patients with flexible flatfoot are unknown. In this study, 15 flexible flatfeet were studied, each plantar fascia was divided into 12 positions, and the morphologies and mechanical properties in the 12 positions were measured *in vivo* with B-mode ultrasound and shear wave elastography (SWE). Peak pressures under the first to fifth metatarsal heads (MH) were measured with FreeStep. Statistical analysis included 95% confidence interval, intragroup correlation coefficient ($ICC_{1,1}$), one-way analysis of variance (one-way ANOVA), and least significant difference. The results showed that thickness and Young's modulus of plantar fascia were the largest at the proximal fascia (PF) and decreased gradually from the proximal end to the distal end. Among the five distal branches (DB) of the fascia, the thickness and Young's modulus of the second and third DB were larger. The peak pressures were also higher under the second and third MH. This study found a gradient distribution in that the thickness and Young's modulus gradient decreased from the proximal end to the distal end of plantar fascia in the longitudinal arch of flexible flatfeet. In the transverse arch, the thickness and Young's modulus under the second and third DB were larger than those under the other three DB in flexible flatfoot, and the peak pressures under the second and third MH were also larger than those under the other three MH in patients with flexible flatfoot. These findings deepen our understanding of the changes of biomechanical properties and may be meaningful for the study of pathological mechanisms and therapy for flexible flatfoot.

Keywords: flexible flatfoot, plantar fascia, shear wave elastography, morphology properties, mechanical properties

INTRODUCTION

Plantar fascia is a ligament that attaches the calcaneus to metatarsals (Orchard, 2012). It plays an important role in passive force transmission (Stecco et al., 2013). Its main task is to stabilize the arch of the foot and reduce the influence of ground reaction force on metatarsal heads (MH) and the longitudinal foot arch (Hicks, 1954; Ker et al., 1987; McKeon et al., 2015). There is a close

---

Abbreviations: SWE, shear wave elastography; PF, proximal fascia; MF, middle fascia; BF, branches of fascia; DB, distal branches; ROI, region of interest; 95% CI, 95% confidence interval; ICC1,1, intragroup correlation coefficient; one-way ANOVA, one-way analysis of variance; MH, metatarsal head; COP, center of pressure.

relationship between plantar fascia and foot function, and studies have shown that when plantar fascia changes, it will produce clinical problems, for example, heel pain (Wearing et al., 2006). Thus, research on plantar fascia has a broad interest.

During the past decades, numerous studies on plantar fascia have been conducted. Guo et al. (2018) found a certain relationship between the mechanical tension of plantar fascia and fiber morphology. Chen et al. (2019a,b) found that people who used forefoot strike were more likely to suffer from plantar fasciitis. Tas and Cetin (2019a) focused on the relationship between plantar pressure distribution and the morphology and mechanical properties of plantar fascia. Welte et al. (2021) revealed the effect of plantar fascia extensibility on the windlass mechanism of plantar fascia. Wang et al. (2019) illustrated the morphology and mechanical properties of plantar fascia in normal feet. These studies strengthen the understanding of the mechanical properties of plantar fascia in normal feet. However, to the author's knowledge, the morphology and mechanical properties of the whole plantar fascia of flexible flatfeet have not been reported to date.

Flatfoot is a common foot posture abnormality, with the highest incidence of 78% (Sung, 2016), and is characterized by a low medial longitudinal arch (Pehlivan et al., 2009). Flatfoot can be divided into rigid flatfoot and flexible flatfoot. Rigid flatfoot means that the medial longitudinal arch is always missing in both load-bearing and nonload-bearing positions. Flexible flatfoot means that the medial longitudinal arch is missing only in the load-bearing position, while in the nonload-bearing position, it is the same as that of a normal foot (Carr et al., 2016). The abnormal structural changes of the flexible flatfoot under load will gradually lead to changes in the morphology and mechanical properties of the plantar fascia, which may lead to plantar fasciitis and other diseases. The changes in the morphology and mechanical properties of plantar fascia will in turn affect the foot kinematics of patients with flatfoot, resulting in clinical symptoms such as patellar tendinopathy and medial tibial stress syndrome (Kohls-Gatzoulis et al., 2004; Van der Worp et al., 2011; Hamstra-Wright et al., 2015). Studies have shown that the potential cause of plantar fasciitis is the abnormal morphology and mechanical properties of plantar fascia (Wearing et al., 2006; Wu et al., 2011).

Therefore, the objective of this study was to investigate the morphology and mechanical properties of plantar fascia of patients with flexible flatfoot by B-mode ultrasound and shear wave elastography (SWE) *in vivo*. A comprehensive analysis was conducted combined with plantar pressure measurement. The results of the study may provide a meaningful reference and basis for analysis of the pathological mechanism and rehabilitation in patients with flexible flatfoot as well as more accurate definitions for foot finite element models.

METHODS

Ethics Statement

This study was based on the principles outlined in the Helsinki Declaration, which was approved by the Ethics Committee of the Second Hospital of Jilin University (No. 2020085). All volunteers who participated in the study signed written informed consent agreements.

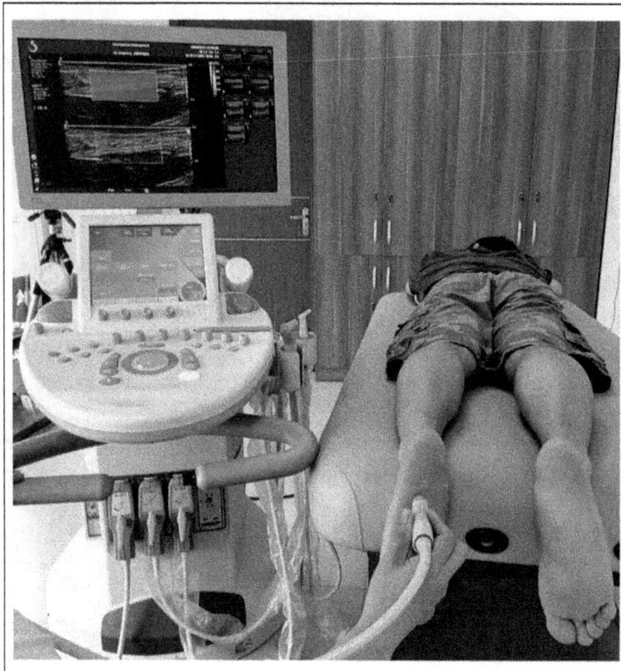

FIGURE 1 | The experimental device and the position of the subjects.

Selection of Research Subjects

The subjects of this experiment were patients with flexible flatfeet. They had the typical characteristics in that the medial longitudinal arch was missing only in the load-bearing position, while in the nonload-bearing position, it was the same as that of a normal foot (Carr et al., 2016). An intelligent scanner was employed to confirm the diagnosis and severity of flatfeet, of which the diagnostic principle was the arch index proposed by Cavanagh et al. (1987). The arch index was widely accepted and adopted (Wearing et al., 2004; Wong et al., 2012; Nirenberg et al., 2020; Wang et al., 2020). The inclusion criteria were as follows: 1) healthy male, 20–30 years old; 2) the diagnosis being flexible flatfeet; and 3) no history of other foot diseases. The exclusion criteria were as follows: 1) rigid flatfeet; 2) a history of foot trauma or surgery; 3) presence of systemic diseases that may affect plantar fascia, such as rheumatoid arthritis, diabetes, and gout; and 4) the presence of diseases that affect local plantar fascia, such as calcaneal spur or nodular fasciitis and plantar fibromatosis. Finally, 10 volunteers with 15 flexible flatfeet were included, and the basic characteristics of the volunteers were age, 26.2 ± 1.6 years; weight, 65.2 ± 2.2 kg; height, 175.2 ± 2.7 cm.

Test Device and Procedure

The subjects were asked to avoid intense sports 1 week before the test. B-mode and SWE mode of an Aixplorer ultrasonic scanner (Aixplorer ultrasonic imager, Aix-en-Provence, France) were used to measure the thickness and Young's modulus of plantar fascia, respectively. The linear transducer frequency was 10–2 MHz

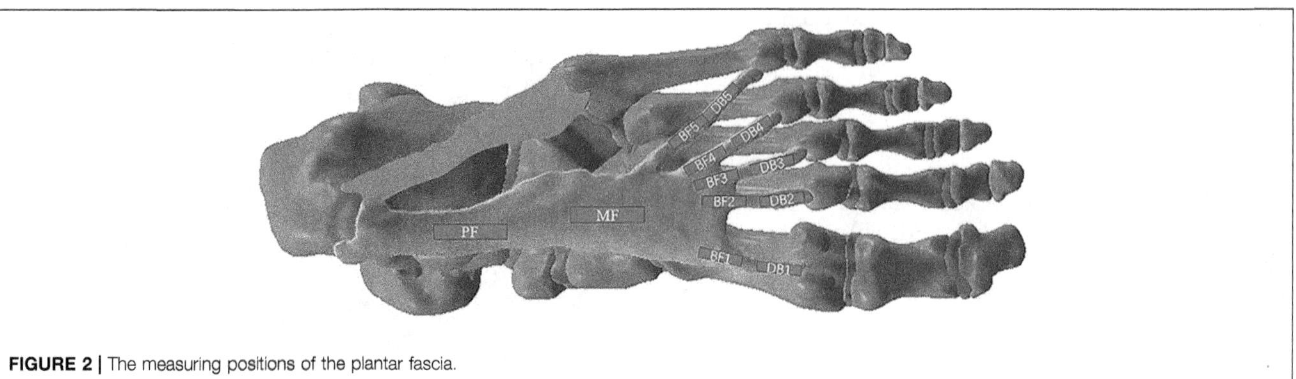

FIGURE 2 | The measuring positions of the plantar fascia.

for this study. The sampling depth was adjusted according to the positions of plantar fascia. It was set at 1.5–2.5 cm to include the whole plantar fascia, and the mechanical index was 1.0 in this study. During measurement, each subject lay prone on the examination bed, with the lower limbs straight and the feet hanging naturally (Haen et al., 2017) on the edge of the examination bed (**Figure 1**). The upper body and legs were relaxed.

In order to observe the entire changes in the plantar fascia, it was divided into four main regions: proximal fascia (PF), middle fascia (MF), five branches of fascia (BF1-BF5), and five distal branches (DB1-DB5), 12 positions in total (**Figure 2**). The PF was measured at a point 1 cm away from the insertion to the calcaneus. The location of the five DBs was defined as the farthest end where the plantar fascia has not been fused with joint capsule. The ultrasonic transducer was parallel to the plantar fascia, and the thickness of plantar fascia was measured in the middle of every position. Subsequently, the elastic measurement via SWE was performed. The width of the square-shaped elastography window (region of interest, ROI) was as large as possible, and the height was set to include the complete plantar fascia. Q-Box^{TM}Trace was used to measure Young's modulus (maximum, minimum, and average, in kPa) of plantar fascia with a length of 1 cm at each position, and Young's modulus scale was adjusted to 0–600 kPa (Wang et al., 2019). Additionally, the mean Young's modulus value was used for the data analysis in the study. At each position, Young's modulus and thickness of plantar fascia were measured three times.

Plantar Pressure Measurement

FreeStep (Sensor Medica, Italy) was employed to detect the plantar pressure of the subjects during level walking. Subjects were requested to walk normally, without rushing, acceleration, or deceleration. Data were collected barefoot at a self-selected speed (Rao et al., 2011; Hillstrom et al., 2013) along a 2 m walkway, and the walking velocity was 1.33 ± 0.97 m/s. The peak pressures under the first to fifth MH were measured during the push-off stage.

Statistical Analysis

IBM Statistical Package for the Social Sciences (SPSS) statistical software version 26.0 (SPSS Inc., Chicago, IL, United States) was used to analyze all the data. The 95% confidence interval (95% CI) and intragroup correlation coefficient ($ICC_{1,1}$) were used to measure and evaluate the reliability of plantar fascia thickness and Young's modulus. Generally, the values of $ICC_{1,1}$ in the ranges of 0–0.40, 0.41–0.6, 0.61–0.79, and 0.8–1.0, respectively, indicate poor, medium, good, and excellent reliability. At the same time, the one-way analysis of variance (one-way ANOVA) was used to compare the differences between different positions of plantar fascia. If the result of one-way ANOVA was $p < 0.05$, least significant difference was used to compare the differences between every two positions of plantar fascia. For least significant difference, P values we used had been corrected by the number of pairwise comparisons. Statistical difference was defined as $p < 0.05$. In order to better understand the spatial distribution in thickness and Young's modulus of plantar fascia, an exponential function (first-order exponential decay) was used to fit and analyze the variation trend of plantar fascia from the calcaneal to the five DB.

TABLE 1 | Intragroup correlation results of thickness and Young's modulus in 15 flexible flatfeet.

Foot identity	Thickness		Young's modulus	
	$ICC_{1,1}$ 95%CI	95%CI	$ICC_{1,1}$	95%CI
#1	0.994	(0.984, 0.998)	0.999	(0.998,1.000)
#2	0.991	(0.977, 0.997)	0.995	(0.987,0.999)
#3	0.994	(0.985, 0.998)	0.996	(0.989,0.999)
#4	0.987	(0.964, 0.996)	0.999	(0.996,1.000)
#5	0.981	(0.950, 0.994)	0.998	(0.994,0.999)
#6	0.986	(0.963, 0.996)	0.997	(0.991, 0.999)
#7	0.977	(0.938, 0.993)	0.996	(0.989,0.999)
#8	0.995	(0.986, 0.998)	0.988	(0.968,0.996)
#9	0.988	(0.969, 0.996)	0.992	(0.979,0.998)
#10	0.979	(0.944, 0.993)	0.996	(0.990, 0.999)
#11	0.979	(0.945, 0.993)	0.995	(0.987, 0.999)
#12	0.976	(0.938, 0.993)	0.996	(0.989, 0.999)
#13	0.981	(0.950, 0.994)	0.985	(0.961, 0.995)
#14	0.981	(0.951, 0.994)	0.993	(0.980, 0.998)
#15	0.988	(0.969, 0.996)	0.999	(0.996,1.000)

RESULTS

Intragroup Correlation Results of Thickness and Young's Modulus

The intragroup correlation results of the thickness and Young's modulus of the 15 flatfeet are listed in **Table 1**. The $ICC_{1,1}$ ranged

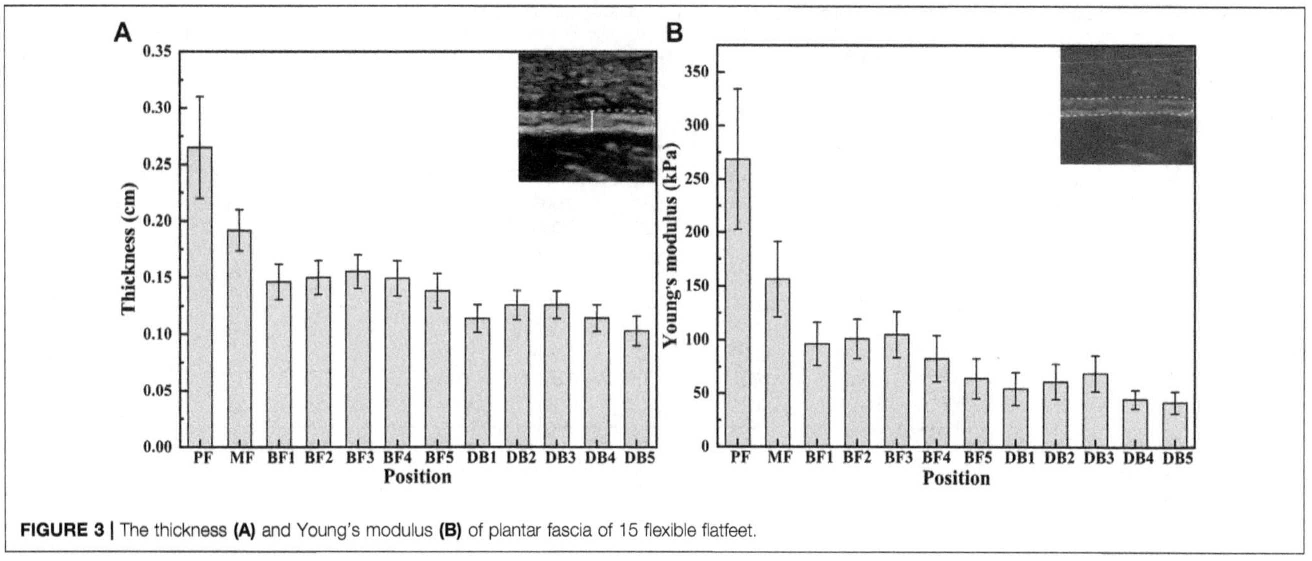

FIGURE 3 | The thickness **(A)** and Young's modulus **(B)** of plantar fascia of 15 flexible flatfeet.

from 0.976 to 0.995 and the corresponding 95% CI was 0.938, 0.998 for thickness of plantar fascia. The $ICC_{1,1}$ ranged from 0.985 to 0.999 and the 95% CI was 0.961, 1.000 for Young's modulus of plantar fascia.

Distribution Pattern of Thickness and Young's Modulus of Plantar Fascia

The results of thickness and Young's modulus of plantar fascia of 15 flexible flatfeet are shown in **Figure 3**. The results showed that both the thickness and Young's modulus of plantar fascia decreased gradually from the proximal end to the distal end. Among the five DB, the thickness and Young's modulus of the second and third branches were larger than the other three.

The one-way ANOVA was used to compare the differences between different positions of plantar fascia. If the result of one-way ANOVA was $p < 0.05$, least significant difference was used to compare the differences between every two positions of plantar fascia. The one-way ANOVA results showed that the differences in thickness and Young's modulus between different positions were statistically significant ($p < 0.05$). Least significant difference results showed that, in terms of plantar fascia thickness, PF > MF > all the five BFs > all the five DBs. Among the five DBs, DB2 and DB3 > DB1 and DB4 > DB5. The differences were statistically significant ($p < 0.05$). There was no statistical difference between DB2 and DB3, and there was also no statistical difference between DB1 and DB4 (**Table 2**). For Young's modulus, PF > MF > all the five BF > the corresponding position of DB. Among the five DBs, DB2 > DB4 and DB5; DB3 > DB1 and DB4 and DB5; DB1 > DB5. All the differences were statistically significant ($p < 0.05$). There was no statistical difference between DB2 and DB3, and no statistical difference was found between DB2 and DB1. There was also no statistical difference between DB4 and DB5 (**Table 3**).

Peak Pressure Distribution Under Five MHs

The peak pressure under five MHs of 15 flexible flatfeet is shown in **Figure 4**. The pressures under the second and third MH were higher than those under the other three MH, and the differences were statistically significant ($p < 0.05$) (**Table 4**). This distribution pattern is similar to the thickness and Young's modulus in the five DBs.

Spatial Distribution of Plantar Fascia Thickness and Young's Modulus

In order to better understand the spatial distribution in thickness and Young's modulus of plantar fascia, an exponential function (first-order exponential decay) was used to fit and analyze the variation trend of plantar fascia from the calcaneal to the five DB.

The spatial distribution of plantar fascia thickness and Young's modulus of foot #1 is shown in **Figure 5**. The results showed that the thickness and Young's modulus of plantar fascia were the largest at the calcaneus tubercle, and the thickness and Young's modulus of five fascial bundles gradually decreased as plantar fascia extended from the calcaneus to the five toes. The spatial distribution of thickness and Young's modulus in the other 14 flexible flatfeet also showed a similar tendency. The thickness and Young's modulus of plantar fascia of 15 flatfeet at PF and five DBs are shown in **Figure 6**.

DISCUSSION

This study investigated the morphology and mechanical properties of plantar fascia of patients with flexible flatfoot by B-mode ultrasound and ultrasonic elastography *in vivo*. A comprehensive analysis was conducted combined with plantar pressure measurements.

In order to evaluate the accuracy of the data, the repeatability of the thickness and Young's modulus data was analyzed in all 15 flexible flatfeet. The results showed that all the values of $ICC_{1,1}$ were more than 0.9, which indicated that the data of the study had good reliability. At the same time, a previous study reported that B-mode ultrasound was a reliable and reproducible method for detecting the thickness of plantar fascia and SWE mode was a reliable and reproducible method for detecting the elasticity of plantar fascia (Wang et al., 2019).

TABLE 2 | *P* value of least significant difference results between different positions in thickness of plantar fascia.

Position/ Thickness (mm)	MF	BF1	BF2	BF3	BF4	BF5	DB1	DB2	DB3	DB4	DB5
PF (0.265 ± 0.045)	0.000[a]	0.000[a]	0.000[a]	0.000[a]	0.000[a]	0.000[a]	0.000[a]	0.000[a]	0.000[a]	0.000[a]	0.000[a]
MF (0.192 ± 0.018)	–	0.000[a]	0.000[a]	0.000[a]	0.000[a]	0.000[a]	0.000[a]	0.000[a]	0.000[a]	0.000[a]	0.000[a]
BF1 (0.146 ± 0.016)	0.000[a]	–	0.33	0.024[a]	0.452	0.048[a]	0.000[a]	0.000[a]	0.000[a]	0.000[a]	0.000[a]
BF2 (0.150 ± 0.015)	0.000[a]	0.33	–	0.2	0.824	0.003[a]	0.000[a]	0.000[a]	0.000[a]	0.000[a]	0.000[a]
BF3 (0.155 ± 0.015)	0.000[a]	0.024[a]	0.2	–	0.133	0.000[a]	0.000[a]	0.000[a]	0.000[a]	0.000[a]	0.000[a]
BF4 (0.149 ± 0.015)	0.000[a]	0.452	0.824	0.133	–	0.006[a]	0.000[a]	0.000[a]	0.000[a]	0.000[a]	0.000[a]
BF5 (0.138 ± 0.015)	0.000[a]	0.048[a]	0.003[a]	0.000[a]	0.006[a]	–	0.000[a]	0.002[a]	0.003[a]	0.000[a]	0.000[a]
DB1 (0.114 ± 0.012)	0.000[a]	0.000[a]	0.000[a]	0.000[a]	0.000[a]	0.000[a]	–	0.003[a]	0.003[a]	0.942	0.000[a]
DB2 (0.126 ± 0.013)	0.000[a]	0.000[a]	0.000[a]	0.000[a]	0.000[a]	0.002[a]	0.003[a]	–	0.96	0.004[a]	0.000[a]
DB3 (0.126 ± 0.012)	0.000[a]	0.000[a]	0.000[a]	0.000[a]	0.000[a]	0.003[a]	0.003[a]	0.96	–	0.003[a]	0.000[a]
DB4 (0.114 ± 0.012)	0.000[a]	0.000[a]	0.000[a]	0.000[a]	0.000[a]	0.000[a]	0.942	0.004[a]	0.003[a]	–	0.004[a]
DB5 (0.103 ± 0.013)	0.000[a]	0.000[a]	0.000[a]	0.000[a]	0.000[a]	0.000[a]	0.006[a]	0.000[a]	0.000[a]	0.004[a]	–

[a]Difference was statistically significant.
P values have been corrected (multiplied by k); k represents the number of pairwise comparisons. There were 12 positions; thus, k = 66.
"/" = the same position.

TABLE 3 | *P* value of least significant difference results between different positions in Young's modulus of plantar fascia.

Position/ Young's modulus (KPa)	MF	BF1	BF2	BF3	BF4	BF5	DB1	DB2	DB3	DB4	DB5
PF (268.662 ± 65.970)	0.000[a]	0.000[a]	0.000[a]	0.000[a]	0.000[a]	0.000[a]	0.000[a]	0.000[a]	0.000[a]	0.000[a]	0.000[a]
MF (156.407 ± 35.046)	–	0.000[a]	0.000[a]	0.000[a]	0.000[a]	0.000[a]	0.000[a]	0.000[a]	0.000[a]	0.000[a]	0.000[a]
BF1 (96.302 ± 20.356)	0.000[a]	–	0.399	0.126	0.015[a]	0.000[a]	0.000[a]	0.000[a]	0.000[a]	0.000[a]	0.000[a]
BF2 (101.060 ± 18.322)	0.000[a]	0.399	–	0.492	0.001[a]	0.000[a]	0.000[a]	0.000[a]	0.000[a]	0.000[a]	0.000[a]
BF3 (104.938 ± 21.512)	0.000[a]	0.126	0.492	–	0.000[a]	0.000[a]	0.000[a]	0.000[a]	0.000[a]	0.000[a]	0.000[a]
BF4 (82.553 ± 21.637)	0.000[a]	0.015[a]	0.001[a]	0.000[a]	–	0.001[a]	0.000[a]	0.000[a]	0.013[a]	0.000[a]	0.000[a]
BF5 (63.860 ± 18.791)	0.000[a]	0.000[a]	0.000[a]	0.000[a]	0.001[a]	–	0.09	0.613	0.404	0.001[a]	0.000[a]
DB1 (54.271 ± 15.303)	0.000[a]	0.000[a]	0.000[a]	0.000[a]	0.000[a]	0.09	–	0.233	0.011[a]	0.084	0.024[a]
DB2 (61.004 ± 16.479)	0.000[a]	0.000[a]	0.000[a]	0.000[a]	0.000[a]	0.613	0.233	–	0.18	0.004[a]	0.001[a]
DB3 (68.567 ± 16.750)	0.000[a]	0.000[a]	0.000[a]	0.000[a]	0.13	0.404	0.011[a]	0.18	–	0.000[a]	0.000[a]
DB4 (44.500 ± 8.578)	0.000[a]	0.000[a]	0.000[a]	0.000[a]	0.000[a]	0.001[a]	0.084	0.004[a]	0.000[a]	–	0.598
DB5 (41.524 ± 10.270)	0.000[a]	0.000[a]	0.000[a]	0.000[a]	0.000[a]	0.000[a]	0.024[a]	0.001[a]	0.000[a]	0.598	–

[a]Difference was statistically significant.
P values have been corrected (multiplied by k); k represents the number of pairwise comparisons. There were 12 positions; thus, k = 66.
"/" = the same position.

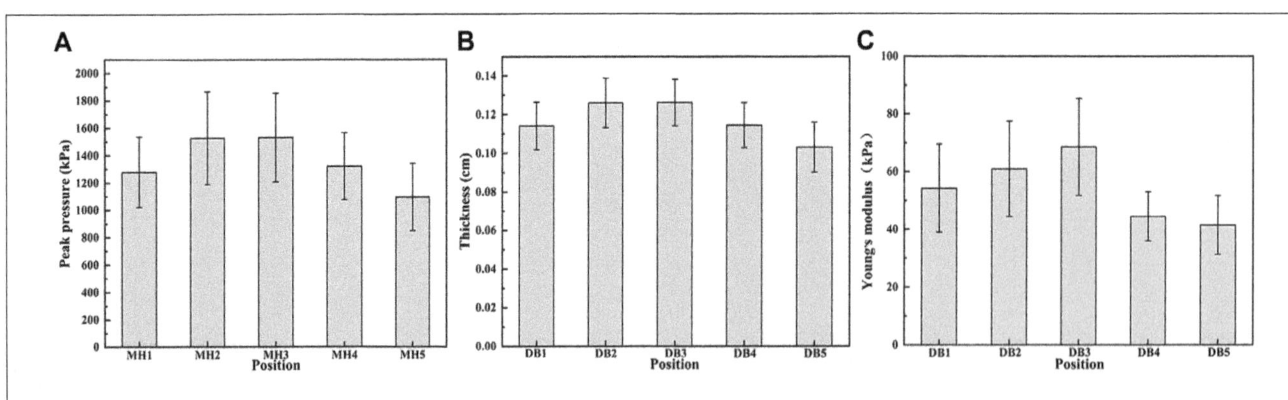

FIGURE 4 | The peak pressure under the five metatarsal heads (MH1–MH5) **(A)**, the thickness **(B)**, and Young's modulus **(C)** in the five distal branches of the plantar fascia in 15 flatfeet.

Plantar fasciitis is one of the most common foot musculoskeletal diseases in primary diagnosis and treatment institutions (Thing et al., 2012; Young, 2012), and it is more likely to occur in patients with flatfoot than with normal foot (Riddle et al., 2003). It is characterized by heel pain after rest because it mainly affects the plantar fascia inserted into the

TABLE 4 | *P* value of least significant difference results between different positions in peak pressure.

Position	MH1	MH2	MH3	MH4	MH5
MH1 (1278.400 ± 258.050)	—	0.000[a]	0.000[a]	0.411	0.000[a]
MH2 (1526.400 ± 338.292)	0.000[a]	—	0.927	0.411	0.000[a]
MH3 (1531.200 ± 323.522)	0.000[a]	0.927	—	0.000[a]	0.000[a]
MH4 (1321.200 ± 243.951)	0.411	0.000[a]	0.000[a]	—	0.000[a]
MH5 (1094.800 ± 246.413)	0.000[a]	0.000[a]	0.000[a]	0.000[a]	—

[a]*Difference was statistically significant.*
P values have been corrected (multiplied by k); k represents the number of pairwise comparisons. There were five positions; thus, k = 10.
"/" = the same position.

calcaneus (Huang et al., 2000). The pain can also extend along the length of the plantar fascia (Thomas et al., 2016; Babatunde et al., 2019). In this study, the maximum Young's modulus of proximal plantar fascia was 387.1kPa, while that of a normal foot was about 300kPa (Wang et al., 2019). Studies showed that there was a positive correlation between Young's modulus and tendon force (Yeh et al., 2013; Yeh et al., 2016). Thus, the increased Young's modulus of the proximal plantar fascia indicates that the plantar fascia bears greater stress, leading more easily to the degeneration of plantar fascia (Huffer et al., 2017). The increase of Young's modulus in plantar fascia near calcaneus attachment in patients with flatfoot may provide a theoretical explanation for the high incidence of plantar fasciitis in patients with flatfoot.

The results of the study showed that the plantar fascia of the flexible flatfoot was spatially dependent from proximal to distal, and the thickness and Young's modulus of the five branches decreased gradually from proximal to distal. The differences between different parts were statistically significant. This feature of gradient changes is consistent with the results in normal plantar fascia (Wang et al., 2019). In the finite element model, the plantar fascia is often regarded as a linear elastic material, and the whole plantar fascia has the same Young's modulus (Phan et al., 2021). Thus, the spatial distribution feature (different Young's modulus in different regions) obtained in this study is helpful to define more accurate material properties for flatfeet finite element models to achieve more meaningful simulation results.

However, among the DB, Wang et al. (2019) showed that the thickness and Young's modulus between the five branches of the normal plantar fascia were the greatest under the first MH, while this study showed that the thickness and Young's modulus under the second and third MH were greater in patients with flexible flatfoot. At the same time, this study showed that the peak pressures under the second and third MH were greater than that under the fourth and fifth MH, which was consistent with the results of Buldt et al. (2018) and Hillstrom et al. (2013). It is speculated that this result may be due to the difference in the degree of collapse of the medial and lateral longitudinal arches in patients with flexible flatfoot. These results indicate that, in patients with flexible flatfoot, the degree of collapse of the medial longitudinal arch is more than that of the lateral arch, resulting in higher force and higher pressure on the medial side in the push-off phase. The stronger pressure stimulates plantar fascia, leading to its degeneration (Wearing et al., 2006). Shiotani et al. (2019) also noted that plantar fascia is mechanically stretched, so the morphology and mechanical properties of plantar fascia may be adapted to stress accumulation.

The center of pressure (COP) is defined as the centroid of the pressure distribution at a series of moments in time as the ground reaction is applied over the plantar surface of the foot (Cho and Choi, 2005). It was found that the peak pressures under the

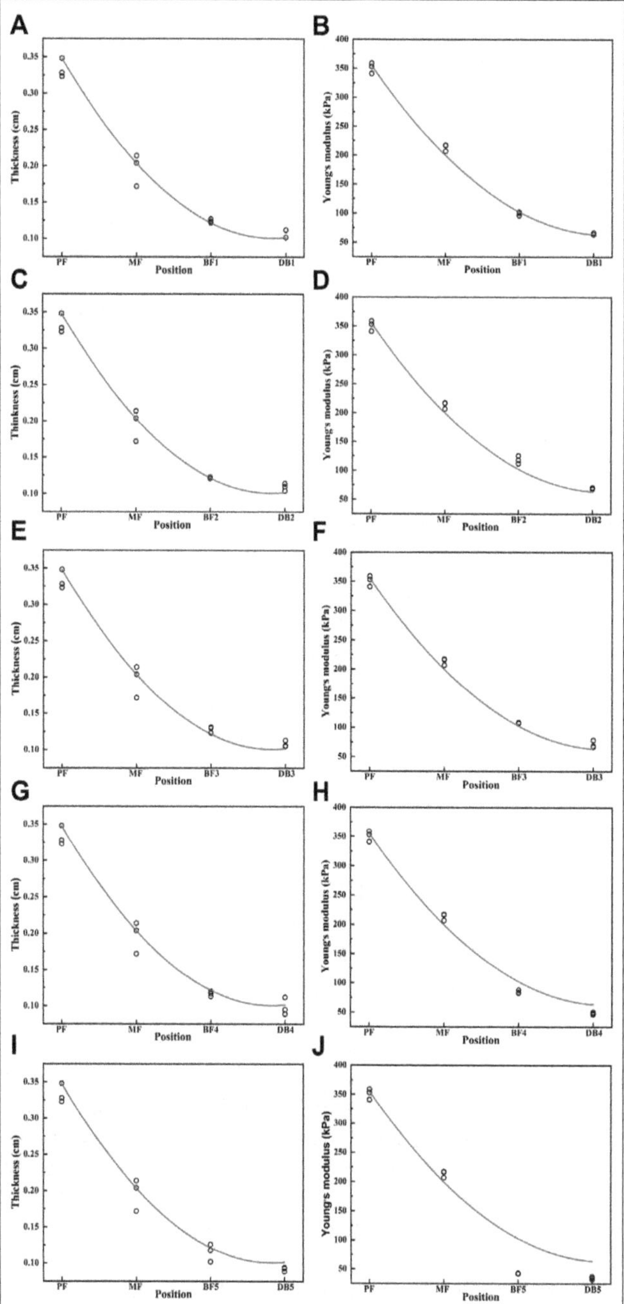

FIGURE 5 | The curve of the thickness and Young's modulus of the plantar fascia from the calcaneus to the five distal branches in foot #1: **(A)** thickness of the first branch, **(B)** Young's modulus of the first branch, **(C)** thickness of the second branch, **(D)** Young's modulus of the second branch, **(E)** thickness of the third branch, **(F)** Young's modulus of the third branch, **(G)** thickness of the forth branch, **(H)** Young's modulus of the forth branch, **(I)** thickness of the fifth branch, and **(J)** Young's modulus of the fifth branch.

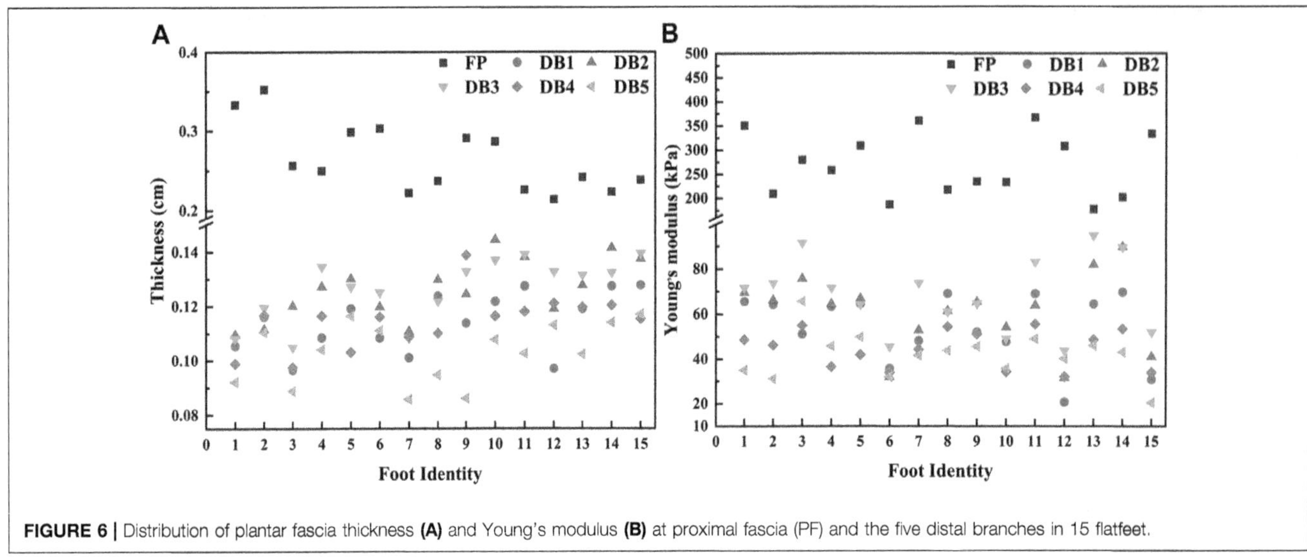

FIGURE 6 | Distribution of plantar fascia thickness **(A)** and Young's modulus **(B)** at proximal fascia (PF) and the five distal branches in 15 flatfeet.

second and third metatarsals were higher than those under the other metatarsals. Thus, the COP would move laterally from the first MH. These results were the same as those of Han et al. (2011). They found that, in the normal foot, the trajectory of the COP moved from the lateral heel, moved medially in forefoot, and then ended at the big toe. In flatfeet, the COP moved straight from the heel to the toe without medial shifting in the forefoot. There was a tendency for the COP in flatfoot to shift laterally in the forefoot than the COP in normal foot. These results also confirm our inference; that is, the medial longitudinal arch collapses more than the lateral arch in flatfoot, which leads to the higher force and higher pressure under the second and third metatarsals and the COP moving outward.

Morphologic and mechanical properties of the plantar fascia may be important factors affecting the plantar pressure distribution because the primary task of the plantar fascia is to stabilize the foot arches (McKeon et al., 2015). Studies (Tas and Cetin, 2019a) also show that there is a significant positive correlation between plantar pressure distribution and the thickness of plantar fascia. Higher plantar pressure may lead to plantar fascia hypertrophy. Foot orthoses could modify tissue loading by altering kinematics, kinetics, muscle activity, and sensory feedback (Mills et al., 2010), and they have been demonstrated to have a good therapeutic effect in plantar fasciitis (Buchbinder, 2004). The changes in morphology and mechanical properties of plantar fascia and peak pressure of the forefoot in patients with flexible flatfoot found in our study may provide the basis for the development of new foot orthoses for flexible flatfoot.

There were limitations in this study. Firstly, the sample size was limited to 15 cases, and there was no grading according to mild, moderate, and severe flexible flatfeet. However, the results showed that although the sample size is small and there may be some differences in disease degree among participants, the spatial distribution characteristics of thickness and Young's modulus of plantar fascia in all 15 flexible flat feet were similar, which indicated that the spatial distribution characteristics are less affected by the disease severity, and the research results may have broad representative significance. Secondly, this study did not include the control group, but our group has previously conducted and published one study on the morphology and mechanical properties of plantar fascia in normal feet (Wang et al., 2019). In addition, the age, height, and body weight of the volunteers who participated in this study are similar to those in our previous published work. Therefore, we cited and employed the published data (normal foot data) as the healthy control group in this study (Wang et al., 2019). Thirdly, though SWE has been used to evaluate the material properties of plantar fascia (Shiotani et al., 2019; Tas and Cetin, 2019b), studies have shown that the shear wave velocity of layered tissue is affected by its thickness and surrounding tissue properties (Helfenstein-Didier et al., 2016; Martin et al., 2018, 2019; Sadeghi and Cortes, 2020); especially when the thickness of the relevant tissue is equal to or less than the wavelength, SWE is no longer applicable (Li et al., 2018). The thickness of plantar fascia measured in this study is millimeter, which is far greater than the wavelength. In addition, the results of Helfenstein-Didier et al. (2016) in measuring the human Achilles tendon show that there is a high correlation between the shear modulus measured by SWE and the new guided wave technology-phase velocity mode, even considering the influence of thickness. Therefore, although the results of the differences between different positions in plantar fascia as well as between patients with flexible flat feet and healthy volunteers in this study may not be affected, it is necessary to explore the influence of thickness on the properties of plantar fascia materials by using guided wave technology in the future.

CONCLUSION

This study found a gradient distribution in that the thickness and Young's modulus gradient decreased from the proximal end to the distal end of plantar fascia in the longitudinal arch of flexible flatfeet. In the transverse arch, the thickness and Young's modulus under the second and third DB were larger than those under the other three DB in flexible flatfoot, and the peak pressures under the second and third MH were also larger than those under the other three MH in patients with flexible flatfoot. These findings deepen our understanding of the changes of biomechanical properties and may be meaningful for the study of pathological mechanisms and therapy for flexible flatfoot.

AUTHOR CONTRIBUTIONS

ZQ and ZJ were responsible for the experiments and manuscript preparation. JW, FC, and LR participated in discussions and revisions. JL and LR worked as supervisors for all procedures.

FUNDING

This research was supported by the project of National Natural Science Foundation of China (No. 52175270), the Key Project of the National Natural Science Foundation of China (No. 91848204), National Natural Science Foundation of China (No. 52005209), the Interdisciplinary Research Funding Program for Doctoral Students of Jilin University (No. 101832020DJX049), and China Postdoctoral Science Foundation (No. 2021T140260 and No. 2021M691206).

ACKNOWLEDGMENTS

The authors would like to thank all the volunteers who contributed to this study.

REFERENCES

Babatunde, O. O., Legha, A., Littlewood, C., Chesterton, L. S., Thomas, M. J., Menz, H. B., et al. (2019). Comparative Effectiveness of Treatment Options for Plantar Heel Pain: a Systematic Review with Network Meta-Analysis. *Br. J. Sports Med.* 53, 182–194. doi:10.1136/bjsports-2017-098998

Buchbinder, R. (2004). Plantar Fasciitis. *N. Engl. J. Med.* 350, 2159–2166. doi:10.1056/NEJMcp032745

Buldt, A. K., Forghany, S., Landorf, K. B., Levinger, P., Murley, G. S., and Menz, H. B. (2018). Foot Posture Is Associated with Plantar Pressure during Gait: A Comparison of normal, Planus and Cavus Feet. *Gait & Posture* 62, 235–240. doi:10.1016/j.gaitpost.2018.03.005

Carr, J. B., 2nd, Yang, S., and Lather, L. A. (2016). Pediatric Pes Planus: A State-Of-The-Art Review. *Pediatrics* 137, e20151230. doi:10.1542/peds.2015-1230

Cavanagh, P. R., Rodgers, M. M., and Iiboshi, A. (1987). Pressure Distribution under Symptom-free Feet during Barefoot Standing. *Foot & Ankle* 7, 262–278. doi:10.1177/107110078700700502

Chen, T. L.-W., Agresta, C. E., Lipps, D. B., Provenzano, S. G., Hafer, J. F., Wong, D. W.-C., et al. (2019a). Ultrasound Elastographic Assessment of Plantar Fascia in Runners Using Rearfoot Strike and Forefoot Strike. *J. Biomech.* 89, 65–71. doi:10.1016/j.jbiomech.2019.04.013

Chen, T. L.-W., Wong, D. W.-C., Wang, Y., Lin, J., and Zhang, M. (2019b). Foot Arch Deformation and Plantar Fascia Loading during Running with Rearfoot Strike and Forefoot Strike: A Dynamic Finite Element Analysis. *J. Biomech.* 83, 260–272. doi:10.1016/j.jbiomech.2018.12.007

Cho, W. H., and Choi, H. (2005). Center of Pressure (COP) during the Postural Balance Control of High-Heeled Woman. *Conf. Proc. IEEE Eng. Med. Biol. Soc.* 2005, 2761–2764. doi:10.1109/IEMBS.2005.1617044

Guo, J., Liu, X., Ding, X., Wang, L., and Fan, Y. (2018). Biomechanical and Mechanical Behavior of the Plantar Fascia in Macro and Micro Structures. *J. Biomech.* 76, 160–166. doi:10.1016/j.jbiomech.2018.05.032

Haen, T. X., Roux, A., Soubeyrand, M., and Laporte, S. (2017). Shear Waves Elastography for Assessment of Human Achilles Tendon's Biomechanical Properties: an Experimental Study. *J. Mech. Behav. Biomed. Mater.* 69, 178–184. doi:10.1016/j.jmbbm.2017.01.007

Hamstra-Wright, K. L., Bliven, K. C. H., and Bay, C. (2015). Risk Factors for Medial Tibial Stress Syndrome in Physically Active Individuals Such as Runners and Military Personnel: a Systematic Review and Meta-Analysis. *Br. J. Sports Med.* 49, 362–369. doi:10.1136/bjsports-2014-093462

Han, J. T., Koo, H. M., Jung, J. M., Kim, Y. J., and Lee, J. H. (2011). Differences in Plantar Foot Pressure and COP between Flat and Normal Feet during Walking. *J. Phys. Ther. Sci.* 23, 683–685. doi:10.1589/jpts.23.683

Helfenstein-Didier, C., Andrade, R. J., Brum, J., Hug, F., Tanter, M., Nordez, A., et al. (2016). In Vivoquantification of the Shear Modulus of the Human Achilles Tendon during Passive Loading Using Shear Wave Dispersion Analysis. *Phys. Med. Biol.* 61, 2485–2496. doi:10.1088/0031-9155/61/6/2485

Hicks, J. H. (1954). The Mechanics of the Foot. II. The Plantar Aponeurosis and the Arch. *J. Anat.* 88, 25–30.

Hillstrom, H. J., Song, J., Kraszewski, A. P., Hafer, J. F., Mootanah, R., Dufour, A. B., et al. (2013). Foot Type Biomechanics Part 1: Structure and Function of the Asymptomatic Foot. *Gait & Posture* 37, 445–451. doi:10.1016/j.gaitpost.2012.09.007

Huang, H. H., Qureshi, A. A., and Biundo, J. J., Jr. (2000). Sports and Other Soft Tissue Injuries, Tendinitis, Bursitis, and Occupation-Related Syndromes. *Curr. Opin. Rheumatol.* 12, 150–154. doi:10.1097/00002281-200003000-00009

Huffer, D., Hing, W., Newton, R., and Clair, M. (2017). Strength Training for Plantar Fasciitis and the Intrinsic Foot Musculature: A Systematic Review. *Phys. Ther. Sport* 24, 44–52. doi:10.1016/j.ptsp.2016.08.008

Ker, R. F., Bennett, M. B., Bibby, S. R., Kester, R. C., and Alexander, R. M. (1987). The spring in the Arch of the Human Foot. *Nature* 325, 147–149. doi:10.1038/325147a0

Kohls-Gatzoulis, J., Angel, J. C., Singh, D., Haddad, F., Livingstone, J., and Berry, G. (2004). Tibialis Posterior Dysfunction: a Common and Treatable Cause of Adult Acquired Flatfoot. *BMJ* 329, 1328–1333. doi:10.1136/bmj.329.7478.1328

Martin, J. A., Brandon, S. C. E., Keuler, E. M., Hermus, J. R., Ehlers, A. C., Segalman, D. J., et al. (2018). Gauging Force by Tapping Tendons. *Nat. Commun.* 9, 1592. doi:10.1038/s41467-018-03797-6

Martin, J. A., Schmitz, D. G., Ehlers, A. C., Allen, M. S., and Thelen, D. G. (2019). Calibration of the Shear Wave Speed-Stress Relationship in *Ex Vivo* Tendons. *J. Biomech.* 90, 9–15. doi:10.1016/j.jbiomech.2019.04.015

Mckeon, P. O., Hertel, J., Bramble, D., and Davis, I. (2015). The Foot Core System: a New Paradigm for Understanding Intrinsic Foot Muscle Function. *Br. J. Sports Med.* 49, 290. doi:10.1136/bjsports-2013-092690

Mills, K., Blanch, P., Chapman, A. R., Mcpoil, T. G., and Vicenzino, B. (2010). Foot Orthoses and Gait: a Systematic Review and Meta-Analysis of Literature

Pertaining to Potential Mechanisms. *Br. J. Sports Med.* 44, 1035–1046. doi:10.1136/bjsm.2009.066977

Nirenberg, M., Ansert, E., Campbell, J., and Curran, M. (2020). Forensic Implications of Foot Arch index Comparison between Dynamic Bare Footprints and Shoe Insole Foot Impressions. *Sci. Justice* 60, 375–380. doi:10.1016/j.scijus.2020.03.001

Orchard, J. (2012). Plantar Fasciitis. *BMJ* 345: e6603. doi:10.1136/bmj.e6603

Pehlivan, O., Cilli, F., Mahirogullari, M., Karabudak, O., and Koksal, O. (2009). Radiographic Correlation of Symptomatic and Asymptomatic Flexible Flatfoot in Young Male Adults. *Int. Orthopaedics (Sicot)* 33, 447–450. doi:10.1007/s00264-007-0508-5

Phan, P. K., Vo, A. T. N., Bakhtiarydavijani, A., Burch, R., Smith, B., Ball, J. E., et al. (2021). In Silico Finite Element Analysis of the Foot Ankle Complex Biomechanics: A Literature Review. *J. Biomech. Eng.* 143. doi:10.1115/1.4050667

Rao, S., Song, J., Kraszewski, A., Backus, S., Ellis, S. J., Md, J. T. D., et al. (2011). The Effect of Foot Structure on 1st Metatarsophalangeal Joint Flexibility and Hallucal Loading. *Gait & Posture* 34, 131–137. doi:10.1016/j.gaitpost.2011.02.028

Riddle, D. L., Pulisic, M., Pidcoe, P., and Johnson, R. E. (2003). Risk Factors for Plantar Fasciitis. *The J. Bone Jt. Surgery-American Volume* 85, 872–877. doi:10.2106/00004623-200305000-00015

Sadeghi, S., and Cortes, D. H. (2020). Measurement of the Shear Modulus in Thin-Layered Tissues Using Numerical Simulations and Shear Wave Elastography. *J. Mech. Behav. Biomed. Mater.* 102, 103502. doi:10.1016/j.jmbbm.2019.103502

Shiotani, H., Yamashita, R., Mizokuchi, T., Naito, M., and Kawakami, Y. (2019). Site- and Sex-Differences in Morphological and Mechanical Properties of the Plantar Fascia: A Supersonic Shear Imaging Study. *J. Biomech.* 85, 198–203. doi:10.1016/j.jbiomech.2019.01.014

Stecco, C., Corradin, M., Macchi, V., Morra, A., Porzionato, A., Biz, C., et al. (2013). Plantar Fascia Anatomy and its Relationship with Achilles Tendon and Paratenon. *J. Anat.* 223, 665–676. doi:10.1111/joa.12111

Sung, P. S. (2016). The Ground Reaction Force Thresholds for Detecting Postural Stability in Participants with and without Flat Foot. *J. Biomech.* 49, 60–65. doi:10.1016/j.jbiomech.2015.11.004

Tas, S., and Cetin, A. (2019a). An Investigation of the Relationship between Plantar Pressure Distribution and the Morphologic and Mechanic Properties of the Intrinsic Foot Muscles and Plantar Fascia. *Gait Posture* 72, 217–221. doi:10.1016/j.jbiomech.2015.11.004

Taş, S., and Çetin, A. (2019b). Mechanical Properties and Morphologic Features of Intrinsic Foot Muscles and Plantar Fascia in Individuals with Hallux Valgus. *Acta Orthopaedica et Traumatologica Turcica* 53, 282–286. doi:10.1016/j.aott.2019.03.009

Thing, J., Maruthappu, M., and Rogers, J. (2012). Diagnosis and Management of Plantar Fasciitis in Primary Care. *Br. J. Gen. Pract.* 62, 443–444. doi:10.3399/bjgp12X653769

Thomas, M. J., Menz, H. B., and Mallen, C. D. (2016). Plantar Heel Pain. *BMJ* 353, i2175. doi:10.1136/bmj.i2175

Van Der Worp, H., Van Ark, M., Roerink, S., Pepping, G.-J., Van Den Akker-Scheek, I., and Zwerver, J. (2011). Risk Factors for Patellar Tendinopathy: a Systematic Review of the Literature. *Br. J. Sports Med.* 45, 446–452. doi:10.1136/bjsm.2011.084079

Wang, K., Liu, J., Wu, J., Qian, Z., Ren, L., and Ren, L. (2019). Noninvasive *In Vivo* Study of the Morphology and Mechanical Properties of Plantar Fascia Based on Ultrasound. *Ieee Access* 7, 53641–53649. doi:10.1109/Access.2019.2909409

Wang, Y.-T., Chen, J.-C., and Lin, Y.-S. (2020). Effects of Artificial Texture Insoles and Foot Arches on Improving Arch Collapse in Flat Feet. *Sensors* 20, 3667. doi:10.3390/s20133667

Wearing, S. C., Hills, A. P., Byrne, N. M., Hennig, E. M., and Mcdonald, M. (2004). The Arch index: a Measure of Flat or Fat Feet? *Foot Ankle Int.* 25, 575–581. doi:10.1177/107110070402500811

Wearing, S. C., Smeathers, J. E., Urry, S. R., Hennig, E. M., and Hills, A. P. (2006). The Pathomechanics of Plantar Fasciitis. *Sports Med.* 36, 585–611. doi:10.2165/00007256-200636070-00004

Welte, L., Kelly, L. A., Kessler, S. E., Lieberman, D. E., D'andrea, S. E., Lichtwark, G. A., et al. (2021). The Extensibility of the Plantar Fascia Influences the Windlass Mechanism during Human Running. *Proc. R. Soc. B.* 288, 20202095. doi:10.1098/rspb.2020.2095

Wong, C. K., Weil, R., and De Boer, E. (2012). Standardizing Foot-type Classification Using Arch index Values. *Physiother. Can.* 64, 280–283. doi:10.3138/ptc.2011-40

Wu, C.-H., Chang, K.-V., Mio, S., Chen, W.-S., and Wang, T.-G. (2011). Sonoelastography of the Plantar Fascia. *Radiology* 259, 502–507. doi:10.1148/radiol.11101665

Yeh, C.-L., Kuo, P.-L., Gennisson, J.-L., Brum, J., Tanter, M., and Li, P.-C. (2016). Shear Wave Measurements for Evaluation of Tendon Diseases. *IEEE Trans. Ultrason. Ferroelect., Freq. Contr.* 63, 1906–1921. doi:10.1109/TUFFC.2016.2591963

Yeh, C.-L., Kuo, P.-L., and Li, P.-C. (2013). Correlation between the Shear Wave Speed in Tendon and its Elasticity Properties. *2013 Ieee Int. Ultrason. Symp. (Ius)*, 9–12. doi:10.1109/Ultsym.2013.0003

Young, C. (2012). Plantar Fasciitis. *Ann. Intern. Med.* 156, ITC1–1. ITC1-2, ITC1-3, ITC1-4, ITC1-5, ITC1-6, ITC1-7, ITC1-8, ITC1-9, ITC1-10, ITC11-11, ITC11-12, ITC11-13, ITC11-14, ITC11-15; quiz ITC11-16. doi:10.7326/0003-4819-156-1-201201030-01001

20

The Correlation between Quality of Life and Acceptability of Disability in Patients with Facial Burn Scars

Xiuni Zhang[1†], Yuan Liu[2†], Xiaohong Deng[2†], Chengsong Deng[2], Yunfeng Pan[2] and Ailing Hu[2*]*

[1] Department of Trauma and Orthopaedics, Guangzhou Panyu Central Hospital, Guangzhou, China, [2] Third Affiliated Hospital of Sun Yat-sen University, Guangzhou, China

***Correspondence:**
Yunfeng Pan
p-yunfeng@163.com
Ailing Hu
h-ailing@163.com*

† These authors have contributed equally to this work and share first authorship

The purpose of our research is to understand the status of the quality of life and level of disability acceptance in patients with facial burn scars and to explore the correlation between quality of life and disability acceptance and how to improve nursing care for these patients. Patients with facial burn scars were investigated in an outpatient clinic of tertiary hospitals from September 2015 to February 2016. A cross-sectional survey was conducted. The questionnaires used included demographic data and investigations using the burn scars table, Burn-Specific Health Scale-Brief (BSHS-B), and acceptance disability scale (ADS). Differences between participants in terms of demographic characteristics, quality of life, and disability acceptance were assessed using two-tailed independent *t*-tests. The total score of quality of life and disability acceptance in facial burn scar patients was 137.06 ± 17.05 and 185.68 ± 23.74, respectively. The results of Spearman correlation analysis showed that the overall quality of life score of facial burn scar patients was positively correlated with disability acceptance ($r = 0.245$, $p = 0.007$). The quality of life of facial burn scar patients will improve with the improvement of disability acceptance level. Therefore, medical staff can improve the quality of life of patients by improving their disability acceptance level.

Keywords: quality of life, acceptability of disability, facial, burn scars, nursing

INTRODUCTION

Burns are generally caused by high-intensity currents, high temperatures, chemicals, physical rays, etc. (Simons et al., 2018; Van Lieshout et al., 2018). With continuous mechanization and urbanization, the incidence of burns continues to increase. Although the government's efforts in prevention and treatment have reduced the mortality of burn, the disability rate of burn patients has not decreased. It is reported that the annual incidence of burns in China is ~2% (Brewin and Homer, 2018), which occupies the second highest mortality rate among accidents. As an obvious exposed part of the body, facial burns account for more than half of all burn incidents.

The loose subcutaneous adipose tissue and complex vascular nerves in facial areas makes it easier for body fluids to accumulate in the interstitial space. At the same time, the body's own oral and nasal secretions increase the incidence of infection in facial burns, resulting in hypertrophic scars or keloids during the tissue repair process (Kowal-Vern and Criswell, 2005). Deep second degree burns usually leave scars of different sizes, and when the wounds are not treated properly, shallow second degree burns or even degree I burns may form scars.

Scars after burns can cause dysfunction and disfigurement, which greatly affects the patient's daily life and social interaction. Patients often feel disappointment, fear, inferiority, anxiety, loneliness, suspiciousness, and mental disorders due to changes in their appearance. Disfigurement can also lead to social escape. Some patients still cannot accept themselves after long-term recovery and even have a suicidal tendency (Yurdalan et al., 2018).

Burns can produce negative emotions such as anxiety and depression, which in turn affect the quality of life (Kowal-Vern and Criswell, 2005; Miller et al., 2013; Cakir et al., 2015; Spronk et al., 2018a). Studies have shown that the quality of life of patients with burn scars is moderate. A survey (Palmu et al., 2015) showed that the quality of life (QOL) in patients with small burns was higher than the QOL in patients with a total burn area of 30%. At the same time, most patients agree that face and hand burns have a greater impact on the patient's QOL than the actual burn area does. Salvador-Aanza et al. found that different burn patients have different changes in their body, in mental function and in other dimensions. There are many studies on the psychological function of patients after burns at home and away, but systematic research on the QOL in patients with facial burn scars is rarely reported. Some current studies have shown that the factors affecting the quality of life of patients with facial burn scars are as follows (Finnerty et al., 2016; Polychronopoulou et al., 2018): social factors [gender, marital status, occupation, and economic status (Levi et al., 2018; Spronk et al., 2018a)] disease-related factors [effects of scarring on facial function, the degree of influence, the degree of burn, and the duration of disease (Watson et al., 2018)] and psychosocial factors (stress, suppression, social support, and disability acceptance) (Garcia et al., 2016).

Disability acceptance refers to the degree to which a patient builds his or her own knowledge by integrating his or her lifestyle into an experience of dealing with disability. Patients with a higher level of disability acceptance can truly understand the meaning of existence and the ability of the group at the present stage by realizing the loss of their own value and group value due to their disabilities (Nicholls et al., 2012). Therefore, the degree of disability acceptance can predict an individual's ability to respond to attitudes against disability. The obvious exposure of facial burn scars and the importance of appearance characteristics may easily lead to a feeling of inferiority in patients with facial burn scars. Additional research efforts should be made toward understanding the relevant psychological changes after discharge from the hospital, such as the acceptance of disability.

Researchers have studied the correlation between quality of life and disability acceptance. Some studies have shown that quality of life is affected by the acceptance of disability. The level of patient disability acceptance increases with the duration of disability, and the patient is better able to adapt to life after the illness, so the quality of life also has a significant upward trend. The quality of life also increases significantly (Garcia et al., 2016). The reasons may be as follows. (a) Patients are more able to adapt to life after a longer duration of disability. (b) The effect of rehabilitation therapy is more obvious over time, and the degree of patient disability also improves. There are also studies (Nicholls et al., 2012; Baldwin et al., 2018) that indicate that there is a positive correlation between quality of life and disability acceptance.

In summary, it may have a special relationship between Quality of life and disability acceptance in patients with facial burn. However, there is no quantitative study between the two factors. Therefore, we conducted a case investigation to understand the status of the quality of life and level of disability acceptance in patients with facial burn scars and to explore the correlation between quality of life and disability acceptance and how to improve nursing care for these patients.

METHODS

Participants

Patients with facial burn scars were investigated in an outpatient clinic of tertiary hospitals from September 2015 to February 2016. All participants are voluntary and signed informed consent before investigation.

The inclusion criteria were as follows:

(1) Patient age $\geq$ 18 years old
(2) Patients with facial damage caused only by heat, current, chemicals, laser exposure, radiation, etc., and the wound had a hypertrophic scar or keloid of >2 cm^2 after healing
(3) Conscious patients
(4) Patients with an educational level of primary school and above

The exclusion criteria were as follows:

(1) Patients with disabilities in other parts of the body
(2) Patients with heart failure, severe liver disease, stroke, and other serious physical illnesses
(3) Patients with a history of mental illness

All participants are voluntary and signed informed consent before investigation.

Investigation

In this study, a cross-sectional survey was conducted to investigate the demographic information, quality of life, disability acceptance, and related factors of patients with facial burn scars after discharge. The questionnaires used included demographic data and investigations using the burn scars table, Burn-Specific Health Scale-Brief (BSHS-B), and acceptance disability scale (ADS). This study was approved by the ethics committee of the central hospital of Panyu District, Guangzhou.

Measures

Demographic Data and Survey on Burn Scarring

An investigation was conducted by a self-designed questionnaire, which includes 10 questions (gender, age, educational level, pre-burn occupation, current occupation, marital status, place of residence, per capita monthly income of the family, average monthly treatment cost, and mode of payment for medical expenses). The disease and treatment-related information questionnaire included eight questions [cause of burn, time of scar formation, scar site, scar area, whether the patient thinks the burn scar affects facial function (e.g., facial function, sweat gland function, etc.), observation of scar by the patient, length of hospitalization, and presence of burns on other body parts].

Burn-Specific Health Scale-Brief (BSHS-B)

The Burn-Specific Health Scale-Brief was used to investigate the quality of life. The scale includes 9 dimensions and 40 items, including body image, work, heat sensitivity, treatment regimens, simple abilities, interpersonal relationships, hand function, affect, and sexuality. Each item of the scale has 5 rating options for each dimension score, and the Likert 5-point scale was adopted. The scale of 1–5 points for items 1–9 represents 5 levels of "failure to achieve." The scale of 1–5 for items 10–40 represent 5 grades of "conformity," from complete conformity to non-conformity. The lower the score of each dimension is, the lower the quality of life (Chin et al., 2018). Previous studies have shown that the scale has good reliability and validity [83], and the Chinese version of the simplified burn health scale BSHS-B has a total Cronbach's α reliability coefficient of 0.968 and Cronbach's α coefficient of 0.795~0.940 after being evaluated by relevant professionals (Gandolfi et al., 2018).

Acceptance Disability Scale (ADS)

The scale includes four dimensions called transformation, enlargement, containment and subordination, with a total of 50 items, in which 35 items are scored in a negative direction (one point representing "agree very much" and six points representing "disagree very much"). The remaining 15 items were scored positively. The total score of the scale ranged from 50 to 300. Low acceptance level is defined as a total score of 50–133, and scores ranging from 134 to 217 and 218 to 300 were for moderate and high acceptance levels, respectively. The subordination dimension ranges from 5 to 30 points, in which the ranges of 5–12, 13–22, and 23–30 are defined as low, moderate and high acceptance levels, respectively. The containment dimension ranges from 16 to 96 points, in which the ranges of 16–42, 43–79, and 80–96 are defined as low, moderate and high acceptance levels, respectively. The transformation dimension ranges from 15 to 90 points, in which the ranges of 15–40, 41–65, and 66–90 are defined as low, moderate and high acceptance levels, respectively. The transformation dimension ranges from 14 to 84 points, in which the ranges of 14–37, 38–61, and 62–84 are defined as low, moderate and high acceptance levels, respectively. The Cronbach's α value of this scale is 0.95 (Nicholls et al., 2012).

Sample Size Calculation

The sample size was calculated according to the total number of scale dimensions used. The empirical formula is sample size = [Max (dimension degree) × (10~20)] × [1 + (10%~15%)]. Among the questionnaires used in this survey, the Chinese version of the BSHS-B has the highest dimensionality coefficient, with a dimensionality of 9; therefore, the dimensionality of this scale is used as the benchmark for the sample size. Considering some invalid questionnaires, the sample size required for this survey is finally defined as 130 patients.

Quality Control

Before the investigation, the specialist nurses were given unified training on the scoring methods of the BSHS-B, ADS and disability acceptance scale, and the contents of the questionnaires were explained in the same words without guidance. Researchers and trained specialist nurses handed out and recycled all questionnaires used at the site. In the process of completing the questionnaires, unclear questions were explained, checked and supplemented in time. During the investigation, the subjects were strictly selected according to the inclusion criteria and exclusion criteria. The content and purpose of the survey were explained to the volunteers first, and then the questionnaires were collected on the premise of their informed consent. The researcher answered the questions one by one within the specified time. The investigators were required to read the answers one by one for those who could not fill in the answers by themselves, and the volunteers made their own choices without intervention.

The questionnaires were evaluated after collection. Invalid questionnaires were removed, and two teams input the data to a computer-independent order to avoid entry error. Ten percent of the data were checked through random inspection, and the unqualified rate of random inspection was controlled below 0.5%. The qualified rate of this sampling inspection was 100%.

Data Analysis

General Demographic and Disease-Related Conditions data about Facial Burn Scar Patients were described by frequency and percentage. The Quality of Life Score was summarized as maximum, minimum, mean, and standard deviation. Each dimension of Acceptance Disability was defined as low, moderate and high acceptance and described by frequency and percentage. Differences between participants in terms of demographic characteristics, quality of life, and disability acceptance were assessed using variance analysis. Spearman correlation analysis was conducted on the quality of life score and disability acceptance.

$$\rho_{Qol,ADS} = \frac{Cov(Qol, ADS)}{\sqrt{D(Qol)}\sqrt{D(ADS)}} \tag{1}$$

In, which, $\rho_{Qol,ADS}$, $Cov(Qol, ADS)$, $\sqrt{D(Qol)}$, $\sqrt{D(ADS)}$ stands for the correlation, covariance between the quality of life score and disability acceptance, and their own standard variance, respectively. $P < 0.05$ was considered as significantly difference, and, all the analysis was performed using R version 3.4.3.

RESULTS

General Demographic Data of Facial Burn Scar Patients

A total of 130 people were investigated in this survey, 121 valid questionnaires were recovered, and the effective questionnaire recovery rate was 93.08%. The age of the facial burn scar patients ranged from 18 to 83 years, with an average age of 42.77 ± 13.82 years old. The majority of patients were male (63.6%) and married (86%). The ratio of males to females was ~1.75:1. The education levels of patients were 12.4, 35.5, 47.9, and 4.1% for primary school, junior high school, senior high school, junior college, and undergraduate or above, respectively. In total, 82.6% of patients live in cities. Unemployed persons before burning accounted for 1.7% of the total number, while the proportion increased to 17.4% after burning. Approximately 63.6% of families have a monthly income of 2,000~4,000 yuan per capita. The average monthly treatment cost was 620.74 yuan. A total of 66.9% of patients did have medical insurance (**Table 1**).

Disease Related Information of Facial Burn Scar Patients

In total, 113 people (93.4%) suffered from thermal burns. The average scar formation time of facial burns was 116.72 days, ranging from 15 to 427 days, of which 96 patients exhibited scars within 6 months and 25 exhibited scars after 6 months. Submandibular scars were the most common scar formation sites among the facial burns, accounting for 71.9% of 87 patients. Fifty-seven patients had a burn scar area ≥5 cm^2, accounting for 47.1% of patients. A total of 7.4% of the patients believed that the impact of their scars was significant. A total of 34.7% of patients often have sensation of their facial burn scars, while only 3.3% of patients have no sensation of facial burn scars. The first hospital stay of facial burn scar patients was 2–74 days in duration, with an average of 20.31 ± 17.82 days. Three (1.7%) patients suffered from facial burns alone; 71 (58.7%) were complicated with trunk burns; 67 (55.4%) were complicated with upper limb burns; and 31 patients (25.6%) were complicated with lower limb burns (**Table 2**).

Quality of Life

Among 121 patients, 28.93% (35/121) had a score of quality of life greater than 145, 47.22% (57/121) had a quality of life between 130–145, and 23.97% (29/121) had a quality of life below 130. The total score of quality of life in facial burn scar patients was 137.06 ± 17.05. The scores of body image, work, heat sensitivity, simple abilities, interpersonal relationships, hand function, affect, and sexuality were 12.31 ± 2.52, 12.60 ± 3.27, 16.01 ± 3.57, 16.31 ± 2.90, 10.61 ± 2.77, 14.29 ± 1.97, 18.00 ± 4.42, 25.49 ± 4.32, and 11.44 ± 1.50, respectively (**Table 3**). There's significantly difference between each dimension of quality of life ($F = 271.53$, $P < 0.01$).

Acceptance Disability Scale (ADS)

The total score of disability acceptance was 185.68 ± 23.74. Among the scoring items, the scores for transformation, enlargement, dimension, containment and subordination were 58.64 ± 9.31, 54.12 ± 7.54, 58.04 ± 8.62, and 14.88 ± 2.75, respectively. The degree of disability acceptance and its dimensions are divided into three levels: low, medium, and high. In the distribution of the total disability acceptance score of the study subjects, 91.7% of patients were at the moderate acceptance level, while 22.3% of patients in the compliance dimension scored at the low acceptance level (**Table 4**).

Correlation Analysis of Quality of Life and Handicap Acceptance

Spearman correlation analysis was conducted on the quality of life score and disability acceptance. The results are shown in **Table 5**. The results showed that the overall quality of life score of

TABLE 1 | General demographic of facial burn scar patients ($n = 121$).

Variable name	Frequency	Percentage (%)
Gender		
Male	77	63.6
Female	44	36.4
Age (years)		
18–30	28	23.1
31–44	43	35.5
45–59	32	26.4
60–83	18	14.9
Education level		
Primary school	15	12.4
Junior high school	43	35.5
High school	58	47.9
College, undergraduate or above	5	4.1
Pre-burn occupation		
Workers	40	33.1
Farmers	23	19.0
Individuals, businessmen, enterprises, government	40	33.1
Housewives	11	9.1
Unemployed	2	1.7
Students	5	4.1
Current occupation		
Workers	28	23.1
Farmers	22	18.2
Individual, business, enterprise, government, service	32	26.4
Housewives	12	9.9
Unemployed	21	17.4
Students	5	4.1
Other	1	0.8
Marital status		
Unmarried	15	12.4
Married	104	86.0
Divorced/separated	2	1.7
Residence		
City	100	82.6
Countryside	21	17.4
Per capita monthly income (yuan)		
<2,000	6	5.0
2,000–4,000	77	63.6
>4,000	38	31.4
Payment method of medical expenses		
At their own expense	81	66.9
Medical insurance	40	33.1

TABLE 2 | Disease-related conditions of facial burn scar patients ($n = 121$).

Variable	Frequency	Percentage (%)
Cause of bum		
Thermal burns	113	93.4
Chemical bums	6	5.0
Others (radiation bums)	2	1.7
Combined with burns on other body parts		
Trunk	71	58.7
Limb	67	55.4
Lower limb	31	25.6
No combined burns	3	2.5
Scar formation time		
Within 6 months	96	79.3
More than 6 months	25	20.7
Facial scar formation site		
Frontal compartment	11	9.1
Face	26	21.5
Submandibular area	87	71.9
Eyelid	18	14.9
Mouth	10	8.3
Nasal area	1	0.8
Scar area of facial burns		
2~4 cm^2	64	52.9
5~15 cm^2	46	38.0
>15 cm2	11	9.1
Number of days of first hospitalization		
>9 days	36	29.8
More than 9 days	61	50.4
≥30 days	24	19.8
Observation of facial scar by patients		
Regular observation	42	34.7
Sometimes observation	36	29.8
Occasional observation	43	35.5
Does the patient think the bum scar will affect his or her facial function		
Basically no	72	59.5
Little influence	40	33.1
Great influence	9	7.4

TABLE 3 | The quality of life score of facial burn scar patients ($n = 121$).

Item	$X \pm s$	Average score of the single entry
Total score	137 06 ± 17.05	3.43
Body image	12.31 ± 2.52	3 08
Work	12.60 ± 3.27	3.15
Heat sensitivity	1601 ± 357	3.2
Treatment regimens	16.31 ± 2.90	3.26
Simple abilities	10.61 ± 2.77	3.54
Interpersonal relationships	14.29 ± 1.97	3.57
Hand function	18 00 ± 4.42	3.6
Affect	25.49 ± 4.32	3.64
Sexuality	11.44 ± 1.50	3.81

facial burn scar patients was positively correlated with disability acceptance ($r = 0.245$, $p = 0.007$).

DISCUSSION

In this survey, the overall quality of life of patients with facial burn scars was divided into 77~160 points with an average score of 137.0 ± 17.05 points, indicating that the quality of life of patients with facial burn scars is at a moderate or low level. However, some researchers scored 182.43 ± 48.6 points in the study on the quality of life of patients in the burn rehabilitation period. This result may be because the face is a special area where once burned, it can easily be observed by other people, so burns on the face have a substantial effect the quality of life of patients. At the same time, facial burn scarring can increase the psychological pressure of the patient and cause great interference to his or her work and life, which may lead to a moderate-to-low quality of life (Spronk et al., 2018b).

According to the Appraisal Standard for Disability Degree of Industrial Injury and Occupational Disease of Workers, the subjects of this study have disabilities ranging from grade 4 to grade 10. The results of this study show that the total score of disability acceptance of facial burn scar patients is 185.68 ± 23.74, which is close to the score of other subjects (181.46 ± 39.45) and higher than score range of the low level of acceptance. This finding indicates that the disability acceptance of burn scar patients is at a medium level and still needs to be improved. According to the grading distribution of the total score of disability acceptance for facial burn scar patients, 91.7% of the patients were at a moderate acceptance level. The low acceptance level was 3.3%. Patients with a high acceptance level only accounted for 5%.

To our knowledge, there's still no report about the relationship between quality of life and the acceptance of disability in facial burn patients, and the acceptance of disability plays a significant role in mediating the correlation between general self-efficacy and depression/general quality of life in mild traumatic brain injury patients (Yehene et al., 2019). The results of this survey show that disability acceptance in facial burn patients is a factor affecting the quality of life of patients, and there is a positive correlation between the two factors. Similar to the research results, the reasons may be as follows. (1) The overall quality of life improvement level in patients is not only affected by the treatment level during hospitalization but also has a great correlation with the attitude in coping with their own disability. Through reasonable cognition, patients can adopt logical thinking to overcome the belittling of self-esteem, create a good life, adapt to their environments with a reasonable outlook on life, and improve their effective adaptability to their disabilities. Patients need reasonable cognition to guide adaptive behavior in the process of social reintegration after burn. Patients can identify new role orientations and self-definitions and then

TABLE 4 | Acceptance disability level of facial burn scar patients ($n = 121$).

Variable quantity	Low acceptance		Moderate acceptance		High acceptance	
	N	Percentage (%)	*N*	Percentage (%)	*N*	Percentage (%)
Transformation	9	7.4	87	71.9	25	20.7
Enlargement	4	3.3	94	77.7	23	19
Containment	7	5.8	114	94.2	0	0
Subordination	27	22.3	91	75.2	3	2.5
Total score of disability acceptance	4	3.3	111	91.7	6	5.0

TABLE 5 | Correlation between quality of life and disability acceptance in patients with facial burn scar ($n = 121$).

BSHS-B dimensions	Transformation	Enlargement	Containment	Subordination	Total score
Total score of quality of life	0.203*	0.277**	0.235**	−0.264**	0.245**
Simple abilities	0.062	0.132	0.059	−0.280**	0.073
Hand function	0.137	0.248**	0.078	−0.331**	0.130
Affect	0.301**	0.347**	0.357**	−0.287**	0.345**
Interpersonal relationships	0.160	0.165	0.184*	−0.299**	0.165
Sexuality	0.276**	0.402**	0.250**	−0.431**	0.279**
Body image	−0.053	0.008	0.051	0.022	0.017
Heat sensitivity	0.138	0.105	0.185*	−0.046	0.170
Treatment regimens	0.155	0.177	0.198*	−0.053	0.190*
Work	0.075	0.301	0.083	0.079	0.619

*$P < 0.05$, **$P < 0.01$.

adopt adaptive behaviors to promote the recovery of body functions and the improvement of various skills and abilities. The improvement of disability acceptance level is conducive to further improving the physical condition of patients. (2) Improvement in the degree of disability acceptance changes patients' cognition to a certain extent, improves patients' control over their own emotions, and allows them to perceive less negative psychological emotions, thus guiding patients to actively change their self-value and attitude toward life. The continuous improvement in disability acceptance indicates that patients can actively change their self-value recognition and self-cognition, thus improving their quality of life.

Our study found that the affect dimension in the quality of life of facial burn scar patients has a correlation with all dimensions of disability acceptance, of which the correlation coefficient with the containment dimension was the largest, suggesting that the affect dimension has the closest relationship with the control dimension. According to Maslow's hierarchy of needs theory, after human beings have satisfied their physiological and safety needs, they will pursue the satisfaction of the needs of emotion and belonging (Kowal-Vern and Criswell, 2005); emotional needs are more delicate than physiological needs are, and at the same time, emotional needs have a certain relationship with individual physiological characteristics, social education, personal experience, and religious beliefs. If patients can rationally view facial burn scars and control the negative effects caused by facial burn scars so that they do not exceed the actual damage range to the body, the patient's emotion can be expressed more smoothly, and the demand level of emotion and belonging can be realized, thus improving the patient's acceptance of his or her disability. The sex life dimension of the quality of life of patients with facial burn scars is correlated with all dimensions of disability acceptance, of which the correlation coefficient with the compliance dimension is the largest, indicating that the sex life dimension is most closely related to the compliance dimension. By analyzing the reasons, patients cannot accept their current appearance changes and do not obey their current physical conditions. They still attach great importance to the facial appearance changes caused by sudden accidents and show higher attention to their own abilities and appearance. Patients will be more inclined to think that burn scars lead to the disability of their bodily functions, thus affecting their sex life (Capek et al., 2018).

CONCLUSION AND CLINICAL SIGNIFICANCE

The quality of life of facial burn scar patients will improve with the improvement of disability acceptance level. Therefore, medical staff can improve the quality of life of patients by improving their disability acceptance level. Medical staff can assist patients to find control and management methods of the body, expand the scope of patients' values, establish a correct evaluation of their appearance, obey the changes brought about by facial burn scars, assist patients to reconstruct their internal aesthetics, and help patients to rediscover their own value orientation and meaning of life by guiding patients to formal medical institutions for scar treatment consultation and follow-up.

AUTHOR CONTRIBUTIONS

XZ, YL, and AH contributed to the conception and design of the study. XZ and XD organized the database. YL, CD, and YP performed the statistical analysis. XZ wrote the first draft of the manuscript. YL, XD, and CD wrote sections of the manuscript. All authors contributed to manuscript revision, read, and approved the submitted version.

REFERENCES

Baldwin, S., Yuan, H., Liao, J., Grieve, B., Heard, J., and Wibbenmeyer, L. A. (2018). Burn survivor quality of life and barriers to support program participation. *J. Burn Care Res.* 5, 823–830. doi: 10.1093/jbcr/irx058

Brewin, M. P., and Homer, S. J. (2018). The lived experience and quality of life with burn scarring-the results from a large-scale online survey. *Burns* 7, 1801–1810. doi: 10.1016/j.burns.2018.04.007

Cakir, U., Terzi, R., Abaci, F., and Aker, T. (2015). The prevalence of post-traumatic stress disorder in patients with burn injuries, and their quality of life. *Int. J. Psychiatry Clin. Pract.* 1, 56–59. doi: 10.3109/13651501.2014.981545

Capek, K. D., Culnan, D. M., Desai, M. H., and Herndon, D. N. (2018). Fifty years of burn care at shriners hospitals for children, Galveston. *Ann. Plast. Surg.* 3 (Suppl. 2), S90–S94. doi: 10.1097/SAP.0000000000001376

Chin, T. L., Carrougher, G. J., Amtmann, D., McMullen, K., Herndon, D. N., Holavanahalli, R., et al. (2018). Trends 10 years after burn injury: a burn model system national database study. *Burns* 8, 1882–1886. doi: 10.1016/j.burns.2018.09.033

Finnerty, C. C., Jeschke, M. G., Branski, L. K., Barret, J. P., Dziewulski, P., Herndon, D. N. (2016). Hypertrophic scarring: the greatest unmet challenge after burn injury. *Lancet* 10052, 1427–1436. doi: 10.1016/S0140-6736(16)31406-4

Gandolfi, S., Carloni, R., Bertheuil, N., Grolleau, J. L., Auquit-Auckbur, I., and Chaput, B. (2018). Assessment of quality-of-life in patients with face-and-neck burns: the burn-specific health scale for face and neck (BSHS-FN). *Burns* 6, 1602–1609. doi: 10.1016/j.burns.2018.03.002

Garcia, L. P., Huang, A., Corlew, D. S., Aeron, K., Aeron, Y., Rai, S. M., et al. (2016). Factors affecting burn contracture outcome in developing countries. *Ann. Plast. Surg.* 3, 290–296. doi: 10.1097/SAP.0000000000000856

Kowal-Vern, A., and Criswell, B. K. (2005). Burn scar neoplasms: a literature review and statistical analysis. *Burns* 4, 403–413. doi: 10.1016/j.burns.2005.02.015

Levi, B., Kraft, C. T., Shapiro, G. D., Trinh, N. T., Dore, E. C., Jeng, J., et al. (2018). The associations of gender with social participation of burn survivors: a life impact burn recovery evaluation profile study. *J. Burn Care Res.* 6, 915–922. doi: 10.1093/jbcr/iry007

Miller, T., Bhattacharya, S., Zamula, W., Lezotte, D., Kowalske, K., Herndon, D., et al. (2013). Quality-of-life loss of people admitted to burn centers, United States. *Qual. Life Res.* 9, 2293–2305. doi: 10.1007/s11136-012-0321-5

Nicholls, E., Lehan, T., Plaza, S. L., Deng, X., Romero, J. L., Pizarro, J. A., et al. (2012). Factors influencing acceptance of disability in individuals with spinal cord injury in Neiva, Colombia, South America. *Disabil. Rehabil.* 13, 1082–1088. doi: 10.3109/09638288.2011.631684

Palmu, R., Partonen, T., Suominen, K., Vuola, J., and Isometsa, E. (2015). Return to work six months after burn: a prospective study at the Helsinki Burn Center. *Burns* 6, 1152–1160. doi: 10.1016/j.burns.2015.06.010

Polychronopoulou, E., Herndon, D. N., and Porter, C. (2018). The long-term impact of severe burn trauma on musculoskeletal health. *J. Burn Care Res.* 6, 869–880. doi: 10.1093/jbcr/iry035

Simons, M., Lim, P. C. C., Kimble, R. M., and Tyack, Z. (2018). Towards a clinical and empirical definition of burn scarring: a template analysis using qualitative data. *Burns* 7, 1811–1819. doi: 10.1016/j.burns.2018.04.006

Spronk, I., Legemate, C., Oen, I., van Loey, N., Polinder, S., van Baar, M. (2018b). Health related quality of life in adults after burn injuries: a systematic review. *PLoS ONE* 5:e0197507. doi: 10.1371/journal.pone.0197507

Spronk, I., Legemate, C. M., Dokter, J., van Loey, N. E. E., van Baar, M. E., Polinder, S. (2018a). Predictors of health-related quality of life after burn injuries: a systematic review. *Crit. Care* 1:160. doi: 10.1186/s13054-018-2071-4

Van Lieshout, E. M., Van Yperen, D. T., Van Baar, M. E., Polinder, S., Boersma, D., Cardon, A. Y., et al. (2018). Epidemiology of injuries, treatment (costs) and outcome in burn patients admitted to a hospital with or without dedicated burn centre (Burn-Pro): protocol for a multicentre prospective observational study. *BMJ Open* 11:e023709. doi: 10.1136/bmjopen-2018-023709

Watson, E. J. R., Nenadlová, K., Clancy, O. H., Farag, M., Nordin, N. A., Nilsen, A., et al. (2018). Perioperative research into memory (PRiMe): cognitive impairment following a severe burn injury and critical care admission, part 1. *Burns* 5, 1167–1178. doi: 10.1016/j.burns.2018.04.011

Yehene, E., Lichtenstern, G., Harel, Y., Druckman, E., and Sacher, Y. (2019). Self-efficacy and acceptance of disability following mild traumatic brain injury: a pilot study. *Appl. Neuropsychol. Adult* 2, 1–10. doi: 10.1080/23279095.2019.1569523

Yurdalan, S. U., Unlu, B., Seyyah, M., Senyildiz, B., Cetin, Y. K., and Cimen, M. (2018). Effects of structured home-based exercise program on depression status and quality of life in burn patients. *Burns* 5, 1287–1293. doi: 10.1016/j.burns.2018.02.015

Permissions

All chapters in this book were first published by Frontiers; hereby published with permission under the Creative Commons Attribution License or equivalent. Every chapter published in this book has been scrutinized by our experts. Their significance has been extensively debated. The topics covered herein carry significant findings which will fuel the growth of the discipline. They may even be implemented as practical applications or may be referred to as a beginning point for another development.

The contributors of this book come from diverse backgrounds, making this book a truly international effort. This book will bring forth new frontiers with its revolutionizing research information and detailed analysis of the nascent developments around the world.

We would like to thank all the contributing authors for lending their expertise to make the book truly unique. They have played a crucial role in the development of this book. Without their invaluable contributions this book wouldn't have been possible. They have made vital efforts to compile up to date information on the varied aspects of this subject to make this book a valuable addition to the collection of many professionals and students.

This book was conceptualized with the vision of imparting up-to-date information and advanced data in this field. To ensure the same, a matchless editorial board was set up. Every individual on the board went through rigorous rounds of assessment to prove their worth. After which they invested a large part of their time researching and compiling the most relevant data for our readers.

The editorial board has been involved in producing this book since its inception. They have spent rigorous hours researching and exploring the diverse topics which have resulted in the successful publishing of this book. They have passed on their knowledge of decades through this book. To expedite this challenging task, the publisher supported the team at every step. A small team of assistant editors was also appointed to further simplify the editing procedure and attain best results for the readers.

Apart from the editorial board, the designing team has also invested a significant amount of their time in understanding the subject and creating the most relevant covers. They scrutinized every image to scout for the most suitable representation of the subject and create an appropriate cover for the book.

The publishing team has been an ardent support to the editorial, designing and production team. Their endless efforts to recruit the best for this project, has resulted in the accomplishment of this book. They are a veteran in the field of academics and their pool of knowledge is as vast as their experience in printing. Their expertise and guidance has proved useful at every step. Their uncompromising quality standards have made this book an exceptional effort. Their encouragement from time to time has been an inspiration for everyone.

The publisher and the editorial board hope that this book will prove to be a valuable piece of knowledge for researchers, students, practitioners and scholars across the globe.

List of Contributors

Chenyu Shi and Jincheng Wang
School of Nursing, Jilin University, Changchun, China
Orthopaedic Medical Center, The Second Hospital of Jilin University, Changchun, China

He Liu, Qiuju Li, Ronghang Li, Yan Zhang and Yuzhe Liu
Orthopaedic Medical Center, The Second Hospital of Jilin University, Changchun, China

Chenyu Wang
Department of Plastic and Reconstructive Surgery, The First Hospital of Jilin University, Changchun, China

Ying Shao
Orthopaedic Medical Center, The Second Hospital of Jilin University, Changchun, China
Department of Plastic and Reconstructive Surgery, The First Hospital of Jilin University, Changchun, China

Iain A. Rankin, Thuy-Tien Nguyen and Spyros D. Masouros
Department of Bioengineering, Imperial College London, London, United Kingdom

Louise McMenemy
Department of Bioengineering, Imperial College London, London, United Kingdom
Academic Department of Military Surgery and Trauma, Royal Centre for Defence Medicine, ICT Centre, Birmingham Research Park, Birmingham, United Kingdom

Jonathan C. Clasper
Department of Bioengineering, Imperial College London, London, United Kingdom
Department of Trauma and Orthopaedic Surgery, Frimley Park Hospital, Surrey, United Kingdom

Yuzhen Wang
Research Center for Tissue Repair and Regeneration Affiliated to the Medical Innovation Research Department and 4th Medical Center, PLA General Hospital and PLA Medical College, Beijing, China
PLA Key Laboratory of Tissue Repair and Regenerative Medicine and Beijing Key Research Laboratory of Skin Injury, Repair and Regeneration, Beijing, China
Research Unit of Trauma Care, Tissue Repair and Regeneration, Chinese Academy of Medical Sciences, 2019RU051, Beijing, China
Department of Burn and Plastic Surgery, Air Force Hospital of PLA Central Theater Command, Datong, China

Ubaldo Armato
Histology and Embryology Section, Department of Surgery, Dentistry, Pediatrics and Gynecology, University of Verona Medical School Verona, Verona, Italy
Department of Burn and Plastic Surgery, Second People's Hospital of Shenzhen, Shenzhen University, Shenzhen, China

Jun Wu
Department of Burn and Plastic Surgery, Second People's Hospital of Shenzhen, Shenzhen University, Shenzhen, China

Harry Ming Chun Choi, Alex Kwok-Kuen Cheung, Michelle Chun Har Ng and Gladys Lai Ying Cheing
Department of Rehabilitation Sciences, The Hong Kong Polytechnic University, Kowloon, Hong Kong

Yongping Zheng
Department of Biomedical Engineering, The Hong Kong Polytechnic University, Kowloon, Hong Kong

Antonio Alessandrino, Marco Biagiotti, Giulia A. Bassani, Valentina Vincoli and Giuliano Freddi
Silk Biomaterials Srl, Lomazzo, Italy

Anna Chiarini, Ilaria Dal Prà and Ubaldo Armato
Human Histology & Embryology Section, Department of Surgery, Dentistry, Pediatrics & Gynecology, University of Verona Medical School, Verona, Italy

Piergiorgio Settembrini
Department of Vascular Surgery, San Carlo Borromeo Hospital, Milan, Italy

Pasquale Pierimarchi
Institute of Translational Pharmacology, National Research Council, Rome, Italy

Wei Liu, Jianchao Li and Fang Pu
Key Laboratory of Biomechanics and Mechanobiology, Ministry of Education, Beijing Advanced Innovation Center for Biomedical Engineering, School of Biological Science and Medical Engineering, Beihang University, Beijing, China

Weiyan Ren
Key Laboratory of Rehabilitation Technical Aids for Old-Age Disability, Key Laboratory of Human Motion Analysis and Rehabilitation Technology of the Ministry of Civil Affairs, National Research Center for Rehabilitation Technical Aids, Beijing, China

Lijun Zhang, Hanxiao Yin, Mingzhou Yuan, Xiaoyan Wang, Fangyingnan Zhang, Fei Zhou, Shaohai Qi, Bin Shu and Jun Wu
Department of Burns, The First Affiliated Hospital, Sun Yat-sen University, Guangzhou, China

Xun Lei
School of Public Health and Management, Chongqing Medical University, Chongqing, China

Johnson N. Y. Lau
University of Hong Kong, Hong Kong Polytechnic University, Kowloon, China

Weiyan Ren and Junchao Guo
Key Laboratory of Rehabilitation Technical Aids for Old-Age Disability, Key Laboratory of Human Motion Analysis and Rehabilitation Technology of the Ministry of Civil Affairs, National Research Center for Rehabilitation Technical Aids, Beijing, China

Wenqiang Ye and Wei Liu
Key Laboratory for Biomechanics and Mechanobiology of Chinese Education Ministry, Beijing Advanced Innovation Center for Biomedical Engineering, School of Biological Science and Medical Engineering, Beihang University, Beijing, China

Yijie Duan
Key Laboratory for Biomechanics and Mechanobiology of Chinese Education Ministry, Beijing Advanced Innovation Center for Biomedical Engineering, School of Biological Science and Medical Engineering, Beihang University, Beijing, China

Hongmei Liu
Key Laboratory of Rehabilitation Technical Aids for Old-Age Disability, Key Laboratory of Human Motion Analysis and Rehabilitation Technology of the Ministry of Civil Affairs, National Research Center for Rehabilitation Technical Aids, Beijing, China
Key Laboratory for Biomechanics and Mechanobiology of Chinese Education Ministry, Beijing Advanced Innovation Center for Biomedical Engineering, School of Biological Science and Medical Engineering, Beihang University, Beijing, China

Yih-Kuen Jan
Department of Kinesiology and Community Health, University of Illinois at Urbana-Champaign, Champaign, IL, United States

Yubo Fan
Key Laboratory for Biomechanics and Mechanobiology of Chinese Education Ministry, Beijing Advanced Innovation Center for Biomedical Engineering, School of Biological Science and Medical Engineering, Beihang University, Beijing, China
School of Engineering Medicine, Beihang University, Beijing, China

Qi Fang
The First Clinical Hospital of Guangzhou Medical University, Guangzhou, China

Xinlu Wang
The First Clinical Hospital of Guangzhou Medical University, Guangzhou, China
Department of Plastic Surgery, General Hospital of Southern Theater Command, PLA, Guangzhou, China

Biao Cheng and Pengcheng Xu
Department of Plastic Surgery, General Hospital of Southern Theater Command, PLA, Guangzhou, China

Zexin Yao
Department of Plastic Surgery, General Hospital of Southern Theater Command, PLA, Guangzhou, China
Department of Public Health, Guangdong Pharmaceutical University, Guangzhou, China

Longbao Feng
Beogene Biotech (Guangzhou) Co, Ltd, Guangzhou, China

Rui Guo
Key Laboratory of Biomaterials of Guangdong Higher Education Institutes, Department of Biomedical Engineering, Guangdong Provincial Engineering and Technological Research Center for Drug Carrier Development, Jinan University, Guangzhou, China

Shoou-Jeng Yeh
Section of Neurology and Neurophysiology, Cheng-Ching General Hospital, Taichung, Taiwan

Chi-Wen Lung
Department of Creative Product Design, Asia University, Taichung, Taiwan
Rehabilitation Engineering Lab, Kinesiology and Community Health, Computational Science and Engineering, University of Illinois at Urbana-Champaign, Champaign, IL, United States

Fang-Chuan Kuo
Department of Physical Therapy, Hungkuang University, Taichung, Taiwan

Ben-Yi Liau
Department of Biomedical Engineering, Hungkuang University, Taichung, Taiwan

Zhicheng Hu, Shaobin Huang, Peng Wang, Yunxian Dong, Pu Cheng, Hailin Xu, Bing Tang and Jiayuan Zhu
Department of Burn Surgery, The First Affiliated Hospital of Sun Yat-sen University, Guangzhou, China

Peng Liu
Department of Burn Surgery, The First Affiliated Hospital of Sun Yat-sen University, Guangzhou, China
Department of Burn and Plastic Surgery, Guangzhou Red Cross Hospital, Medical College, Jinan University, Guangzhou, China

Gayathri Victoria Balasubramanian, Nachiappan Chockalingam and Roozbeh Naemi
Centre for Biomechanics and Rehabilitation Technologies, Staffordshire University, Stoke-on-Trent, United Kingdom

Eoghan J. Mulholland
Gastrointestinal Stem Cell Biology Laboratory, Wellcome Trust Centre for Human Genetics, University of Oxford, Oxford, United Kingdom

Rita E. Roberts and Timothy J. Koh
Department of Kinesiology and Nutrition, University of Illinois at Chicago, Chicago, IL, United States
Center for Tissue Repair and Regeneration, University of Illinois at Chicago, Chicago, IL, United States
Jesse Brown VA Medical Center, Chicago, IL, United States

Rhonda D. Kineman
Jesse Brown VA Medical Center, Chicago, IL, United States
Department of Medicine, Section of Endocrinology, Diabetes and Metabolism, University of Illinois at Chicago, Chicago, IL, United States

Onur Bilgen
Department of Mechanical and Aerospace Engineering, Rutgers University, Piscataway, NJ, United States

Yue-Ping Wang, Rui-Hao Cheng, Ying He and Li-Zhong Mu
School of Energy and Power Engineering, Dalian University of Technology, Dalian, China

Teresa C. O. Marsi, Ritchelli Ricci and Tatiane V. Toniato
Institute of Research and Development, University of Vale Do Paraiba, São Josė dos Campos, Brazil

Luana M. R. Vasconcellos
Department of Bioscience and Oral Diagnosis, Institute of Science and Technology, São Paulo State University, São Paulo, Brazil

Conceição de Maria Vaz Elias
Scientific and Technological Institute, Brasil University, São Paulo, Brazil

Andre D. R. Silva
Air Force Academy, Brazilian Air Force, Pirassununga, Brazil

Andre S. A. Furtado, Leila S. S. M. Magalhães, Edson C. Silva-Filho and Anderson O. Lobo
LIMAV - Interdisciplinary Laboratory for Advanced Materials, Materials Science & Engineering Graduate Program, UFPI-Federal University of Piaui, Teresina, Brazil

Fernanda R. Marciano
Department of Physics, Federal University of Piaui, Teresina, Brazil

Andrea Zille
Department of Textile Engineering, Centre for Textile Science and Technology, University of Minho, Guimarães, Portugal

Thomas J. Webster
Department of Chemical Engineering, Northeastern University, Boston, MA, United States

Sharon Eve Sonenblum
Rehabilitation Engineering and Applied Research Laboratory, The George W. Woodruff School of Mechanical Engineering, Georgia Institute of Technology, Atlanta, GA, United States

Stephen H. Sprigle
Rehabilitation Engineering and Applied Research Laboratory, The George W. Woodruff School of Mechanical Engineering, Georgia Institute of Technology, Atlanta, GA, United States
College of Design, Georgia Institute of Technology, Atlanta, GA, United States

Megan Measel
Wallace H. Coulter Department of Biomedical Engineering, Georgia Institute of Technology, Atlanta, GA, United States

John Greenhalgh
FONAR Corporation, Melville, NY, United States

John McKay Cathcart
School of Health Sciences, Ulster University, Northern Ireland, Coleraine, United Kingdom

Zhongyuan Deng, Tao Zhang and Xiaojian Li
Department of Burn and Plastic, Guangzhou Red Cross Hospital, Medical College, Jinan University, Guangzhou, China

Zhihui Qian, Zhende Jiang, Jianan Wu, Jing Liu and Luquan Ren
1Key Laboratory of Bionic Engineering, Jilin University, Changchun, China

Fei Chang
Orthopaedic Medical Center, The Second Hospital of Jilin University, Changchun, China

Lei Ren
Key Laboratory of Bionic Engineering, Jilin University, Changchun, China
School of Mechanical, Aerospace and Civil Engineering, University of Manchester, Manchester, United Kingdom

Xiuni Zhang
Department of Trauma and Orthopaedics, Guangzhou Panyu Central Hospital, Guangzhou, China

Yuan Liu, Xiaohong Deng, Chengsong Deng, Yunfeng Pan and Ailing Hu
Third Affiliated Hospital of Sun Yat-sen University, Guangzhou, China

Index

Printed in the USA
CPSIA information can be obtained
at www.ICGtesting.com
JSHW051623061123
51533JS00005B/80